HEALTH CARE
ECONOMICS

WIL

S

Intr

He

R

HEALTH CARE ECONOMICS

THIRD EDITION

Paul J. Feldstein, Ph.D.

Professor
FHP Foundation Chair in Health Care Management
Graduate School of Management
University of California
Irvine, California

WILEY

A WILEY MEDICAL PUBLICATION
JOHN WILEY & SONS
New York • Chichester • Brisbane • Toronto • Singapore

To Anna

Library of Congress Cataloging in Publication Data:

Feldstein, Paul J.
    Health care economics/Paul J. Feldstein.—3rd ed.
        p. cm.—(Wiley series in health services, ISSN 0195-3907)
    (A Wiley medical publication)
    Includes bibliographical references and index.
    ISBN 0-471-86031-X
    1. Medical economics.   2. Medical economics—United States.
I. Title.   II. Series.   III. Series: A Wiley medical publication.
    [DNLM: 1. Economics, Medical—United States.   W74 F312h]
RA410.F44 1988
338.4′736210973—dc19
DNLM/DLC
for Library of Congress   88-273
                                                                          CIP

Printed in the United States of America
10 9 8 7 6 5 4 3 2

Preface
to the Third Edition

This book grew out of a course on the economics of health services that I have taught at
the University of Michigan for many years. During this period the health economics
literature increased rapidly, resulting in a course reading list sufficiently large to cause
my students concern. As the literature increased, so did its technical content, often
assuming a background students lacked. In addition, the literature developed un-
evenly, leaving gaps which this book is designed to fill. This introductory text attempts
to provide an analytical approach to the study of medical care and, through the use of
numerous applications, to illustrate the usefulness of economics to the understanding
of public policy issues in medical care.

The material in this book presumes familiarity with some of the economic concepts
presented in a microeconomics course at the undergraduate level. I have, therefore,
tried to refresh students' memory of these concepts when discussing the applicability
of economics to health care. Since institutional knowledge of medical care issues is
generally not uniform among students, particularly undergraduates, I have defined
concepts and described legislation that would be more familiar to students in a School
of Public Health.

This book is meant to be used for a one-semester course in health economics. Realizing that instructors' preferences for topics to include in such a course may differ,
more material is included than would normally be covered in one semester. For the
interested student, both recent and historical references are provided should the student wish to pursue a particular subject in greater depth.

While writing this book and the subsequent revisions, I have tried to clarify those
subjects found by my students to be most difficult and most inadequately explained in
the classroom. If the reader has difficulty understanding certain sections, he or she
will have developed a better appreciation for my students' experience. For example, as
a result of student comments I became aware of the need to make explicit the relationship between economic analysis and the value judgments underlying different public
policies. For this reason, I have tried to stress these issues in the various subjects
discussed.

The emphasis of this book is on the financing and delivery of personal medical services, rather than on the broader issues of health and health services. This narrower

focus reflects the extensive emphasis of federal and state legislation and of current policy issues, such as financing medical services and concern with efficiency in the delivery of services, on personal medical services rather than health or health services, which might be well more appropriate. The relationship of personal medical services to health is discussed in an early chapter; thereafter, the text emphasizes the definition, measurement, and selection of public policies to achieve economic efficiency and equity in the financing and delivery of personal medical services.

Since the time the first edition appeared, in 1979, the medical sector has undergone dramatic changes. Health policy is constantly changing. The emphasis on national health insurance has declined; the concern over a shortage of physicians has changed to a concern over a surplus of physicians. From being reimbursed on a cost-plus basis, hospitals now face prospective, fixed prices. The provision of hospital services by independent community hospitals has changed, with hospital mergers being more frequent and multihospital systems being more common. Also, the movement toward increased regulation of medical services has changed to market competition along with the development of new alternative delivery systems, advertising, and hospital discounts.

This latest revision retains a historical perspective on how and why the medical sector has changed. Economic analysis is useful for understanding the effects on equity and efficiency of previous methods of financing and delivering medical services as well as current approaches. Economics is also helpful for understanding why these various changes have occurred.

In addition to updating tables and the text, a number of additional changes have been made in this latest revision. Chapter 21, "The Market for Long-Term Care Services" has been added. Several chapters have been extensively revised. New sections, such as comparable worth, physician payment methods, adverse selection, cost shifting, and who bears the burden of the social security tax, have been included in existing chapters. A large number of review questions have been included as an appendix. I hand these questions out to my students at the beginning of the semester, and as an incentive for the students to think about them I select several for the midterm and final exams. Hopefully, others might find them useful.

In writing this book and in teaching my course I have benefited from the work of other health economists. Some measure of that debt is indicated by the numerous references to others' work found throughout the book. In preparing this edition, Ron Vogel provided helpful comments and Thomas Wickizer and Robert Miller were able research assistants. I wish to acknowledge the valuable assistance of Jack Tobias, the Reference Librarian in the School of Public Health, University of Michigan, who is one of the great resources of that school. Jeremiah German gave me extensive suggestions for the second edition and Darrell Graham provided invaluable research assistance. For the first edition, Irene Butter, John Kuder, Geoffrey Shepherd, Kenneth Warner, Carolyn Watts, and Jack Wheeler provided many helpful comments and suggestions. John Goddeeris provided excellent research assistance.

PAUL J. FELDSTEIN

Contents

viii Contents

Tables

xiii

Figures

CHAPTER 1

An Introduction to the Economics of Medical Care

TRENDS IN MEDICAL EXPENDITURES

Expenditures on personal medical services have risen more rapidly than expenditures on most other goods and services in the economy. Annual expenditures on personal medical services have increased from $35.8 billion in 1965 to $371.4 billion in 1985. In 1965, 5.2 percent of the gross national product (GNP) was being spent on *personal* medical services (see Table 1-1). By 1985, 9.3 percent of the GNP was being allocated to *personal* medical services. (Total medical expenditures were $425 billion in 1985 and comprised 10.7 percent of GNP.) Spending on medical care services, which increased 9 percent in 1985, continues to increase at a faster rate than GNP, which increased at 5.7 percent over the same period. If the rate of increase in medical care expenditures continues to expand more rapidly than GNP, personal medical services will continue to consume an increasing portion of all goods and services produced in the United States.

Part of the increase in personal medical care expenditures is the result of increases in the population receiving such services. The population, however, has been growing at less than 1 percent (.9) per year. Thus when we adjust for such population increases by examining expenditures on a per capita basis, we find that the annual percentage increase in per capita medical expenditures over the past 20 years is still very close to the annual percentage increase in total personal medical expenditures. Per capita medical expenditures have risen from $180.73 in 1965 to $1,504.25 in 1985.

Not all of the increase in medical expenditures represents an increase in the quantity of services per capita. A substantial part of the expenditure increase has been due to an increase in prices for the same services, as well as a change in the type of services provided. The price of medical care, as measured by the Consumer Price Index, has been increasing quite rapidly. Starting in 1966, the price of medical care began to increase at a faster pace than it had in the past; this acceleration in medical prices

1

TABLE 1-1. Trends in Personal Medical Care Expenditures

(1) Calendar Year	(2) Total (Billions)	(3) Annual % Increase Total	(4) % of GNP	(5) Per Capita Total	(6) Annual % Inc. Per Capita Total	(7) Annual % Inc. in CPI Medical Care	(8) Private Expend. (Billions)	(9) Annual % Increase Private	(10) % of Total	(11) Per Capita Private	(12) Annual % Inc. Per Capita Private	(13) Public Expend.	(14) Annual % Inc. Public	(15) % of Total	(16) Per Capita Public	(17) Annual % Inc. Per Capita Public	(18) Federal Expend. (Billions)	(19) Annual % Inc. Per Capita Federal	(20) State and Local Expend. (Billions)	(21) Annual % Inc. State
1950	$ 10.9		3.8	$ 70.37			$ 8.5		77.6	$ 54.59		$ 2.4		22.4	$ 15.78		$ 1.1		$ 1.3	
1955	15.7	7.6	3.9	93.29	5.8	3.8	12.1	7.3	77.0	71.86	5.7	3.6	8.5	23.0	21.43	6.3	1.6	5.9	2.0	9.0
1960	23.7	8.6	4.7	128.81	6.7	4.1	18.5	8.9	78.2	100.76	7.0	5.2	7.6	21.8	28.05	5.5	2.2	4.1	3.0	8.5
1965	35.8	8.6	5.2	180.73	7.0	2.5	28.1	8.7	78.4	141.75	7.1	7.7	8.2	21.6	38.98	6.8	3.6	8.9	4.1	6.5
1966	39.6	10.6	5.2	197.61	9.3	4.4	29.5	5.0	74.3	146.92	3.7	10.1	31.2	25.7	50.69	30.0	5.3	43.3	4.9	19.5
1967	44.4	12.1	5.6	219.29	11.0	7.1	29.3	-.7	66.0	144.71	-1.5	15.1	49.5	34.0	74.58	47.1	9.5	78.6	5.6	14.3
1968	50.2	13.1	5.7	245.50	12.0	6.1	32.5	10.9	64.6	158.66	9.6	17.7	17.2	35.4	86.84	16.4	11.4	18.7	6.4	14.3
1969	56.9	13.4	6.0	275.64	12.3	6.9	36.8	13.2	64.6	178.05	12.2	20.1	13.6	35.4	97.59	12.4	13.2	14.6	7.0	9.4
1970	65.1	14.4	6.6	312.29	13.3	6.4	42.6	15.8	65.5	204.57	14.9	22.5	11.9	34.5	107.72	10.4	14.5	9.2	7.9	12.9
1971	72.0	10.6	6.7	340.64	9.1	6.5	46.4	8.9	64.4	219.50	7.3	25.6	13.8	35.6	121.14	12.5	16.8	13.9	8.8	11.4
1972	80.2	11.4	6.7	375.53	10.2	3.2	51.4	10.8	64.0	240.47	9.6	28.8	12.5	36.0	135.06	11.5	18.9	11.7	9.9	12.5
1973	88.7	10.6	6.7	411.20	9.5	3.9	56.7	10.3	63.9	262.62	9.2	32.0	11.1	36.1	148.58	10.0	21.1	10.2	11.0	11.1
1974	101.0	13.9	7.0	463.84	12.8	9.3	62.4	10.1	61.8	286.69	9.2	38.6	20.6	38.2	177.15	19.2	25.8	12.1	12.8	16.4
1975	116.8	15.6	7.5	530.97	14.5	12.0	70.7	13.3	60.5	321.20	12.0	46.1	19.4	39.5	209.77	18.4	31.4	20.8	14.7	14.8
1976	131.8	12.8	7.7	593.67	11.8	9.6	80.3	13.6	60.9	361.60	12.6	51.5	11.7	39.1	232.07	10.6	36.1	13.9	15.4	4.8
1977	148.7	12.8	7.8	663.16	11.7	9.6	90.8	13.1	61.1	404.96	12.0	57.9	12.4	38.9	258.20	11.3	41.0	12.2	16.9	9.7
1978	166.7	12.1	7.7	735.57	10.9	8.4	101.5	11.8	60.9	447.86	10.6	65.2	12.6	39.1	287.71	11.4	46.4	12.1	18.8	11.2
1979	189.1	13.4	7.8	825.68	12.3	9.3	114.7	13.0	60.7	500.95	11.9	74.4	14.1	39.3	324.73	12.9	53.1	13.2	21.3	13.3
1980	217.9	15.2	8.3	940.62	13.9	10.9	131.5	14.7	60.4	567.66	13.3	86.4	16.1	39.6	372.96	14.9	62.5	16.5	23.9	12.2
1981	255.0	17.0	8.7	1,089.93	15.9	10.7	152.1	15.7	59.6	649.68	14.5	102.9	19.1	40.4	439.82	17.9	74.6	18.1	28.3	18.4
1982	284.9	11.7	9.0	1,186.10	8.8	11.6	171.5	12.8	60.2	713.99	9.9	113.4	10.2	39.8	472.11	7.3	83.9	9.6	29.5	4.2
1983	315.2	10.6	9.3	1,299.79	9.6	8.7	190.4	11.0	60.4	785.16	10.1	124.8	10.1	39.6	514.64	9.0	92.9	9.7	31.9	8.1
1984	341.8	8.4	9.1	1,396.68	7.5	6.2	206.5	8.5	60.4	843.89	9.4	135.45	8.5	39.6	553.33	7.5	101.1	7.8	34.3	7.5
1985	371.4	8.7	9.3	1,504.25	7.7	9.4	224.0	8.5	60.3	907.25	7.5	147.5	8.9	39.7	597.41	8.0	112.6	10.4	34.8	1.5

SOURCES: Daniel R. Waldo et al., "National Health Expenditures," *Health Care Financial Review*, Fall issues, 3, 7 and 8, Tables 1–3; U.S. Bureau of the Census, *Statistical Abstract of the United States*, (1981 and 1986), 102nd and 106th eds. (Washington, D.C.: U.S. Government Printing Office, 1981 and 1986), Tables 779 and 796.

Note: "Personal medical care expenditure" is equal to total health care expenditures less expenditures for prepayment and administration, government public health activities, and research and construction of medical facilities.

continued until the early 1970s, when federal price controls were imposed on the economy. The Economic Stabilization Program lasted longer for the medical sector than for the rest of the economy, from 1971 until 1974. With the removal of those price controls, medical prices rose rapidly. As the rate of inflation in the economy increased in the late 1970s, so did the rise in medical prices. Similarly, as inflation declined in the early 1980s, so did the rise in medical prices. However, the increase in medical prices has continued to outstrip the rise in the economy's inflation rate. This rapid rate of increase in medical prices over time has resulted in medical price increases consisting of approximately two-thirds of the annual percentage increase in total medical expenditures.

In 1966, the passage of Medicare and Medicaid produced dramatic changes in the medical sector. Medicare is a federal program for financing the medical services of the aged; Medicaid is a federal-state financing program for the medically indigent. Prior to 1966, the medical sector was predominately private. In 1965, 80 percent of medical expenditures were privately financed. The introduction of Medicare and Medicaid had both short- and long-run consequences for the medical care sector. By 1985, although the private sector had increased its total expenditures (from $28 billion in 1965 to $224 billion in 1985), this total represented a declining share of total personal medical expenditures, 60 percent. The federal rather than state government is paying an increasing share (30 percent) of total personal medical expenditures. In 1965, the federal government spent $3.6 billion on personal medical services, while the states spent $4.1 billion. By 1985, the federal government was spending $112.6 billion a year and the states were spending $34.8 billion.

With the enactment of Medicare and Medicaid, the aged and the poor had increased access to medical care. Hospitals were paid according to their costs and physicians received their usual and customary fees. Private medical insurance was also becoming more widespread during this period. The consequence was that provider prices began to increase more rapidly, as did expenditures on medical services. As both private insurance and government payments lessened the financial burden on the patient, there were few constraints remaining to hold down the use of services and prices charged by providers. The federal and state governments became alarmed as they saw their expenditures under Medicare and Medicaid exceed their budgets for these two programs. There were concerns about the reasons for the continual rapid increases in medical prices and the efficiency of the medical sector. Regulatory programs, such as utilization review and controls on hospital capital, were enacted to hold down the rise in medical expenditures. Business and labor also became concerned with the rapid increases in employees' health insurance premiums. By the late 1970s, it was clear that the regulatory programs were not working. And then in the early 1980s, to the surprise of most health care experts, the medical market started becoming competitive. As market competition became more widespread, concerns about access to medical care by the poor and aged arose once again.

The rapid and continuing increase in the amount of our nation's resources being devoted to personal medical services and the increasing role of government in financing personal medical services (over 40 percent of total medical care expenditures) raise important policy questions.[1] For example, are the large annual percentage increases in

---

[1]Public expenditures on health and medical care services as a percentage of all federal and of all governmental (including state and local) expenditures have been increasing rapidly since 1966. Prior to 1966, government medical expenditures, as a percentage of all governmental expenditures, remained steady at approximately 3.7

medical prices, which contribute to the increase in expenditures, justified? Could a greater amount of medical services be provided, for the same amount of expenditures, if those resources were allocated differently? To analyze these type of issues, we must examine the efficiency with which the medical sector produces its output.

We may further ask: Should the government be spending an increasing share of its limited resources on personal medical services when there are competing needs, such as for education and welfare reform? To answer this question, it is necessary first to determine the amount of medical services redistribution that should occur and the population groups to be served. Once these value judgments have been stated explicitly, economics can determine the most efficient way to achieve a given equity goal.

Economics offers two basic tools and a set of criteria with which to analyze issues of efficiency and distribution. The first tool is techniques of optimization. Optimization techniques specify the appropriate criteria to be used when allocating scarce resources so as to minimize the cost of achieving a given objective. We can use techniques of optimization to evaluate the efficiency of the current system of medical services delivery. Similarly, optimization techniques can be used by governments and other organizations to determine the most efficient allocation of medical and nonmedical resources to achieve a given objective, such as an increase in the health status of the population.

The second economic tool is the determination of equilibrium situations, by which, for example, economists can predict the final result of a change in demand for a service. Predicting new equilibrium situations involves the use of the familiar tools of supply and demand analysis. The use of supply and demand analysis should point to the causes for the rapid increases in medical care prices and expenditures and should enable us to predict prices and expenditures in the years ahead. Supply and demand analysis is also used for estimating the consequences, in price, quantity of service, and total expenditure, of policies governing the redistribution of medical services in the population, such as through national health insurance.

Implicit in the use of the foregoing analytical tools is a set of criteria for evaluating economic welfare. These welfare criteria are used to determine whether someone is made better or worse off as a result of a particular action or policy and to evaluate the performance of an industry. Welfare criteria and the explicit statement of the assumptions that underlie their use contribute to the study of medical care. Much public policy is based on the values held by individuals and their perception of the most efficient method for achieving the given set of values. A specific set of welfare criteria provides the means by which differences in values and differences in methods for achieving a set of values can be separately evaluated.

BASIC CHOICES THAT MUST BE MADE WITH REGARD TO MEDICAL SERVICES

Problems of scarcity are the basis for the development and use of the economist's tools and criteria. The economist's skill in using optimization techniques, forecasting, and

---

percent. Federal medical expenditures, as a percentage of all federal expenditures, remained steady at approximately 3.0 percent. By 1983 the percentages were 11.0 percent and 12.6 percent, respectively. U.S. Bureau of the Census, *Statistical Abstract of the United States, 1986* (Washington, D.C.: U.S. Government Printing Office, 1986); Daniel R. Waldo, Katherine R. Levit, and Helen Lazenby, "National Health Expenditures, 1985," *Health Care Financing Review*, 8(1), Fall 1986.

criteria for evaluating economic performance is useful and necessary regardless of how medical care is organized and provided in a country. The decisions that must be made in any medical system are the same whether they are made by consumers or by government.

Three basic choices determine the organization of health and medical services (and other sectors of the economy). The first choice is determination of both the amount to be spent on health and medical services and the composition of those services. The second choice is a selection of the best method for producing medical services; two such methods are health maintenance organizations (HMOs) and fee-for-service. Even within a given delivery system, choices must be made regarding the amounts of capital and equipment to use relative to the amounts and types of labor in providing a service. The third choice is a selection of the method for distributing health services among the population. The first two choices are concerned with issues of economic efficiency, the third with equity in use of health services.

Every country must decide on how much it wants to spend on medical services and the best methods for producing and distributing them. A crucial assumption underlying the application of economics to this decisionmaking process is that alternatives exist for each of the three basic decisions to be made. If there were no alternatives, economics would not be of use to decisionmaking in a situation of resource scarcity. It is important to determine whether or not there are choices in medical care for making the decisions noted above. A discussion of choices in medical care should also clarify whether differences in selecting the choices to be made result from differences in values or a disagreement over the method of achieving an agreed-on set of values. In the following discussion of these three sets of medical care decisions, the economic tools discussed above will be used to illustrate the usefulness of economics both in clarifying and in making choices.

Determining the Output of Medical Services

The first set of medical care decisions to be made is referred to as the determination of output: How much should be allocated to, and what should be the composition of, medical services? In a medical system using a price system for resource allocation, consumer and physician decisions determine the quantity and quality of medical services. Theoretically, the consumer will select those services which, given his or her income and the prices of different services, maximize satisfaction. It is assumed that consumers make such choices rationally and that they have information on both the benefits derived from different services and the prices of those services. If these assumptions are correct, consumers will allocate their scarce resources (both time and income) to those services and activities that provide them with the greatest amount of benefits. The accuracy of these assumptions with respect to medical services are discussed below.

To understand the allocation process used by consumers when selecting among various commodities, including both goods and services, and also be able to predict changes in consumer allocation, it is necessary to understand marginal analysis, which is the basis of the optimization technique. Consumers' purchases provide them with benefits, or utility; additional purchases of those same services provide additional benefits, but these additional benefits decline as more units are purchased. The benefits derived from consuming the first unit of a commodity are high; subsequent units of

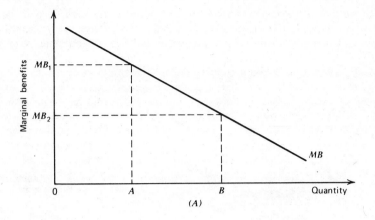

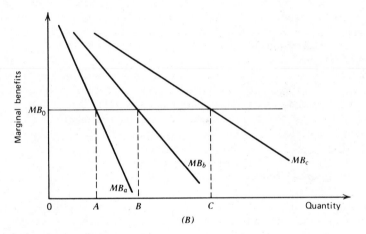

Figure 1-1. Marginal benefit curves of (A) a single commodity, (B) different commodities.

that same commodity provide smaller benefits. Although total benefits increase with additional units of the same commodity, the marginal benefit of additional units declines. This relationship between marginal benefits and additional units of a service is shown in Figure 1–1A. The marginal benefit from consuming OA units of the particular commodity represented in Figure 1–1A is MB_1. If additional units are consumed, the marginal benefit received from those additional units declines, from MB_1 to MB_2.

The consumer receives benefits from many different commodities. To maximize the total benefits from all commodities purchased, the consumer will allocate his or her limited resources to ensure that the marginal benefits received from all commodities purchased are equal.[2] This optimization rule for equating the marginal benefits of the last units of different commodities does not mean that the same number of units of each commodity will be consumed. It is more likely that when the marginal benefits of

---

[2] For the sake of simplicity, it is here assumed that the prices of the different commodities are equal.

different commodities are equal, the buyer will be consuming differing quantities of the commodities purchased. The reason is that the marginal benefits decline at different rates for different commodities. The consumer is likely to purchase more units of those commodities with a gradual decline in marginal benefits than of those with a very sharp decline. As shown in Figure 1-1B, the marginal benefits are equal at MB_0 for different commodities when the consumer is purchasing OA units, OB units, and OC units of three different commodities. Any other allocation process would result in a lower total level of benefits. The consumer therefore maximizes the amount of benefits for a given income by allocating it across commodities to ensure that the marginal benefits from the last units are equal.

To allow for differences in commodity prices, the consumer must compare not only the marginal benefits of different commodities but also the ratio of the marginal benefit to the price of each commodity (MB/P). When this is done, *the marginal benefit per dollar spent will be equal for all commodities.* (It should be noted that the marginal benefits received from the purchase of a commodity vary among consumers. These differences may be illustrated with reference to Figure 1-1B. The marginal benefit curves of Figure 1-1B in this case represent the marginal benefits received from the same commodity by different consumers.)

The consumer evaluates the marginal benefits of a purchase in relation to its price, or stated differently, the consumer compares the ratio of marginal benefit to marginal cost for each purchase with the ratio of every other purchase. The marginal cost to the consumer is the price he or she must pay for that commodity. When the consumer has equated the marginal benefits and the marginal costs of each purchase, his or her scarce resources have been allocated to maximize total benefits. In an equilibrium situation, when that quantity demanded equals the quantity supplied, the equilibrium price reflects the value placed on the last units purchased by all consumers since all consumers face the same price in a given market. In a competitive market, prices represent the costs of production. The costs of production in turn reflect the value of other goods and services that might have been produced with the same resources. When an efficient price system is used for allocating resources, the marginal benefits to consumers of purchasing the last unit equal the marginal costs of the resources used to produce it.

Any of the following changes in factors affecting consumers' allocation decisions would cause a change in their purchasing behavior: a change in the price of one commodity relative to that of other commodities, a change in income, or a change in perception of the benefits to be derived from consuming additional units. Economic tools (i.e., optimization techniques), which provide criteria that enable a consumer to allocate resources so as the maximize benefits, also provide the basis for understanding changes in consumer demand. It is in this way that the two tools of economics—optimization techniques and the determination of equilibrium situations—are related.[3]

---

[3]This discussion of marginal analysis is not meant to imply that *every* consumer continuously undertakes an exact system of calculation for purchasing all commodities. Consumers, on the average, do consider such factors as marginal benefits, relative prices, and their level of income when making their purchase decisions. Psychological and sociological variables are also included in economic models as predictors of consumer behavior. However, to the extent that consumers have information and act to maximize their total benefits, predictions based on changes in relative prices and income will result in more accurate predictions of consumer demand than will other (e.g., psychological or sociological) models of consumer behavior that exclude such economic variables.

The description above of the consumer choice process in a market system illustrates the importance of price in making choices. A nonmarket approach toward determining the amount of resources to be allocated to medical care requires a substitute mechanism that will perform the price function—that is, that will provide an incentive to consumers to limit their use of services to the point at which the cost of those services equals their value. Such a mechanism must also ration that available quantity of services among consumers and provide information to providers of changes in their demand. Although the functions that prices perform must still be performed under a nonmarket system, alternative mechanisms to perform these functions have generally been found to be unsatisfactory.

How Best to Produce Medical Services

The second set of decisions that must be made in any health system is selection of the best method for producing the amount of medical services to be provided. Medical services can be provided in different organizational settings, including health maintenance organizations or solo practitioners practicing under a fee-for-service arrangement. Even within a particular delivery system, the combinations of health personnel and equipment can vary. If the providers of medical services have the incentive to minimize their costs, they will use the various inputs—health personnel and capital—according to their relative costs and productivity. The method of optimization used by the provider will be similar to that used by the consumer of medical services. In place of marginal benefits and relative prices on the consumer side, marginal productivity of inputs and their relative costs will be used by providers to determine the least costly method of providing a service. The decision rule will also be the same. When the ratio of the marginal productivity of an input to its wage is equal to that of other inputs, the firm is minimizing its costs of providing medical services.

When the provider's costs are minimized, the combination of services (hospital and physician care) and the inputs (types of health personnel and capital) used to provide medical care will be both technically and economically efficient. Technical efficiency means that the medical services will be produced using the minimum number of inputs of any given proportion. However, several different combinations of inputs may be technically efficient. To minimize the cost of providing medical services, it is necessary to be not only technically but also economically efficient. The decisionmaker must choose among the several combinations of inputs, each of which is technically efficient, to determine which combination is also economically efficient—that is, least costly. To do so, the decisionmaker must consider the relative costs of the different inputs as well as their productivities.

When the economist applies the tools for optimization to the set of choices governing the production of medical services, several problems of medical services delivery are brought into sharper focus. Some medical care professionals have proposed the use of certain standards in the delivery of medical services: four hospital beds per 1,000 population is one such standard; specified lengths of stay, by diagnosis, for hospitalized patients is another example; and ratios of the number of registered nurses per hospitalized patient is a third. Standards such as these imply that medical services can or should be produced by only one method. If the provision of medical services were actually subject to such fixed proportions, no choice of production methods would exist, and the effectiveness of the economist's tools for minimizing medical care costs would be very limited. It is, however, unlikely that the choices for producing medical care are so limited. Depending upon the illness being treated, ambulatory care and nursing home services can be substituted for hospital care, with no decrease in the quality of treatment. Lengths of stay can be varied depending upon the availability of other facilities in the community and someone to care for the patient at home. Other kinds of nursing personnel can substitute for registered nurses in the care of the hospitalized patient. Presently, wide variations exist across communities in lengths of stay by diagnosis, in use of registered nurses, and in number of hospital beds per 1,000 population. Substituting medical services and personnel without decreasing their quality is more possible than some would have us believe.

If greater substitution in the production and delivery of medical services is possible, using the standards described above will hinder economic efficiency in providing medical care. Using inputs without regard to their relative costs is unlikely to result in the least-cost combination. The cost of hospital care relative to the cost of ambulatory and nursing home services has been increasing very rapidly. If four hospital beds per 1,000 population was the least costly input ratio 30 years ago, changes in the relative costs of hospital care and other services would seem to require that inputs be combined differently to achieve the least costly method today. A similar analysis could determine the optimum number of registered nurses per patient relative to other types of nursing personnel. As the relative costs (and productivities) of inputs change over time, it is to be expected that the combination of inputs that is least costly for providing medical services will change also. The economist's tools of optimization can determine which combination of services and inputs is most efficient for providing medical care. Similarly, the concepts embodied in these tools provide a decisionmaker with vital information about the costs of different choices, which can be used to decide how best to deliver medical services.

The second of the economist's tools, the prediction of new equilibrium levels of prices and quantities, can be used to anticipate changes required in the production of medical services. A change in the price of an input will, as discussed above, result in a change in the combination of inputs that is least costly to use in producing medical care. It is also possible to analyze the new equilibrium situation that will result from the change. An increase in the price of an input will cause a reduction in the quantity demanded of it and an increase in demand for those inputs whose prices have not changed. If the higher-priced inputs are used mainly in the provision of one type of service, such as hospital care, we would then expect to observe a reduction in the quantity demanded of that service because its price has risen as its inputs have become more costly. As the cost of medical services increases, the supply curve of medical care will shift upward. Assuming no change in the demand for medical services, the price of medical care will increase and the quantity demanded will decrease. The extent of the actual change in prices and quantities of medical care will depend upon the elasticities of supply and demand.

The tools of demand and supply can be used to trace the consequences of a change in input prices throughout the medical system. They can also be used to anticipate the effects of changes in medical technology on productivity, medical prices, and quantities of services. Such equilibrium analyses are particularly helpful in anticipating future expenditures for medical care to be borne either by patients or by the government, such as those that would occur under a system of national health insurance.

The Distribution of Medical Services

The third set of decisions that must be made in any medical system govern the distribution of the system's output. We must select from a number of alternatives when making this decision. We can provide medical care free of charge to all persons; we can distribute medical care in accordance with consumers' willingness to spend their incomes for it. We can also increase the medical care use of those consumers with incomes that are insufficient to purchase the amount of medical care society deems appropriate and necessary.

Economics can clarify the issues involved in the distribution of medical services by providing a set of criteria for determining whether or not a person's welfare is improved by a particular policy. If the purpose of that policy is to improve the person's welfare, economic criteria will suggest the most efficient means for accomplishing that goal. Two value judgments govern the distribution of medical services. The first is whether or not consumers should determine the amount they wish to spend on medical services. The second concerns the method and size of subsidy to be extended to those low-income consumers whose use of medical services is below what society believes it should be. The economist cannot decide which values are preferable; however, economics can help make the process of choosing more rational by providing information on the costs and the implications of different sets of values, and also by providing criteria for determining the most efficient method for achieving a given set of values.

Chapter 20 contains a more complete discussion of the different values underlying the subsidies designed to redistribute medical services in the population. It also contains an analysis of the economic efficiency of existing methods of financing medical services as well as of those proposed under alternative approaches to national health insurance.

THE APPLICABILITY OF ECONOMICS TO THE STUDY OF MEDICAL CARE

Critics have questioned the applicability of economics to the study of medical services on two levels: first, they have questioned the accuracy of assumptions underlying economic behavior of consumers and medical providers, and second, they have challenged the implicit values, such as consumer sovereignty, that influence the goal to be achieved (i.e., consumer satisfaction). For example, critics have claimed that it is inaccurate to assume that the consumer of health services is rational, and that he or she has sufficient information when deciding on use of services. Such critics also claim that the purchaser of medical services is not the consumer, as in nonmedical markets, but the physician, who also has a financial interest in the services to be purchased. With regard to economists' traditional assumptions about providers of medical services, critics claim that these providers are organized as nonprofit organizations and therefore do not have the same motivations as for-profit firms in other industries. Further, since consumers may be irreparably harmed by incompetent providers, more stringent controls must be exercised over the provision of medical services than over nonmedical goods and services. Finally, such critics claim that access to medical services is considered a right by society and its distribution cannot be left solely to the marketplace.

It is important to distinguish between criticism directed at the validity of economic assumptions and criticism of the use of economic criteria for evaluating medical system performance. If economic analyses are undertaken, they will be based upon a given set of assumptions, which will lead us to predict a certain outcome. If the observed behavior is different from what was expected, the assumptions are reexamined to determine whether a different assumption could explain the divergence between the expected and observed behavior. For example, one factor affecting the performance of an industry is whether entry is permitted into that industry. An economic analysis would initially assume that entry into a market, such as the physician market, is free. Based on this assumption, we expect to observe certain measures of performance in that market; high physician incomes relative to other occupations would lead to increased enrollment in medical schools. If what we observe is different from what we have predicted, we then examine whether the free-entry assumption is accurate. Thus economic analysis isolates those assumptions to be reexamined when a divergence occurs between expected and observed behavior.

If the observed performance of an industry is different from what we would expect in a competitive market, public policy may be required to change that industry's performance. Some public policy prescriptions attempt to make structural changes that will bring an industry's actual performance into greater conformity with its expected performance. If, for example, an industry is observed to provide its services inefficiently, we examine whether efficiency incentives exist in that industry. If such incentives are lacking, one appropriate policy prescription would be to improve the incentives for efficient operation.

For each of the aspects of medical care to be analyzed, the expected performance of consumers and providers will be contrasted with the observed performance. When a divergence is discovered between the two, the underlying assumptions will be reexamined to account for the observed behavior. The specific assumptions regarding consumer information, incentives for efficiency, and barriers to entry can thus be examined to determine what effect these factors have on the economic performance of the medical care sector when they differ from their theoretical assumptions.

The medical care market is also acknowledged to be different from other markets because it includes a greater demand for consumer protection. However, different approaches to providing consumer protection are available. These alternative approaches, together with other, possibly unique aspects of medical care, will be analyzed with respect to their impact on the performance of the medical care sector.

Criticisms of the values underlying the use of economic criteria for evaluating medical system performance are more difficult to resolve. Given a scarcity in the availability of resources for providing medical services, what criteria should society use for making the three basic medical care decisions? A medical system that values economic efficiency in consumption and production will base its choice of the amount to spend on medical services on the criteria of satisfying consumer preferences; it will base its method of providing services on the criteria of least cost; and it will base its choice of the amount and method of medical services redistribution on the criteria of consumer preference. Under this value system, medical service benefits are defined by consumer preference rather than by government or health agency perception of consumer preference.

If decisionmakers reject the foregoing criteria, new criteria must be specified. The criterion of efficiency in production is more likely to be acceptable than is the criterion of satisfying consumer preferences. In the latter case, the alternative that proponents are likely to substitute is a "needs" approach to the allocation of medical services. Under a needs approach, the value placed on medical services and the resources necessary to satisfy those needs are centrally determined. Because resources are insufficient to satisfy all medical needs, an additional decision rule must be developed that will enable the decisionmakers to choose which needs and which population groups will be given highest priority.

The replacement of one set of values by another does not influence the usefulness of economics in the decisionmaking process; its value lies in its ability to make that process more rational by showing what the costs of different choices are. To the extent that economic analysis can clarify the costs of alternatives and make the values underlying those alternatives explicit, it is a useful approach to the study of medical care.

THE TRADE-OFF BETWEEN QUANTITY AND QUALITY IN THE PROVISION OF MEDICAL SERVICES

The following example of the trade-off between quantity and quality illustrates the kinds of choices that must be made with regard to medical services. One of the choices that any medical system must make in determining the use of its limited resources is the combination of quantity and quality of medical services it wishes to provide. If the length of training of health professionals is long, and if the equipment and facilities used are the most technically advanced, fewer services will be available to the entire population. This trade-off between quantity and quality (which actually refers to the level of training of health professionals—a process measure, not an outcome measure, of quality) is shown in Figure 1–2. Point A represents a combination where quality is relatively high and is received by a small percentage of the population. Point B represents a different combination: a large percentage of the population receives some medical services, while the quality of those services is relatively low. The quantity-quality trade-off curve in Figure 1–2 is referred to as a production possibilities curve.[4]

What criterion should determine the combination of quality and quantity of medical services that a society should choose? If the criterion were the maximizing of consumer preferences, then, assuming adequate information and proper safeguards, consumers would be the appropriate group to select the quantity-quality combination that should prevail.[5] Alternatively, health professionals can select the quantity-quality trade-off, as they have done in the United States. For example, health professionals establish the educational requirements and determine the number of educational institutions through their accreditation policies. There are fewer health professionals than there would be if educational requirements were more flexible and if fewer re-

---

[4]The curve is shaped as it is (concave to the origin) because the resources used in producing quantity and quality (which are equivalent to two different outputs) are not completely substitutable for one another. As more of one combination of services is produced (as represented by point A or B), the resources are switched from producing one type of services to the other. The released resources are more specialized, hence more efficient, in producing their previous output. Moving those same resources into the production of a different good or service will cause them to be less efficient in the production of that new service. Thus the costs of producing more of the new output are increased.

[5]The resultant quantity-quality combination would maximize consumer satisfaction because the marginal benefits of those services (to the consumer) would equal the marginal cost of resources used in their production.

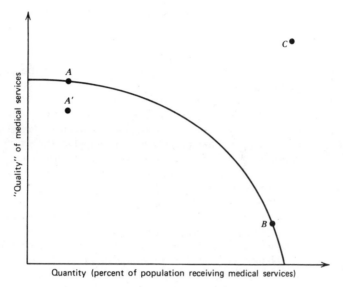

Figure 1-2. The quantity–quality trade-off in medical care.

strictions were placed on entry into the health professions and on the tasks that professionals are permitted to perform.

The discussion of the quantity-quality trade-off can also be used to illustrate the
second set of choices that must be made in any medical care system—namely, how
best to produce medical services. Any quantity-quality combination on the production
possibilities curve is assumed to have been produced in the least costly manner. The
amount of resources devoted to medical services is represented by the area under the
curve. If, owing to the placement of restrictions on the least costly manner of production or the use of a method of provider reimbursement that removes efficiency incentives, the providers of medical services are not as efficient as they might be, then fewer
medical services will be produced for the same amount of resources. This situation is
shown in Figure 1-2, where A′ represents the same amount of resources as used at
point A but the output is less than that achieved at point A. A′ is obviously inefficient
in that resources are being wasted; either more medical services or medical services of
higher quality could be produced with the same quantity of resources. It is important
to determine whether the current medical care system is at point A or A′ and, if so, the
reasons why it is.

The third set of choices concerning medical services distribution might be illustrated by a quantity-quality analysis of the statement, "All Americans should receive
the highest quality of medical care." The highest quality of medical care to all would
be represented by point C in Figure 1-2, which is equivalent to 100 percent of the
population (farthest to the right on the horizontal axis), and by the highest point on
the quality axis. To achieve such a goal, additional resources equivalent to the distance between point C and the current production possibilities curve would be required. These additional resources would be financed either by an increase in taxes or
by decreased expenditures on other programs. These choices provide differing marginal benefits. Who is to decide their relative benefits? Health professionals attach

greater benefits to medical as opposed to other services; however, they do not bear the costs of their decisions. Consumers, who will bear the costs, may not share professional estimates of the relative benefits.

Each medical system must make choices in three areas: how much to spend on medical services, how best to produce those services, and how to distribute them. People differ in their values as to how those choices should be made. To evaluate how the medical system performs with respect to each of those choices, it is necessary to establish criteria for what is considered good performance. The performance criteria used by economists are based upon a set of values incorporated into their definition of economic efficiency—namely, maximizing consumer satisfaction and using the least costly method of production. If decisionmakers disagree over these values, it is necessary to state explicitly an alternative set of values. People can then decide whether they prefer one set of values over another. For any alternative set of values, it is also necessary to state the criteria to be used for evaluating the performance of the medical system. The debate over appropriate public policy in medical care is often confused because a clear distinction is not made between differences in values and differences in the best way to achieve a particular set of values. Clarification of these differences should sharpen the debate over the most appropriate public policies for medical care.

CHAPTER 2

The Production of Health: The Impact of Medical Services on Health

MEDICAL CARE AS AN OUTPUT OF THE MEDICAL SERVICES INDUSTRY AND AS AN INPUT TO HEALTH

The first of two alternative ways of looking at medical care is to regard it as the final output of the medical care industry. When viewing medical care as an output, it is important to determine how efficiently it is produced. Industry analyses of the factors affecting the supply of and demand for physician services, hospital care, and the various manpower markets enables us to infer the performance of the medical care industry; that is, we can compare the price and output of the industry as it now exists with the price and quantity (as well as quality) that might exist if the medical care industry underwent a structural change. A structural change would be said to have occurred if physicians, who were predominately in solo practice and were reimbursed under a fee-for-service arrangement, organized into larger groups, such as prepaid group practices, that included other providers, such as hospitals. Many lesser structural changes can also occur, such as changing the state practice acts, which determine the tasks that different health professionals can perform, or changing the requirements for entering a health profession. All of these proposals affect the structure, hence the performance, of the medical services industry. When medical care is viewed as the output of the medical services industry, our understanding of the structure of that industry (and of its component industries) enables us to evaluate its performance.

The second way of looking at medical care is to view it, not as a final output, but rather as one input among many, all of which contribute to an output referred to as "good health." Improvements in health status may be achieved by providing medical services, undertaking medical research, instituting environmental health programs,

15

such as those which control air pollution, and by conducting health education programs aimed at changing the lifestyle of consumers.

When determining the amount of resources to be allocated to the medical services sector if the objective is to ensure an increase in health, it is best to view medical care as one of many factors that can improve health status. This approach helps us to determine those program inputs to which resources should be allocated in order to improve health. This allocation question is different from that contained in the first view, which is concerned with the appropriate structure of the medical services industry and the allocation of resources for producing medical care itself. These two different ways of viewing medical care should be recognized explicitly, as each is useful for different public policies. To determine whether medical care is being produced efficiently, one must examine it as a final output; to determine the most efficient way to allocate resources to increase health, one must view medical services as one of several inputs for achieving that goal.

The second, or input, view will be adopted in the remainder of this chapter, which will first present a theoretical approach for determining how many resources should be allocated to medical care; second, empirical estimates of medical care's marginal contribution to increased health will be reviewed; and third, applications and implications of those findings will be discussed.

DETERMINING THE ALLOCATION OF RESOURCES TO MEDICAL CARE USING A HEALTH PRODUCTION FUNCTION

To determine among which inputs the allocation of resources would be least costly for achieving an increase in health levels, it is necessary to understand the concept of a "health production function." A production function describes the relationship between combinations of inputs and the resulting output; it is to be distinguished from a production possibility curve which describes the trade-off between different outputs from a given set of resources. Health can be produced using different combinations of inputs. (It is assumed in empirical studies of health production functions that the estimated relationships are technically efficient; that is, the inputs produce the maximum possible output.) The economist (and the policymaker) is interested in determining which combination of inputs is economically efficient—that is, least costly, for producing the output, health. Before we can determine the least costly combination of inputs for producing a given level of health, we must determine the production function for health. Once it has been determined, and estimates have been developed for the marginal effects of each of the inputs on health, comparisons can then be made between increasing expenditures on different inputs. The process of allocating resources to increase health can be improved once information becomes available on both the relative costs of different programs and their effects on health status. Often the real intent of a program's expenditures may be inferred by determining the effect of its resources.

Several studies have attempted to estimate a health production function. However, before reviewing the results and limitations of these studies, it would be useful to discuss the concept itself. A health production function is an analytical method for determining how to allocate resources among alternative programs to achieve an increase in health. The analytical method involves two steps: specifying, first, what information is required, and second, how that information is to be used for allocating resources. Once the empirical studies of health production functions have been reviewed, those results will be used to determine whether increased expenditures on medical services offer a greater or lesser return for achieving an increase in health levels than would expenditures on alternative programs.

The first step in using a health production function for making allocation decisions is to state a specific function—that is, to define the output (or objective) to be achieved and the alternative approaches for achieving it. To arrive at alternative approaches, the desired output must be explicitly defined. For example, if the objective is increased health of the population, the alternatives will also be fairly general: a better environment, improved nutrition, greater emphasis on preventive care, improved access to medical services, and better personal health habits. For policymakers, however, these alternative policies are not sufficiently specific to indicate which environmental, preventative, or medical care programs to undertake so as to have an impact on the health levels of specified population groups. Unless the health objective is defined by age and sex groupings (and probably location), it will not be possible to determine which project—a cancer screening program or a maternal and child health project—will have the greatest effect on health status.

Health professionals and others knowledgeable about health programs are best able to specify which programs are alternatives for increasing the health status of a particular age–sex population group. By using optimization tools, the economist can determine how to allocate limited health funds among alternative programs to achieve the largest possible increase in health status.

The discussion that follows illustrates the approach that should be used to allocate expenditures among alternative programs to achieve the maximum possible increase in the policy objective. Assuming that the policy objective is to decrease the infant mortality rate, on which type of programs should additional funds be spent? For illustrative purposes, let it be assumed that only two programs exist for reducing infant mortality rates: one is to establish additional intensive care units in selected hospitals for infants of high risk; the other is to increase funding for maternal and child health programs (to expectant mothers and children up to 5 years of age) in health shortage areas. The following approach demonstrates the type of information and analysis required to determine how best to allocate limited funds between these two programs (1).

The relationship between spending additional funds on each program and their impact on infant mortality rates is shown in Figure 2–1. When a program is relatively small, additional inputs devoted to that program are likely to result in relatively large increases in the program's output (decreased infant mortality rates). As additional resources are allocated to that program, the output will continue to increase, but at a more gradual rate. Finally, increases in output will become negligible even though the program's inputs continue to increase. The relationship between program inputs and program output has a curvilinear shape because eventually it becomes more difficult to find high-risk infants, as is illustrated by the establishment of additional intensive care units (ICUs). Placing a third intensive care unit for infants in an area may result in a decrease in use of all three units, even when formerly two units had been fully utilized. Thus, with a third unit, the output per ICU unit falls. Or, if use does not decrease, it will expand to include infants of lower risk than those admitted when there were fewer such units. With maternal and child health programs, initial pro-

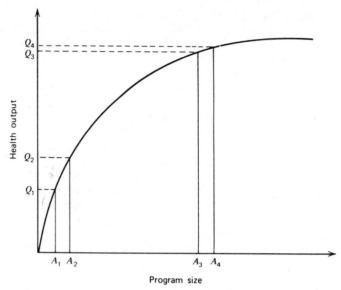

Figure 2-1. The relationship between total output and program size.

grams are likely to provide care for those patients most likely to benefit from them. As additional resources are devoted to maternal and child health, it either becomes more costly to find recipients who will benefit most from these programs, or recipients whose need is not as great begin to use the program. In either case, the output of the program per unit of input begins to decline as the size of the program is increased. It is thus inappropriate to assume that there is a constant (i.e., linear) relationship between a program's inputs and its output. Additional resources spent on health programs are unlikely to produce the same increase in output as did previous increases in the program's expenditures.

Since the relationship between total program output and program input is curvilinear, as shown in Figure 2-1, it must be determined at which point on that total output curve a particular program is operating. If the size of the program is relatively large, as shown by point A_3, then adding resources equivalent to A_3–A_4 will result in an increase in total output of the magnitude Q_3–Q_4. If the program is smaller-for example, at size A_1—the same increase in program resources will result in a larger increase in total program output, from Q_1 to Q_2.

Still using the simplified example, if it costs the same to increase the inputs in two health programs, but one program (e.g., the intensive care unit program) is at size A_3, while the other (i.e., the maternal and child health program) is at size A_1, to which of the two programs should additional resources be allocated? Given the output and input relationship for both, as shown in Figure 2-1, the allocation of a given amount of resources to the program at point A_1 would result in the largest change in health output. Thus the decision rule for allocating resources between the two programs (when the cost of changing either program is the same) is to select that program whose change in total output would be greatest.

It has sometimes been suggested that additional resources should be allocated to those programs whose total output is the largest. Such a decision rule, however, would

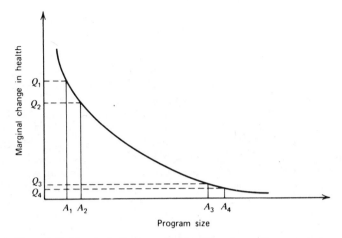

Figure 2-2. Marginal effects on health with a change in program size.

not necessarily result in the largest increase in output for a given expenditure. Allocating additional resources among programs does not mean that those receiving little or no increase in their resources have to close down, thereby losing their entire output. Allocation decisions are based not on the total output of competing programs, but rather on *changes* in total output of competing programs. The total output achievable from all programs will be at its maximum only when additional resources are allocated to programs whose increase in total output is greatest.

Another way of illustrating how the allocation technique above results in the largest increase in total output is to examine the marginal relationships between inputs and outputs of the various programs. The marginal changes between total inputs and total outputs of each program are shown in Figure 2-2. These marginal relationships, which reflect the change in total output resulting from a unit increase in a program's inputs, eventually decline with increased program size for the same reason that the total output curve shown in Figure 2-1 increases at a decreasing rate. The marginal relationship shown in Figure 2-2 is the slope of the curve shown in Figure 2-1.

Once it is understood that marginal analysis is the tool for maximizing total output, the implications of allocation decisions based on a need criterion become clear. If additional resources were devoted to intensive care units, an increase in infant health levels from Q_3 to Q_4 would result. As long as further increases in total output beyond Q_4 could be achieved, its advocates, using the need criterion, would recommend additional resources for such programs. Scarce resources, however, have a "cost." The additional resources required to increase the ICU program beyond size A_4 could be spent on programs whose change in total output would have been greater. The real cost of the resources devoted to increasing the size of the ICU program is the benefit (output) that could have been achieved if those resources had been spent on alternative programs.

Resources will be allocated in an optimal manner when the additional output produced by resources in one program equals the forgone benefits of using those same resources on alternative programs. This approach toward allocating resources differs from that of health professionals, who generally see only the unmet needs that could be eliminated by devoting still more resources to their own programs.

Since empirical studies on the relationship between total program output and program inputs are not always available, it is difficult to develop estimates of the marginal effect of increased program resources. Data are more likely to be available on the program's total output and total expenditures. Analysts are therefore able to calculate the *average* benefits of the program (total output/total inputs). Because of the greater availability of average measures, they are often used as the basis for comparing the benefits of and allocating resources to competing programs. The use of such average measures, however, can result in an incorrect allocation of resources among health programs.

The average and marginal benefits of two programs are shown in Figure 2–3. At point Z (equivalent to a certain program size) the two programs could appear to be identical because their average benefits are equal. However, at point Z, the marginal benefits of program B are greater than those of program A. Since resource allocations made on the basis of marginal benefits result in the greatest increases in total output, using average benefits (perhaps as a proxy for marginal benefits) can result in error, as this example illustrates.

In Figure 2–1 it was assumed for the sake of simplicity that the cost of increasing the size of the two programs was the same. This is generally not the case. When the costs of increasing a program's size are not equal, the comparison cannot simply be made between the changes in the output of the two programs. The relevant criterion for allocating resources to programs having different benefits and costs is to select those programs whose marginal benefit per dollar spent is greatest. For example, assume that an increase in program A would result in a decrease in infant mortality of 30 infants. The marginal costs of achieving that increased benefit is $300,000. An increase in program B yields, as a marginal benefit, a decrease in infant mortality of 20 infants at a marginal cost of $100,000. The marginal benefits per dollar spent are larger for program B; a decrease in infant mortality of two per $10,000 as compared with one per $10,000 under program A.[1]

Based upon the foregoing discussion, we can summarize the type of information needed to allocate scarce resources among alternative health programs. First, the particular population group whose health is to be affected must be specified. The disease category for that given population group must also be specified so as to be able to form a health production function. Third, the marginal effect on health of each of the health programs should be empirically estimated. Unfortunately, very little information exists among health professionals or economists about the marginal impacts of alternative health programs. Thus allocation decisions are currently being made with little or no information about their marginal effects. Determining the marginal impact on health of increased expenditures on medical services and on alternative health

---

[1]For the sake of simplicity, this discussion has assumed that the input–output relationship for each program is independent of changes in scale in the other programs. In actuality, this is not so. For example, if one health program emphasizes prevention, then an increase in resources for this program is likely to affect the productivity of others, such as acute care services. These interrelationships between health programs may cause the input–output curve of particular programs to shift either to the left or to the right; that is, the marginal benefits of the affected program may be increased or decreased without changing expenditures for that program.

In some cases acute care programs may become more productive, as for example after an increase in knowledge or technology (perhaps resulting from increased expenditures on research programs). An increase in knowledge or technology may enable a provider to see more patients or to have a more favorable effect on the outcome of the treatment provided. Alternatively, an increase in preventive programs may decrease the need for acute treatment in the population, thereby lowering the number of patients treated in existing acute care programs. The productivity of existing programs would therefore be lessened.

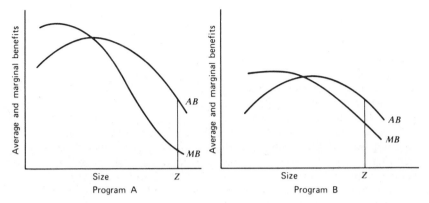

Figure 2-3. Average and marginal benefits from alternative health programs.

programs is an important area for research. Some general information is available on the overall marginal effect of medical services on health. For decisionmaking, however, information is required on the marginal effect that specific medical and other health programs have on disease-specific illness rates for particular population groups.[2]

If decisionmakers are to allocate scarce resources so as to produce the maximum possible increase in health levels, they must understand the economic concepts underlying their allocation; they must also generate the information needed to enable appropriate analyses to be undertaken (2). Program managers often avoid generating useful information because they do not want their program to be compared with competing health programs. They believe that the uncertainty of their program's effects will enhance their bargaining position.

The foregoing description of the information requirements of a health production function and the application of that information for allocating resources among alternative health programs provides a background for evaluating the empirical studies to be discussed.

EMPIRICAL STUDIES OF A HEALTH PRODUCTION FUNCTION

The justification often given for government intervention to provide more medical services to the population in general and to underserved population groups in particular is the desire to improve health status. If the objective of government expenditures is to increase health levels, it is important to derive empirical estimates of the net impact that medical care has on health.

---

[2]Given the very limited data on the marginal effects of alternative health programs, only the grossest comparisons can be made. Ideally, with more appropriate data, additional refinements can be incorporated into the comparisons. For example, differences over time in both the stream of benefits and costs of alternative programs should be discounted. Unfortunately, the analyst may place too great an emphasis on such refinements when the basic data used in the analysis are subject to strong limitations. This results in attributing an unwarranted degree of credibility to the analytical results. The large variability in estimates of a program's effects may outweigh the consequences of those refinements.

Empirical studies attempting to estimate the marginal contribution of medical services to increased health have been conducted at two levels of aggregation. The more aggregate studies of health production have used counties, states, and even countries as the basis of analysis (3). In these studies, the empirical analysis attempted to estimate the independent effect that each of the various factors, including medical services, has had on health levels. Each of the factors affecting health, including measures of health itself, were based on averages of the level of aggregation (i.e., state or county) used as the unit of observation. The less aggregate studies of health production, "microanalyses," used individuals as the unit of measurement (4).

The important distinction between the macro and micro studies of health production lies in the variables used to measure health status. No single measure of health can adequately represent the concept of health status; instead, it is described by certain of its quantifiable aspects. It is always implicitly assumed that these quantifiable measures are closely related to other aspects of health. On an aggregate level, available health measures are those collected by government agencies as part of vital statistics. These measures, such as births and deaths, also tend to be more accurate than others. Morbidity and disability measures of health are generally unavailable on an aggregate level, and they are not likely to be as reliable as mortality data. When mortality rates are used as the measure of health, the simplest such index is the crude death rate, which is the number of deaths per 1,000 population. More useful health indices are those that are age–sex specific. Such population-specific death rates, unlike the crude death rate, would not be affected by changes in the overall composition of the population (5). When studies of health production use individuals as the unit of observation, mortality rates cannot be used meaningfully, unless a longitudinal analysis is used. Instead, the measures of health used are generally time-loss indicators, such as the number of work-loss days, the individual's own evaluation of health status, and the number of chronic conditions.[3] The unavailability of data needed to measure health status adequately has led to the practice of measuring health by the use of negative health indices. These measures are obviously incomplete in their assessment of what is believed to constitute good health.

In addition to medical services, other factors affecting age-sex specific mortality rates in studies of health production include lifestyle variables, such as income, occupation, cigarette smoking, and alcohol consumption; environmental variables, such as the quality of housing and urbanization (which, in addition to capturing the effect of pollution, might also represent such offsetting factors as increased access to medical care); and an efficiency factor, measured by the number of years of formal education, which assumes that persons who are more efficient at producing health can do so at a lower cost. The better-educated person may not only be able to recognize symptoms and seek treatment earlier than others, but may also be more likely to use preventive services.

Health production studies generally measure the contribution of medical services to health in several ways: by quantities of the individual components of medical services,

---

[3]In his study on work-loss rates, M. Silver found that work loss was positively correlated with income but negatively correlated with the earnings rate (a weekly wage measure). Although Silver acknowledges that this finding may be caused by a combination of incentives and causations—higher earnings make work loss more expensive, while higher income may carry with it some health risks—he claims that recovery at home is a "superior" good. Therefore, the positive association of income with work loss represents normal economic behavior rather than a health risk. Silver therefore concludes that work loss may be an unreliable measure of true health status because it is too greatly affected by economic behavior.

such as the number of physicians and hospital beds per thousand population; by the utilization of medical services, such as the number of physicians visits or hospital patient days; or by aggregate expenditures on medical services, which include changes in prices, utilization of services, and differences in quality of services.

Auster, Leveson, and Sarachek analyzed interstate differences in age-sex adjusted mortality rates for 1960 (6). Their principal purpose was to estimate the elasticity of health with respect to medical services, which is the percentage change in mortality rates that would occur as a result of a 1 percent change in medical services. The authors used multivariate analysis and included measures of medical services, as well as a number of environmental factors, believed to affect health.[4] The medical services input was measured in two ways: as expenditures on medical services and as a separate production function for medical services (which included as inputs into that production function the number of physicians per capita, the number of paramedical persons per capita, and so on).

The statistical results of the Auster, Leveson, and Sarachek study, which accounted for more than 50 percent of the interstate differences in mortality rates, indicated that environmental and personal factors had a greater effect than medical services on mortality rates. The specific findings for some of the more important factors affecting interstate differences in mortality rates were: (a) expenditures on medical care had an elasticity of approximately – .1, meaning that a 1 percent increase in medical expenditures would lead to a .1 percent decrease in age-sex adjusted mortality rates; (b) the elasticity of mortality rates with respect to education was almost twice as large as for medical services, – .2; (c) cigarette consumption per capita resulted in a positive increase in mortality rates (i.e., the elasticity estimate was +.1, meaning that a 1 percent increase in cigarette consumption per capita results in a .1 percent increase in mortality rates); and (d) family income also had a positive effect on mortality rates (i.e., the income elasticity was +.2). The authors explain the positive effect of income on mortality rates in 1960 by the association of high income with a lifestyle that includes adverse diets and fast cars. Occupations with higher incomes might also be associated with more stress and less exercise. The effect of income on health status probably differs according to level of income. At low levels, a rise in income would have a positive effect on health status; persons could afford more nutritious diets, improved housing, and better sanitation facilities. After a certain level of income has been reached, according to the results above, the effect of income on health probably becomes negative. Adverse diet, lack of exercise, and increased stress decrease health status. In the Auster, Leveson, and Sarachek study, the total effect of environmental and personal factors (e.g., income, education, and cigarette consumption) outweighed the marginal contribution of medical services to health status.[5]

---

[4]An important assumption in such cross-sectional studies, of which the authors are well aware, is that the mortality rate is related only to the quantity of medical services used in the particular year for which the study was undertaken. In reality, it is likely that the amount of medical services and influence of environmental factors over the lifetime of the population, rather than just the current period, will affect the population's health status in a given year.

[5]Since smoking generally begins early in life, Grossman, Lewit, and Coate have estimated the price elasticity of demand for teenage smoking. With respect to teenage smoking participation, the price elasticity is – 1.2 and is – 1.4 with respect to the quantity of cigarettes smoked. Thus increasing cigarette taxes can have an important effect on reducing smoking by teenagers. This study is summarized, along with others, in Michael Grossman, "Government and Health Outcomes," *American Economic Review*, May 1980: p. 194.

Hadley studied the impact of medical care, education, and income on both general and disease-specific mortality rates (7). His purpose was to estimate the elasticity of health with respect to medical services. Separate production functions were estimated for 12 age–race–sex cohorts; eight for adults 45 years of age and over and four for infants. The data were from 1968 to 1972 and were based on counties with a minimum population size. Although the results differed somewhat from cohort to cohort, Hadley found that the elasticity of the mortality rate, from all causes, with respect to medical care expenditures is approximately $-.15$; that is, a 10 percent increase in medical care expenditures would lead to a 1.5 percent decrease in the mortality rate. The effect was much greater for white males than for black males. Income and education were also found to have a negative effect on mortality rates.

Using individuals as the unit of measurement, Michael Grossman estimated the individual's demand for healthy time. Good health, or healthy time, in Grossman's model is demanded both because it enters the individual's utility function directly for its consumption value and because, as an investment, it increases the time available for other activities. Grossman found that education increases efficiency in producing health and that the elasticity of health with respect to medical services varies between .1 and .3. Grossman also found that the income elasticity of health is negative, in spite of a positive income elasticity with respect to medical services (8).

A problem with cross-sectional studies that attempt to measure the effect of medical services on health status is that, at any point in time, greater use of medical services may represent increased use by those whose health is poor. Further, increased use of medical services may have an effect on health status over a period longer than that in which they are used. To correct for these problems in interpreting the effect of increased use of medical services on health status, Lee Benham and Alexandra Benham studied the change in health status of groups of individuals during the period 1963–1970 (9). Using data from two different surveys, the authors classified individuals into 28 education–age categories (consisting of four education and seven age groupings) and attempted to determine the impact that increased use of medical services had on the health status of each education–age category between 1963 and 1970. (Education was considered as a proxy measure for permanent income.)

During the period studied, 1963–1970, two large government programs were started (Medicare and Medicaid) to finance increased use of medical services for the poor and elderly. The measures of health status used were: health status reported, the number of symptoms reported, and disability days reported during the previous year. The contribution of medical services was measured by the number of nonobstetric physician visits and nonobstetric hospital utilization.

The authors' statistical analysis related the (average) health status of each education–age group in 1970 to the (average) health status of that same group in 1963 and to changes in that group's utilization of medical services between 1963 and 1970. The authors assumed that increased utilization of medical services between 1963 and 1970 was primarily the result of an increase in government financing of medical services to the poor and elderly rather than a response to changes in that group's health status. The results of the Benham and Benham study were consistent with the previous studies. Increased use of medical services did not result in an improvement in health status during the period studied.

Results from the RAND Health Insurance Experiment provide more evidence regarding the effect of an increase in medical care on health outcomes (10). Participants were assigned to alternative health insurance plans for a period of three to five years.

The plans varied in the amount that the participant had to pay out of pocket for their medical care. Participants in plans with less cost sharing had higher utilization, with the highest utilization of medical services occurring in the insurance plan where the participant did not have to pay anything out of pocket. In addition to studying the effect that out-of-pocket payment has on medical use and expenditures, the study also analyzed the effect of greater use of medical services on the participants' health status.

The health of adults were compared according to whether they were in a plan in which utilization was greater (i.e., no out-of-pocket payment) or smaller (those plans where the patients paid various amounts for their medical services). General health measures, such as physical and role functioning, mental health, social contacts, and health perceptions, were used as well as measures of physiologic health, such as diastolic blood pressure and functional far vision. Of the numerous health status measures used, the health benefits of increased use of medical services were quite limited; greater use of medical services resulted in lower diastolic blood pressure for those initially diagnosed as hypertensive and improved far vision for those with initial far-vision problems. Further, increased medical use had no statistically significant impact on the general health of subgroups, which differed according to their incomes and their initial health status. The researchers concluded that, for the average participant, greater medical care use had no statistically significant effect on health habits associated with cardiovascular disease and certain kinds of cancer, nor on five general measures of health. However, "people with specific conditions that physicians have been trained to diagnose and treat (myopia, hypertension) benefit from free care" (11).

A separate analysis of the RAND data on increased use of medical services on the health of children found that it had no impact on the health outcome of the average child. Moreover, increased use did not have any effect on children who were "at risk" of illness because of an existing condition (12).

Perhaps more persuasive than these statistical attempts to determine the contribution of additional medical services to increased health is Victor Fuchs's excellent discussion of causes of death by age (13). Fuchs examines the contribution of living standards, lifestyle, and medical services to the decline in infant mortality rates since 1900 and to causes of adult deaths. The large decline in infant mortality rates from 1900 to the present [6] has been due largely to rising living standards, the spread of literacy and education, a large decline in the birthrate, possibly chlorination of the water supply and pasteurization of milk, and the introduction of antimicrobial drugs in the 1930s. "It is important to realize that medical care played almost no role in this decline" (14). It was not until fairly recently (late 1960s) that maternal and infant services were extended to underserved families and intensive care units were provided for premature infants who were at high risk. Fuchs also points out that in other developed countries with fewer medical services than the United States and a large proportion of home births delivered by a midwife, infant mortality rates are lower than in the United States. Specific medical service programs targeted to high-risk pregnancies are likely to make a larger contribution to decreases in infant mortality rates than merely making more medical services generally available to the entire population. For example, in countries where medical services are provided free, as in Great Britain, the infant mortality rate is still not as low as that achieved in other developed countries. The

---

[6]For example, the infant mortality rate in New York City declined from 140 per 1,000 live births in 1900 to 21.9 per 1,000 in 1968. By 1984 the mortality rate had declined to 12.8 per 1,000 live births.

lowest infant mortality rates in 1977 (between 8.0 and 8.9 per 1,000 live births) were those of Sweden, Switzerland, Denmark, and Japan.

When Fuchs examined mortality rates by cause of death for different age groups—adolescents and young adults (15–24 years of age), middle-aged persons (35–44), and late-middle-aged persons (55–64)—he again concluded that increased use of medical services has a smaller impact on health than the way in which people live. In the younger age groups, accidents (particularly from use of automobiles), suicides, and homicides are the major causes of death. In middle age, heart disease is the leading cause of death; accidents, suicides, cirrhosis of the liver (caused by alcoholism), and lung cancer are the other major contributors. Among nonwhites, homicides are the second leading cause of death. Again, the major causes of death may be attributed to behavioral factors. For persons in their late middle age, heart disease is again the leading cause of death; neoplasms are second.

Fuchs compares causes of death by age group in the United States and Sweden, with interesting results (15). The major factors explaining the lower Swedish mortality rates in each of the various age groups are again determined to be behavioral (Swedes are less violent and have fewer accidents) and attributed to lifestyle (diet, exercise, smoking, and stress). "At present . . . the greatest potential for reducing coronary disease, cancer, and the other major killers still lies in altering personal behavior." Fuchs further notes: "Given our present state of knowledge, even the most lavish use of medical care would not bring the U.S. rate more than a small step closer to the Swedish rate" (16).

The studies employing statistical techniques to estimate a health production function and the discussion by Fuchs on the leading causes of death both suggest that health status is more importantly related to lifestyle factors than to increments of medical services. Although the total benefit of medical services may be large, allocation decisions are rarely all-or-nothing decisions; instead, they are incremental. If policymakers have an increase in health status as their objective, an increased provision of medical services is likely to have a relatively smaller impact on health than will alternative policies. Further, these additional expenditures on medical services are not without a cost; greater increases in health status could be achieved if these same funds were spent on other programs.

APPLICATIONS OF A HEALTH PRODUCTION FUNCTION (17)

One type of analysis that can be undertaken using information developed from a health production function is to determine from among which alternative health programs to allocate additional resources. For example, the empirical study by Auster, Leveson, and Sarachek discussed earlier estimated the elasticity of health with respect to medical services at approximately .1; with respect to education it was estimated at .2. The 1980 economic cost of mortality in the population was estimated at $176 billion, while the economic cost of morbidity was estimated at $68 billion (18). If we assume that these costs have risen by the amount of the CPI between 1980 and 1985, or 30.5 percent, then in 1985, the economic cost of mortality was $229.7 billion and the economic cost of morbidity was $88.7 billion. If a 1 percent increase in medical expenditures resulted in a decrease of .1 percent in mortality, and presumably also in morbidity, then such an expenditure would save $318.4 million ($229.7 million from a decrease in mortality and $88.7 million from a decrease in morbidity). The cost of a 1 percent increase in medical expenditures that totaled $371.4 billion in 1985 would be $3.714 billion.

To determine whether to allocate funds to medical services or to alternative health programs, it is necessary to compare the costs of increasing other health programs to achieve the same economic benefits. Since the elasticity of health with respect to education is twice as large as it is for medical services (.2 as compared with .1), education expenditures would have to be increased by only .5 percent to achieve the same economic benefits as medical services.

In 1985, expenditures on education totaled $244.4 billion (19). One-half percent of that amount would be $1.222 billion. To achieve an increase in health output equal to $318.4 million would have required a $3.714 billion medical expenditure and only a $1.222 billion educational expenditure. Allocating additional funds to education would, at the margin, appear to be preferable to spending those funds on medical services.

The foregoing discussion illustrates the type of analysis to perform when determining how to allocate additional funds. This cost-benefit analysis assumes that no additional economic effects result from an increase in health and that no other reasons exist for undertaking the investment expenditure. It also assumes that the economic value of an increase in health is conceptually correct and accurately measured. All of these caveats are meant to indicate the limitations of such gross cost-benefit analyses. Before one actually allocated funds among education and medical services programs, it would be necessary to have more precise information as to which educational programs have an impact on health levels; the same would be true for medical services programs. Such broad categorizations as education or medical services are not useful for making allocation decisions.

Another application of a health production function is to explain the decline in age-adjusted mortality rates over time. As shown in Table 2–1, age-adjusted mortality rates declined 23.6 percent between 1970 and 1985. Using the empirical estimates developed in the Auster, Leveson, and Sarachek article, the decline in mortality over this period can be accounted for by the following factors. Expenditures per capita for medical services (adjusted for price increases) increased 48 percent during the period 1970–1985. Based on an elasticity estimate of $-.1$, the effect of such increased expenditures is an estimated reduction in mortality of 4.8 percent during this period. The increase in real family income was negligible during this period, so despite an elasticity estimate of .2, income should have no impact on the decline in mortality rates. An increase in education in the population of 4.1 percent, based on an elasticity of $-.2$, was expected to result in a decline in mortality of .8 percent. Per capita cigarette consumption declined by 26 percent, leading to a 2.6 percent decline in mortality rates, based on an elasticity estimate of .1 percent.

The percentage decline in mortality rates during this period not accounted for by the factors above is relatively large: 15.4 percent, or approximately 1 percent per year. During the period for which Auster, Leveson, and Sarachek calculated their results, 1955–1965, the unexplained percentage decline in the mortality rate was 5.0 percent. Auster et al. attributed the unexplained portion of the decreased mortality rate to technological change. The 23.6 percent decline in mortality rate during the period 1970–1985 was much greater per year (1.57 percent) than for the period 1955–1965, when it was only 3.9 percent, or .39 per year.

TABLE 2-1. Contribution of Selected Medical Services and Environmental Factors to Changes in the Age-Adjusted Death Rate, 1970–1985

	Percentage Change in Variable	Percentage Change in Mortality per Percentage Change in Variable	Percentage Change in Mortality
Actual change in U.S. death rate[a]			− 23.6
Health care expenditures per capita, deflated by CPI for medical care[b]	48	− .1	− 4.8
Median family income, deflated by CPI for all items[c]	0	.2	0
Education (median number of school years completed 25 and over)[d]	4.1	− .2	− .8
Cigarette consumption per capita[e]	− 26	.1	− 2.6

SOURCES:

[a]National Center for Health Statistics, *Monthly Vital Statistics Report*, 34(13), September 19, 1986: 15, Table 5.

[b]Daniel R. Waldo et al., "National Health Expenditures, 1985," *Health Care Financing Review*, 8(1), Fall 1986: 13, Table 1; U.S. Bureau of the Census, *Statistical Abstract of the United States*, 1986, 106th ed. (Washington, D.C., U.S. Government Printing Office, 1985), p. 100, Table 155; *Monthly Labor Review*, 110(3): 83, Table 32. Nominal expenditures rose from $304 to $1,504 per capita (Waldo et al., "National Health Expenditures, 1985," *op. cit.*, p. 13, Table 1); in 1970, the medical care CPI was 120.6 (U.S. Bureau of the Census, *Statistical Abstract of the United States, op. cit.*, p. 100, Table 155), while in 1985, it was 403.1 (*Monthly Labor Review, op. cit.*, p. 83, Table 32).

[c]Income, number of years of education, and smoking figures are for 1984. Real per family income in 1984 dollars was $26,394 in 1970 and $26,433 in 1984 (in 1984 dollars) (U.S. Bureau of the Census, *Statistical Abstract of the United States, 1986, op. cit.*, p. 450, Table 752.

[d]*Ibid.*, p. 133, Table 216.

[e]*Ibid.*, p. 760, Table 1356.

The decline in mortality over this period is generally attributed to two components: declines in infant mortality rates and in deaths from heart disease.

The largest declines in mortality rates during the period 1965–1985 occurred in infant mortality rates, which decreased from 26.4 per 1,000 live births in 1955, to 24.7 in 1965, to 16.1 in 1975, to 10.5 in 1985 (20). It has been suggested that this more rapid decline in infant mortality rates is, for the most part, the result of factors other than increased medical care expenditures, particularly liberalized abortion laws.

Between 1955 and 1964 the infant mortality rate declined by .6 percent per year. After 1964, however, the infant mortality rate fell more rapidly, approximately 4.5 percent a year. The most important portion of the decline in infant mortality (77 percent) was the decline in the neonatal rate (i.e., infant deaths within the first 27 days of life per 1,000 live births), which is twice as large as and fell more rapidly than the postneonatal mortality rate (i.e., infant deaths occurring between 28 and 364 days). Attempts to explain the decline in infant mortality must therefore understand the reasons for the decline in the neonatal rate.

Grossman and others conducted several studies to determine the causes of the decline in neonatal mortality rates. In one study, using county-level aggregate data, Corman and Grossman examined the determinants of neonatal mortality rates for a three-year period centered on 1977 (21). Specifically, the authors examined the impact on neonatal mortality of the availability of neonatal intensive care, the legalization of abortion, subsidized family planning services for low-income women, community health centers, maternal and infant nutrition programs, and Medicaid. Separate analyses were conducted for white and black women to determine the effects of each of the above on the neonatal mortality rate. The various factors affecting neonatal mortality differed in their effects on white and black women. The authors then used the results of their analysis to explain the decline in infant mortality between the years 1964 and 1977. During that time, the white neonatal mortality rate declined from 16.2 to 8.7 per 1,000 live births, whereas the black neonatal rate declined from 27.6 to 16.1. The authors determined that for blacks the most important factor causing a reduction in the neonatal rate was the availability of abortion; its effect, 1.2 deaths per 1,000 live births, was almost twice as large as the next most important contributor. Next in importance was availability of neonatal intensive care units and the increase in female schooling, each reducing the rate by .7 death per 1,000 live births. Medicaid expenditures was fourth at .5 death per 1,000 live births. For whites, schooling was most important, followed by subsidized nutrition programs, Medicaid, and the availability of neonatal intensive care units; the availability of abortion was fifth. The abortion effect on blacks was four times greater than on whites, and the effect of neonatal intensive care units was twice as large.

Increased availability of abortion, neonatal intensive care units, and increased female schooling continued to contribute to the decline in infant mortality after 1980. On a cautious note, however, the authors comment that budget cutbacks in poverty-related programs may have a deleterious effect on the neonatal rate. More important, if prohibitions on abortion were enacted, there could be a large adverse impact on the neonatal mortality rate.

Grossman has conducted several other studies on the determinants of health and the importance of nonmedical variables. In a study of child and adolescent health, Grossman and others found that the home environment in general and mother's schooling in particular played an extremely important role. . . ." Holding other factors constant, "children and teenagers of more-educated mothers have better oral health, are less likely to be obese, and less likely to have anemia than children of less-educated mothers. Father's schooling plays a much less important role" (22).

Also contributing to the sharp decline in the overall mortality rate since 1965 have been reductions in heart disease. According to several studies, the main contributing factors to the decline in heart disease, and in its mortality, have been changes in lifestyle factors, such as reduced smoking, lower serum cholesterol levels, control of hypertension, and improvements in the number and quality of coronary care units (23). For example, Goldman and Cook attempted to quantify the relative contribution of lifestyle changes and medical interventions in explaining the 21 percent decline in ischemic heart disease mortality that occurred between 1968 and 1976. They concluded that lifestyle changes accounted for 54 percent of the decline (reduced serum cholesterol levels contributed 30 percent and reduced cigarette smoking, 24 percent). Over the nine-year period studied, medical interventions accounted for less than 40 percent of the decline. The authors note that while the medical interventions, such as coronary care units, are expensive innovations, lifestyle changes, aside from government-financed publicity, are relatively costless and contributed more to the decline in ischemic heart disease mortality.

The cost-benefit application and the analysis of mortality rates over time illustrate the types of analyses that could be undertaken based on knowledge of a health production function. To be useful for policymakers, more specific information on health production functions, by disease categories and for different population groups, is required. Before more precise estimates of health production functions can be derived, however, it is necessary for policy analysts to understand the types of data that need to be collected and how they will be useful for decisionmaking.

The remainder of this book will examine the efficiency with which medical care is produced by the medical care industry. Even though the marginal impact of medical services on health may be relatively small, the increase in private and governmental financing of medical services has been large. The contribution to health of such expenditures will be reduced even further if increased prices of medical services absorb most of the increase in expenditures. The need to examine the efficiency of medical services and the equity of their distribution is addressed in the remaining chapters.

REFERENCES

1. For a more complete discussion of how economic analysis has been used by the government for the allocation of resources between health programs, see Robert N. Grosse, "Cost Benefit Analysis of Health Services," *Annals of the American Academy of Political and Social Science*, 399, January 1972: 89–99. For a more complete discussion of the principles and applications of cost-benefit analysis, see Kenneth E. Warner and Bryan R. Luce, *Cost-Benefit and Cost-Effectiveness Analysis in Health Care* (Ann Arbor, Mich.: Health Administration Press, 1982). For an excellent discussion of cost-effectiveness applied to illustrative health care issues, see Louise B. Russell, *Is Prevention Better than Cure?* (Washington, D.C.: Brookings Institution, 1986).

2. Joseph Lipscomb has developed a resource allocation model that can be used for determining the optimal allocation of resources among various medical care programs so as to maximize a society's health status. He uses linear and integer programming methods to solve the model. For a detailed explanation of the model, see Joseph Lipscomb, "Health Resource Allocations and Quality of Care Measurement in a Social Policy Framework," *Policy Sciences*, 9, 1978: 19–43; and Joseph Lipscomb et al., "Health Status Maximization and Manpower Allocations," in Richard Scheffler, ed., *Research in Health Economics*, Vol. 1 (Greenwich, Conn.: JAI Press, 1979), pp. 301–401.

3. Examples of health production functions using macro data are given by Richard Auster, Irving Leveson, and Deborah Sarachek, "The Production of Health, an Exploratory Study," *Journal of Human Resources*, IV, Fall 1969: 411–436; Charles T. Stewart, Jr., "The Allocation of Resources to Health," *Journal of Human Resources*, VI, Winter 1971; and Jack Hadley, *More Medical Care, Better Health?* (Washington, D.C.: The Urban Institute, 1982). See also a critique of the Stewart article by Edward Meeker, "Allocation of Resources to Health Revisited," *Journal of Human Resources*, VIII, Spring 1973: 257–259.

4. Joseph P. Newhouse, "Determinants of Days Lost from Work Due to Sickness," in Herbert E. Klarman, ed., *Empirical Studies in Health Economics*, Proceedings of the 2nd Conference on the Economics of Health (Baltimore: Johns Hopkins University Press, 1970), pp. 59–70; Morris Silver, "An Economic Analysis of Variations in Medical Expenses and Work-Loss Rates," in Klarman, ed., *ibid.*, pp.

121–140; Michael Grossman, "On the Concept of Health Capital and the Demand for Health," *Journal of Political Economy*, March-April 1972; Lee Benham and Alexandra Benham, "The Impact of Incremental Medical Services on Health Status, 1963–1970," in R. Andersen, J. Kravitz, and O. Anderson, eds., *Equity in Health Services: Empirical Analysis of Social Policy* (Cambridge, Mass.: Ballinger, 1975); Joseph P. Newhouse and Lindy J. Friedlander, "The Relationship Between Medical Resources and Measures of Health: Some Additional Evidence," *Journal of Human Resources*, 15(2), 1980; Harriet O. Duleep, "Measuring the Effect of Income on Adult Mortality Using Longitudinal Administrative Record Data," *Journal of Human Resources*, 21(2), 1986; David J. Knesper et al., "Preliminary Production Functions Describing Change in Mental Health Status," *Medical Care*, 25(3), March 1987.

5. For a more complete review of health measures, their definitions, and attendant difficulties, see Daniel F. Sullivan, *Conceptual Problems in Developing an Index of Health*, Public Health Service Publication 1000, Series 2, No. 17 (Washington, D.C.: U.S. Government Printing Office, May 1966). Also see Milton M. Chenn and James W. Bush, "Health Status Measures, Policy, and Biomedical Research," in Selma J. Mushkin and David W. Dunlap, eds., *Health: What Is It Worth? Measures of Health Benefits* (Elmsford, N.Y.: Pergamon Press, 1979), pp. 15–41; Robert H. Brook et al., "Overview of Adult Health Status Measures Fielded in RAND's Health Insurance Study," *Medical Care*, 17(7), Supplement, July 1979; and A. J. Culyer, ed., *Health Indicators* (New York: St. Martin's Press, 1983). For health measures specifically for the elderly, see Robert L. Kane and Rosalie R. Kane et al., *Assessing the Elderly: A Practical Guide to Measurement* (Lexington, Mass.: Lexington Books, 1981).

6. Auster, Leveson, and Sarachek, *op. cit.*

7. Hadley, *op. cit.*

8. Grossman, *op. cit.*

9. Benham and Benham, *op. cit.*

10. Robert H. Brook et al., "Does Free Care Improve Adults' Health? Results from a Randomized Controlled Trial," *New England Journal of Medicine*, 309(23), December 1983: 1426–1434.

11. *Ibid.*, p. 1432.

12. Burciaga R. Valdez et al., "Consequences of Cost-Sharing for Children's Health," *Pediatrics*. 75(5), May 1985: 952–961.

13. Victor R. Fuchs, *Who Shall Live?* (New York: Basic Books, 1974), 30–55. The data presented by Fuchs represent average relationships and do not indicate the relative marginal costs of achieving changes in health status. For policy purposes, it would be desirable to know the marginal effects of each of the variables on health status.

14. *Ibid.*, p. 32.

15. *Ibid.*, p. 45.

16. *Ibid.*, p. 46.

17. The applications in this section are based on the article by Auster, Leveson, and Sarachek *op. cit.*; the data, however, have been updated.

18. The 1980 estimates of economic cost of mortality and morbidity (which represents the discounted value of future earnings) are from Dorothy P. Rice, Thomas A. Hodgson, and Andrea N. Kopstein, "The Economic Cost of Illness: A Replication and Update," *Health Care Financing Review*, 7(1), Fall 1985: 61–80.

19. U.S. Bureau of the Census, *Statistical Abstract of the United States, 1986*, 106th ed. (Washington, D.C.: U.S. Government Printing Office, 1986), p. 128, Table 206.

20. National Center for Health Statistics, *Monthly Vital Statistics Report*, 34(13), September 19, 1986: p. 15, Table 5.

21. Hope Corman and Michael Grossman, "Determinants of Neonatal Mortality Rates in the U.S.: A Reduced Form Model," *Journal of Health Economics*, 4(3), September 1985: 213–236. For additional discussion of the reasons for the decline in infant mortality, see Jeffrey E. Harris, "Prenatal Medical Care and Infant Mortality," and Mark R. Rosenzweig and T. Paul Schultz, "The Behavior of Mothers as Inputs to Child Health: The Determinants of Birth Weight, Gestation and Rate of Fetal Growth," in Victor R. Fuchs, ed., *Economic Aspects of Health* (Chicago: University of Chicago Press, 1982).

22. Michael Grossman, "Government and Health Outcomes," *American Economic Review*, May 1982: p. 192.

23. Michael Stern, "The Recent Decline in Ischemic Heart Disease Mortality," *Annals of Internal Medicine*, 91, October 1979: 630–640; Joel Kleinman, Jacob Feldman, and Mary Monk, "The Effects of Changes in Smoking Habits on Coronary Heart Disease Mortality," *American Journal of Public Health*, 69, August 1979: 795–802; Lee Goldman and Francis Cook, "The Decline in Ischemic Heart Disease Mortality Rates: An Analysis of the Comparative Effects of Medical Interventions and Changes in Lifestyle," *Annals of Internal Medicine*, 101(6), December 1984: 825–836.

CHAPTER 3

An Overview of the Medical Care Sector

DESCRIPTION OF THE MEDICAL CARE MARKETS

Expenditures on the Major Components of Medical Care

As an introduction to the medical care sector, let us examine the magnitude and changing composition of expenditures on the major components of medical care. As shown in Table 3–1, the two largest components of medical care, hospital and physician services, accounted for 42 and 21 percent of the $371.4 billion of total personal medical expenditures in calendar year 1985.[1] Current expenditures on hospital care, $166.7 billion, are twice as large as those for physician services, $82.8 billion. The relative proportions of expenditures on hospital, physician, and other medical services have not been constant over time. In 1965, before the large-scale involvement of government in financing medical care for the indigent and elderly, total personal medical expenditures were $35.9 billion and expenditures for hospital care represented 33 percent of that amount; at that time hospital expenditures were only 64 percent greater than those for physician services. By 1985, the expenditures for hospital care had increased more rapidly than expenditures for all of the remaining components of medical services.

Patients' and physicians' lessening concern with the price of hospital care contributed to the more rapid increase in hospital expenditures. Government expenditures on total medical services increased from $8.4 billion in 1965 to $152.6 billion in 1985. Of the $152.6 billion, 58.8 percent went for hospital services—an $84 billion increase over 1965. The largest portion of this increase can be attributed to Medicare and Medicaid payments for personal health care. In 1965, before the introduction of Medicare and Medicaid, government expenditures for personal health care were only 23.5 percent of total personal health care expenditures, but in 1985, almost 20 years after

---

[1] Personal health care expenditures were approximately $53.6 billion less than total health expenditures in 1985. The difference between the two (in billions) are expenses for prepayment and administration ($26.2), government public health activities ($11.9), and research and construction of medical facilities ($15.4).

TABLE 3-1. Total Private and Public Expenditures for Personal Health Care Services by Type of Expenditure and Source of Funds, Calendar Years 1965, 1975, and 1985

	1965			1975			1985		
	Total (Billions)	Private Percentage	Public Percentage	Total (Billions)	Private Percentage	Public Percentage	Total (Billions)	Private Percentage	Public Percentage
Hospital care	$13.9	61.2	38.8	$ 52.1	44.7	55.3	$166.7	46.1	53.9
Physician services	8.5	92.9	7.1	24.9	73.9	26.1	82.8	70.9	29.1
Dentist services	2.8	100.0	.0	8.2	95.1	6.1	27.1	97.8	2.2
Drug/drug sundries	5.2	96.2	3.8	11.9	91.6	8.4	28.5	90.5	9.5
Other[a]	5.5	59.3	40.7	20.0	52.1	47.8	66.3	45.6	54.4
Total	35.9	76.5	23.5	117.1	60.5	39.6	371.4	58.8	41.1

SOURCES: Robert Gibson and Daniel Waldo, "National Health Expenditures, 1980," *Health Care Financing Review*, 3, September 1981: 20–30, Table 2; U.S. Department of Health and Human Services, *HHS News*, newsletter dated July 26, 1982, Table II; Daniel Waldo, Katharine R. Levit, and Helen Lazenby, "National Health Expenditures, 1985," *Health Care Financing Review*, 8(1), Fall 1986: 15–18, Tables 3, 8.

Note: The individual categories may not add up to their totals because of rounding.

[a] "Other" includes other professional services, eyeglasses and appliances, nursing home care, and other personal health care.

the initiation of these two programs, the government share of personal health care expenditures climbed to 41.1 percent, nearly doubling its 1965 percentage.

By 1985, patient payments accounted for only 9.4 percent of the total hospital bill, as shown in Table 3–2, the remainder of which was paid either by government (53.9 percent) or by private insurance (35.6 percent). Direct patient payments were smaller for hospital care than for any other medical service. On the average, patients are responsible for 26 percent of expenditures for physician services and 76 percent of expenditures for drugs. As the portion of the hospital bill paid for directly by the patient declines, so does the patient's or physician's incentive to question the prices charged by hospitals.

The patient's use of the hospital is generally believed to be less responsive to the price charged than is the use of most other medical services. The declining portion of the hospital bill for which the patient is responsible, together with the small effect that price has on hospital use, have removed patient and physician incentives to be concerned with how rapidly hospital prices are increasing or with relative costs of hospitals. Under these circumstances, a more rapid increase in hospital expenditures would be expected. Conversely, a slower rate of increase in expenditures would be expected for medical services whose use is more affected by higher prices and for which patients pay a larger fraction of the bill. These factors are important for understanding the changing composition of medical expenditures.

Over time, as shown in Table 3–3, direct patient payments for all medical services have declined from 51.6 percent in 1965 to 32.5 percent in 1975 to 28.4 percent in 1985. The government portion of personal health care expenditures has risen over that same period from 22 percent in 1965 to 34.3 percent in 1975 to 39.7 percent in 1985. As more of the bill for medical services is paid for by government and private insurance, the influence of price on the patients' use of the service and choice of a provider from whom to purchase that service diminishes. The removal of price incentives from patients and the increase in the ability of providers to pass on higher prices to third-party payors and government have important implications for the performance of the medical care market.

The government's financing of medical services is not uniform for each of the components of medical care; it is most concerned with cost containment in those areas to which it is financially committed. Higher prices for hospital services are of greater financial consequence and therefore of greater concern to the government than are similar price increases for dental services, whose financing is predominantly private.

The sharp increase and change in composition of medical care expenditures indicate a need for a set of economic tools to predict equilibrium situations. To understand why expenditures have increased so rapidly, it is necessary to determine why prices and quantities of medical care have been changing. Understanding the reasons for such changes is essential for forecasting and for anticipating the effects of public policy on prices, quantities, and expenditures in each of the medical markets.

The Interrelationship of the Different Medical Care Markets

Medical care, which is the output of the overall medical care market, is, in fact, the outcome of several interrelated markets. These include the markets for registered nurses, hospital services, physician services, and even the market for health professional education. To be able to forecast the effects of a change in government policy on

TABLE 3-2. Amount and Percentage of Personal Health Care Expenditures Met by Third Parties, by Type of Expenditure, Calendar Year 1985 (Billions of Dollars)

Type of Expenditure	Total	Direct Payments	Third-Party Payments							
			Total	Private Health Insurance	Government Expenditures					
					Total	Federal			State[b]	Other[c]
						Medicare	Medicaid	Other[a]		
Amount										
Total	371.4	105.6	265.8	113.5	147.4	70.5	21.9	20.2	34.8	4.9
Hospital care	166.7	15.6	151.1	59.3	89.9	48.5	8.1	15.1	18.2	2.1
Physicians' services	82.8	21.8	61.0	36.8	24.1	17.1	1.9	.7	4.4	.0
Dentists' services	27.1	17.2	9.9	9.3	.8	—	.3	.2	.3	—
Drug/drug sundries	28.5	21.7	6.8	4.0	2.7	—	1.4	.0	1.3	—
All other services[d]	66.3	29.3	37.0	4.0	30.2	4.9	10.3	4.3	10.7	2.7
Percentage Distribution										
Total	100.0	28.4	71.6	30.5	39.7	19.0	5.9	5.4	9.4	1.4
Hospital care	100.0	9.4	90.6	35.6	53.9	29.1	4.9	9.1	10.9	1.1
Physicians' services	100.0	26.3	73.7	44.4	29.3	20.7	2.3	.1	5.3	.0
Dentists' services	100.0	63.5	36.5	34.4	2.3	—	1.1	.1	1.1	—
Drug/drug sundries	100.0	76.1	23.9	14.0	9.9	—	4.9	—	4.6	—
All other services[d]	100.0	44.2	55.8	6.0	45.7	7.4	15.5	6.5	16.1	4.1

SOURCE: Daniel Waldo, Katherine R. Levit, and Helen Lazenby, "National Health Expenditures, 1985," *Health Care Financing Review*, 8(1), Fall 1986: 15–19, Tables 3, 9.

Note: Excludes expenses for prepayment and administration, government public health activities, and research and medical facilities construction.

[a]Includes expenditures for maternal and child health programs, vocational rehabilitation programs, temporary disability insurance, Public Health Service activities, Indian Health Service programs, workers' compensation programs, Veterans Administration Services, Alcohol, Drug Abuse and Mental Health Administration programs, and Defense Department programs.

[b]Includes state and local Medicaid payments.

[c]Includes expenditures for industrial in-plant health services and contributions from private philanthropic organizations.

[d]Includes other professional services, eyeglasses and appliances, nursing home care, and other personal health care.

TABLE 3-3. Percentage Distribution by Source of Personal Health Expenditures in the United States, 1965, 1970, 1975, 1980, and 1985

Source	1965	1970	1975	1980	1985
	Amount (Billions of Dollars)				
	35.9	65.4	117.1	219.7	371.4
	Percent[a]				
Private	78.0	65.6	60.5	60.6	60.3
Direct payments	51.6	40.5	32.5	28.7	28.4
Insurance benefits	24.2	23.4	26.7	30.7	30.6
All other	2.2	1.7	1.3	1.2	1.3
Public	22.0	34.3	39.5	39.4	39.7
Federal	10.1	22.2	26.8	28.4	30.3
State and local	11.9	12.1	12.7	10.9	9.4

SOURCE: Daniel Waldo, Katherine R. Levit and Helen Lazenby, "National Health Expenditures, 1985," *Health Care Financing Review*, 8(1), Fall 1986: 16.

[a]The percentages may not add up to 100 percent because of rounding.

the medical care sector or to determine the effects of a natural change such as an increase in the aged population, it is necessary to have a model of the medical care sector that describes the relationship of various submarkets and components of medical care to each other. The model which follows describes the various submarkets that comprise the medical care sector, demonstrates the way in which these different sectors are interrelated, and illustrates the usefulness of such a framework for forecasting and policy analysis (1). This overview of the medical care sector will also indicate the various subject areas to be covered in this book.

Three types of markets are present in the medical care sector, as shown in Figure 3-1. The patient's demand for a medical treatment (for a particular diagnostic category) is expressed by going to a physician whose determination of how to treat the patient is based on both economic and noneconomic factors. The physician's selection of one or more of several institutional settings—hospitals, outpatient facilities, nursing homes, the physician's office, or even home care—is based on the relative prices of each of those settings, the relative cost of each to the physician, and the efficacy of each in treatment. The demand for institutional care will depend on patient demand factors, physician considerations, and the relative price and efficacy of treatment in the different institutional settings. These institutional settings may thus be seen both as complements to and substitutes for one another.

A change in the demand for different institutional settings that is the result of, for example, a change in the age of the population, will be reflected in institutional demands for manpower and other factor inputs (e.g., capital and supplies). These comprise the second set of markets to be analyzed. Such institutional demands for manpower and other inputs represent the demand side of the health manpower (and inputs) markets. The demand for a particular health manpower category, for example, will depend upon factors relating to the patient's (and/or their physicians') demand for the institutional settings in which that manpower group is employed,

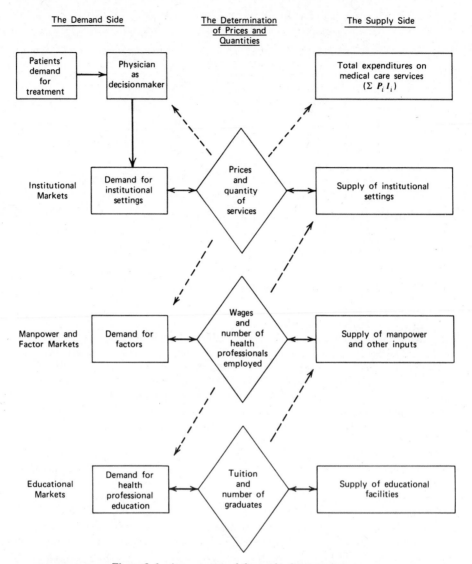

The Demand Side   The Determination   The Supply Side
                          of Prices and
                          Quantities

Figure 3-1. An overview of the medical care sector.

the wages of the group, and the relationship of their wages to those of other health workers.

The demand for an education by prospective health professionals will depend upon the demand for health professionals in the market just described. The demand for a health professional education, which is the amount that a person is willing to pay in terms of tuition and forgone income, is determined by the expected income and wages that might be earned (as determined in the manpower market) and by noneconomic motivating factors.

The supply side of each of these markets works as follows. The supply of health professional educational institutions (in terms, for example, of institutional capacity and faculty) and the demands for such education determine the number of graduates and the tuition rate to be charged. The number of graduates (the time required to educate each category of health manpower will, of course, vary) plus the existing stock of health manpower (less deaths and retirements) comprise the supply of health manpower at any given time. The supply of each category of health manpower in conjunction with the demands for such manpower will determine incomes and wages as well as employment (the participation rate). The outcomes of the health manpower (and other input) markets will affect the supply of services offered in different institutional settings. The cost of providing care in a given institutional setting will rise as the wages for a given manpower group rise and as more members of that manpower category are used to provide care. In each institutional setting, the costs of providing care together with the demands for care will determine how much care is provided; this is the outcome of the institutional markets. Total expenditures for personal medical care consist, then, of the prices of each institutional setting multiplied by the quantity of care provided in each setting.

To summarize the demand side of each of these separate markets, the demand for institutional care is derived from the initial demands for medical treatments. The demand for health manpower is similarly derived from the demand for institutional care, and the demand for a health professional education is derived from the demand for each health manpower profession. Similarly, the supply of medical services is based upon the availability of the supplies in each of these other markets and upon their costs.

To forecast the consequences of change in the demand or supply side of any part of this model, it is necessary to understand how the markets in each of the sectors operate. For example, legal restrictions on the tasks that health professionals are permitted to perform affect the demand for different health professionals, the wages they are paid, and consequently, the price and availability of medical service. Similarly, past subsidies to medical schools that have enabled the schools to set low tuition levels and fix the number of educational spaces irrespective of the demand for those spaces has affected the availability of physicians, their incomes, and the fees they charge. The performance of each of the separate markets in the medical care sector—the different institutional markets, manpower markets, and educational markets—will influence each of the other markets and the final price and expenditures for medical care. A market in which price is higher and output is less than if it were functioning properly is subject to proposals for improving its performance.

Under the traditional fee-for-service system, the physician is assumed to act as the patient's agent in determining which set of institutional settings would be used for providing care to the patient. Under traditional insurance coverage, each provider is paid separately. As managed care systems have developed, such as health maintenance organizations (HMOs), the HMO receives an annual capitation fee and is responsible for providing all the medical services the patient may require. In both cases, the physician continues to determine the combination of institutional settings that would be used in patient treatment. The incentives facing the physician, patient, and the HMO, however, may differ. This issue will be discussed in greater depth; nevertheless, the model described is relevant for understanding and forecasting change under each of these different delivery systems.

APPLICATIONS OF A MODEL OF THE MEDICAL CARE SECTOR

The effects of alternative public policies on the final market—that is, on the price and availability of medical services—can be predicted, using the tools of supply and demand analysis, on the basis of an understanding of the different medical care markets and their interrelationships.

Our ability to forecast the likely consequences of changes in demand or supply conditions in medical care also requires an accurate overview of the medical care sector. Figure 3–2 describes the same markets discussed above by means of a different set of diagrams, showing each of the separate markets within the institutional, manpower, and educational markets in terms of a traditional supply and demand relationship.

A Demand Policy

As a result of an increase in health insurance in the population, we would expect to observe an increase in the demand for medical care (as would be shown by a shift in demand in Figure 3–2A). How much the demand for medical care will increase will depend, in part, on the importance of price to increased utilization (i.e., the price elasticity of demand for medical care). As a result of an increase in demand, depending upon supply conditions in medical care, we would expect an increase in prices as well as an increase in medical care utilization. To forecast what will happen to prices and utilization for each component of medical care, we must examine how this increase in medical care demand is transmitted to each of the other markets. As a result of lower out-of-pocket prices to consumers for medical care, following greater insurance coverage, the demand for different institutional settings will increase; certain institutional settings will experience a larger increase in demand than others, depending, in part, upon which population groups will increase their demand, what types of medical treatments will be demanded, and how important price is to utilization in each market. As a result of the increased institutional demand, prices in these settings will increase, as will the quantity of services provided. The institutions affected will demand more inputs to supply that increased demand.

Various health professions will therefore experience an increase in demand for their services. Within each health manpower market, the employing institution's demand for a given health profession will be affected by the wages it would have to pay, the relative wages of other manpower groups that may be substituted for them, their relative productivity, the price of the output, and any legal restrictions that may prevent the use of certain personnel in performing specified tasks. With the increase in demand for health manpower and given the existing stock (i.e., currently trained professionals) of that manpower group, wages and the employment rate in each of the health manpower markets will increase. Exactly how much each will increase will depend upon the supply conditions (elasticity) and performance of each health manpower market. The resulting higher incomes will eventually increase the demand for an education leading to entrance into that profession. Thus, lowering an economic barrier to the use of medical care services by providing health insurance has increased demand for different institutional settings, manpower professions, and a health professional education.

The demand increase in each of the different markets will be followed by increases in prices as well as output. The size of the price and output increases in each market

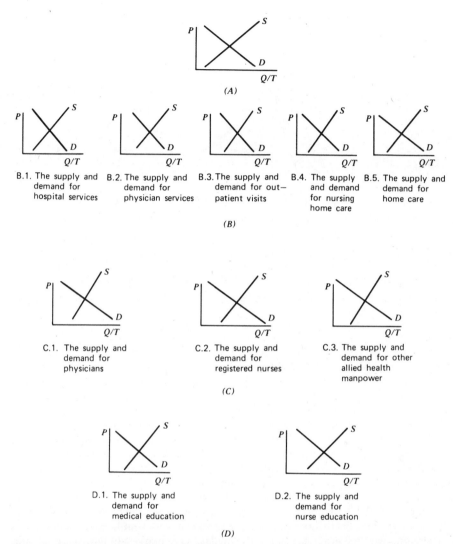

Figure 3–2. An economic model of the medical care sector: *(A)* the market for medical care services; *(B)* the markets for institutional services *(C)* the markets for health manpower, *(D)* the markets for health professional education.

resulting from that initial increase in demand will depend upon the size of the demand increase and the responsiveness of supply (supply elasticity) within each market. The less elastic supply is, the greater the price increase and the smaller will be the increase in output. It is precisely because of this effect on prices and output that an analysis of the efficiency of the supply side of each of the medical care markets becomes so important. If the supply side of the market is relatively inelastic—that is, if it takes a relatively large price increase to bring about an increase in output—then demand programs will result in large price increases and small output increases; consequently, it

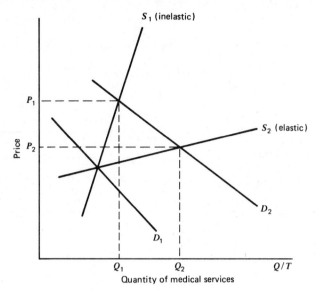

Figure 3–3. The effect on prices and medical services of an increase in demand when there are different supply elasticities.

will cost a great deal of money to achieve an increase in output. For example, according to Figure 3–3, an increase in demand will affect prices and quantity of services differently, depending upon the elasticity of supply. If supply is relatively elastic (S_2), then an increase in demand, from D_1 to D_2, will be accompanied by a price increase, but it will be much less (P_2) than if supply were inelastic (S_1), in which case the new price would be (P_1). Similarly, a much greater increase in services provided will occur under conditions of elastic supply (Q_2 versus Q_1). If the increase in demand were to occur as a result of a government subsidy program, and if supply were inelastic (S_1), the increased government expenditures for that program would pay for higher prices (P_1) and less output (Q_1) than if supply were more elastic (S_2).

It is thus important to understand what the supply elasticity is for each of the medical care markets. If markets with relatively inelastic supply can be made more elastic, the potential benefits in terms of lower prices and increased output can be very great. Therefore, we shall examine each of the medical care markets in terms of economic efficiency to determine how well each performs. We shall ask, how does each of these markets respond to changes in demand? Could their prices be lower and outputs greater if changes were made in their structure? By examining each of the medical care markets in terms of structure and performance, we can determine whether the efficiency of those markets can be improved and what mechanisms will be most useful for improving economic performance.

Other demand policies will also be examined using the framework noted above. For example, one way in which the government can reduce its expenditures on hospital services to the aged is to provide coverage for care in a less costly setting. Providing insurance coverage to the aged for services provided by a hospice would, assuming that the hospice is a substitute for at least some care that would otherwise be provided in a hospital, decrease the demand for hospital care (a shift to the left in the demand for hospitals). As the demand for hospital services decrease, the hospital's derived demand for its inputs and staff would similarly decrease. As the out-of-pocket price to the aged for hospice services was reduced as a result of the government insurance coverage, there would be an increase in the quantity demanded of hospice services, with a consequent increase in the derived demand for inputs used by the hospice. Whether or not covering a lower-cost substitute to hospitals reduces the overall expenditure on services for that medical treatment depends on the relative cost of those services and changes in use of each of those services. (A detailed example of how to determine the savings of insuring a lower-cost substitute is provided in Appendix 3, Chapter 6.)

A Supply Policy

A model of the medical care sector as described above is also useful for explaining how a supply subsidy might work. Typical governmental supply subsidies provide funds to educational institutions for increasing the number of health professionals. Such programs cause a shift to the right in the supply of the educational institutions and increase the schools' enrollment capacity. The effect is to increase the number of graduates in the educational market. As the number of graduates (e.g., physicians or nurses) increases and the supply of those particular health professionals in the health manpower market shifts to the right, the wages or incomes of the subsidized health professionals become lower than they might otherwise have been. The larger number of health professionals (those that were subsidized) and their relatively lower wages will result in an increase in demand for them in the institutional market (a movement down the institutions' demand for such personnel); since they will be substituted for other health professionals whose wages and numbers were not affected by supply subsidies. The effect on the institutional sector will be a shift to the right in their supply curve, since they can presumably produce the same quantity of services at a lower price (or a greater quantity of services at the same price). This is because the price of one of their inputs has been reduced as a result of the subsidy. Institutions will be affected differently by such a subsidy, since some institutions use relatively more of the subsidized input (e.g., hospitals use relatively more registered nurses) than others. The subsidy program's overall effect on the final price and quantity of medical care will vary, depending upon how much of an increase in the input occurs as a result of that supply subsidy, how much of a decrease in the price of that input occurs, how much of that subsidized input is used in the production of medical care, and so on.

A completely specified model of the medical care sector should enable us to trace the effects of a supply subsidy program throughout each of the different medical care markets. We can then compare several supply subsidy programs on the basis of what it costs them to achieve a change in the final price and quantity of medical care services. Thus such a model of the medical care sector allows us to compare alternative government supply subsidies, each of which is designed to increase the availability of medical care. Such subsidy programs need not be directed solely at a manpower category; they may be directed at any number of inputs, such as less-trained personnel who increase the productivity of more highly trained professionals, or they may provide subsidies for hospital construction. An overall model of medical care thus allows any number of supply subsidy programs to be evaluated on the basis of the cost of the subsidy and its final effect on the price and availability of medical care.

CONCLUDING COMMENTS

The model of the medical care sector just described also serves to enumerate the differ-ent subject areas of this book. To understand the medical care sector it is necessary to learn about the theory of demand for medical care and the consequent derived de-mands within each of the other markets. In the demand section, as in all other sec-tions, the theoretical discussion of demand will be followed by a review of studies that have attempted to estimate the theoretical variables discussed; the review will be fol-lowed by a summary of empirical estimates of the factors that affect demand.

After explaining the demand side of the medical care sector we will examine the supply side of the different markets. In this way we hope to be able to judge the effi-ciency of each of the different medical care markets: hospital services, physician ser-vices, the market for physicians, the market for registered nurses, and the market for medical education. In addition to judging the efficiency of each of these markets, we will evaluate the relevant government policies that have an impact on these separate markets, such as health manpower legislation in the manpower markets. Finally, we will make public policy recommendations for improving efficiency within each of these markets, based upon our analysis of their inadequate market performance.

This overview of medical care will also be used to discuss alternative approaches to its redistribution. Even though inefficiencies continue to exist in the medical care mar-ket, society may decide to increase the consumption of medical care to the population or to selected population groups. Such an overview suggests that it is possible to achieve an increase in consumption of medical care services either by shifting the de-mands for care or by increasing the quantity of a particular input on the supply side (i.e., shifting supply). Each of these policies will result in an increase in the quantity of medical care services consumed, as shown in Figure 3–4. For example, to increase the quantity of medical services consumed from Q_0 to Q_1 (based upon a normative judg-ment that it is desirable to do so), either the demand for medical care can be increased from D_1 to D_2, or the supply can be increased from S_1 to S_2. Either of these policies

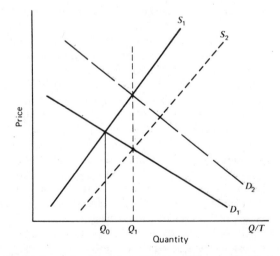

Figure 3–4. Alternative demand and supply policies to achieve a redistribution of medical care.

will achieve the objective of increasing the use of medical care from Q_0 to Q_1. However, these different redistributive policies will differ in their costs and their effects on other population groups.

Public policies designed to redistribute care by means of supply subsidies will be analyzed in each of the sections devoted to particular markets. The last chapters in this book will analyze various demand subsidy programs, such as proposals for national health insurance.

The overview presented here illustrates why medical care is said to be the output of the medical care sector. The efficiency of the separate markets and their interrelationship affects the efficiency with which medical care is produced, the cost at which it is produced, and the growth of expenditures in this sector. The evaluation of the efficiency of each of these markets is, therefore, of prime concern for public policy.

The foregoing model of medical care also illustrates the alternative approaches that may be used to redistribute medical services and the means for evaluating them. These two concepts, efficiency and redistribution (equity), will be the basis upon which both the separate markets and government policies will be analyzed throughout this book.

REFERENCES

1. The description of the medical care sector in this section is based upon an article by Paul J. Feldstein and Sander Kelman, "An Econometric Model of the Medical Care Sector," in H. Klarman, ed., *Empirical Studies in Health Economics* (Baltimore: Johns Hopkins University Press, 1970). Economists have developed other econometric models of the medical care sector. Perhaps the most ambitious of these is the one by D. E. Yett, L. Drabek, M. S. Intriligator, and L. J. Kimbell, *A Forecasting and Policy Simulation Model of the Health Care Sector* (Lexington, Mass.: Lexington Books, 1979).

CHAPTER 4

Measuring Changes in the Price of Medical Care

THE USES OF A DEFINITION OF THE PRODUCT OF THE MEDICAL CARE INDUSTRY

How has the price of medical care changed over time? Under what systems of reimbursement and what kinds of institutional arrangements is medical care produced most efficiently? What factors account for the differences in utilization of medical care among individuals and over time? These questions define major areas of research in the economics of medical care. They are of interest to policymakers as well, given the current public concern with rising medical costs and inefficiencies and inequities in the production and distribution of medical care. To answer any of these questions, we must define the product of the medical care industry implicitly if not explicitly. Any discussion of medical care prices presupposes some choice of units. Similarly, any comparison of the productive efficiency of two medical care providers presupposes some standard for measuring their outputs.

The units in which medical care is traditionally measured, such as the different items that appear on a patient's bill after a stay in the hospital, are far from ideal indicators of health costs and efficiency. Some of them are not really homogeneous measures of anything. Exactly what a hospital patient purchases for the daily room charge, for instance, may vary with diagnosis, choice of hospital, and most certainly will vary over time. But more important, the traditional units used for payment purposes do not seem to be true units of output, if we define output as that which yields satisfaction or utility to consumers. The physician's visit, the hospital bed day, the diagnostic test, and the prescription drug are perhaps more properly viewed as inputs into the production of medical care than as final outputs themselves. After all, the typical consumer of medical care does not set out to purchase a specific bundle of services. From the patient's point of view, the demand for medical care is ordinarily the demand for a treatment for some perceived physical or mental disorder. After the patient consults a physician, a treatment is prescribed that often uses various inputs in combination.

If it were feasible, it would be more useful to measure the costs or prices of medical care in terms of final outputs rather than in terms of the inputs to the treatment process. Such an approach would reflect the effects on medical costs both of increases and decreases in input productivity and of technological advances. Similarly, efficiency studies and policies designed to promote efficiency ought to focus more on efficiently satisfying consumers' medical needs and wants than on the efficient production of particular medical inputs. When it is possible to substitute less costly inputs for more costly ones, without changing the treatment outcome—such as treating patients with relatively simple cases on an ambulatory rather than an inpatient basis, or using nursing home care or the services of a visiting nurse in place of the last few days of a hospital stay—such substitutions ought to be encouraged.

Viewing medical goods and services as inputs in the production of care is also useful in studying medical care utilization. For purposes such as manpower planning and investment in hospitals, it is important to forecast the utilization of particular components of medical care. Looking at these different segments of the industry as suppliers of inputs emphasizes their interrelationship. The availability and price of hospital services is likely to influence, and in turn be influenced by, the utilization of outpatient or ambulatory services and long-term care. Ideally, of course, equity in medical care should be defined by how well individuals' medical needs are met rather than by the number of physicians' visits or hospital days consumed by different segments of the population.

A measure of the output produced by the medical care industry could also be used to measure the price of medical care over time, to evaluate the efficiency of alternative methods of delivering medical care, and to explain variations in the use of specific medical services; however, medical economics has not yet satisfactorily devised such a measure. The word "health" is inevitably used to describe the output of the medical industry, but health, which is itself a difficult concept to measure, is not determined solely or even primarily by medical care consumption. The health of a population is not really a fair measure of the success of its medical care system.

Some have suggested that treatment ought to be considered the unit of output, since individuals ordinarily seek medical care to obtain treatment for actual or perceived, current or potential illnesses. Total output would then be a weighted sum of the number of cases of different types treated. In this way, we could make meaningful comparisons of the cost of medical care over time and could assess the relative efficiency of different medical care providers.

There are, however, several difficulties in measuring medical care output by the number of treatments. Because the quality of treatments of particular conditions may vary, institutions providing high-quality care at high unit costs might be automatically judged to be inefficient unless quality is included in the output measurements. Although not part of the treatment of existing illnesses, preventive care can affect the likelihood of future illnesses and the costs of treatment, and therefore should somehow also be included in an output measure. Although such problems have yet to be resolved, treatment is a better indicator of medical output than are the specific goods and services by which it is usually measured, as it indicates both the interrelationships within medical care and how reimbursement policies for its improvement should be designed.

The rest of this chapter analyzes the measurement of prices, particularly in the field of medical care, beginning with a description of the functions and limitations of the Consumer Price Index (CPI). This is followed by a detailed discussion of the medical care component of the CPI, which is still the most widely used index of medical care prices. The final section describes and evaluates another approach to measuring the price of medical care—one that is based on the use of medical treatment as the most appropriate unit of medical care output.

THE CONSUMER PRICE INDEX

What Should the CPI Measure?

The CPI is generally viewed as an index of the cost of living. The percentage change in the CPI from one year to the next is taken as a measure of the rate of inflation—that is, of the rate at which a family's income would have had to increase just to keep up with rising prices. Many union contracts contain provisions for automatically increasing wages in line with increases in the CPI. Social security benefit levels are now keyed to it as well, as are the pensions of retired federal employees. Private pension plans, however, are rarely affected by changes in the CPI. In all, the incomes of about half of the U.S. population are directly affected by changes in the CPI. By 1986, a 1 percent change in the CPI was triggering an increase in payments under these various escalation provisions of at least $2.8 billion. Besides these direct effects on the economy, the CPI is viewed by makers of monetary and fiscal policy as an important indicator of the nation's inflation rate. It is also frequently used in social science research to deflate time series of money values, such as the average wage in a particular occupation over a period of years, and to express them in constant dollars.

These are some of the most prominent uses to which the CPI is put, but they do not exactly define what it is. The Bureau of Labor Statistics (BLS) calculates the CPI in an attempt to measure changes in the price of that bundle of goods and services which was purchased on the average by members of a well-defined segment of the American population in a certain base year. A price index of this type, in which individual prices are weighted by base-year quantities, is called a Laspeyres index.[1] Thus the CPI aims to measure how much the average household in its surveyed population will have to spend to buy the same market basket in the current year it bought in the base year. At first glance this might seem to be a logical measure of the change in the cost of living.

---

[1]It can be expressed by the following formula:

$$I_t = \frac{\Sigma_i Q_{bi} P_{ti}}{\Sigma_i Q_{bi} P_{bi}}$$

where I_t = value of the index in year t
  Q_{bi} = quantity of good i purchased in the base year
  P_{bi} = price of good i in the base year
  P_{ti} = price of good i in the year t

Such an index is often multiplied by some scaling factor so that it equals 100 in some particular year. Of course, if the index is multiplied by the same scaling factor in each year, percentage changes from year to year are not affected.

For several reasons, however, pricing a fixed market basket is not quite the same thing as measuring the cost of living. For one thing, the additional income required to purchase the base-year market basket in a later year will generally exceed the increase necessary to buy a market basket that is *equivalent in the eyes of the consumer* to that purchased in the base year. This is because consumers will substitute away from those items for which price is rising more rapidly and thus will lessen, to some extent, the impact of the general price increase.[2] If the price of beef rises particularly rapidly, for example, consumers will tend to buy less beef and more pork, chicken, or other meats. Because of this substitution bias, the Laspeyres index method of measurement tends to overstate cost of living increases.

More fundamentally, one may ask what a true cost-of-living index ought to measure. Economists often speak of a cost-of-living index as a measure of the cost of maintaining a given level of welfare or utility, of remaining on a certain indifference curve. If we take this point of view, the cost of living is influenced by much more than the prices of goods and services that consumers buy. Tax rates influence the amount of gross income needed to maintain a certain level of welfare. Taxes that directly influence the prices of products, such as sales taxes, are reflected in the index; income taxes are not. On the other hand, governmental provision of more free-of-charge services, such as better highways or better fire departments, may increase the standard of living achievable at any level of income. One might argue that standards of living are also affected by changes in crime rates, environmental pollution, and other such factors essentially beyond the individual's control. It is not necessarily true that a household is better off when its gross income increases faster than the prices of the goods and services it buys (1).

Aware of the difficulty of measuring the cost of maintaining a level of welfare, the BLS attempts the more modest task of measuring the price of a fixed bundle of goods and services. Even this job, however, is not simple. The market basket purchased by the average household in the surveyed population is constantly changing, not only in response to price changes, but also in response to changes in incomes, tastes, and other factors as well. The quality of existing goods and services changes, and new products that had no counterparts in the past are introduced. It would be meaningless to go on pricing the same goods and services without making an allowance for these changes. In the succeeding section, we discuss how the BLS resolves some of the major issues involved in constructing the CPI, and what the effects of these decisions on the performance of the index are likely to be.

---

[2]An index that used current-year quantities as weights would understate cost-of-living increases because it would put too much weight on items whose prices had increased relatively slowly. Such an index is called a Paasche index. Clearly, some sort of average of a Laspeyres and Paasche index will yield a better measure of cost-of-living changes than either one individually. The Laspeyres formula is used primarily because of the high cost of continually collecting information on weights. Also, past studies have shown that the substitution bias has only a small effect on the CPI. For example, the substitution bias between 1972 and 1980 accounted for only 6 percent of inflation over that eight-year period. For a discussion of this issue, see Jack Triplett, "Reconciling the CPI and the PCE Deflator," *Monthly Labor Review*, 104(9), September 1981. For a good discussion of index-number theory, see Kenneth Arrow, "The Measurement of Price Changes," in *The Relationship of Prices to Economic Stability and Growth*, compendium of papers submitted by panelists appearing before the U.S. Congress Joint Economic Committee, March 31, 1958: 77–87.

Issues and Problems in Constructing the CPI

Population Coverage

The CPI has traditionally been designed with urban wage earners and clerical workers in mind, but the precise definition of the covered population has changed over time (2). Until 1964, only families were included. At that time, single persons were added and the stipulation that household income should be less than $10,000 was dropped. After the 1964 revision of the CPI, its coverage included about 45 percent of the total U.S. population.

In the latest revision, the results of which were incorporated in the published CPI in January 1978, the BLS has expanded the CPI population to include all urban households in Standard Metropolitan Statistical Areas (SMSAs) (3). Since 1981 there have been 323 SMSAs. An SMSA is a large population center and neighboring communities that are highly integrated economically and socially with that center. This represents an addition of professional, managerial, and technical workers, self-employed and short-term workers, the unemployed, and those not in the labor force (including retired people). Population coverage now includes about 80 percent of the total noninstitutional population. Those not covered by the CPI are rural households, nonprofit organizations, and the military. A separate index for wage earners and clerical workers has been continued. Because it claims that the more comprehensive index will rise more slowly than the traditional CPI, organized labor has supported the continued use of the traditional index in contract escalation provisions (4).

Sampling Problems

Although it currently makes greater use of them since the 1978 revision, the BLS has not always used probability sampling techniques in constructing the CPI. Several aspects of their sampling methodology may bias the CPI (5). The BLS assigns weights to different items in the CPI based on data from periodic consumer expenditure surveys.[3] The previous survey involved interviewing 20,000 households in 216 areas to determine the items (and quantity) that people consume. Also, 20,000 people were asked to record a two-week diary of small, frequently purchased items. The major criticism of these surveys has been that at 10-year intervals, they are not conducted frequently enough. The BLS's weighting system was, until 1978, still based on 1960–1961 information rather than on data from the 1972–1973 survey. The next ten-year revision of the CPI was released in 1987 and uses data from the 1980 census and the 1982–1983 Consumer Expenditure Survey. Up until 1987, the weights for the CPI were based on the 15-year-old Consumer Expenditure Survey.

Table 4–1 indicates changes in the relative weights of major groups of items over the years. The years 1935–1939, 1952, 1963, 1981, and 1986 were chosen because they correspond to major revisions in the CPI growing out of new consumer expenditure surveys. The 1981 weights are based on the 1972–1973 survey and were first incorporated in the CPI in January 1978. December 1986 was chosen because it was the most recent data available; 1986 also includes in the CPI the new rental equivalence treatment of home ownership (6). It is interesting to note the similarity between the impor-

---

[3]The national CPI is built up from indexes calculated for a sample of cities. Separate city indexes are published. Differences between city indexes, however, do not measure price differences between cities, but only indicate price changes for each city since the base period.

TABLE 4-1. Relative Importance of Major Components of the CPI, Selected Years (Percent)

Group	1935–1939	December 1952	December 1963	December 1981 CPI-U	December 1981 CPI-W	December 1986[a] CPI-U	December 1986[a] CPI-W
All items	100.0	100.0	100.0	100.0	100.0	100.0	100.0
Food and beverages	35.4	32.2	25.2	17.5	19.1	17.8	19.7
Housing	33.7	33.5	34.0	46.0	42.7	42.9[b]	40.5[b]
Apparel and upkeep	11.0	9.4	10.6	4.6	4.6	6.3	6.4
Transportation	8.1	11.3	14.0	19.3	21.8	17.2	19.1
Medical care	4.1	4.8	5.7	4.9	4.4	5.4	4.5
Entertainment[c]	2.8	4.0	3.9	3.6	3.4	4.4	4.1
Other goods and services[d]	4.9	4.8	5.7	4.0	4.0	5.9	5.1

SOURCES: U.S. Department of Labor, Bureau of Labor Statistics, *Handbook of Labor Statistics, 1980*, p. 331: and *CPI Detailed Report*, Table 1, pp. 10–11, and Table 7, pp. 31–32.

[a]BLS unpublished data, new series.

[b]The rental equivalence approach to homeowner's costs: effective January 1985.

[c]Called "reading and recreation" before December 1977.

[d]Includes "personal care," usually shown separately before December 1977.

TABLE 4-2. CPI and Major Groups, 1935–1986 (1967 = 100)

Year	All Items	Food	Housing	Apparel and Upkeep	Transpor- tation	Medical Care	Entertain- ment[a]	Other[b]
1935	41.1	36.5	49.3	40.8	42.6	36.1	41.8	44.8
1945	53.9	50.7	59.1	61.7	47.8	42.1	62.4	56.9
1955	80.2	81.6	82.3	84.1	77.4	64.8	76.7	79.8
1965	94.5	94.4	94.9	93.7	95.9	89.5	95.9	94.2
1970	116.3	114.9	118.9	116.1	112.7	120.6	113.4	116.0
1972	125.3	123.5	129.2	122.3	119.9	132.5	122.8	125.5
1974	147.4	161.7	150.6	136.2	137.7	202.4	133.8	137.2
1976	170.5	180.8	177.2	147.6	165.5	184.7	151.2	153.5
1977	181.5	192.2	189.6	154.2	177.2	150.5	157.9	159.2
1978[c]	195.4	211.4	202.8	159.6	·185.5	219.4	176.6	183.3
1979[c]	217.4	234.5	227.6	166.6	212.0	239.7	188.5	196.7
1980[c]	246.8	254.6	263.3	178.4	249.7	265.9	205.3	214.5
1981[c]	272.4	274.6	293.5	186.9	280.0	294.5	221.4	235.7
1982[c]	289.1	285.7	314.7	191.8	291.5	328.7	235.8	259.9
1983[c]	298.4	291.7	323.1	196.5	298.4	357.3	246.0	288.3
1984[c]	311.1	302.9	336.5	200.2	311.7	379.5	255.1	307.7
1985[c]	322.2	309.8	349.9	206.0	319.9	403.1	265.0	326.6
1986[c]	328.4	319.7	360.2	207.8	307.5	433.5	274.1	346.4

SOURCES: U.S. Department of Labor, Bureau of Labor Statistics, *Handbook of Labor Statistics, 1975–1980*; *CPI Detailed Report*, various issues; BLS unpublished data for 1986.

Note: The 1978 revision brought about several definitional changes, which have made it impossible to directly link pre- and post-1978 indexes for "entertainment" and "other."

[a]Entertainment includes most of what was called "reading and recreation"; Entertainment excludes certain subcomponents found in "reading and recreation," such as TV and sound equipment, TV repair, and educational expenses.

[b]"Other" now includes educational and "personal care" expenses, which were previously found under other categories. It also includes tobacco products, and personal and educational expenses; it no longer includes alcoholic beverages.

[c]CPI for All Urban Consumers.

tance of the different components of the CPI for All Urban Consumers and CPI for Urban Wage Earners and Clerical Workers. The similar weights indicate that the expenditure patterns of the two groups are relatively similar. This is expected since urban wage earners and clerical workers represent a large portion of urban consumers.

The most striking trends in Table 4–1 are the declines in importance of food and the increase in transportation in consumer budgets. The weight assigned to food has fallen considerably despite the fact that, as Table 4–2 shows, its price has risen as fast as the all-items index. The decline in the importance of food in consumer budgets probably reflects low income elasticity rather than high price elasticity. As per capita incomes have increased, a smaller fraction has been used to buy food. According to Table 4–1, the transportation component of expenditures has increased in relation to the food component as the latter has become less important. Food and housing remain, however, the most important elements in consumer budgets, together accounting for well over half of expenditures on the average.

Price data cannot be gathered on every purchased item represented in the consumer expenditure surveys. The CPI classifies goods and services into successively smaller subgroups, down to what is referred to as an expenditure class (EC), of which there are currently 68. The EC is further subdivided into groups known as item strata. Finally, the item strata are divided into categories called entry-level items. An example of an entry-level item is a color television set. However, since there are many different models of color TV sets, the exact model to be priced is determined through a process which involves probability sampling, which was a change introduced in the 1972–1973 CPI revision. The assumption is that the other items in the EC are changing in price, on the average, at the same rate as the item or items actually priced.

It is less expensive to collect price information from sellers rather than from consumers. But this introduces another sampling problem: From what outlets should price information be gathered? In this area, as well as for subcategories within an expenditure category, little attempt was made to apply probability sampling prior to the 1972–1973 revision. A major difficulty was the absence of data on the outlets from which consumers purchased goods and services. Currently, a Point-of-Purchase Survey is used to aid in choosing "price reporters" on a probability basis.

The Point-of-Purchase Survey and store-specific pricing, because they have introduced probability sampling to the CPI, have increased the likelihood that the prices used in determining the CPI represent the actual distribution of prices in the market. However, there is still the problem of outdated weights. Up until 1978 the weights for the CPI were based on the 15-year-old, 1962–1963 Consumer Expenditure Survey. Even the latest weights were not current at their time of introduction. They were based on a survey that was already five years old. These outdated weights, because of the substitution effect, may lead to an upward bias, as has already been explained. To monitor and possibly correct any biases in the current weights, BLS has maintained continuing Consumer Expenditure and Point-of-Purchase Surveys, which are much smaller versions of the 1972–1973 surveys. These surveys may eventually lead to a more timely and inexpensive means of updating the CPI weights.

Quality Changes and New Products

As stated above, the BLS regards the CPI not as a true cost-of-living index, but as a price index for a bundle of goods and services. Even as an indicator of the rate of price increase in the economy, however, the contents of the bundle must be kept up to date with actual consumer purchases. For this purpose price changes that directly result from changes in product quality should be omitted from the index. For example, if a color television set is substituted for a black-and-white set, the index should not reflect the full price difference between the two, since most of it will be due to product quality differences. If the BLS considers the change in quality to be small, there is no adjustment for quality improvement; this causes an upward bias in the CPI. Otherwise, substitutions of new for old items are normally accomplished by linking. When the substitution is made, both the old and the new market baskets are priced. Percentage changes in the index prior to the link reflect percentage changes in the price of the old market basket; percentage changes after the link reflect percentage changes in the price of the new market basket. Thus, the price difference between the two market baskets at the time of the link is not reflected at all in the index.[4]

In many cases linking appears to be a good method of changing the CPI market basket. If the link is made at a time when one product is beginning to replace another in the market, but both are available and are purchased by some consumers, then the higher-priced one is worth the difference in price. The BLS has been criticized primarily for introducing new items too slowly (7); introductions occur at major revisions and when old items go off the market entirely. Based on the following description of events, it has been argued that the reluctance to introduce the new products imparts an upward bias on the CPI. Initially, a new item tends to have a relatively high price. This price falls as production expands, and an increase in the number of producers leads to greater price competition. Then, as newer products come to replace it in the market, its relative price may rise as the scale of production contracts. If consumers accept a new item while its price is relatively high, and if the item is absent from the index until after its price has fallen, the index will fail to register that fall in price of an item already important in consumer budgets. This problem occurs, as will be discussed, with the introduction of new drugs.

A change in the quality of an existing product is similar in conception to the introduction of a new product. A problem arises, however, in the attempt to separate price change from quality change when an improved model of a commodity such as an automobile or refrigerator replaces the older model on the market. In practice, the BLS usually adopts one extreme measure or the other: in cases where price changes occur simultaneously with quality changes, it ignores the quality change or the price change entirely (8). In the latter case, the quality-improved product is in effect treated as a new product and linked into the index in place of the old one.[5] In the automobile industry, the BLS obtains the cost of quality improvements from the manufacturer. If the BLS decides that the change increases the consumers' utility, they accept the manufacturer's estimate of the cost of the improvement. The possibility that manufactur-

---

[4]The following is a simple hypothetical example of linking. Suppose that an EC has been represented by one item, black-and-white TV sets, and a decision has been made to price color sets instead. Let us say that the index for this EC was equal to 100 in year 1. The price of black-and-white sets rises from $150 to $165, from year 1 to year 2, which is an increase of 10 percent. The index, still based on black-and-white sets, rises to 110. At that point the link is made. Color sets go from $400 to $420, from year 2 to year 3, a 5 percent increase. The index, now based on the price of color sets, increases 5 percent to 115.5 in year 3. The $235 difference between the prices of color and black-and-white sets in year 2 never shows up in the index at all.

AN EXAMPLE OF LINKING

Year	B&W TV Sets	Index	Color TV Sets
1	$150	100	—
2	165	110	$400
3	—	115.5	420

[5]The issue of adjusting for quality changes in a price index has received a great deal of attention from economists and statisticians. One proposed method for making such adjustments is the so-called hedonic technique. It can be applied to products for which many types are available at any one time; automobiles are perhaps the best example. Data are collected on the prices and characteristics of a number of different models at a point in time. Regression analysis is then used to estimate the contribution of different characteristics (in the case of the automobile, horsepower, fuel economy, interior room) to price. We can use this information to estimate what current models would have cost in the base year, based on their characteristics. The difference between these prices

ers overstate the costs of improvements to hide price increases may cause a downward bias in the CPI.

Table 4–2 presents values for the CPI and its major component groups during the 1935–1986 period. Since all the component indexes are scaled to equal 100 in 1967, those with the smallest values in 1935 increased the fastest in the period 1935–1967. The major component groups with the highest values in 1986 have increased the fastest since 1967. A one-point increase in an index is, of course, a smaller percentage increase today than it was in 1935. Table 4–2 shows that the indexes for the different major groups have had quite different patterns of increase over the years. Over the period as a whole, medical care has risen most rapidly.

THE MEDICAL CARE COMPONENT OF THE CPI (MCPI)

Background of the MCPI

In 1985, medical care had a weight of 6.5 percent in the CPI, up from 4.7 percent in 1981. Most of this increase in weight may be attributed to the change to the rental equivalent method of measuring the home ownership component of the CPI. This change caused home ownership to have a smaller weight, thereby increasing the weight of other components. The increased weight of medical care was also a result of its more rapidly rising price. An increase of about 15.4 percent in the MCPI would, in and of itself, increase the CPI by 1 percent. Through its effect on the overall CPI, the MCPI influences not only wages and other payments to a large fraction of the population, but also public perceptions of the inflation rate in the economy. As the only major index of medical care prices, it is often cited as a measure of inflation in that sector.

The BLS views the MCPI, like the CPI, as an index of the price of a fixed bundle of goods and services. Periodic consumer expenditure surveys, the basic source of information for determining the CPI weights, provide information on the weights of particular items in the medical market basket of the relevant population; it is the movement in the price of this basket that the MCPI attempts to trace. Our discussion will center on how well this objective is carried out in practice, and on how well the MCPI approximates an index of the price of medical care.

Table 4–3 presents an overview of movements in the MCPI and its component items since 1940. A glance at the table reveals that the "Medical Services" category has increased much more rapidly than the "Medical Care Commodities" category. More specifically, while the "Medical Service" items have increased somewhat more rapidly than the overall MCPI, the "Hospital Room Rate" has been the fastest-rising component of the MCPI.

Table 4–4 gives a breakdown of the relative weights of the items included in the MCPI as of December 1986. These weights are based on the 1982–1983 Consumer Expenditure Survey data on quantities of medical goods and services consumed, up-

---

and the current-year prices would be estimates of the pure price change. To date, this method has not been used by the BLS. For a more complete discussion of this subject, see John Muelbauer, "Household Production Theory, Quality, and the Hedonic Technique," *American Economic Review*, 64, December 1974: 977–994, and Zvi Griliches, "Hedonic Price Indexes for Automobiles: An Econometric Analysis of Quality Change," in *The Price Statistics of the Federal Government*, (Cambridge, Mass.: National Bureau of Economic Research, 1961), 173–196.

TABLE 4-3. Trends in the MCPI, Selected Years, 1940–1986 (1967 = 100 unless noted)

Item	1940	1950	1960	1965	1970	1975	1980	1981	1982	1983	1984	1985	1986
Medical care	36.8	53.7	79.1	89.5	120.6	168.6	265.9	294.5	328.7	357.3	379.5	403.1	433.5
Medical care commodities[a]	70.8	88.5	104.5	100.2	103.6	118.8	168.1	186.5	205.7	223.3	239.7	256.7	273.6
Prescription drugs	66.2	92.6	115.3	102.0	101.2	109.3	154.8	172.5	192.7	213.8	234.3	256.5	278.6
Nonprescription drugs and medical supplies (1977 = 100)[b]							120.9	133.6	145.8	155.2	163.3	171.2	179.1
Over-the-counter items[b]					106.2	130.1							
Medical care services	32.5	49.2	74.9	87.3	124.2	179.1	287.4	318.2	356.0	387.0	410.3	435.1	468.6
Professional services							252.0	277.9	301.5	323.0	346.1	367.3	390.9
Physicians' services	39.6	55.2	77.0	88.3	121.4	169.4	269.3	299.0	327.1	352.3	376.8	398.8	427.7
Dentists' services	42.0	63.9	82.1	92.2	119.4	161.9	240.2	263.3	283.6	302.7	327.3	347.9	367.3
Other professional services (1977 = 100)							123.6	135.2	144.3	153.0	159.9	171.0	180.3
Examination, prescription, and dispensing of eyeglasses[c]	58.1		85.1	92.8	113.5	149.6							
Other medical care services							330.1	366.9	421.9	464.4	488.0	517.0	562.6
Hospital and other medical services (1977 = 100)						132.2	133.5	152.5	174.1	193.9	210.6	224.0	237.4
Hospital service charge[d]													
Hospital room	13.7	30.3	57.3	75.9	145.4	236.1	418.9	481.1	556.7	619.7	670.9	710.5	753.1
Other hospital and medical care services (1977 = 100)							132.8	151.2	170.5	190.0	207.0	220.9	234.2

SOURCES: U.S. Department of Labor, Bureau of Labor Statistics, *Handbook of Labor Statistics*, 1975 and 1981 editions; *CPI Detailed Report*, various issues; BLS unpublished data for 1986.

Note: The only indexes available prior to 1978 are for urban wage earners and clerical workers. However, the table uses the more comprehensive All Urban Consumer indexes, which were introduced in 1978, for the years 1978–1981.

[a] "Medical care commodities" was introduced as a new category in 1978. It took the place of the category "drugs and prescriptions." The index values for "medical care commodities" from 1940 to 1977 are actually for the old "drugs and prescriptions" category.

[b] "Over-the-counter items" became part of the broader category "nonprescription drugs and medical supplies" in 1978.

[c] "Examination, prescription, and dispensing of eyeglasses" was discontinued in 1978. The examination portion of this category was absorbed by the new category "other professional services."

[d] "Hospital service charge" was replaced by the newly devised and more comprehensive "hospital and other medical services" category in 1978.

TABLE 4-4. Relative Weights of Items in the MCPI
(as of December 1986)

	U(%)	W(%)
MEDICAL CARE	100.0	100.0
Medical Care Commodities	19.5	19.5
Prescription Drugs	12.4	12.0
Nonprescription Drugs and Supplies	7.1	7.5
Medical Care Services	80.6	80.5
Professional Services	41.9	42.3
Physicians' Services	18.7	18.7
Dental Services	14.6	15.7
Other Professional Services	8.6	7.9
Other Medical Care Services	38.7	38.2
Hospital and Related Services	11.5	11.6
Health Insurance	27.2	26.6

SOURCE: U.S. Department of Labor, Bureau of Labor Statistics, unpublished data.

Note: The weights in the table are current to December 1986. They are
based on 1977 weights, but they have been adjusted for differences in
the rates of increase of prices of the MCPI components with which they
correspond. U, All Urban Consumers Index; W, Wage Earners and
Clerical Workers Index.

dated to 1986 prices. Notice once again that the weights for the All Urban Consumer
Index and the Wage Earners and Clerical Workers Index are very similar. The significance of this similarity will become apparent in the next section.

Constructing the MCPI

Population Coverage

The population covered by the MCPI and the overall CPI is, of course, the same. Since
1978 when the population coverage was extended to include the elderly, the population included in the MCPI has become more representative of the general population.
Previously, when the aged, who are large consumers of medical services, were excluded, the weight assigned to medical care in the traditional CPI understated its importance in total consumption for the entire population; the relative weights of particular services within the MCPI were also different from the relative weights of those
items in total U.S. medical care consumption. Hospital services, for example, are relatively more important for the elderly and unemployed than for urban wage earners
and clerical workers. Dentists' fees are relatively less important. The MCPI has therefore become more representative of the general population.

There are still a number of shortcomings to the MCPI, however, which limit its
usefulness as a general price index for medical care consumed in the United States,
although it is often used as though it were. As a matter of policy, the BLS does not
include changes in income taxes as changes in the cost of living, and it does not include
governmental service provided free of charge as elements of consumer budgets. In expanding the population coverage of the CPI, the BLS has added groups for whom the

government, through Medicare and Medicaid, pays a large portion of their medical care service. In keeping with its general policy, the BLS does not attempt to reflect these governmental expenditures in the CPI weights. The MCPI is not designed as an index of the price of the bundle of medical care services *consumed* by its target population, but of those services *purchased* by it.

The importance of some of these points is illustrated in Tables 4–5 and 4–6. Table 4–5 compares the weights of particular services in the MCPI [6] with the weights of similar services in consumer expenditures on health services and supplies. The weights are compared for 1964, 1975, 1981, and 1985 and the MCPI is compared both with consumer expenditures and with total national expenditures on health services and supplies.

There are two major reasons why the weight of medical care differs in the MCPI and in total medical expenditures. The differences between the MCPI [the first column for each year (e.g., 1, 4, 7, and 10)] and Consumer Expenditures (the second column in each year) is probably the difference in population included. These differences were larger in 1964 than in later years when the aged were included in the CPI in 1978. The larger weight for hospital services in Consumer Expenditures reflected the relatively high consumption of such services by the groups previously excluded from the CPI. Total health expenditures (the third column in each year) also includes government expenditures, which are deliberately excluded from the CPI. Thus even though differences between the MCPI and Consumer Expenditures have narrowed as the populations have become similar, government expenditures for medical care have increased and were weighted heavily toward hospital services. Thus the weight for hospital care is greater in total expenditures than in the MCPI and Consumer Expenditures. Correspondingly, the weights of dentists' fees and drugs fall as we move across the three columns. Dental services and drugs are predominately paid for by consumers and not the government; thus these components have a much larger weight with respect to what consumers spend but they represent a smaller portion of total medical expenditures, including government purchases. Note that nursing home services had no weight in the MCPI prior to the 1978 revision, which is not surprising given that the CPI was limited to wage earners and clerical workers and excluded the elderly; the government is also a large payor of nursing home services.

If the medical care price index was based on actual consumer expenditures or on total medical expenditures, the MCPI would have increased faster than it did in the past decade, since consumer and total expenditures give a heavier weight to the fastest-rising component, hospital care.

Table 4–6 demonstrates that the weight of medical care within the CPI index itself would be different if the index covered the entire population and total consumption rather than consumer purchases. For 1965, 1975, 1980, and 1985 the CPI weight of medical care is compared with the weight of *consumer* expenditures on health services and supplies in personal consumption and with the weight of *total* expenditures on personal health care *plus* government purchases. Notice that in 1965, both of the latter weights are larger than the weight of medical care in the CPI, indicating that groups excluded from the CPI consumed more medical care relative to their total consumption than did those covered by the index. In later years the populations in the different

---

[6]The weight given to hospital services includes the portion of the health insurance component representing hospital services. The weight given to physician fees includes the nonhospital services part of the health insurance component.

TABLE 4-5. Relative Weights of Items in MCPI, in Consumer Expenditures on Health Services and Supplies, and in Total National Expenditures on Health Services and Supplies, Calendar Years 1964, 1975, 1981, and 1985

	1964			1975			1981			1985		
	MCPI (December 1963) (1)	Consumer Expenditures (2)	Total Expenditures (3)	MCPI (December 1975) (4)	Consumer Expenditures (5)	Total Expenditures (6)	MCPI[a] (December 1981) (7)	Consumer Expenditures (8)	Total Expenditures (9)	MCPI[a] (December 1986) (10)	Consumer Expenditures (11)	Total Expenditures (12)
Hospital services[b]	17.9	29.4	37.4	28.5	31.7	42.0	27.6	33.6	43.1	24.6	31.3	40.7
Physicians' services	28.1	29.1	23.9	28.5	25.7	20.3	28.6	25.7	20.0	27.1	24.6	20.2
Dentists' services	15.1	10.1	7.8	14.0	10.9	6.7	14.4	10.7	6.3	15.8	11.1	6.6
Medical care commodities (drugs and prescriptions)[c]	20.0	20.8	16.4	12.0	19.3	12.3	16.4	15.8	9.9	12.9	10.8	7.0
Nursing and convalescent homes	0.0	3.0	3.5	0.0	6.0	8.2	<1.0	6.8	8.8	0.0	7.7	8.6

SOURCES: Robert Gibson, "National Health Expenditures, 1980," *Health Care Financing Review*, September 1981 and Fall 1986; R. Hanft, "National Health Expenditures, 1950–65," *Social Security Bulletin*, February 1967: 5; Department of Health and Human Services, *HHS News*, newsletter dated July 26, 1982: 00, Table 11; U.S. Department of Labor, Bureau of Labor Statistics, *The Consumer Price Index: History and Techniques*, Bulletin 1517, 1966, p. 47: U.S. Department of Labor, Bureau of Labor Statistics, *Relative Importance of Components in the Consumer Price Index, December 1975, 1977, 1986.*

[a]The index for All Urban Consumers is used.

[b]Because of definitional changes, "hospital services" does not include the same services in the 1978 revision that it did in the 1964 revision of the MCPI. The 1978 revision made "hospital services" a more comprehensive category. Although the room charge is still the major subcomponent, it includes a much broader range of hospital services than the 1964 revision. In addition, it includes other medical care services. These other services comprise only a small fraction of this index. One of the "other services" is "nursing and convalescent home care," which was not included in the MCPI before the 1978 revision.

[c]"Medical care commodities" was first reported in 1978. See the footnotes to Table 4-3 for a description of how it has changed from the 1964 to the 1978 revision.

59

TABLE 4-6. Weights of Medical Care in CPI, in Personal Consumption, Plus Government Purchases, Calendar Years 1965, 1975, 1980, and 1985

	1965	1975	1980	1985
Weight of medical care in CPI[a]	5.7	6.4	4.9	6.5
Weight of consumer expenditure on health services and supplies in personal consumption[b]	6.5	7.2	7.9	8.2
Weight of total expenditures on health services and supplies in personal consumption plus government purchases[b]	8.3	12.0	13.1	14.1

SOURCES: U.S. Bureau of the Census, *Statistical Abstract of the United States, 1986;* U.S. Department of Commerce, Bureau of Economic Analysis, *Survey of Current Business,* July 1986; Daniel Waldo et al., "National Health Expenditures, 1985," *Health Care Financing Review*, September 1986: 15, Table 3; U.S. Department of Labor, Bureau of Labor Statistics, *Relative Importance of Components in the Consumer Price Index*, various issues.

[a]The CPI weight is for All Urban Consumers.

[b]Health expenditures data are for fiscal years, while total consumption figures are for calendar years.

expenditure categories became similar. However, the divergence between the different weights becomes much greater in the later years. This reflects the increasing role of government in financing medical care. It appears that the CPI weight of medical care will continue to understate the importance of medical care in total consumption, particularly if the role of government in this sector continues to expand and the CPI fails to include such expenditures in determining its weights.

Sampling and the MCPI

The particular sampling problems of the all-items CPI already discussed are, of course, troublesome for the MCPI as well. We now discuss the systematic biases between the calculated MCPI and the true one that the BLS attempts to measure. Until the 1978 revision, only a small sample of the wide variety of medical goods and services purchased by consumers was actually priced in the MCPI.[7]

The BLS did not choose the items priced by probability sampling; they were selected "with the assistance of appropriate professional associations" (9). It is clear that the relatively simple, inexpensive, and frequently purchased goods and services were

---

[7]From 1939 to 1947, prices were obtained for the following items: physician home and office visits; obstetrical cases; surgical fees for appendectomy and tonsillectomy; several dental services; hospital ward; private room, and semiprivate room rates; private nurse rates; eye examinations and glasses; and several drugs and prescriptions. In 1947, a budget cut forced the BLS to discontinue pricing dental charges for cleaning teeth, replacement lenses for eyeglasses, women's pay ward rates, and private nurse rates. Group hospitalization insurance was added in 1952, as was surgical insurance in 1958.

Although this sample provided some representation for a variety of services, it could not be considered comprehensive. For example, the only physician services priced were an office visit, a home visit, an obstetrical case, and two surgical procedures. The first three (including the obstetrical case until 1961) were priced for general practitioners only, despite the fact that one-third of all private practice physicians in 1950 and over half in 1960 were specialists. For a more complete discussion of sampling, see Elizabeth Langford, "Medical Prices in the Consumer Price Index," *Monthly Labor Review*, 80, September 1957: 1953–1958; and Jeremiah German, "Some Uses and Limitations of the Consumer Price Index," *Inquiry*, 1, July 1964: 149–150.

chosen for pricing, and the less common and more expensive ones were not. The extent to which this sampling procedure may have biased the index is not known, nor is the direction of the bias obvious. It is clear that the omitted goods and services were, on the average, more expensive than those priced, but it is the *rate of change* in price that the index measures, and it is not clear how this differed for omitted and included items.

The 1964 CPI revision expanded the number of items priced. The number of physician services priced, for example, was expanded to seven. The drugs and prescriptions sample was expanded from three to 16 (10). Hospital ward rates were dropped, but some additional hospital services were priced for use in computing the health insurance component.

Still, probability sampling techniques were not applied systematically in choosing the items for pricing until the 1978 revision (11). In this revision, BLS specified a much larger sample of medical care items for pricing. At each particular outlet, or provider of medical care, the item(s) to be priced are chosen by probability sampling from this larger group. Thus, contrary to past practice, not all general practitioners sampled are asked for their fees for the same services, nor are all drug outlets asked for the prices of the same drugs. In the case of physicians' fees, 10 physician service categories or specialties have been identified, as have a number of services in each category. The items for which prices are obtained from any particular physician in the outlet sample are chosen from the list of services corresponding to his or her specialty. Similar procedures are used in sampling the prices of drugs, hospital services, and other components of the MCPI. By choosing items for pricing by probability sampling from a large group, the BLS increases the probability that the calculated index will approximate the true one.

A problem in the area of physicians' fees has been how to record a single provider's charges for a single service that may vary according to the patient's ability to pay (12). The BLS gathers data from physicians on their usual or customary charges for particular services, but the average fee received by the physician is a more relevant price, since it is also the average price paid by the consumer. Customary charges may differ from average prices *received* because customary charges may differ from average charges and because not all charges are collected. For example, a physician participating in Blue Shield may receive less than their billed charges. The physicians' fees component of the MCPI, based as it is on customary charges, may change at a different rate than the fees actually received by the physician.

Quality Changes and New Products

In the MCPI, as throughout the CPI, the BLS intends to trace movements in the price of a *constant-quality* market basket of goods and services. It is particularly difficult, however, to measure the quality of most of the medical services priced. For example, how can we separate quality changes from price changes when a physician's office visit fee, a hospital's semiprivate room charge, or the premium on a health insurance policy changes? It is difficult to know when or how to introduce product and quality changes into the MCPI. In response to index critics who cite its handling of quality changes and new products as its most serious weakness, let us examine the problems of adjusting for such changes as they relate to the different components of the MCPI.

Drugs and Prescriptions. It is widely agreed that, relative to their rapid development and adoption, the BLS has been slow to introduce new drugs into the MCPI. Critics also agree that a more rapid introduction of new products into this component would make the MCPI more representative of the market basket actually purchased (13). Until changes were made in 1960, the entire drugs and prescriptions component consisted of only six items: aspirin, milk of magnesia, and multivitamins among nonprescriptions, and penicillin, a narcotic, and a nonnarcotic among prescriptions (14).

Skeptics have noted the disparity between movements in this index and price changes in drugs and prescriptions. Once again, no systematic bias in a particular direction is clearly evident. Some have argued that since new drugs initially tend to have relatively high prices, the failure of the MCPI to include them results in an understatement of price increases. But this is incorrect. For example, when a hospital purchases drugs, the prices it pays probably increase faster than the drug component of the MCPI because of the continuous introduction of relatively highly priced new drugs. The fact that the new drugs are purchased while the old ones are still available would seem to indicate that the price increases are offset by quality improvements. If so, the BLS's practice of linking new drugs and prescriptions into the MCPI after a considerable lag may actually lead to a slight *overstatement* of drug price increases. New drugs frequently come down in price after their introduction, as production expands and competition among sellers increases. An index that only picks them up slowly may do so after they have come down in price, and thus the index will rise more rapidly (or fall more slowly) than one which links in new drugs shortly after they are introduced.

Hospital Services. It is difficult to separate price from quality changes in hospital services. Prior to 1972, hospital services were represented in the MCPI by daily room charges only.[8] The index of semiprivate room charges was frequently cited as an index of the price of hospital care. This use of the semiprivate room charge not only ignored problems of quality change but also presumed that the prices of other services not included in the basic room charge were changing at the same rate.[9] In 1972, an expanded hospital service charge index was introduced. It included the semiprivate room charge, the operating room charge, and the charges for eight specific ancillary services. The 1978 revision specified a much larger number of services for pricing. There are now 12 items in addition to hospital rooms for which data are gathered. At each hospital in the outlet sample, one or more items are chosen from this larger group for pricing by probability sampling.

Nonetheless, the most important component in the hospital service charge index is the basic room charge, which is not a constant-quality item. Adjusting for changes in the quantity of services provided under the daily room charge would seem consistent with the BLS's philosophy of attempting to price a constant-quality market basket. A study by the American Hospital Association suggested an approach for adjusting for quality change in a price index for hospital care (15). Instead of looking at charges, the investigators used cost data from the budgets of a fairly large but nonrandom sample of hospitals. They determined how many times, on the average, 37 different services were performed per patient day. By weighting the unit costs of these services by the

---

[8]In the 1964 revision, operating room and x-ray diagnostic series charges were priced and used in the computation of the health insurance component.

[9]The room charge index is also sensitive to changes in hospital pricing policies that may not affect the overall level of hospital charges. The extremely rapid increase in the semiprivate room charge index immediately after the introduction of Medicare was probably due to a movement away from the traditional policy of keeping room rates below actual costs and overcharging on ancillary services.

frequency with which they were performed in a base year, the investigators arrived at what they considered a cost index for a constant bundle of services. That is, they estimated how much it would have cost to produce the 1969 patient day in 1974, based on the 1974 unit costs of services. As might have been expected, their index rose much more slowly (36.9 percent) than the hospital semiprivate room charge component of the MCPI (56.4 percent) during the period under study (1969–1974). These findings suggest that failure to account for quality improvements in computing the index of semiprivate room charges may lead to an index of hospital prices that is biased upward.

There are problems in interpreting the results of the AHA study. For example, should all increases in service intensity be interpreted as quality improvements and therefore not be reflected in a pure price index? Or, what is essentially the same question, are all increases in the number of nursing hours, diagnostic tests, and other services provided routinely by hospitals worth their price to consumers? If the market for hospital services conformed closely to the competitive model, the answer would be yes, since if the increased service intensity were not worth its price, consumers would not pay for it. But imperfections in this market—including the limited ability of consumers to judge the quality of hospital care and the incentive distorting effects of hospital insurance—make this conclusion less obvious.

Health Insurance. The treatment of health insurance in the MCPI provides another example of the conceptual problems involved in adjusting for quality changes. Health insurance premiums may change in response to any of four types of changes: (a) changes in the price of medical services covered by the policy, (b) changes in the ratio of premiums collected to benefits paid out (the difference between the two is overhead expense), (c) changes in the comprehensiveness of the policy, and (d) changes in the average utilization of services by policyholders (16). Types a and b are clearly price changes and should be reflected in an index of the price of health insurance. A change of type c represents a change in the nature or quality of the policy and thus ought not to be reflected in the index. It is less clear how to classify type d. Changes in the average utilization of services by policyholders might occur in response to any number of things, such as changes in the incidence of illnesses (e.g., Aids), advances in medical knowledge or technology, and the introduction of cost-containment policies that place restrictions on use of services. One might argue that premium changes of type d are pure price changes, since the policy itself is unchanged. For the uninsured, however, increases in medical expenses due to increased consumption of services would not be considered price increases. Also, a patient facing restrictions on their use of services is worse off than without such restrictions.

On balance, it is reasonable to make some adjustment for premium changes resulting from changes in average utilization of services, but how to make it is unclear. If premium increases due to utilization increases are not reflected at all in an index of health insurance prices, we are assuming that such increases are always worth their full price to policyholders. Conversely, if we treat all premium increases due to utilization changes as as mere price increases, we are assuming that increased utilization is worth nothing.

From 1950 to 1964, the BLS included health insurance in the MCPI by pricing the most widely held Blue Cross-Blue Shield family plan in each sample area (note that the premiums of health insurance plans not priced were assumed to change at the same rate as those that were priced). All premium changes in the priced plans were reflected in the index, except those judged to be the result of changes in the comprehensiveness of policies, type c above. No attempt was made to adjust for premium changes of type d, those due to changes in average utilization.

In the 1964 revision, the BLS discontinued a direct pricing of health insurance policies. Instead, BLS decided to price a bundle of services representing those covered by health insurance, and to make periodic adjustments for changes in the weight of the overhead component of health insurance premiums. These steps were designed to account for premium changes of types a and b and to eliminate the need to adjust for premium changes of types c and d, since these are not reflected in the index in the first place. Of the two methods that have been used, the former will show a more rapid increase during times of increasing health services utilization; the latter will show a more rapid increase when utilization is decreasing. Neither method is more obviously correct. The same method used in the 1964 revision has been carried over to the 1978 revision with only slight modification. The BLS is experimenting with different and hopefully better ways of calculating the price of health insurance.

Professional Services. Doctors frequently complain that the MCPI overstates the rate at which their fees are increasing because it does not account for quality improvements. They argue that physicians today are generally better trained than they were in the past and that, with the aid of an expanded body of knowledge and improved technology, they are providing better quality services. From their point of view, an office visit today cannot be considered the same product as an office visit of 20 years ago.

Such physicians may have a valid point. The quality of their services is difficult to judge, and the BLS has generally ignored the possibility of quality change in pricing the services of medical professionals.[10] Regardless of whether or not BLS believes that physician fees should be quality adjusted, no method exists to measure and adjust for such changes.

In summarizing our discussion of the MCPI, we might emphasize three points. First, the MCPI is not designed as a comprehensive price index for all medical care consumed in the United States. Although it was originally targeted to a population that was not representative of the entire United States in terms of medical care consumption, its representativeness has improved since 1978. However, the MCPI still neglects the increasingly important share of medical care purchased by government. Second, the sampling procedures used have become more sophisticated, so that the MCPI is likely to resemble more closely the index that would have been calculated if all the relevant data (rather than samples) had been used. However, it is again questionable whether the price data collected from providers are representative of what patients, insurance companies, and other organizations actually pay the provider. Third, the difficulty in accounting for quality change and the introduction of new products raises questions about what the MCPI does and what it ought to measure. These questions lead us into the next section, which is a discussion of an alternative measure of the price of medical care.

---

[10]Except, apparently, when an obvious method of adjustment is available. For example, in 1961 obstetricians' fees for obstetrical cases were substituted for general practitioners' fees for the same service. The obstetricians' fees were linked in—that is, the difference between their fees and those of general practitioners was attributed entirely to a quality difference.

AN ALTERNATIVE MEDICAL CARE PRICE INDEX: THE COSTS OF TREATMENT OF A REPRESENTATIVE GROUP OF ILLNESSES

The Concept

Many of us choose intuitively to measure the product of the medical care industry by the number of episodes of illness treated rather than by the number of specific goods and services provided. When some mental or physical disorder is perceived, a consumer is prompted to seek medical care. The specific goods and services—physician visits, hospital bed days, prescription drugs, and so forth—function as inputs that are combined to produce treatments for such conditions. It is therefore reasonable to measure the cost of medical care by looking at specific illnesses and seeing how the average treatment costs per episode change over time. Many economists have found this cost-of-treatment approach to measuring medical care costs conceptually appealing.

In 1962, Anne Scitovsky detailed a proposal for an index of this type that would combine separate indexes of the treatment costs for specific illnesses into a composite index, weighting each component by the percentage of total medical expenditures spent on that illness in a base year (17). This procedure is analogous to the method by which the various component indexes are aggregated into the all-items CPI.[11]

While conceding that a costs-of-treatment index might be more expensive to construct, Scitovsky contended that its concept would be far superior to the traditional MCPI, since, unlike the MCPI, it could reflect quality changes in medical care and the introduction of new medical products and techniques. Since new goods and services are introduced over time and influence the costs of treating illnesses, their influence would automatically be reflected in a cost-of-treatment index. Similarly, if the quality of services—hospital bed days or physician visits, for example—improved over time, reducing the time and/or medical industry inputs required to treat illnesses, this change in input(s) quality would automatically be adjusted to the extent that it influenced costs of treatments. To compare the costs-of-treatment and MCPI approaches, suppose that hospital room charges increased, but that the increase was accompanied by a quality change that shortened hospital stays without requiring increases in the use of other inputs. The MCPI would show an increase because of the increase in room charges. The costs-of-treatment index would increase less and perhaps even decline, depending on the net effect of the changes on costs of treatments. It would thus adjust for this sort of quality change, whereas the traditional MCPI would not.

As long as the quality of *treatments* remained constant over time, this cost-of-treatment approach would appear to be a simple and direct method of adjusting for the effects on medical care price of changes in the quality of *inputs*. But not all changes in the amount or kinds of inputs used in providing treatments merely change the cost of producing an equivalent product. Many, perhaps most, such changes in methods of treatment change the product as well. They might change the probability of recovery or the amount of pain experienced in the course of the treatment, thus effectively changing the quality of the treatment itself. Even changes that alter the length of

---

[11]Scitovsky suggested that in order to minimize the costs of compiling such an index, illnesses might be grouped by similarity of treatment, with one or several illnesses chosen for actual pricing from each group. Such a procedure would involve an assumption that within groups, the costs of treatment of different illnesses would change at about the same rate over time.

treatment affect not only treatment costs but quality too, since patients prefer shorter treatments to longer ones.

Recognizing that her proposed index would not adjust automatically for such changes in the quality of treatments, Scitovsky suggested that for each illness included in the calculation of the index, a single objective indicator of quality be chosen. The average number of disability days might be appropriate for some infectious diseases or conditions requiring surgery; the number of live births per 100 pregnancies might be the quality measure for maternity cases. Using these quality indicators to adjust the individual costs-of-treatment indexes would have "the great merit of making possible more complete and systematic correction for quality changes," Scitovsky argued (18). As we shall see, however, the issue of how to deal with changes in the quality of treatments has remained a major point of contention in the debate over the merits of this approach to measuring the cost of medical care.

A modification of the original Scitovsky idea arose out of a comment by Yoram Barzel. Using the example of polio, he argued that although the costs of treating individual cases of polio may have remained constant or possibly increased, the introduction of polio vaccine has led to a drop in the total cost of polio because its incidence has been curtailed. Barzel contended that it is more appropriate to look at the *expected* treatment costs of an illness rather than at the treatment costs of cases that actually occur (19). His suggestion has considerable merit. The prevention of a case or illness clearly represents an output that is superior to the successful treatment of a similar case, but if we concentrate on the costs per case of treating specific illnesses when they occur, we ignore the influence of preventive medical care. An index that measures the costs of medical treatments should reflect the role of preventive care, otherwise it gives a misleading view of changes in the price of care and the productivity of the industry.

In replying to Barzel, Scitovsky essentially agreed with him on this point and proposed a slight modification of her original approach (20). Instead of looking only at average treatment costs of illnesses when they occur, she proposed averaging all medical costs associated with particular illnesses, including the costs of preventive care, over the number of cases treated *plus* the number prevented. In theory, this would seem a reasonable way of accounting for preventive care in a costs of treatment index.

The Scitovsky Findings

An actual costs-of-treatment index has not been constructed. However, in several separate studies Scitovsky, Scitovsky and McCall, and Scitovsky examined the treatment costs of a selected group of illnesses covering the periods 1951–1964, 1964–1971, and most recently, 1971–1981. These studies made no adjustments for changes in treatment quality (21). The study was limited to cases treated by physicians at the Palo Alto Medical Clinic (PAMC)—a multispecialty, largely fee-for-service group practice of about 140 physicians in Palo Alto, California. Data on treatment costs were obtained from the records of PAMC and Stanford University Hospital, where nearly all patients requiring hospitalization were treated. Data on costs of treatment rendered outside PAMC or Stanford Hospital were obtained from the patients directly. Before attempting generally to evaluate the costs-of-treatment approach to measuring the costs of medical care, let us examine the Scitovsky and Scitovsky-McCall findings. Table 4–7 presents a summary of the findings on the changes in treatment costs for the conditions studied. It is striking that in so many cases the percentage increases in treatment costs

TABLE 4-7. Percentage Increase in the Costs of Treatment of Selected
Illnesses, 1951–1981

	1951–1964	1964–1971	1971–1981
Otitis media	69	31	113
Appendicitis			
Simple	73	79	254
Perforated	86	115	235
Maternity care	73	56	257
Cancer of the breast	103	70	254
Forearm fractures (children)			
Cast only	52	17	183
Closed reduction no general anesthetic	85	102	173
Closed reduction, general or regional anesthetic	355	62	253
Myocardial infarction	NA	126	294
Pneumonia (nonhospitalized)	NA	31	114
Duodenal ulcer (nonhospitalized)	NA	12	184
MCPI	55	47	129

SOURCES: Anne A. Scitovsky and Nelda McCall, "Changes in the Cost of Treatment of Selected Illnesses, 1951–1964–1971," Health Policy Program, Palo Alto Medical Research Program, August 1975, pp. 10, 17; Anne A. Scitovsky, "Changes in the Costs of Treatment of
Selected Illnesses, 1971–1981," *Medical Care*, 23(12), December 1985: 1347.

exceeded the percentage increases in the MCPI. In the 1951–1964 period, the percentage increase in treatment cost exceeded the increase in the MCPI in all but one case. In
the 1964–1971 period, the percentage increase in the MCPI exceeded the percentage
increase in treatment costs in approximately one-quarter of the cases, while in the
latest period, 1971–1981, the percentage increase in treatment costs exceeded the increase in the MCPI in all but two cases. These results are at least a little surprising.
Unless it can be shown that the quality of treatments for these illnesses improved substantially over the period, these results seem to belie the allegation that the MCPI
overstates increases in the price of medical care by failing to account for productivity
improvements.

In fact, however, a number of possible explanations can be made for the differences
between the rates of increase in the estimates of treatment costs and the MCPI. For
example, Scitovsky found that the prices of ancillary hospital services were rising particularly rapidly. These services were not even priced by the BLS at that time, and the
MCPI may have been biased downward by their omission. It is also possible that for
the sample of illnesses chosen, treatment costs rose faster than the cost of medical care
in general.[12] Further, medical care prices tend to be higher in larger cities, and since
Palo Alto doubled in size and became part of the San Francisco metropolitan area
during the 1951–1964 period, part of the higher costs for the treatment approach may

---

[12]The cost of treatment estimates are also based on small samples (ranging in size in 1951 from only three cases of
forearm fractures, closed reduction, no general anesthetic, to 99 cases of simple appendicitis), and thus may
contain some random error.

be a result of more rapid medical price increases in Palo Alto. The MCPI for San Francisco also increased faster than the national MCPI during this period (22).

The greater increase shown in the costs-of-treatment approach can also be attributed to a closing of the gap between customary and average charges for physicians' services. Scitovsky used data on actual charges for services rather than customary charges as the BLS does.[13] If it is true that average actual charges were increasing faster than customary charges—that the practice of cutting fees for low-income patients were becoming less prevalent—this might account for part of the differences in results. Scitovsky found some evidence to this effect. Scitovsky found, for example, that for pediatricians in PAMC from 1951 to 1964, the average charge increased 54 percent more than the customary charge for an office visit, and 31 percent more for a home visit (23).

A final reason why the costs-of-treatment approach rose more rapidly than the BLS index for medical care is that the latter measures only the price of an input, while the cost-of-treatment approach also includes the quantities of inputs used. Those diseases for which the treatments remained basically the same increased less than the MCPI. For example, treatment for an ulcer during the period 1964–1971 did not change very much, however, during the 1971–1981 period there were important diagnostic and treatment changes. During the earlier period ulcer treatment costs rose less rapidly than the MCPI while in the latter period it rose more rapidly. There has also been an important quality change as a result of these treatment changes, with respect to healing and prevention of a recurrence.

Table 4–8 presents a more detailed breakdown of changes in the methods of treatment in the illnesses that were studied. Not all inputs, such as drugs, have been included. The following are some general trends. The number of physician visits used in treating cases tended to increase. (1981 data on physician visits and other input data were unavailable in the latest study.) The average length of stay in the hospital generally declined. However, total use of ancillary services increased dramatically, particularly for those cases requiring hospitalization. Clearly, important changes in methods of treatment have affected costs in each direction, and cost-increasing changes have been quite common.

Evaluating the Cost-of-Treatment Approach

The results of the Scitovsky studies clearly show that in the absence of adjustments for changes in treatment quality, a costs-of-treatment index might well rise even faster than the MCPI. However, if such adjustments were made, the index might rise more slowly than the BLS index. In evaluating the merits of the costs-of-treatment approach to measuring the costs of medical care, it is important to consider whether or not a legitimate basis and a practical method exist for making adjustments for changes in treatment quality.

Some argue that any increase in treatment costs that result directly from changes in the amounts or types of inputs used in treatments ought to be regarded entirely as quality improvements, not as price increases. This point of view assumes that if the old treatment method for an illness is still available, consumers will not purchase a more

---

[13]Actual charges billed, not those collected, were used. Scitovsky suggests that because collection ratios were improving, the gap between customary charges and average charges collected was narrowing even faster than that between customary charges and actual charges billed.

TABLE 4-8. Number of Physician Visits, Average Length of Stay, Diagnostic and Other Services per case, Selected Illnesses, 1951–1981

	1951	1964	1971	1981
Otitis media				
Physician visits	1.8	1.7	1.9	
Appendicitis simple				
Physician visits	2.9	5.6	5.5	
ALOS (days)	4.3	4.2	3.8	3.5
Laboratory tests	4.7	7.3	14.3	19.2
IV solutions	.1	2.4	4.6	
Appendicitis perforated				
Physician visits	6.8	9.1	11.8	
ALOS (days)	10.8	10.7	10.1	8.1
Laboratory tests	5.3	14.5	53.9	58.2
IV solutions	6.7	12.7	14.2	
Maternity care				
Physician visits	12.7	14.5	14.9	
ALOS (days)	4.6	3.8	2.8	1.9
Laboratory tests	4.8	11.5	14.8	21.6
Breast cancer (mastectomy treated only)				
Physician visits	13.9	17.8	14.9	
ALOS	12.7	10.2	9.5	3.3
Laboratory tests	5.9	14.8	16.6	32.9
X-rays				
Diagnostic	.7	2.0	1.8	2.2
Radiotherapy	1.7	11.0	10.6	
IV solutions	1.0	1.7	1.7	

	1951	1964	1971	1981
Forearm fractures				
Cast only				
Physician visits	5.3	4.5	4.4	
X-rays	2.3	2.3	2.2	2.1
Closed reduction, no general anesthesia				
Physician visits	6.7	6.1	7.0	
X-rays	3.7	2.7	4.1	3.6
Closed reduction, general or regional anesthetic				
Physician visits	5.8	7.9	8.1	
X-rays	2.0	5.4	5.3	4.3
ALOS (days)	1.0	1.2		
Myocardial infarction				
Physician visits	NA	27.6	26.0	
ALOS	NA	19.7	18.8	10.6
Laboratory tests	NA	37.9	81.3	124.8
X-rays	NA	1.3	3.5	2.5
IV solutions	NA	1.6	10.6	
Electrocardiograms	NA	5.4	9.0	
Inhalation therapy	NA	12.8	37.5	
Pneumonia				
Physician visits	NA	3.0	2.6	
Laboratory tests	NA	3.0	3.0	4.2
X-rays	NA	2.0	1.3	0.5
Duodenal ulcer				
Physician visits	NA	4.7	3.8	
Laboratory Tests	NA	5.4	7.9	11.0
X-rays	NA	2.4	2.3	1.5

SOURCES: Anne A. Scitovsky and Nelda McCall, "Changes in the Cost of Treatment of Selected Illnesses, 1951–1964–1971," Health Policy Program, Palo Alto Medical Research Program, August 1975, pp. 27, 28; Anne A. Scitovsky, "Changes in the Costs of Treatment of Selected Illnesses, 1971–1981," Medical Care, 23(12), December 1985: 1347, 1348.

input-intensive method of treatment unless the increase in quality is at least worth the increase in costs. Citing the Scitovsky data on the treatment of forearm fractures, Barzel points out that even though the differential in fees between general practitioner treatment and orthopedic surgeon treatment widened between 1951 and 1964, the percentage of cases treated by orthopedic surgeons increased. He interprets this as a shift in demand, and argues that it indicates that consumers value the additional quality of treatment by an orthopedic surgeon at its additional cost at least.

Others are skeptical of whether medical care markets respond to consumer preferences so perfectly. Scitovsky claims that changes in methods of treatment are generally forced on consumers. She suggests, for example, that "the primary reason for the increased use of specialists is physicians' reluctance, not to say unwillingness, to treat cases outside their special field" (24). She does not deny that changes in methods of treatment are generally quality improvements, but (and here she reverses the position taken in her earlier paper) argues that since quality is forced on the consumer and since he or she does not really have the option of choosing the old treatment methods, an index of the cost of medical care should not be adjusted for such improvements in quality.

These two points of view—complete adjustment for cost-increasing changes in methods of treatment or no adjustment whatever—are the extremes on this issue, and neither of them seems entirely correct. Forced or not, if a change in treatment methods really improves the quality of care, then the new treatment is a different and better product than the old. Comparing its price with the price of the old treatment overstates the increase in the price of a constant amount of medical care.

On the other hand, is it correct to assume that changes in treatment methods are always worth their full costs? This would be a reasonable assumption if medical care markets conformed closely to the competitive model. However, given that substantial third-party coverage for medical expenses exists and that consumers have little knowledge of medicine, patients are likely to accept the judgments of physicians as to what treatment methods are appropriate. Physicians, for their part, are not trained (and until recently have had little incentive) to weigh the benefits and costs of prescribing new methods of treatment; they apparently believe that any treatment change with an expected positive incremental benefit is justified, regardless of its additional costs. If patients pay little or nothing for care at the time they receive it, why should they not choose the method of treatment their physician believes is best, whatever its true cost? If medical care markets work in the manner just described, we would expect that innovations in methods of treatment will tend to be quality improving and that improvements in quality may not always justify their true costs.[14] Thus, to adjust entirely for such cost-increasing changes in treatment methods in a medical care price index may be seriously misleading. Some middle ground between the two extremes of ignoring changes in treatment quality completely and assuming that they are always worth their full costs is more desirable than adopting either one.

---

[14]This does not imply that the consumer is irrational. Each policyholder's individual consumption of medical care has a negligible effect on insurance premiums, and thus regardless of what others do, each maximizes utility of consuming medical care to the point where to him or her, marginal benefit equals marginal costs (which is zero—neglecting time costs—if the insurance policy is comprehensive). When everyone acts in this way, premiums rise, and the whole group may be worse off than before the introduction of new methods of treatment.

Scitovsky's original suggestion that indexes of the treatment costs of specific ill-nesses be adjusted by some objective indicator of outcome quality is correct. However, three very serious problems still hinder the implementation of this approach. One problem is that the quality of a medical treatment is truly multidimensional; Sci-tovsky's suggestion that a single quality indicator for each illness be adopted might be too simplistic. Would it be proper to judge the quality of an automobile on its miles-per-gallon rating, or on any other single statistic? The probability of recovery, the expected number of disability days, the probable extent of physical impairments once recovery is completed, the painfulness of the treatment, and the amenities provided along with it are only some of the relevant aspects of the quality of a treatment. Deter-mining how different treatment methods affect these different aspects of quality might be very costly, although such information would obviously be useful for other purposes besides the construction of a medical care price index.

The second problem, which would still be troublesome even if complete informa-tion existed on the technical aspects of the outcomes of different treatment methods, arises when placing values on differences in treatment quality. What value, for exam-ple, should be placed on a slightly lower probability of death from a particular dis-ease, or on a little less pain? The problem of determining such values is as much con-ceptual as technical; its solution is not clear. For example, consider the suggestion by Scitovsky that, to hold quality constant, the costs of maternity care might be measured by the costs of handling all the pregnancies necessary to produce a certain number of live births (25). A reduction in the frequency of miscarriages certainly represents an improvement in the quality of maternity care, but should the cost-quality relationship be the one Scitovsky postulates? On what grounds can we assume that an obstetrician who is 99.9 percent successful in delivering babies is exactly twice as good as one who delivers only one live birth for every two cases handled? A doubling of the success rate in delivering babies or in treating an illness might imply more than a twofold increase in quality. But exactly how much more? This is the kind of question that must be answered if a cost-of-treatment index is to be adjusted correctly for changes in quality of treatments.

Third, it was suggested that the *expected* treatment cost of an illness is a more rele-vant measure than the average costs of cases actually treated. Since the expected costs is the probability of contracting an illness times the average costs of treatment, it can be influenced by preventive medical care. In principle, an expected-costs-of-treat-ment index could be calculated in the manner described earlier. For each illness, the total costs of treatment would be averaged over the number of cases treated plus the number of cases prevented. However, it is not simple to distinguish the number of cases eliminated by preventive medical care alone. Incidence rates of illnesses are in-fluenced by many factors, including nutrition, personal health habits, lifestyle, and environmental factors such as pollution levels. The simple method of comparing the incidence of an illness in a base year with that in a later year and taking the difference as a measure of the effects of preventive care is not satisfactory. Other factors may be responsible for the difference. If birthrates go down and less is spent on maternity care, for example, does this mean that the medical care industry is more productive? Is it less productive if the nation increases its consumption of cigarettes and the incidence of lung cancer goes up? Surely the answer is no in both cases. Ideally, then, the effects of preventive care on incidence rates should be computed separately from those of other factors when preparing an index of expected treatment costs. Multivariate statistical techniques might be used for this task, but it is questionable whether precise estimates could be obtained.

Despite its limitations, the costs-of-treatment approach retains a theoretical appeal; it would enable more meaningful comparisons to be made of the cost of medical care, both cross sectionally and over time. The fixed-bundle-of-goods-and-services method of pricing medical care used by the BLS yields results that are difficult to interpret meaningfully. The treatment of an illness seems a more appropriate notion of medical care output than the physician's visit, the hospital patient day, or the other more conventional units used by the BLS. Still, enormous practical difficulties and perhaps considerable cost would be involved in actually constructing a costs-of-treatment index as a substitute for the MCPI. In addition, some conceptual problems involved in this approach have not been solved adequately, most notably the issues of how to deal with changes in the quality of medical treatments and how to take account of the preventive aspects of medical care. However, the BLS is unlikely to embrace the costs-of-treatment approach in the near future.

APPENDIX: HEALTH INSURANCE PREMIUMS AS A MEASURE OF THE PRICE OF MEDICAL CARE

Another alternative approach to assessing the price of medical care, suggested by some economists, is to measure it in terms of health insurance premiums. Melvin Reder reasons that "if medical care is that which can be purchased by means of medical insurance, then its 'price' varies proportionately with the price of such insurance."[15] The apparent advantages of this price-of-insurance approach are its simplicity and the fact that productivity changes that influence the cost of providing care would automatically be reflected in the index. For example, technical changes that lower the costs of providing treatments would lead to downward pressure on insurance premiums and thus hold down the index of the price of medical care. Improvements in preventive care, which we have seen would be difficult to assess in a costs-of-treatment index, would also show up automatically in a price-of-insurance index. Preventive measures, to the extent that they lowered the expected cost of medical care, would also lower the costs of providing health insurance and would thus be reflected in this kind of index.

However, users of this approach will encounter the familiar conceptual problems involving the issue of quality change. A health insurance policy need not remain a

---

[15]Melvin Reder, "Some Problems in the Measurement of Productivity in the Medical Care Industry," in V. Fuchs, ed., *Production and Productivity in the Service Industries* (New York: Columbia University Press, 1969), p. 98. In "Productivity and the Price of Medical Services," *Journal of Political Economy*, 77, November-December 1969: 1014–1027, Barzel also makes a case for this kind of index. In this same paper Barzel calculates an index of Blue Shield policy premiums for 1945 to 1964 and attempts to test the hypothesis that the physicians' fee component of the CPI overstates price increases for physicians' services by failing to adjust for improvements in the quality of services. He does find that premiums for Blue Shield group medical and surgical insurance policies increased on the average by only 66.5 percent from 1945 to 1964 compared with 85.3 percent for the physicians' fee component of the CPI. The implications of this finding are not clear, however. The entire difference in percentage increases between the two indexes is accounted for in the first three years (both increase about 60 percent between 1948 and 1964). Were Blue Shield plans capturing economies of scale in claims processing from 1945 to 1948 (their membership tripled during that time)? Did Blue Shield plans obtain preferential prices for their members, who were at that time mainly low-income families? It should be noted that an index of Blue Shield premiums cannot be considered a comprehensive price index for medical care, since Blue Shield covers physicians' services almost exclusively.

constant-quality good over time, even if the language of the policy remains unchanged. Changes in the incidence of illnesses may occur, for example, for reasons beyond the control of the medical care industry. Such changes may affect the utilization of medical services and thereby raise or lower health insurance premiums. Alternatively, physicians may develop more input-intensive treatment methods over time, improving the quality of care but also raising insurance premiums. In neither case would it be correct to price the insurance policy as though it were a constant-quality item. Consider a third example: Suppose that there were increases in hospital capacity and physicians in a previously underserved area. It is likely that the amount of illness left untreated would drop, that treatments would generally be more complete, and that travel time and waiting time would decrease. Health insurance premiums would have to increase, but surely such premium increases would not be pure price changes. The improvement in care may more than compensate the population for the increase in premiums.

It appears, then, that the price-of-insurance approach is subject to the same basic problem that plagues the other methods of pricing medical care that we have examined: How can we quantify that component of price change that represents the value consumers place on increased quality (or loss they attach to lower quality)? Adjusting a price-of-insurance index for quality change would be at least as conceptually and practically difficult as adjusting a costs-of-treatment index.

Another kind of difficulty would arise by focusing exclusively on health insurance premiums. Since most individuals do not have complete insurance coverage for medical care, changes in insurance premiums are not the only factors that affect their cost of care. Many policies, for example, contain ceilings on the amounts the insurer will pay for specific services. If the service costs exceed those ceilings and continue to increase, medical care costs will increase for the insured, since they will be forced to make up out-of-pocket what the policy does not cover. In the meantime, the insurance premium may not change. To avoid this kind of difficulty, the index might be based entirely on the premiums of very comprehensive prepaid insurance plans, without deductibles, coinsurance provisions, or ceilings. Since only a small percentage of the population is covered by such insurance plans, however, it is not clear how meaningful the index would be. There is little justification for assuming that the costs of medical care for those with no insurance coverage, for those with coverage for only specific types of services, and for those with less-than-complete coverage would always change in the same manner as the costs for those with comprehensive prepaid coverage.

REFERENCES

1. For a further discussion of the appropriateness of the CPI as a cost-of-living index, see Janet L. Norwood, "Indexing Federal Programs: The CPI and Other Indexes," *Monthly Labor Review*, 104, March 1981: 60–65.

2. See U.S. Department of Labor, *The Consumer Price Index: History and Techniques*, Bulletin 1517, 1966, especially p. 84.

3. For a general discussion of the 1978 revision of the CPI, see the following: U.S. Department of Labor, Bureau of Labor Statistics, *Concepts and Content over the Years*, Report 517, May 1978; and *The CPI—How Will the 1977 Revision Affect*

It?, Report 449, 1975. See also John Laying, "The Revisions of the CPI," *Statistical Reporter*, February 1978: 140–148.

4. Julius Shiskin, "Updating the Consumer Price Index—an Overview," *Monthly Labor Review*, 97, July 1974: 3–4.

5. Philip McCarthy, "Sampling Consideration in the Construction of Price Indexes with Particular Reference to the United States Consumer Price Index," in *The Price Statistics of the Federal Government* (Cambridge, Mass.: National Bureau of Research, 1961), pp. 197–232.

6. Prior to the 1983 revision of the CPI-U and the 1985 revision of the CPI-W, the homeownership component of the CPI was determined by the asset and shelter value of the home, based on the price of the house, mortgage interest rates, property taxes, insurance, and maintenance costs. The problem with this method was that about 3 percent of households bought a new house during the 1972–1973 Consumer Expenditure Survey. The entire weight of home ownership was determined by the house price and mortgage payment by only 3 percent of the population in one year, even though the number of home purchases varies greatly from year to year. Further, the standard long term fixed interest rate mortgage no longer represented the typical mortgage because of the introduction of variable interest rates. The rental equivalence of home ownership uses rental market information in places where housing is mostly owner occupied so that the rental units are more similar to owner-occupied units. Robert Gillingham and Walter Lane, "Changing the Treatment of Shelter Costs for Homeowners in the CPI," *Monthly Labor Review*, 105(6), June 1982.

7. *The Price Statistics of the Federal Government*, pp. 37–39. (This useful report, prepared by a Price Statistics Review Committee of the National Bureau of Economic Research, is often referred to as the Stigler Report, after the committee chairman, George Stigler.)

8. Shiskin, *op. cit.*, p. 18.

9. Elizabeth Langford, "Medical Prices in the Consumer Price Index," *Monthly Labor Review*, 80, September 1957: p. 1056.

10. J. German, "Some Uses and Limitations of the Consumer Price Index," *Inquiry*, July 1964.

11. Daniel Ginsburg, "Revisions in the Medical Care Component of the Consumer Price Index," remarks delivered to the Blue Cross Conference on "Health Care in the American Economy: Issues and Forecasts," Hilton Head Island, S.C., January 18, 1977.

12. See, for example, Anne Scitovsky, "Changes in the Costs of Treatment of Selected Illnesses," *American Economic Review*, 57. December 1967: 1188–1189.

13. *The Price Statistics of the Federal Government*, 37–39.

14. German, *op. cit.*, 149–150.

15. P. Joseph Phillip, James Jeffers, and Abdul Hai, "Indexes of Factor Input Price, Service Intensity, and Productivity of the Hospital Industry," in *The Nature of Hospital Costs: Three Studies* (Chicago: Hospital Research and Educational Trust, 1976), 201–262.

16. Ginsburg, *op. cit.* The description of the handling of health insurance in the MCPI that follows is also based on information from this source.

17. Anne Scitovsky, "An Index of the Cost of Medical Care—A Proposed New Approach," in Solomon J. Axelrod, ed., *The Economics of Health and Medical Care* (Ann Arbor, Mich.: Bureau of Public Health Economics, University of Michigan, 1964), 128–147.

18. Scitovsky, *Ibid.*, p. 139.

19. Yoram Barzel, "Cost of Medical Treatment: Comment," *American Economic Review*, 58, September 1968: 937–938.

20. Anne Scitovsky, "Cost of Medical Treatment: Comment," *American Economic Review*, 58, September 1968: 939–940.

21. Anne Scitovsky, "Changes in the Costs of Treatment of Selected Illnesses, 1951–65," *American Economic Review*, 57, December 1967: 1182–1195; Anne Scitovsky and Nelda McCall, "Changes in the Costs of Treatment of Selected Illnesses, 1951–1971," Health Policy Discussion Paper, University of California School of Medicine, San Francisco, September 1975; and Anne Scitovsky, "Changes in the Costs of Treatment of Selected Illness, 1971–1981," *Medical Care*, 23(12), December 1985: 1345–1357.

22. Scitovsky, "Costs of Treatment, 1951–65," p. 1190.

23. *Ibid.*, p. 1188.

24. Scitovsky, "Costs of Medical Treatment: Comment," 938–939.

25. Scitovsky, "Costs of Medical Treatment: Comment," p. 939.

CHAPTER 5

The Demand for Medical Care

THE PURPOSE OF DEMAND ANALYSIS

One of the purposes of an analysis of the demand for medical care is to determine those factors which, on the average, most affect a person's utilization of medical services. At any point in time many factors influence the consumer's choice to seek medical treatment of a given intensity. It would be virtually impossible to explain completely every individual's utilization of medical services, but certain factors are important for most persons. Demand analysis seeks to identify which factors are most influential in determining how much care people are willing to purchase. The better our understanding of those factors, the better we will be able to explain variations in utilization among population groups and between areas.

Such an understanding will also enable us to forecast future utilization more accurately; to do so, each of the factors affecting demand is forecasted separately. If, for reasons of social policy, it were desirable to change a certain population group's utilization of medical care, then by our understanding of which factors affect demand, such a change could be wrought. Thus an understanding of which factors affect demand, and to what extent, will enable us to explain variations in use of medical services. That knowledge can be used to forecast demand more accurately and to bring about changes in utilization if we desire.

DEMAND VERSUS NEED AS A BASIS FOR POLICY AND PLANNING

At various times it has been proposed that the planning of health facilities and health manpower be based solely upon estimates of need for medical care in the population. Need has generally been defined as the amount of medical care that medical experts believe a person should have to remain or become as healthy as possible, based on current medical knowledge.[1] The Lee and Jones research of the 1930s (1) was one of the classic studies using medical need as the basis for determining physician requirements in the country. The Hill-Burton formula for planning hospital facilities also used need as the criterion for the number of beds required in an area. Four and one-half beds per thousand population was the standard adopted for determining whether additional beds should be built in an area. The only adjustment to this ratio was the population density in an area. If the density was fewer than six persons per square mile, then the standard became 5.5 beds per thousand population.

The assumption underlying the use of need as a basis for public policy in medical care is that need itself is, or should be, the main determinant of hospital and physician use. However, since need is only one factor affecting demand for care, basing resource allocation decisions solely on medical need is likely to result in misallocation. If the estimated amount of services required to meet medical need exceeds the amount that people will actually use, then an allocation of facilities and manpower on the basis of need alone will result in an underutilization of those resources that could have been used elsewhere or in another manner. If, on the other hand, people use more medical care than would be provided based solely on a need criterion, then there will be an excess demand and increased waiting times. Shortages of facilities and manpower are costly because they waste a patient's time—time that could have been spent in a more productive manner.

Thus planning based solely on medical need is likely to result in the use of either too few or too many resources. These consequences are shown in Figure 5-1. Planning according to medical need is shown by a vertical line, since need is independent of price. (Need is also independent of the prices of other services, of income, and of insurance coverage. Changes in these other factors would not change need, as medically defined.) The number of medical facilities determined by need is shown along the horizontal axis (e.g., Q_0 equals four beds per 1,000 population). If utilization is less than need (Q_1) or greater than need (Q_2) at a given price (P_0), then either too many (Q_0-Q_1) or too few (Q_2-Q_0) resources will be allocated to medical facilities.

When need is viewed as one factor affecting demand, then greater or lesser needs for care would be represented by different demand curves; for example, D_2 may include a greater amount of need than D_1. Changes in medical need cause a shift in the demand for care. If preventive care reduces the future need for acute medical services, this may be shown by a shift to the left in the demand for acute care (e.g., from D_2 to D_1).

Planning according to demand would at least ensure against the wasting of resources and patients' time. If utilization is less than medical need (e.g., utilization equals Q_1), then by understanding which factors affect demand and by knowing how much demand can be changed when one of these factors is changed, we can increase demand so that quantity demanded at the market price equals medical need. Conversely, if a decrease in utilization is desired where it exceeds need (e.g., utilization

[1]J. Jeffers et al. state: "An accurate specification of a population's 'needs' for medical services requires perfect knowledge of the state of its members' health, the existence of a well-defined standard of what constitutes 'good health,' and perfect knowledge of what modern medicine can do to improve ill (or below standard) health. It must be acknowledged that existing diagnostic procedures are not capable of providing perfect knowledge of the state of any population's, or even an individual's health. It also must be acknowledged that a clear-cut consensus as to what constitutes 'good health' does not exist among health professionals." James R. Jeffers, Mario F. Bognanno, and John C. Bartlett, "On the Demand Versus Need for Medical Services and the Concept of 'Shortage,'" *American Journal of Public Health*, 61(1), January 1971: p. 47.

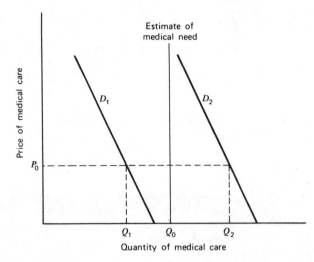

Figure 5-1. Need versus demand as the basis for planning in medical care.

equals Q_2), utilization can also be decreased by influencing one of the factors affecting demand. Using a demand analysis does not mean that medical need is disregarded in planning, only that other demand factors are incorporated in estimating what use will be. The emphasis, then, is on accurately forecasting demand. Once demand has been forecast, we can decide, based on reasons of social policy, whether demand should be increased or decreased. Planning according to medical need alone is based on the assumption that medical need should be the only criterion for determining utilization, which is a value judgment that not everyone would share. Everyone may not place the same value on fulfilling all or even a certain percentage of their medical needs. Some may not be willing to pay the necessary price or to spend the necessary time to receive all the medical care that medical experts believe they should receive. Disregarding demand factors is likely to result in a waste of resources as well as a failure to ensure that those persons with the greatest need receive care.

If not need, should demand be the criterion for determining the quantity of medical services to be used? An assumption underlying all demand analysis is that people allocate their scarce resources among different goods and services in a way that maximizes their utility. Some persons might say, however, that medical care does not provide any utility, since the patient does not desire to purchase it. Many goods fall into this category: auto repair services, legal services, and home repairs. The desirability of the service is not relevant to the applicability of demand analysis. "Undesirable" services could simply be redefined, as in the case of medical care, to mean those services that provide benefits by alleviating or eliminating illness.

The marginal benefits derived from additional units of medical care differ. For example, diagnostic uncertainty declines as more specialists' services and tests are used. In addition, the probability of recovery from particular illnesses varies depending upon the quantity of medical care used. Some units of medical care provide large amounts of reassurance to patients; others provide the amenities. Some medical services are a substitute for services performed by the family in the home. Patients and their families differ in their perception of the value of these different aspects of medical care, which accounts for differences in the amounts they are willing to pay for these perceived benefits. Similarly, if the price of medical care were reduced, more people might be willing to buy more services of the above-mentioned types.[2]

Since patients perceive the benefits from additional units of medical care differently, and since they are willing to pay different amounts for those additional services, who is to judge how much medical care should be used? If the patient makes this determination, then, as is the case in a market-oriented economy, he or she would use medical services to the point where the marginal benefit of the last unit equals the price he must pay for those units. If, however, medical need is the criterion for rationing medical care, then regardless of the patient's willingness to pay, he or she would not be allowed to receive more medical care than others believe they need.

In most markets in the United States, output quantity and quality are based upon the concept of consumer sovereignty. The assumption is that consumers are the best judges of how to use their resources to increase their own utility; how they choose to spend their money, together with the cost of producing those goods, will determine the variety and quality of the goods and services being produced.[3] The concept of consumer sovereignty in medical care is not uniformly accepted by health professionals, whose task it then becomes to develop an alternative set of criteria sufficiently specific to determine not only the quantity of resources to be spent on medical care but also the method by which these limited resources are to be allocated among different patients and institutional settings. These alternative criteria must substitute for all those allocative functions that would, in a system of consumer sovereignty, be performed by prices and differing consumer demands. In addition, an alternative system should make explicit the values underlying its distribution of medical care.

The determination of optimal output in a market, whether it is made with respect to medical care demand, the manpower markets, or the health education markets, is based upon the concept of marginal benefits and marginal costs. When the marginal benefits of a service are equal to the marginal costs of producing that service, the amount of that service is considered to be optimal. If the marginal benefits are either less than or greater than the marginal costs of producing a service, consumption in that market is considered to be economically inefficient (i.e., resources are misallocated in that they are not placed in their highest-valued uses). Efficiency in consumption, therefore, is one criterion by which the output of different medical care markets will be evaluated. The other criterion is efficiency in production: whether the output is produced at minimum cost. Economic efficiency in consumption and in production are criteria that economists use to evaluate the performance of different markets. In medical care, the criterion of efficiency in production is more widely accepted than is the criterion of efficiency in consumption, for which some persons would prefer to substitute a need criterion. Applying the criterion of efficiency in consumption to each medical care market, however, should sharpen the debate on the underlying values

---

[2]The great variability in the use of medical care due to the unpredictability of the individual incidence of illness should not lessen the usefulness of demand analysis. If we are interested in prediction, the variability in medical care use and in the incidence of illness will average out over large groups of individuals. It will be possible to forecast the average demand for care, as opposed to the demand by any particular individual or family. The demand curve represents the average of many individuals' perceived benefits from additional units of medical care in relation to the price they are willing to pay for those additional benefits.

[3]Deciding whether incomes should be redistributed is independent of deciding who should determine the goods and services to be produced in society. If society determines that certain population groups do not have sufficient incomes, their incomes can be supplemented.

and criteria for defining optimal output in each market; should consumers' or health professionals' perception of marginal benefits prevail?

Whether or not people accept the criterion of efficiency in consumption, demand for medical services must still be analyzed if we are to be able to forecast use of services more accurately.

A MODEL OF THE DEMAND FOR MEDICAL CARE

The Demand for Medical Care Derived from The Demand For Health

The traditional theory of consumer demand assumes that consumers purchase goods and services for the utility provided by those specific purchases. A more recent formulation of consumer demand, however, draws a distinction between goods and services purchased in the market and more fundamental objects of choice, referred to as commodities (2). If the commodity demanded by consumers is good health, then health can be produced by goods and services purchased in the market as well as by the time devoted to preventive measures. Within this framework, the demand for medical care is derived from the more basic demand for health.

According to Michael Grossman (3), consumers have a demand for health for two reasons: (a) it is a consumption commodity—it makes the consumer feel better, and (b) it is an investment commodity—a state of health will determine the amount of time available to the consumer. A decrease in the number of sick days will increase the time available for work and leisure activities; the return to an investment in health is the monetary value of the decrease in sick days.

A view of medical care demand as being derived from the demand for health implies the following. First, increases in age result in an increase in the rate at which a person's stock of health depreciates. Over the life cycle, people will attempt to offset part of the increased rate of depreciation in their stock of health by increasing their expenditures on, and use of, medical care. Second, the demand for medical care will increase with increases in a person's wage. The higher their wage, the greater the value of an increase in the number of healthy days. A consumer who is paid a high wage rate will also substitute purchases of medical care services for his or her own time when producing the commodity health. We would thus expect to observe a positive relationship between increased wages and greater expenditures on the demand for medical care. Third, it is hypothesized that education has a negative effect on the demand for medical care. More highly educated people are presumed to be more efficient in producing health. They are, therefore, likely to purchase fewer medical care services.

This view of medical care demand provides a rationale for including in the demand model certain factors believed to affect demand, traditionally known as taste variables, because they influence the individual's demand for health. The importance of the patient's time in relation to the demand for medical care will also be included in the demand model. Analyzing the demand for medical care as being derived from the individual's demand for health provides a better basis for determining which factors should be included in a model of demand for medical care, and for hypothesizing their effects.

Determinants of the Demand for Medical Care

A discussion of the demand for medical care requires an economic framework not only for surveying the literature on factors affecting demand, but also for evaluating empirical research on demand (4). If a demand study excludes relevant factors affecting demand, perhaps because they are not easily measured, or because the investigator is unaware of their importance, then its results are likely to be inaccurate.

Variations in the demand for medical care are determined by a set of patient and physician factors. The patient's demand for medical care is essentially the demand for a treatment, and variations in demand are a result of variations in the number, type, or quality of treatments demanded. This demand is typically initiated by the patient. The physician then combines various inputs to provide a treatment of a given quality. The patient's determinants of demand are his or her incidence of illness or need for care, a set of cultural-demographic factors, and economic factors. The roles of the physician as advisor to the patient and as a supplier of a service are discussed separately below.

Empirical studies on the demand for medical care should thus describe, first, how different factors affect the patient's demand for medical care, and second, what determines how the physician will provide care for a given treatment. For purposes of clarity, the patient and physician phases will be described sequentially, although they occur simultaneously. The aim of empirical research, then, is to derive an estimate of the relationship between patient and physician factors and use of medical care.

The assumption of choice is implicit in studies of demand. Choices are made both of amounts of medical care purchased and of combinations of the components of care that produce a treatment. If choice in these areas were not possible, much less variation in medical care use would be observed when nonmedical factors, such as cultural and economic background, are analyzed. Less variation would also exist in the manner in which a treatment is provided. The patient's and physician's degree of choice depends on two factors: knowledge and the availability of substitutes. It is often assumed that no close substitutes within the field of medical care exist. Even if this were true, which it is not, families might still differ in their demand for medical services because they attach different values to the expected benefits of increased use or because their knowledge of these benefits varies. Within the field of medical care itself, the substitutability of components in providing a treatment appears to be increasing. Not only are ambulatory services and nursing home care partial substitutes for hospitalization, but the increased use of outpatient surgery provides an additional substitute for hospital care. These, then, are the reasons underlying the assumption that the patient exercises choice in his or her demand for medical care and the physician exercises it in the treatment provided.

Factors Affecting the Patient's Demand for Medical Care

As we have noted, the factors affecting a patient's demand for medical care are incidence of illness, cultural-demographic characteristics, and economic factors. The first two, stemming from the family's perception of a medical problem and their belief in the efficacy of medical treatment, shape the consumer's desire for medical care. When translating this desire into an expenditure, the family is limited by the extent of its available resources. Determining the amount to be spent on medical care becomes a part of the problem of allocating scarce resources among alternative desires. Each of these general factors affecting a patient's demand for care is discussed below.

Actual or perceived illness or desire for preventive medicine will determine whether or not an individual is in the market for medical care at any point in time. The onset of illness and the use of a hospital is for many people an unexpected occurrence. Thus, for individuals, illness may be considered a random event, but with respect to the age and sex of the population as a whole, illness has a fair degree of predictability. As individuals age, the incidence of illness increases and morbidity patterns change; chronic diseases become a more important determinant of the need for medical care. Although medical expenditures are approximately the same for both sexes in the early years, there is a difference in the need for medical care among men and women, holding constant marital status and age. Later in life, expenditures incurred by women exceed those incurred by men primarily because of obstetrical charges, although the difference persists beyond the childbearing ages. The relationship between age and use of medical services, however, is not simply linear nor is it the same for each type of medical service. For example, the relationship between age and use of hospital services is different from that which exists between age and the use of dental services. Even for hospital care, there are differences in admissions and in length of stay by age group. Although these population characteristics may not affect each of the components of medical care in the same manner, they are important in explaining variations in the use of these services.

Marital status and number of persons in the family also affect the demand for medical care. Single persons generally use more hospital care than do married persons. The availability of people at home to care for an individual may substitute for additional days in the hospital. Family size also affects demand; a larger family has less income per capita (although not necessarily proportionately less) than does a small family with the same income.

Education is also believed to affect the demand for medical services. A greater amount of education in the household may enable a family to recognize the early symptoms of illness, resulting in a greater willingness to seek early treatment. We might expect to observe such a family spending more for preventive services and less for more acute illnesses later. Higher levels of education may also lead to increased efficiency in a family's purchase and use of medical services. Years of education in a household may be a proxy measure for a greater awareness of the need for medical care, for different attitudes toward seeking care, and for greater efficiency in its purchase and production. Differences in education among families are expected to result in differences in use and expenditures for medical services.

Although it is important to our understanding to determine the effect that cultural-demographic factors have on the demand for medical services, such factors are not subject to sudden changes, nor are they generally the instrument of public policy. The age structure changes gradually, as do attitudes. The effect that economic factors have on the demand for medical services is of more immediate value for purposes of forecasting and policy.

The economic factors contributing to medical services demand are income, prices, and the value of the patient's time. They affect not only whether a patient will seek medical care but also the extent of the care once treatment is undertaken. Economic factors may not have much of an effect on whether a maternity patient goes to a hospital (although they may influence the choice of hospital), but once she has been admitted, they may affect her length of stay. Each of these economic factors is briefly discussed.

A number of studies have examined the relationship between family income and expenditures on medical care and also the effect of income on use of medical care. When these studies are based on survey data, it is often found that families with higher incomes have greater expenditures for medical care, although the percentages of income spent on medical care declines as income increases. In other words, the income elasticity of medical care expenditures is less than 1; that is, the percentage increase in medical care expenditures is less than the percentage increase in income (5). The manner in which family income is measured must be understood if the effect of income, as it is derived from medical care surveys, is to be interpreted correctly. A family's income in any given year may be abnormally low or high because of the temporary loss of employment, windfall gains, or other unexpected events. Empirical evidence suggests that total consumption is not raised or lowered to correspond with temporary changes in income. Rather, a family's level of consumption is determined primarily by its expected normal or permanent income (6). If transitory income has little or no effect on total expenditures, and families that are sick are likely to be below their normal incomes, then survey data that merely show the relationship between income and expenditures include both permanent and transitory income. Since transitory income is included in the income reported by the survey, although it presumably has little effect on expenditures, the reported survey relationship between income and expenditure is likely to be understated. If the effects of transitory income can be removed, the income elasticity of medical expenditures will be increased. Thus one reason why estimates of the effect of income on medical care expenditures are low is that it is difficult to determine the relationship between permanent income and medical care expenditures from survey data.

Another reason why estimates of income elasticity derived from survey data is biased downward is that employer contributions to health insurance premiums are not normally included in survey data. Such employer contributions do not constitute taxable income for employee recipients. The higher the income tax bracket, the larger the potential tax saving to the employee and the greater is the incentive to have the employer pay for health insurance. If, for persons with higher incomes, a greater proportion of medical expenditures is reimbursed by third-party payors, then survey data showing the relationship between family income and out-of-pocket expenditures will understate the true income elasticity.

Once survey data are corrected for transitory income and employer-paid health insurance premiums, it appears that the income elasticity of medical care expenditures is approximately 1; that is, a 10 percent increase in income will lead to a 10 percent increase in expenditures on medical care.

The price of a service and the use of that service are, according to economic theory, inversely related: as the price is reduced, purchase or use of the service will increase. Knowledge of price elasticity of demand for medical services is therefore of great importance for public policy. Many persons have generally assumed, however, that prices have very little effect on use of medical services. If national health insurance is to result in greater use of medical services, its proponents must assume that the use of medical services is responsive to changes in price; if not, national health insurance will not result in any changes in use but merely in a redistribution of income. Before discussing estimates of price elasticity of demand for medical services, it would be useful to discuss what the relevant price variable should represent.

Patients do not usually pay the medical provider's stated price or charges. Part or all of the price (as in the case of Medicaid patients) is paid by a third-party payor or by the government on the patient's behalf. Any estimate of price elasticity of demand should be based upon the net or the out-of-pocket price paid by the patient. Health insurance is one of the most important factors reducing the patient's price. Insurance coverage represents a movement down the individual patient's demand curve, which increases the quantity of services demanded. For all individuals, the existence of insurance coverage represents a *shift* in the overall demand for medical care. The effect of insurance on the individual's demand for care and on the aggregate demand for care is explained graphically and more completely in the appendix to this chapter. Although, as will be discussed, estimates of price and insurance elasticities have generally been found to be inelastic with respect to demand for medical services, these estimates vary by type of medical service and by seriousness of illness.

Certain institutional settings can substitute for others in treatment of an illness. An analysis of the demand for any one component is incomplete if it omits the substitutability and demand for other components. Because a patient can be treated for an illness with different combinations of hospital care, outpatient services, and nursing home care, different lengths of stay in the hospital may reflect differences in the use of other institutional settings. Therefore, a demand analysis of any one component of care should include net prices to the patient of substitutes and complements. Again, the relevant price to the patient of these substitutes and complements is the out-of-pocket, not the stated, price.

One important reason why estimated price elasticities of demand for medical care are expected to be low is that time costs may represent a relatively large portion of the total price of medical care. In addition to prices and income, the consumer's time is a constraint that affects the type of goods and services purchased. Consumer time may be considered an input into the production of a good or service. Cooking a meal and consuming it at home, for example, requires more consumer time than does eating in a restaurant. When time costs are high, people will substitute purchased services for their own time. Since time has an opportunity cost, it is also scarce and should be viewed as one of the resource constraints facing the consumer. The importance of including time costs, as well as the money costs of consuming a good or service, is that it enables us to explain and predict consumer demand more accurately. If either time or money costs of a service decrease, the quantity demanded would be expected to increase. For example, people with higher earned incomes, such as businessmen, typically have a higher cost of time; consequently, they have a higher demand for air travel than do those with low time costs, such as students.

In medical care, time is used in traveling to a provider and in waiting to be treated. The following example illustrates how differences in time costs affect the price elasticity of demand for a service. Assume that the patient's out-of-pocket price for visiting a medical provider is $10 and that the time costs are equal to $20; the total price of the visit is therefore $30. If the elasticity of the medical service with respect to the total price were − 1.0, meaning that a 10 percent change in the total price results in a 10 percent change in use, and if the out-of-pocket price dropped 50 percent (from $10 to $5), the result would be only a 20 percent decrease in the total price of care (from $30 to $25). This 20 percent change in the total price would lead to a 20 percent change in use because the price elasticity is − 1.0. Thus, when an out-of-pocket price is reduced by 50 percent and use increases only 20 percent, the calculated price elasticity is − .4. The demand for that service is thereby estimated to be price inelastic. Thus, as time costs contribute a larger proportion of the total price, the calculated price elasticity of demand becomes smaller, while the time price elasticity increases (7).

In the past, as third-party coverage and government reimbursement covered a greater portion of the bill, time costs represented a greater proportion of the patient's total cost. Changes in money and time costs have important implications for the consumption of medical services. Analyses of the impact on the demand for physician services of a change in insurance coverage, from no out-of-pocket price to the introduction of a 25 percent coinsurance provision, found that the use of such services substantially decreased, primarily among those enrollees with the lowest time costs (8). This increase in the money price of the service, to a 25 percent co-pay, represented a much larger increase in total price to persons with low time costs than it did for those with higher time costs. For example, home visits, which involve the lowest time costs, experienced twice as large a decline as other types of visits. Further, enrollees decreased "their demand for care of minor illnesses considerably more than their demand for medical care of other conditions" (9). Nonprofessionals (i.e., those with lower time costs) had a much greater reduction in the number of annual examinations as their out-of-pocket price increased. Female dependents, who have lower time costs than female subscribers, had a larger reduction in visits when the money price of a visit was increased.

The researchers reexamined use rates from the above study four years later to determine whether the effect on physician visits of a 25 percent copayment rate was temporary. The authors found that the 24 percent decline in per capita use of physician visits did not change four years later (10).

Three policy implications follow from the findings that time costs have an important effect on the demand for medical services. First, as out-of- pocket prices to patients decrease, demand for medical care becomes more responsive to the cost of time. If the quantity supplied of medical care does not increase sufficiently to meet increased demands, as is the case under a system similar to the British National Health Service, then the likely method of rationing is to allocate care to those who can afford to wait. Those with a low time cost are more likely to receive care than are those with a high opportunity cost of time. Second, society has determined that certain population groups should receive an increase in their use of medical services. Although the money prices to these groups have been reduced, it may be desirable to reduce their time costs to increase further their use of services. Locating clinics closer to these population groups will lower their travel costs and increase utilization. Third, when planners determine the number and size of hospitals, the patients' time costs should be considered, together with institutional costs, as the relevant costs for planners to minimize. Consumers are willing to pay higher money prices to decrease their time costs. Unless time and money costs are both included in the planning of medical facilities, planners might attempt to lower the costs of hospital or other facility costs by building fewer though larger units, thereby increasing travel time costs to patients.

The Role of the Physician in the Demand for Medical Care

In nonmedical markets the consumer, with varying degrees of knowledge, selects the goods and services that he or she desires. In medical care, however, the patient does not decide, for example, what hospital to enter or the form of treatment he or she is to receive; instead, the patient selects a physician who then makes these choices. In acting on the patient's behalf, the physician uses his or her awareness of the patient's financial resources and medical needs to act as the patient would if he or she had the knowledge and medical authority to make the decision.[4] When choosing the components of care to be used in treatment, the physician will be guided not only by their efficacy but also by their relative prices to the patient (11). For example, if a patient can be treated either as an outpatient or as an inpatient, but the patient's insurance coverage covers only inpatient hospitalization, it would be less costly *to the patient* to be hospitalized. This choice of treatment settings by the physician on the patient's behalf, however, would result in higher total health care costs.

Evidence that physicians make such choices on the patient's behalf is contained in the many studies that relate hospital utilization to the patient's insurance coverage. Although physicians' behavior will also be affected by other factors discussed below, we can use the fact that they often act in the patient's financial and medical interests to predict medical and hospital use according to the patient's financial, sociodemographic, and medical characteristics. The more likely a physician is to be aware of and to act in accordance with the patient's needs, desires, and financial interests, the stronger will be the empirical relationship between such patient characteristics and use of medical services.

With the growth of more comprehensive hospital insurance, financial constraints became less important, and physicians prescribed the highest quality of medical care for their patients. This was rational behavior on the part of the physician and the patient, since the marginal benefit of additional tests and other services, no matter how small, was probably greater than the out-of-pocket price the patient had to pay. The physician was able to practice what Victor Fuchs has referred to as the technologic imperative. In other words, medicine was able to prescribe the best care that was technically possible (12). No consideration was given as to whether the marginal benefits of that additional care exceeded the marginal costs of producing it.

However, other factors may prevent the physician from acting solely in the patient's interest. A physician may not have staff appointments at all of the hospitals in the community. If two hospitals provide similar care for their obstetrics patients, but one of them is more expensive than the other, then, unless the physician has a staff appointment at the less expensive hospital, his or her patient will be admitted to the more expensive hospital.

Also, some hospitals may have utilization review committees that review the appropriateness of admissions and length of stay. In the face of an effective committee, a physician may find it difficult to prescribe hospital care and/or a length of stay that satisfies the patient's preferences. To the extent that such institutional arrangements and sanctions exist, the relationship between utilization and patient characteristics (both economic and noneconomic) will be less clear.

There is a more important reason why the physician may not act solely in the patient's interest. As one of the inputs into the patient's medical treatment, the physician has an economic interest in the manner in which a treatment is provided. In prescribing care to a patient, the physician is acting not only in the patient's interest as an advisor, but also in his or her own interest as a supplier of services. One of the more obvious examples of the effect of this dual role is the decrease in home visits. It is more convenient for a patient who is not seriously ill to be examined and treated by a physician at home. The physician, however, can achieve greater productivity, hence in-

---

[4]The physician has been referred to in this role as a manager or agent for the patient. See *Report of the Commission on Cost of Medical Care*, Vol. I, (Chicago: American Medical Association, 1964), pp. 9–21.

come, by staying in the office and seeing more patients instead of spending time in traveling. It is in the physician's economic interests to shift the travel costs to the patient. Similarly, a physician shifts certain costs to the patient and the patient's third-party payor when they prescribe additional tests for the purpose of protecting themselves against a possible malpractice suit.

Two controversial issues in the medical care literature, together with their policy implications, can be clarified when the dual role of the physician, as an advisor and as a supplier of a service, is used to explain them. The first relates to the idea that the supply of beds creates a demand for those beds, the second to the idea that physicians create demand. The ideas are related, but it is useful to separate them for purpose of analysis.

"A Built Bed Is a Filled Bed." The hypothesis that the supply of beds creates a demand for those beds is associated with the work of Roemer and Shain (13). This belief has long been accepted by persons in the medical care field. Stated in its simplest fashion, it asserts that an increase in the supply of beds in an area will result in their being used. The empirical support for this hypothesis is the close statistical relationship between hospital beds and hospital utilization in an area.

According to this hypothesis, building beds eventually results in their being filled with patients whose hospitalization is not "medically" indicated. The resulting policy implication is that the number of beds in an area should be based upon a medical determination of the need for beds. Since medical need is believed to be similar in all areas, it suggests the establishment of hospital bed limits for each area in the form of bed/population ratios.

The supply-creates-demand hypothesis and its far-ranging policy implications contains a number of conceptual and empirical problems. A simple correlation between beds and hospital use does not constitute empirical verification that they are causally related. The fact that the measures are correlated with one another might simply indicate that they are both affected by the same factors. Presumably, areas with a high demand for hospital care will generate an increase in supply to satisfy that demand; it would thus appear that areas with high demand will have a larger number of beds per capita than will areas with low demand.

It is more difficult to explain why increased demand appears to *follow* increases in bed supply. There are three possible explanations for this observed phenomenon. First, the current demand for hospital care may exceed supply, in which case increasing the supply of beds satisfies existing demand. This situation is shown in Figure 5–2A. If the price of hospital care were set below the equilibrium level, at P_0, and the supply of beds were shown by S_0, hospital use would be Q_0. At a price of P_0, there is an excess demand of $Q_3 - Q_0$. If the supply of beds were increased from S_0 to S_1, and subsequently to S_2 and S_3, hospital use would similarly increase from Q_0 and, eventually, to Q_3. Similar to the situation of continual excess demand is a situation in which supply expands in anticipation of increased demand. This situation is shown in Figure 5–2B. Initially, demand is represented by D_0 and supply by S_0; utilization is Q_0. If the supply of beds were increased to S_1 and then utilization increased to Q_1, it does not mean that supply created a new demand of D_1; rather, the supply of beds was built in anticipation of increased demand.

A second explanation for the apparent relationship between an increase in the bed supply and a subsequent increase in demand is that patients' travel costs have changed. If the additional beds are established in new, smaller, hospitals that are

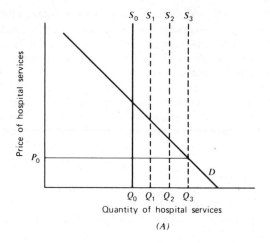

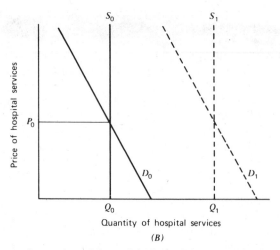

Figure 5-2. Change in the supply and demand for beds: *(A)* an example of excess demand for beds, *(B)* an increase in supply of beds in anticipation of an increase in demand.

closer to prospective patients, then travel costs to the hospital will decrease. Rather than creating a new demand (i.e., a shift of demand to the right), the increase in the supply of beds lowers the total price of hospital care to the patient by lowering the nonmonetary costs and is thus a movement down the patient's demand curve.

The third explanation focuses on the effect that an increase in beds has on the physician. A physician can increase his or her productivity by hospitalizing patients instead of visiting them in their homes. Particularly in rural areas and in areas where physicians are few relative to the population, a physician is likely to admit more patients and keep them in the hospital longer because it is easier to monitor their illnesses while seeing more patients.

The hypothesis that an increase in the bed supply creates its own demand thus appears to be the recognition of a close relationship between beds and their use rather than the discovery of a causal relationship. To understand the reason for this close relationship and for the possibility that a bed increase may precede a use increase, it is necessary to examine what factors are affecting the patient's demand for care and what incentives are facing the patient's physician. Public policy that merely addresses the supply of beds without considering patient demand or physician incentives is likely to result in hospital use that is inequitable and inefficient. When hospital beds are purposely limited, the patients who receive care may not be those who are most in need of care. The value the patient places on hospital care should be related to the cost of providing that care. Arbitrary limits on hospital beds in an area are unlikely to be related either to demand factors or to the value a community has placed on its bed capacity.

In recent years, interest in the supply of beds as the major determinant of use of those beds has declined. As payment for hospital and medical services has changed, so have patient and provider incentives. As a consequence, hospital use has sharply declined, leaving hospitals with many empty beds. (The reasons for these changes are discussed below.) The statistical link between beds and use is no longer in evidence.

Demand Creation. The second way in which the physician's role as the patient's advisor places the physician in conflict with his or her interests as a supplier of medical services has been referred to as *demand creation*. (This subject is also discussed in Chapter 9.) As a supplier of a service, the physician has a financial stake in the services used in treatment. It has been observed that with an increase in the supply of physicians in an area, both the price and quantity of physician services increase. Such a relationship would suggest a positively sloped demand curve. An alternative explanation of the relationship between the number of physicians and the price and quantity of their services suggests that consumers, lacking information on their diagnosis and treatment needs, are prescribed additional, unnecessary services (14). When faced with a relatively high demand, a physician will have little incentive to prescribe additional treatments that may or may not be needed; however, when the supply of physicians increases, the demand facing each one of them decreases. Given the lack of patient information regarding treatment needs, the physician can exploit this ignorance by recommending additional services. This situation is shown graphically in Figure 5–3. The initial supply, demand, price, and quantity of physician services are indicated by S_0, D_0, P_0, and Q_0, respectively. With an increase in the number of physicians, the supply shifts to S_1. Rather than face a decrease in demand for their services (and a consequent fall in income), the physician, as the patient's advisor, recommends additional services. The new demand curve, D_1, shifts to the right. Thus the price and quantity of services have increased with the increase in supply.

Part of the problem in determining the extent of physician-induced demand is statistical; physicians may move to areas where there is a higher rate of illness, better insurance coverage, or higher income, all of which would increase demand for physician services. In estimating the impact of the physician/population ratio on demand, the latter factors must be held constant or else the physician/population ratio will serve as a proxy for these omitted factors as well as a measure of physician density. The correlation of the physician/population ratio with the omitted variables will lead to an upward bias in the estimates of the impact of an increase in the supply of physicians on the demand for medical services.

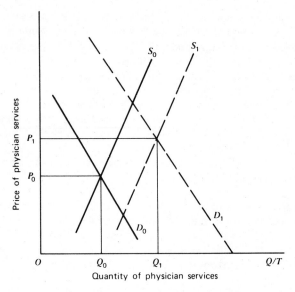

Figure 5–3. Demand creation with an increase in the number of physicians.

A study by Rossiter and Wilensky included the often excluded variables—rate of illness, insurance coverage, and income—and thus were able to estimate the effects on number of visits of the physician/population ratio (15). The authors used individual patient data from the National Medical Care Expenditure Survey (NMCES), which contains detailed health care utilization and expenditure information for 40,000 persons in 1977. It was also possible to distinguish between patient-initiated ambulatory visits (57 percent of all visits) and physician-initiated ambulatory visits (43 percent of all visits), thereby permitting separate estimates of the impact of the physician/population ratio on each type of visit.

The authors concluded that an increased physician/population ratio had no impact on patient-initiated visits. The physician/population ratio did have a positive impact on physician-initiated visits, although the impact was very small, that is, a doubling of the physician/population ratio, which would be a huge increase, would lead to only an 11 percent increase in physician-initiated visits.

For physician-initiated visits, the study found that the out-of-pocket money price and time price (time in the physician's office) had the expected negative effect on number of physician-initiated visits. That is, either patients or physicians or both are somewhat sensitive to the out-of-pocket price of services, while patients are sensitive to time prices. Visits for chronic conditions and other measures of disability were positively related to physician-initiated visits; this is consistent with a model of the physician as the patient's agent.

A recent study by McCarthy on the demand for physician services also casts doubt on the hypothesis of physician-induced demand (16). McCarthy used data from a 1974 American Medical Association Survey of 187 individual primary care physician firms in large metropolitan areas. McCarthy found that the physician/population ratio (squared) had a negative impact on the number of physician office visits. Patients were found to be sensitive to both time (in- office waiting) and money prices, both of which had negative relationships to office visits. The elasticity of both time and money price was greater than 1. Moreover, the number of organized outpatient departments and emergency rooms per 100,000 population, which are measures of substitute sources of care, also had large negative impacts on physician office visits. (These results also support the premise of a monopolistically competitive market for physician services.)

While concluding that there is an absence of physician-induced demand *at the margin*, McCarthy also correctly concludes that demand can no longer be induced further by physicians, although there may have been demand inducement in the past.

Reinhardt underscored this qualification, emphasizing that if an increase in the physician/population ratio leads to a decline in visits per physician, this simply indicates that physicians cannot *at the margin* induce demand to raise their incomes (17). This finding says nothing about what physician- induced demand occurred in the past and therefore how much money is currently being spent on physician-induced visits and tests.

In fact, the finding by McCarthy of a large negative relationship between the physician/population ratio and visits could be interpreted to mean that greater competition, in the form of a higher physician/population ratio, may *undo* past demand creation; for example, physicians could compete on the basis of reducing unnecessary tests and visits (e.g., phone consultations may supplant an in-person visit).

T. Rice asked a different question: What is the impact of a change in Medicare reimbursement on demand for physician services? He finds strong evidence supporting the existence of physician-induced demand in response to Medicare payment changes (18). The study by Rice was similar to an earlier one which looked at the impact on physician output of the price controls of the Economic Stabilization Program, in effect between 1971 and 1974 (19). The latter study found that while controlled prices rose by less than 3 percent per year, the quantity of services provided rose by 9–11 percent in the first year, and 8–15 percent in the second year. Moreover, in the year after the expiration of the price controls, physician prices rose 23 percent, while quantity of services provided by general practitioners *dropped* 9 percent.

Rice examined a change in the reimbursement mechanism in Colorado between 1976 and 1977, which resulted in a relative decrease in fees paid to urban physicians (their reimbursements rose by less than 5 percent) and a relative increase in fees paid to nonurban physicians (their reimbursements rose by approximately 20 percent). Rice found that the lower the reimbursement rate for different services (medical, surgical, laboratory, and radiology), the greater was the intensity of the service provided. For example, a 10 percent decrease in the reimbursement rate for medical services led to a 6.1 percent increase in medical service intensity; a 10 percent decrease in the surgical reimbursement rate led to a 1.5 percent increase in the intensity of surgical services.

The impact of the reimbursement change on quantity of services was less dramatic. While there was no effect on the quantity of medical services provided, there was a relationship between a lower reimbursement rate and an increased quantity of surgical services provided. The change in the reimbursement rate for laboratory services also had a strong impact on the quantity of laboratory services provided; that is, the lower the payment rate for laboratory tests, the greater the number of tests ordered by the physician.

To summarize briefly the studies discussed above, while changes in Medicare reimbursement do not affect market competition among physicians, there appears to be some evidence that demand inducement occurs in terms of both the quantity and intensity of services with a change in reimbursement. Alternatively, increases in the supply of physicians per capita in an area do appear to increase competition among physicians, thereby limiting physician-induced demand or even reducing it.

It may be rationalized that the additional demand created by the physician provides beneficial services; however, these additional services may be unnecessary and would not be provided were there sufficient demands of a more serious nature. One example of a physician-created demand is the recommendation that a patient return the week following an initial visit to enable the physician to determine that progress is satisfactory. A more serious example of demand creation is unnecessary surgery. Patients are least able to judge whether or not a surgical procedure is necessary. The patient may be able to determine whether additional home and office visits are providing any benefits, but in the case of surgery, the consequences to the patient of being mistaken may be more serious. The types of surgery that are likely to result from demand creation are tonsillectomies, appendectomies, and hysterectomies. The physician might rationalize that these surgical procedures are beneficial and do not affect the patient's ability to function. The patient would have no way of determining whether such surgery was useful, since his or her well-being would probably be unchanged after recovering from it.

A number of studies have shown that the rate of surgical procedures is higher when the physician is reimbursed on a fee-for-service basis. Between two population groups, with similar characteristics and similar physician and hospital coverage, the rate of surgical procedures varied according to the method of physician reimbursement: In one group, Health Insurance Plan of Greater New York (HIP), the physician is reimbursed on a capitation basis (the same rate of reimbursement regardless of the number of procedures performed); for the other group of patients, covered by Group Health Insurance in Washington, D.C. (GHI), the physician is reimbursed on a fee-for-service basis. The rate of hospitalized surgical procedures for HIP enrollees was 4.38 per hundred persons per year; for GHI it was 7.18. In another study of GHI and HIP populations no significant difference was found in surgical procedures between adult males, but they were found between adult females—6.56 in GHI and 4.97 in HIP. In a third comparative study of physician reimbursement under a capitation system (Kaiser) and a fee-for-service method (Blue Cross-Blue Shield and commercial insurance), when patients had identical benefit coverage under all three plans, it was found that the hospitalized surgical procedure ratios per hundred persons per year were 3.3, 6.9, and 6.3, respectively. A fourth comparison was of two groups of federal employees with the same benefits, where one group belonged to a capitation plan while the other group belonged to a fee-for-service system. It was found that the rate of hospitalized surgical procedures was 3.9 in the capitation plan and 7.0 in the fee-for-service system. One-third of this difference in the rate of surgical procedures was a result of differences in the rate of surgical procedures for appendectomies (1.4 versus 2.6), tonsillectomies (4.0 versus 10.6), and "female surgery" (5.4 versus 8.2) (20). The evidence above appears to support the hypothesis that when patients lack knowledge and when the physician is both an advisor and a supplier of a service in which he or she has a financial interest, the physician can take advantage of the advisory role by creating additional demand.

This hypothesis has several implications for policymaking. First, increased patient knowledge would lessen the physician's ability to create additional demand. Pauly and Satterthwaite have found that the effect of increased physician supply in an area on patient's use of medical services declines with higher levels of patient education (21). As an alternative to education, the patient can obtain additional information by receiving a second opinion from another physician whenever surgery is recommended. When second opinions are used, it has been found that there is a lower surgical procedure rate (22). The second approach that has been suggested for reducing the amount of unnecessary surgery is to develop institutional arrangements such as tissue review committees. The problem with such review committees is that as long as other physicians in the hospital are financially unaffected by the medical practice of their colleagues, they have little incentive to become concerned with their colleagues' behavior. A third approach is to provide the physician with a financial incentive to avoid unnecessary surgery. One such financial incentive is the fear of a malpractice suit in cases of unnecessary surgery. Another approach is to encourage other methods of physician reimbursement. Capitation-based reimbursement would be one such method, and is discussed more completely in Chapter 12 in the section on health maintenance organizations.

In summary, the physician's role as it affects the demand for medical care is potentially conflicting, as he or she is both an advisor to the patient and a supplier of a medical service.[5] To the extent that the physician acts in the advisory role, considering the patient's needs as well as resources, we would expect to find a strong relationship between the patient's characteristics and his or her demand for medical care. On the other hand, when the use of medical services differs from what we might initially expect, instead of abandoning the economic model of demand, we must examine the reasons for the unexpected use in terms of its effect on physician productivity and income. The important role of the physician in translating the patient's demand for care into use of medical services should not be forgotten in public-policy attempts to control medical costs and utilization. The fee-for-service physician determines the use of all medical resources, yet the physician does not bear fiscal responsibility for those decisions.

A Review of Selected Empirical Demand Studies

A number of studies have attempted to estimate price and income elasticities of demand for medical services. These studies have differed with regard to the theoretical variables included in the demand model, the measurement of the theoretical variables, data, statistical techniques, and methods used for analysis. Most of the demand studies have attempted to estimate the relationship between economic factors and either total medical care expenditures and separately for expenditures on hospital and physician services, while holding constant the effect of other, noneconomic, factors. Very few studies have been able to measure the effect of economic factors by type of medical diagnosis or by seriousness of illness. Ideally, it would be desirable to know price elasticities at different deductible and coinsurance levels, holding constant such factors as health status, time prices, and noneconomic factors. It would then be possible to forecast more accurately changes in utilization if prices were increased or decreased, as under different national health insurance plans.

When expenditures, rather than visits or hospital utilization, are used as the dependent variable, estimated price and income elasticities are generally higher, presum-

---

[5]Many similar advisor-supplier relationships exist with purveyors of other goods and services that consumers purchase—for example, real estate agents and auto mechanics.

ably because expenditures include some measures of quality. Physician visits, hospital admissions, and patient days do not enable the investigator to differentiate between visits that include a greater intensity of services, use of specialists, or changes in the length of the visit. Expenditure data reflect quality as well as quantity of services; therefore, price and income elasticity estimates based on expenditure data partly measure the demand for quality as well as the demand for quantity of services. When expenditure data are used, however, it is particularly important that prices be accurately measured. If, for example, a physician charges a higher price to higher-income persons, part of the difference in expenditures between high- and low-income persons is a result of price differences and not of differences in quantity or quality.

The measurement of price has been troublesome for all demand studies. Ideally, the price should reflect the out-of-pocket price the patient pays, but estimates of out-of-pocket prices for each service are generally unavailable. Instead, the stated price or an average price for all services is used, and whether or not the patient has any insurance coverage is included separately in the statistical analysis. For policy purposes it is desirable to know the effect of deductibles and copayments (of different magnitudes) on utilization. The effect of a copayment will also vary depending upon the size of the patient's income.

The importance of time costs on demand has been included in statistical demand studies only recently. Only a few studies have estimated time price elasticities. Failure to include time explicitly as a factor affecting demand for services may result in incorrectly attributing its effect to other factors.

Demand studies have also differed with respect to the inclusion of substitutes and complements in the demand model. The demand for hospital care will depend, in part, on the price of ambulatory services. The availability of data on substitutes and complements has generally been limited. Excluding such factors from the statistical estimation of demand may affect the price elasticities of demand for hospital services or for other services whose demand is being analyzed.

The measurement of income has also distorted the results of demand studies. Ideally, it is desirable to measure the effect of usual or permanent income, but when surveys collect income data, the incomes of those surveyed may be temporarily high or low. If, for example, a person is sick and his or her income is temporarily low, but his expenditures are related to his usual income, the person will show up in the survey as having a low income but a high expenditure. Thus, if demands for medical services are related to usual and not temporary income, the estimate of income elasticity will be too low when it is measured using temporary incomes.

Data used in demand studies have also differed by level of aggregation. Some studies have been based on state averages; others have used individuals as the unit of observation. In those studies where the level of aggregation encompasses a state, certain factors known to affect demand, such as age, may turn out to be statistically insignificant because there is insufficient variation between states according to age. Use of individual data, however, has generally resulted in lower elasticity estimates. When individual data are used, many individuals in the sample may not have had any utilization during the period covered and it is often difficult to separate the effect of economic factors from all other variables that are included and that have an effect on demand.

The data bases from which elasticity estimates were derived have changed over time. Initially, researchers used state data, which included only gross measures of prices and the degree of availability of insurance coverage. There were then a number of studies which used claims and premium data from specific insurance companies. Occasionally, there were instances of a natural experiment, as when a copayment was introduced in the insurance plan for a particular group of people. Comparisons have also been made between individuals having different insurance policies. More recently, as in the RAND Health Insurance Study, a designed experiment was made possible. As the data have improved, it has become possible to develop better measures of prices, as well as to show the effect of income-related copayments and health status.

The foregoing discussion of empirical demand studies provides some indication of the great variety of variables used, how economic factors are measured, and of the sources of data. Such studies have also used different methods of statistical estimation. Most studies have used a single-equation approach, although some have used simultaneous equations. Differences in statistical estimation methods could also result in different elasticity estimates. Given these differences in approach, data, and methods, it is not surprising that large variations exist in the statistical estimates of price and income elasticities.

The following is a brief summary of the results of statistical demand studies. Generally, hospital and physician services are price inelastic (23). The price elasticity for patient days varies from $-.2$ to $-.7$; for admissions the variation in price elasticity is from $-.03$ to $-.5$; and for physician visits the price elasticity varies from $-.1$ to $-.2$. Insurance coverage for hospital services is currently quite high, approximately 90 percent of the hospital bill is paid for by private or public insurance. It is therefore unlikely that hospital use will increase rapidly if the remaining out-of-pocket prices were to be paid for under any form of comprehensive national health insurance plan. Physician in-hospital services also have a relatively high degree of insurance coverage. Physician office visits, however, have less-complete coverage. Any policy that lowers the price of physician office visits could result in a substantial increase in demand for physician services.

The estimates of elasticity of demand with respect to time are surprisingly high: $-.6$ to -1 with respect to travel time to a public outpatient department and $-.2$ to $-.3$ to a private physician's office. With respect to waiting time, the elasticity of demand for private office visits are $-.05$ and $-.12$ to a public outpatient department (24).

The estimate of income elasticity for medical care expenditures is approximately unity ($+1.0$) (25). The statistical effect of income appears to have declined over time as more of the patient's bill is paid for by third-party payors. The growth in insurance coverage, both as a percentage of the bill paid and in terms of the type of medical services covered, is income related.

The demand for nursing home care appears to be price elastic, approximately -2 (26). Thus policies to include nursing home care under Medicare could result in large increases in use and expenditures on such care. The income elasticity of demand for nursing home care by private-pay patients was estimated to be between 2.3 and 2.8 (27).

To date, too little is known of the effect on hospital use of a decrease in the price of substitute sources of care. One way in which the cost of medical services can be reduced is to provide insurance coverage (thereby lowering the out-of-pocket price) for lower-cost substitutes (e.g., outpatient surgery and home care). The success of such policies depends on both the cross-elasticity of demand for hospital care to the price of such lower costs substitutes and the price elasticity of demand for the substitute whose price is reduced.

TABLE 5-1. Differences Between Plans in Predicted Total Expenditures per Person and in the
Probability of One or More Physician Visits or Hospital Admissions (All Participants)

	Expenditures	Physician Visits (Probability as a Percent of Free Plan)	Hospital Admissions (Probability as a Percent of Free Plan)
Free care	$430	100	100
25-percent coinsurance	81%	93	79
50-percent coinsurance	67%	89	71
95-percent coinsurance	69%	82	75
Individual deductible plan, 95-percent coinsurance	77%	87	88

SOURCE: Adapted from Joseph P. Newhouse et al., *Some Interim Results from a Controlled Trial of Cost Sharing in Health Insurance*, R-2847-HHS, January 1982. The RAND Corporation, 1700 Main Street, P.O. Box 2138, Santa Monica, CA 90406-2138.

The RAND Health Insurance Experiment (RAND) has greatly increased our knowledge of the effect of deductibles and income-related cost sharing on the demand for medical services (28). Under the experiment, participants were randomly assigned to one of 14 insurance plans for three to five years. One of the insurance plans provided free care (no deductibles or cost sharing), while the others involved different cost-sharing percentages. The cost-sharing plans differed according to the family's co-insurance rate, which was either 25, 50, or 95 percent. The 95 percent plan was the same as an income-related catastrophic plan. The maximum annual dollar expenditure of the family under these plans was income related; it was either 5, 10, or 15 percent of income, up to a maximum of $1,000.

The RAND study concluded that as the coinsurance rate rose, overall use and expenditure fell, for adults and children combined. These results are presented in Table 5-1. Compared to the free care plan, a coinsurance rate of 25 percent resulted in a 19 percent decline in expenditures; higher coinsurance rates, 50 and 95 percent, resulted in over 30 percent declines in expenditures. In other words, per person expenditures in the free care plan was 23 percent higher than in the 25 percent plan and 50 percent higher than in the 50 percent coinsurance plan. Price elasticities for the 0–25 and 25–95 percent ranges of coinsurance were calculated according to the type of care received by the patient (e.g., outpatient, hospital, and all care). For the 0–25 percent plan, the price elasticity was $-.17$ for each of the above types of care. Under the 25–95 percent plan, the elasticity estimates were $-.31$, $-.14$, and $-.22$ for outpatient, and all care, respectively. For outpatient care under the 25–95 percent plan, these estimates varied according to whether the treatment was for well care ($-.43$) or for chronic care ($-.23$) (29). We also see that the probability of a physician visit in a year was 7 to 18 percent lower in the cost-sharing plans than in the free care plan, while hospital admissions were 21 to 29 percent lower. For the Individual Deductible Plan, which had coinsurance for ambulatory services (95 percent) and free inpatient services, the respective probabilities were 13 and 11 percent lower than the free plan.

Cost sharing also reduced medical care expenditures and use for children. Annual medical expenditures per child were 10, 19, and 25 percent lower in the 25, 50, and 95 percent coinsurance plans. Further, children in the 95 percent plan had 41 percent fewer outpatient episodes of treatment than did children in the free plan (30).

The results for prescription drugs, outpatient mental health, dental care, and emergency room use were similarly reduced in the coinsurance plans than in the free plan. For example, when comparing the 95 percent plan to the free plan, the respective reductions for the categories above were 43, 57, 32, and 30 percent less (31).

The impact of cost sharing was found to have a larger effect on lower-income persons, particularly children (32). A panel of experts divided episodes of care into those in which medical care produces usually effective treatments and usually less effective treatments. It was determined that for those conditions in which medical care is highly effective, the probability of poor children in the cost-sharing plan having an episode of treatment was 44 percent less than children in the free plan; for nonpoor children the probability was only 15 percent less. For adults, poor adults in the cost-sharing plan had a 41 percent lower probability of seeking treatment than adults in the free plan, while for nonpoor adults it was 29 percent lower.

There is not much difference among poor and nonpoor adults in the cost-sharing plans when it comes to seeking treatment for conditions for which there is rarely an effective treatment. However, for poor and nonpoor children, there is again a substantial difference.

The authors note (33):

> Not all complaints and symptoms require medical attention, so cost sharing does reduce ostensibly inappropriate use of ambulatory care. For some problems, such as a cold, medical care may bring little, if any, tangible benefit because self-care would be equally effective. This favorable outcome of cost-sharing comes at the price, however, of reductions in appropriate care; that is, it appears to invoke a considerable risk of foreclosing medical diagnosis and treatment for conditions in which such intervention can be expected to be effective and to benefit the patient.

The poor are at greater risk of not receiving treatment when such treatment would be effective than are the nonpoor, particularly poor children. This finding should be kept in mind with regard to any government proposals for national health insurance in which cost sharing is not income related.

APPLICATIONS OF DEMAND ANALYSIS

The Allocation of Hospital Beds

Starting in 1948 and lasting for approximately 20 years, the Hill-Burton program, a federal act, subsidized the construction of thousands of hospital beds, costing billions of dollars. The Hill-Burton criterion for supporting hospital bed construction was that 4.5 hospital beds should be available per 1,000 population in areas with more than 12 persons per square mile; that 5.0 beds per 1,000 population should exist in areas with between 6 and 12 persons per square mile; and that 5.5 beds per 1,000 population should exist in areas with fewer than 6 persons per square mile. According to the Hill-Burton formula, population density was the sole determinant of beds per 1,000 population.

In one of the earliest hospital demand studies, Gerald Rosenthal contrasted the Hill-Burton standard with a demand-based approach to determining the number of hospital beds in an area (34). Rosenthal first constructed a model of the demand for hospital utilization. He included both economic (price, insurance, and income) and noneconomic (age, martial status, sex, percent urbanization, race, education, and number of persons per dwelling unit) variables in the demand model. The data were based on state averages for 1950 and 1960. His dependent variables, by state, were patient days, admissions per thousand population, and average length of stay. Separate regressions were estimated for each of the dependent variables for 1950 and then again for 1960. To calculate the expected number of beds per thousand population in any state based on demand factors, Rosenthal inserted the average value for each of the independent variables in each state into the regression model. The number of patient days was estimated for each state on the basis of that state's demand characteristics. The average-sized hospital in a state was used in conjunction with the probability (uniform across states) that it would be filled when translating the estimate of patient days into the number of beds for that state. To make sure that the pressure on facilities in each state was uniform, the same probability of being full (one day in 100) was used; further, since the average-sized hospital varies between states, the substitution of one state's size for another's was avoided.[6]

Based on each state's demand characteristics, the average size of its hospitals, and the same probability of being full, the number of beds per thousand population was estimated for each state for 1950 and 1960. The number of beds per thousand varied from less than two to more than four, with each state having the same pressure on its facilities. The results of this demand-oriented approach were then compared state by state with those yielded by the Hill-Burton formula. Since the Hill-Burton formula does not consider any demand characteristics, only population density, the pressure on facilities varied greatly between states: those with low demand factors had lower occupancy rates and excess hospital beds; those with high demand factors had greater pressure on their facilities through higher occupancy rates, and consequently a greater likelihood of their not having a bed when needed. To equalize out the pressure on facilities, Rosenthal recommended using a demand model to allocate beds among areas.

Rosenthal also demonstrated how the demand model could be used for social policy. If a state desired to increase its utilization, it could lower the price of care and increase insurance coverage in the population. (The number of beds necessary to meet this higher estimate can then be calculated in the same way as described previously.) Manipulating demand factors to bring about a change in utilization was shown to be a

---

[6]If admissions to a hospital have a Poisson distribution, then, given the same probability of being full, smaller hospitals will have a lower average occupancy rate than larger hospitals. For example, if it is estimated that on any given day in a community there will be a demand for 400 patient days, these patient days may be translated into beds in the following manner:

The mean is equal to the variance in a Poisson distribution. Thus $\bar{x} = 400$, $\bar{x} = \sigma^2$, therefore the standard deviation $(\sigma) = 20$. If it is desired to have a bed available 99 times out of 100, that would encompass three standard deviations of the distribution. Thus the number of beds is determined by

$$\bar{x} + 3\,(\sigma) \text{ or } 400 + 3(20) = 460 \text{ beds}$$

and the average occupancy would be 86 percent (400/600).

If the estimate of demand were to be equally shared among 10 independent hospitals, the number of beds required would be $40 + 3(6) = 58$ multiplied by 10 hospitals, for a total of 580 beds. Each 58-bed hospital would have an average occupancy rate of approximately 68 percent (40/58).

more efficient policy instrument than relying on a set number of beds to satisfy legitimate needs for care.

Proponents of the thesis that the bed supply creates a bed demand implicitly assume that the pressure on facilities (not necessarily the occupancy rate) will be the same across all facilities. To test this hypothesis, Rosenthal calculated a pressure index for each state, which was the actual occupancy rate as a percentage of its maximum occupancy. This pressure index varied from a low of 80 to more than 100. The fact that different facilities had different pressures as well as occupancy rates suggested that supply did not create demand. In addition, high pressure indices correlated positively with demand variables and correlated negatively with supply variables. Rosenthal concluded that high demand led to greater pressure on facilities, while an increased bed supply led to lower pressure on facilities.

The study concluded that the allocation of beds should be based upon relative demands in an area rather than upon an arbitrary standard.[7] If it is desired to change utilization rates for a particular population group, it can be achieved more directly and efficiently by changing demand factors rather than simply by changing the number of beds.

Using a Demand Model to Explain Annual Changes in Personal Health Care Expenditures

Personal health care expenditures have increased from $10.9 billion in 1950 to $371.4 billion in 1985. The average annual rates of increase have, however, varied over time. During the period 1950–1960 personal health care expenditures increased at an annual rate of 8.1 percent. After the introduction of Medicare and Medicaid in 1966, annual percentage increases became more rapid. Between 1965 and 1975 it was 12.6 percent per year. The rapid increases in medical care expenditures during these various periods have been the result of increased demands for medical care, the increasingly large involvement of government in the financing of medical care, and increases in the costs of providing such services. Together, these changes in demand and supply have resulted in increased prices and quantities for medical services, both of which constitute a part of the increases in expenditures for medical care.

Although many of the factors affecting both demand and supply have changed during these periods, most factors have been changing gradually. The price of medical services is perhaps the most important factor that has sharply increased. In addition to increases in the price of medical care, there have been increases in the population, changes in its age distribution, and increases in personal incomes, all of which have led to increased demands for medical care. A more detailed analysis of changes in medical care expenditures would examine additional demand factors, but the changes in prices, incomes, and population can be used to provide a rough approximation of the importance of these demand factors in contributing to increases in medical care expenditures during these periods (35).

---

[7]The Rosenthal study should be considered illustrative of the type of demand study to be undertaken for purposes of policy and planning. For actual planning of facilities in an area, a less aggregative demand model would be needed. Estimates of the demand for beds by service—obstetrics, pediatrics, medical-surgery—would also be more useful. Inclusion of substitutes for hospital care and greater stability of the parameters of the model would provide greater confidence in the application of such a model.

As shown in Table 5-2, the rise in the price of medical care as measured by the Medical Care Price Index, which is part of the Consumer Price Index, contributed substantially to each period's increase in medical care expenditures. Before 1965, medical prices contributed less than one-half of the annual percentage increase; during the period preceding Medicare and Medicaid, 1960–1965, medical prices contributed less than 30 percent to the average annual increase in expenditures. However, in the post-1965 period the increase in medical prices contributed more than one-half of the annual percentage increase in medical expenditures, contributing 75 percent of the increase during the 1975–1985 period. When the rate of increase in medical prices is subtracted from the rate of increase in medical expenditures, the result is the average annual percentage increase in the *real* quantity of medical care purchased.

To explain changes in the quantity of medical care purchased during this period, we must first adjust for changes in the population, which will give us the annual percentage increase in the quantity of medical care per person. Subtracting the rate of increase in population from the rate of increase in real medical output yields the annual percentage increase in quantity of medical care per person during this period. As shown in Table 5-2, population changes explain only a small percentage of the overall rate of increase in medical expenditures, particularly in the post-1965 period. During the latter period, population was increasing at a declining rate, approximately 1 percent per year, while medical expenditures was increasing more rapidly than in the past.

Per capita incomes were rising (although at different annual rates of increase) during the different periods examined. If an income elasticity of 1.0 is assumed—that is, the increase in consumer demand for medical care will increase at the same rate as the increase in income—then part of the annual percentage increase in medical care can be accounted for by increased per capita incomes. In the post-1965 period, real (adjusted for inflation) per capita incomes were rising less rapidly than previously.

Medical care prices have been increasing at a faster rate than prices in the rest of the economy. Thus, in addition to the use of the annual rate of increase in medical prices to determine the rate of increase in *real* medical care purchases, the rate of increase in medical prices relative to the prices of other consumer goods and services can be used to represent an increase in the price of real medical care services. With an increase in the price of a service we would expect a decrease in demand for that service; the size of the decrease in demand for medical care depends upon its price elasticity of demand. Assuming that the price elasticity of demand for medical services is − .2, which means that the demand for medical care is relatively price inelastic, a 1 percent increase in price would lead to a .2 percent decrease in quantity demanded. With reference to Table 5-2, the rate of increase in the quantity of medical care will decline by .2 multiplied by the relative rate of increase in the price of medical care.

When these factors affecting demand are summed up for the different periods, most of the annual percentage increase in medical expenditures can be accounted for. The amount of the unexplained residual is smaller for the pre- 1965 periods than for the more recent periods: .9 and 1.6 percent per year for 1950–1960 and 1960–1965, respectively; 2.9 and 1.3 percent per year for 1965–1975 and 1975–1985, respectively.

It is likely that the large unexplained residual, from 1965–1975, which is the percentage increase in real medical care output that cannot be explained by the demand factors we have described, represents changes in the *type* of medical services produced. When medical prices were used to adjust expenditures to determine real output increases, it was assumed that the output produced was similar over time. Innovations

TABLE 5-2. Factors Affecting Changes in Personal Health Care Expenditures

Factor	Average Annual Rate of Change (%)					
	1950–1960	1960–1965	1965–1975	1975–1985	1965–1985	
Personal health care expenditures	8.1	8.7	12.6	12.2	12.4	
Accounted for by:						
Rise in price of medical care (CPI Medical Care)	3.9	2.5	6.5	9.1	7.8	
Population increase (resident population)	1.7	1.5	1.1	1.0	1.0	
Rise in real personal income per capita, increasing medical expenditures by an equal percentage (income elasticity = 1.0)	2.0	3.3	2.1	1.4	1.8	
Decline in quantity demanded because of rise in relative price of medical care (price elasticity = −.2)	−.4	−.2	.0	−.6	−.3	
Total accounted for	7.2	7.1	9.7	10.9	10.3	
Unexplained residual	.9	1.6	2.9	1.3	2.1	

SOURCES: Robert Gibson, "National Health Expenditures, 1980," *Health Care Financing Review*, 2(1), Summer 1980: 21–22; D. Waldo, K. Levit, and H. Lazenby, "National Health Expenditures, 1985," *Health Care Financing Review*, 8(1), Fall 1986, p. 14; U.S. Department of Health, Education, and Welfare, *Social Security Bulletin*, 48(12), December 1985: 51–53.

in medical technology have, however, changed the medical product over time. Further, after Medicare was introduced, the age distribution of hospital patients changed; the aged constituted a larger proportion of the patients. The aged require more costly types of service than do the nonaged. Also, after Medicare, hospitals increased their service quality by adding more facilities and services and increasing ratios of personnel per patient, both of which would contribute to an increase in real expenditures per person in the post-Medicare period. It is likely that if the foregoing analysis included these additional factors, the size of the unexplained residual would be much lower.

THE DEMAND FOR MEDICAL CARE FACED BY THE FIRM

Up to this point we have discussed the determinants of demand for medical services. The demands for hospital care, physician services, nursing, and home care are derived from the demand for a treatment. Based upon estimates derived from empirical studies, the demand for hospital and physician services was determined to be relatively inelastic with respect to price. However, it is important to distinguish between the overall market demand for a service such as hospital care, and the demand facing an individual provider. While the overall demand for hospital care may be relatively inelastic with respect to price, the demand facing an individual hospital, especially in a community with several hospitals, is likely to be more price elastic, since any one hospital is a possible substitute for another.

To determine the demand facing an individual firm, a two-step approach is needed. First, the provider (e.g., a hospital) must estimate the overall market demand for hospital care. To do so, it is necessary to estimate demand by type of service, such as obstetrics, and by market area. For each service, the factors affecting demand must be specified and some estimate derived of the relative importance of each factor (e.g., its elasticity with respect to hospital care). Factors that should be included in an overall demand forecast include, as discussed in the demand model, measures of need, sociodemographic variables, and economic measures. Since the first two sets of variables change gradually, short-range forecasts must place greater emphasis on the economic variables. Substitutes for hospital care, particularly outpatient surgery and health maintenance organizations, can have dramatic decreases on use of the hospital. A forecast of hospital demand must include some estimate of how each of the factors affecting demand will change over time. For example, the likely growth of HMOs in a market area must be estimated. Once an estimate of the population enrolled in an HMO is determined, then the effect of HMOs on hospital use is required, again by type of service. For each of the factors affecting demand, an estimate of how such factors will change over time, together with their likely effect on demand, is required. This approach should provide an overall estimate of demand by type of service.

The second step in a demand forecast for an individual provider is to determine what proportion of the overall market demand will be received by the individual provider. This step involves estimating the market share (the proportion of the total demand) going to the individual provider. The market share, by type of service and by geographic area, will depend upon such factors as the hospital's price relative to other hospitals' prices; the reputation of the hospital relative to those of its competitors;

whether or not the hospital participates in HMOs that its competitor hospitals do not; and the number and location of its primary care physicians, again relative to other hospitals.

By forecasting demand in this two-step process, a provider can determine whether a decrease in its demand was the result of a decrease in overall market demand or a decrease in its market share. It is possible that the overall demand for hospital care has been declining but that a hospital's market share has been increasing. A provider can not only better understand what is occurring in its market, but also determine what competitive actions it might undertake to increase its individual demand.

Having some understanding as to the factors that affect a hospital's market share can suggest how that hospital should allocate resources to increase its market share. By making rough calculations as to the effect of each of the factors affecting market share, the hospital can conduct cost-benefit analyses; the hospital can allocate resources to recruitment of primary care physicians, advertising to enhance its reputation, and so on, so that the effect on market share *per dollar spent* on each of these activities is equal. Although it is difficult to derive precise estimates of such allocations, merely thinking in terms of marginal costs and marginal benefits of alternative allocations should improve the decisionmaking process.

Forecasting demand has become more important to providers in an increasingly competitive environment. Not only must providers forecast their demands so as to establish their staffing patterns, but providers must be able to determine how to increase their market shares relative to their competitors. Demand and market share forecasts are important not only to hospitals, medical groups, and other medical providers, but also to health insurance companies and health maintenance organizations. An understanding of demand analysis should improve one's ability to forecast demand in the foregoing situations.

APPENDIX: THE EFFECT OF COINSURANCE ON THE DEMAND FOR MEDICAL CARE

A diagram may clarify the effect of coinsurance on the demand for medical care. Figure 5–4 shows the relationship between the price of medical care and the quantity demanded, with all of the other determinants of demand being held constant. When the price is P_1, the quantity demanded will be Q_1. If insurance were provided that carried a coinsurance feature, the person using it would have to pay the remainder of the price. The price paid by the patient would be P_2, which is, for example, 80 percent of P_1; the third-party payor would pay the remainder of the price, P_1-P_2. As a result of the 20 percent price reduction, the patient will now demand Q_2 of medical services. (The actual increase in quantity demanded as a result of the decrease in price due to coinsurance will depend upon the size of the coinsurance and the price elasticity of demand.) As long as there is some responsiveness of price to quantity demanded, coinsurance will increase demand by lowering the price the patient will pay for medical care.

Although insurance coverage represents a *movement* down an individual's demand curve, the aggregate effect of an increase in coverage is to cause a *shift* in the demand for medical care. For example, according to the demand curve represented by D_1 in Figure 5–5, an individual would demand Q_1 units of medical care if the out-of-pocket

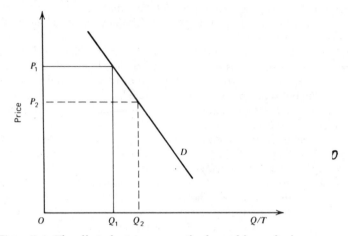

Figure 5-4. The effect of coinsurance on the demand for medical care.

price was $10 per unit. If the individual were now provided with insurance requiring that only 80 percent of the total price be paid, then at a price of $10 per unit the individual need only pay $8. Therefore, the individual would move down his demand curve and consume Q_2 units at a price of $8 per unit. The actual price of Q_2 units is not $8 per unit but $10 per unit; the third-party payor pays 20 percent, or $2 per unit. Thus, the actual demand curve for medical care has shifted to the right. Similarly, if the initial price were $14, the patient with demand curve D_1 would consume Q_3 units of medical care. With the introduction of an 80 percent coinsurance program, the patient would move down his demand curve and consume Q_4 units at a price of $11.20 per unit. The total price per unit at Q_4 is, however, $14 per unit. Each of the points on the original demand curve (D_1) now represent only 80 percent of the total price. The new demand curve (D_2) represents the relationship between the total price

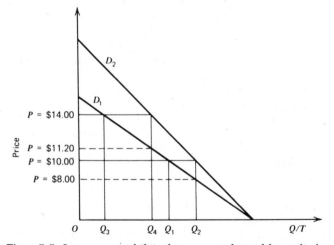

Figure 5-5. Insurance as a shift in the aggregate demand for medical care.

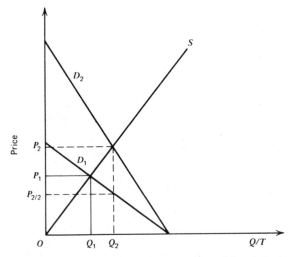

Figure 5-6. The effect of coinsurance on the aggregate demand for medical care with a rising supply curve.

per unit (80 percent of which is paid for by the patient and 20 percent by the third-party payor) and the quantities demanded at these different prices.

The analysis of the effect of insurance becomes more complicated when there is a coinsurance provision *and* a rising supply curve for medical care. For example, according to Figure 5-6, the patient's original demand curve is D_1. The provision of health insurance with a coinsurance feature (for simplicity, it is assumed to be 50 percent with the remainder being paid by the government) will result in a shift in demand to D_2, which represents the amount that both the patient and the government will pay for medical care. Every point on demand curve D_2 represents a doubling of the price for a given quantity over D_1, since it is a 50 percent coinsurance program. So far the analysis is similar to the previous example. However, since the new demand curve (D_2) intersects the supply curve at a higher price than previously, a new equilibrium price and quantity of medical care, P_2 and Q_2, will be established. Q_2 is thus the only quantity at which the public pays one-half the price of the medical care ($P_{2/2}$) that is also an equilibrium position. Thus the price the consumer will pay with a 50 percent coinsurance is greater than 50 percent of the original market price ($P_{1/2}$). The introduction of a percentage copayment feature does not mean that the consumer's price will be a similar percentage of the original market price. Nor does it mean that the amount of care used will increase by that same proportion. The greater the coinsurance paid for by the government (or other third party), the greater the consumer's use of medical services will be, but the actual price the consumer must pay and the amount actually consumed will depend upon the elasticity of both demand and supply. The more elastic demand and supply are, the greater will be the increase in quantity and the less the rise in price.

REFERENCES

1. Roger Lee and Lewis Jones, *The Fundamentals of Good Medical Care* (Chicago: University of Chicago Press, 1933).

2. Kevin J. Lancaster, "A New Approach to Consumer Theory," *Journal of Political Economy*, April 1966.

3. Michael Grossman, "On the Concept of Health Capital and the Demand for Health," *Journal of Political Economy*, March-April 1972.

4. Two valuable reviews of the early literature in this area are Martin S. Feldstein, "Econometric Studies of Health Economics," in M. D. Intriligator and D. A. Kendrick, eds., *Frontiers of Quantitative Economics*, Vol. II (Amsterdam: North-Holland, 1974); and Herbert E. Klarman, *The Economics of Health* (New York: Columbia University Press, 1965).

5. A number of surveys have collected data on family income and expenditures on medical care. A few of the better-known surveys are those conducted by the National Center for Health Statistics as part of the Health Interview Survey and published in Series 10, *Vital and Health Statistics* (Washington, D.C.: U.S. Department of Health, Education, and Welfare, various years.) The National Opinion Research Center, University of Chicago, has also conducted national surveys on medical expenditures. These surveys, which have been conducted at five-year intervals beginning in 1953, have been presented in various publications, such as Odin W. Anderson, Patricia Collette, and Jacob Feldman, *Changes in Family Medical Care Expenditures: A Five Year Resurvey* (Cambridge, Mass.: Harvard University Press, 1963). A more recent national survey (1977) of medical care expenditures was undertaken by the National Center for Health Services Research, and is referred to as the National Medical Care Expenditure Survey.

6. The distinction between permanent and transitory components of income and their relationship to consumption are discussed by Friedman in terms of his permanent income theory of consumption in Milton Friedman, *A Theory of the Consumption Function* (Princeton, N.J.: Princeton University Press, 1957).

7. For a more complete discussion of the role of time in the demand for medical care, see Charles E. Phelps and Joseph P. Newhouse, "Coinsurance, the Price of Time, and the Demand for Medical Services," *Review of Economics and Statistics*, August 1974: See also Jan P. Acton, "Demand for Health Care Among the Urban Poor, with Special Emphasis on the Role of Time," in Richard Rosett, ed., *The Role of Health Insurance in the Health Services Sector* (New York: National Bureau of Economic Research, 1976).

8. The same data were analyzed by Anne A. Scitovsky and Nelda M. Snyder, "Effect of Coinsurance on Use of Physician Services," and Charles E. Phelps and Joseph P. Newhouse, "Effect of Coinsurance: A Multivariate Analysis," in *Social Security Bulletin*, June 1972.

9. Scitovsky and Snyder, *op. cit.*, p. 15.

10. Anne A. Scitovsky and Nelda McCall, "Coinsurance and the Demand for Physician Services: Four Years Later," *Social Security Bulletin*, May 1977.

11. Several articles have discussed the role of the physician in the manner described above. Several of the earlier ones are Robert Rice, "Analysis of the Hospital as an Economic Organism," *Modern Hospital*, 106(4), April 1966; Paul J. Feldstein,

"Research on the Demand for Health Services," *Milbank Memorial Fund Quarterly*, July 1966; and M. S. Feldstein, "Econometric Studies of Health Economics."

12. Victor Fuchs, "The Growing Demand for Medical Care," *New England Journal of Medicine*, July 25, 1968: p. 192.

13. Max Shain and Milton Roemer, "Hospital Costs Relate to the Supply of Beds," *Modern Hospital*, April 1959, and Milton Roemer, "Bed Supply and Hospital Utilization: A Natural Experiment," *Hospitals*, November 1, 1961.

14. The discussion that follows is based on the article by George Monsma, "Marginal Revenue and Demand for Physicians' Services," in H. Klarman, ed., *Empirical Studies in Health Economics*, (Baltimore: Johns Hopkins University Press, 1970); and the article by Mark Pauly and Mark Satterthwaite, "The Pricing of Primary Care Physicians' Services: A Test of the Role of Consumer Information," *Bell Journal of Economics*, Autumn 1981.

15. Louis F. Rossiter and Gail Wilensky, "A Reexamination of the Use of Physician Services: The Role of Physician-Initiated Demand," *Inquiry*, 20, Summer 1983; and "Identification of Physician-Induced Demand," *Journal of Human Resources*, 19(2), Spring 1984.

16. Thomas R. McCarthy, "The Competitive Nature of the Primary Care Physician Services Market," *Journal of Health Economics*, 4, June 1985.

17. Uwe Reinhardt, "The Theory of Physician-Induced Demand: Reflections After a Decade," *Journal of Health Economics*, 4, 1985.

18. Thomas H. Rice, "The Impact of Changing Medicare Reimbursement Rates on Physician-Induced Demand," *Medical Care*, 21(8), August 1983.

19. John Holahan and William Scanlon, *Physician Pricing in California: Price Controls, Physician Fees, and Physician Incomes from Medicare*, HCFA Publication 03006 (Rockville, Md.: Health Care Financing Administration, 1979)

20. For a more complete discussion of the foregoing studies and their sources, see the article by Monsma, *op. cit.*

21. Pauly and Satterthwaite, *op. cit.*

22. Hirsch S. Ruchlin et al., "The Efficacy of Second-Opinion Consultation Programs: A Cost-Benefit Perspective," *Medical Care*, January 1982.

23. For a comprehensive review of demand studies up to the mid-1970s, see Larry J. Kimbell and Donald E. Yett, *An Evaluation of Policy Research on the Effect of Alternative Health Care Reimbursement Systems*, mimeographed (Los Angeles: Human Resources Research Center, University of Southern California, undated). See also Joseph P. Newhouse, "Insurance Benefits, Out-of-Pocket Payments, and the Demand for Medical Care: A Review of the Recent Literature," *Health and Medical Care Services Review*, July-August 1978; and Joseph P. Newhouse, "The Demand for Medical Care Services: A Retrospect and Prospect," in Jacques Van Der Gaag and Mark Perlman, eds., *Health, Economics, and Health Economics* (Amsterdam: North-Holland, 1981).

24. J. Acton, "Demand for Health Care Among the Urban Poor with Special Emphasis on the Role of Time," in R. Rosett, ed., *The Role of Health Insurance in the Health Services Sector* (New York: National Bureau of Economic Research, 1976).

25. There have been a number of studies on the income elasticity of demand for medical expenditures and for physician services. Several such studies and their elasticity estimates are: F. Goldman and M. Grossman, "The Demand for Pediatric Care: An Hedonic Approach," *Journal of Political Economy*, April 1978, estimated an income elasticity for pediatric visits of + 1.32; R. Rosett and L. Huang, "The Effect of Health Insurance on the Demand for Medical Care," *Journal of Political Economy*, March-April 1973, estimated an income elasticity for medical expenditures of + .25 and + .45; V. Fuchs and M. Kramer, *Determinants of Expenditures for Physician Services in the United States, 1948–1968*, Occasional Paper 117 (New York: National Bureau of Economic Research, 1973) estimated an income elasticity of + .57 for physician services; R. Anderson and L. Benham, "Factors Affecting the Relationship Between Family Income and Medical Care Consumption," in H. Klarman, ed., *Empirical Studies in Health Economics* (Baltimore: Johns Hopkins University Press, 1970) estimated an income elasticity of + .63 for physician expenditures; M. Silver, "An Economic Analysis of Variations in Medical Expenses and Work Loss Rates", in Klarman, *ibid.*, estimated an income elasticity of + .85 with respect to physician expenditures and + 1.2 for medical care expenditures; P. Feldstein and J. Carr, "The Effect of Income on Medical Care Spending," *Proceedings of the Social Statistics Section of the American Statistical Association*, 1964, estimated an income elasticity of + 1.0 with respect to medical care expenditures.

26. B. Chiswick, "The Demand for Nursing Home Care: An Analysis of the Substitution Between Institutional and Noninstitutional Care," *Journal of Human Resources*, 11, Summer 1976. See also William J. Scanlon, "A Theory of the Nursing Home Market," *Inquiry*, 17(1), Spring 1980. According to Scanlon, the price elasticity for private pay patients is approximately − 1.

27. Scanlon, *op. cit.*

28. Joseph P. Newhouse, et al., *Some Interim Results from a Controlled Trial of Cost Sharing in Health Insurance* (Santa Monica, Calif.: Rand Corporation, 1982). A shorter version without appendices is contained in *New England Journal of Medicine*, 305(25), December 17, 1981. See also Emmett B. Keeler and John E. Rolph, "How Cost Sharing Reduced Medical Spending of Participants in the Health Insurance Experiment," *Journal of the American Medical Association*, 249(16), April 22, 1983. For a series of criticisms of the Rand experiment, see Bruce L. Welch et al., "The Rand Health Insurance Study: A Summary Critique," *Medical Care*, 25(2), February 1987. For a reply, see Joseph P. Newhouse et al., "The Findings of the Rand Health Insurance Experiment—A Response to Welch et al.," *Medical Care*, 25(2), February 1987.

29. Willard G. Manning, Joseph P. Newhouse, Naihua Duan, Emmett B. Keeler, Arleen Leibowitz, and Susan Marquis, "Health Insurance and the Demand for Medical Care: Evidence from a Random Experiment," *American Economic Review*, 77(3), June 1987, p. 268.

30. Arleen Leibowitz et al., "Effect of Cost Sharing on the Use of Medical Services by Children: Interim Results from a Randomized Controlled Trial," *Pediatrics*, 75(5), May 1985.

31. For the impact of cost sharing on the use of particular types of services, see Kevin F. O'Grady et al., "The Impact of Cost Sharing on Emergency Department Use,"

New England Journal of Medicine, 313(8), August 22, 1985; Willard Manning et al., "The Demand for Dental Care: Evidence from a Randomized Controlled Trial in Health Insurance," *Journal of the American Dental Association*, 110(6), June 1985; Willard Manning et al., "How Cost Sharing Affects the Use of Ambulatory Mental Health Services," *Journal of the American Medical Association*, October 10, 1986; and Arleen Leibowitz et al., "The Demand for Prescription Drugs as a Function of Cost Sharing," *Social Science and Medicine*, 21(10), 1985.

32. Kathleen N. Lohr et al., "Use of Medical Care in the Rand Health Insurance Experiment, Diagnosis and Service-Specific Analyses in a Randomized Controlled Trial," *Medical Care*, 24(9), Supplement, September 1986.

33. *Ibid.*, p. 78.

34. Gerald Rosenthal, *The Demand for General Hospital Facilities*, Monograph 14 (Chicago: American Hospital Association, 1964).

35. The discussion in this section is similar to that presented in an earlier article by Victor Fuchs, "The Growing Demand for Medical Care," *New England Journal of Medicine*, 192, July 25, 1968.

CHAPTER 6

The Demand for Health Insurance

Although the number of services covered and the percentage of the bill paid by health insurance have been increasing over time, insurance coverage still varies greatly by population group, by services covered, and by percentage of the medical bill covered. In pointing to the percentage of the medical bill covered by insurance as a measure of its "adequacy," anything less than 100 percent coverage (or at least a "high" percentage) is deemed by some to be "inadequate." The policy recommendations that follow from such a normative judgment are based either upon the assumption that inadequacy is a result of insufficient financial means on the part of consumers for purchasing the appropriate amount of insurance, or that the inadequacy is a result of the health insurance industry's failure to provide more appropriate coverage. The recommendations based upon this normative judgment of inadequate health insurance are that the government should either provide comprehensive coverage under its own auspices or subsidize the purchase of health insurance.

To determine the "appropriateness" of health insurance coverage in the United States, appropriateness in an economic sense must be defined. It is also important to determine whether there are market conditions that distort the consumer's ability to select the economically appropriate quantity of health insurance coverage. In this chapter, therefore, we examine the determinants of the demand for health insurance. In a subsequent chapter we examine the economic efficiency of the health insurance market to determine whether there are (or have been) distortions on the demand or supply side of that market that result in either "too much" or "too little" (or insufficient varieties) of health insurance being offered. The conclusions with respect to the supply side of that market should indicate the appropriate role of government, if any, as a provider of health insurance.

HEALTH INSURANCE TERMINOLOGY

As a preface to the analysis of the demand for health insurance, a brief discussion of a number of concepts used in health insurance is in order.

Deductibles

When consumers pay a flat dollar amount for medical services before their insurance picks up all or part of the remainder of the price of that service, this is referred to as a deductible. Deductibles may be set in a number of ways: they may apply to each unit of service, or they may be cumulative—for example, once $100 has been paid by the consumer for physician services within a year, the third-party payor will contribute to the price of additional visits. Deductibles may also be established either on a family basis or for each individual. Deductibles may also be related to family income, with higher deductibles being required of persons with higher family incomes, as has been proposed under certain national health insurance schemes.

There are several reasons for using deductibles. One is that it lowers the administrative costs of claims processing in a situation where there are many small claims and the cost of handling these claims is high. In such a situation, the transaction costs might exceed the amount the people are willing to pay for insurance; a deductible provision lowers the transaction costs and enables consumers to purchase insurance for the remainder of their medical expenses at an amount that they are willing to pay that is greater than the transaction costs. Another reason that is offered by proponents for having deductibles is that the insurance premium can be reduced while still providing protection against large medical expenditures. A large percentage of families incur small medical expenditures within a year, while a small percentage of families incur very large expenditures. This phenomenon is illustrated in Figure 6–1A. The insurance costs of covering medical expenditures would obviously be lowered if a deductible were placed at the low end of the expenditure spectrum, as indicated by line A in Figure 6–1A. A third reason is that if the deductible is greater than the price of the service, an incentive is provided for the consumer to shop around.

The case against deductibles is generally made on the grounds that the deductible, no matter how small, may be a deterrent to needed care. Further, a flat deductible, irrespective of family income, represents a greater burden to low-income families than to high-income families.

The effect of the deductible on use of services is complex. If there is a deductible, once the deductible is exceeded and additional services are free, the deductible will have no effect on decreasing the use of services. Once the deductible has been paid, the patient will use the services as though their price were "zero." If the deductible has not been exceeded, the price of the services will determine (other things being held constant) how much they will be used. A deductible by itself, therefore, will either tend to result in greater use of services (similar to a zero price) when a low deductible is used, or if the deductible is high, it will tend to make insurance coverage irrelevant to many users of care. How effective a deductible will be depends upon the size of the deductible, the expected medical expenditures of the family (if on a family basis), and on family income.

Coinsurance

When the third-party payor reimburses the patient for a certain fraction of the price of the service, the arrangement is termed coinsurance. A coinsurance level of 80 percent in effect lowers the price to the patient of those covered services by 80 percent. The patient pays the remaining 20 percent themself. If the price of the services should rise,

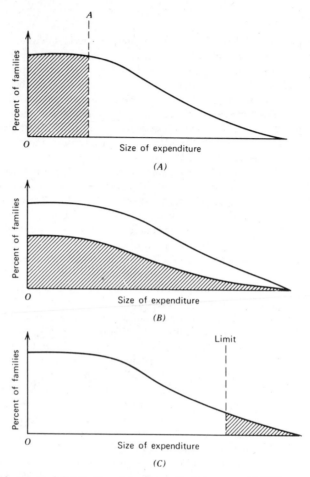

Figure 6-1. The expected distribution of family medical expenses with different types of copayments: *(A)* the imposition of a deductible, *(B)* a coinsurance provision, *(C)* a maximum or limit to coverage.

the insurance would pay 80 percent of the new, higher price. Coinsurance levels can also vary by service covered and by family income. The advantage of coinsurance is that it reduces the price of the service and still provides the patient with an incentive to seek out less costly providers. The effectiveness of a coinsurance feature will depend upon how responsive utilization is to lower prices, which is the price elasticity of demand. If use is not responsive to price, coinsurance will merely be a way of reducing the cost of the insurance package to the consumer. Depending upon the level of coinsurance and the price elasticity of demand, coinsurance can change the distribution of medical expenditures, as shown in Figure 6-1 *B*. Coinsurance would result in the consumer's paying for the shaded portion of Figure 6-1 *B*, while the third-party payor would pay for the remainder of the medical expenses.

Limits and Maximums

One method of reducing the cost of providing insurance coverage to the consumer is to reimburse patients for medical expenses up to a maximum dollar amount or a maximum amount of services; any expenditures above that limit become the responsibility of the patient. This approach shifts the cost of large expenditures, generally considered to be catastrophic, to the patient incurring them instead of distributing them among all insured persons. Limits have been used in the past by Blue Cross, such as when it covered hospital services up to a maximum of 30 days in the hospital. The part of medical expenditures that is excluded by limits and maximums is generally the tail of the distribution, as shown in Figure 6-1 C. Large expenditures, incurred by a small percentage of families, are generally not responsive to prices; to exclude this part of the distribution from coverage appears to be particularly unwise, since large, unexpected losses to a small percentage of the population meet the criteria defining insurance risks. If the objective of using limits is to enable the insurance company to lower its insurance premium to consumers, an alternative approach would be to use a small deductible for the many families that have small expenditures. This front-end deductible, when applied to many families, would be less of a financial hardship than would a catastrophic expense befalling a small percentage of the population.

Insurance coverage for the tail of the distribution (i.e., the large expenditures incurred by a small percentage of the population) is generally referred to as major medical or catastrophic insurance. Major medical coverage was an innovation introduced by the commercial insurance companies in the late 1940s to compete with Blue Cross, which until that time was the dominant third-party underwriter, and which sold hospitalization insurance only up to a maximum limit.

Other Forms of Coverage

Insurance contracts may include any or all of the above in various combinations of deductibles, coinsurance, and limits. Other aspects of insurance coverage should also be briefly mentioned. Some coverage may specifically exclude certain diseases that are preexisting conditions of illness in a potential insurance purchaser. Allowing such purchases would be like allowing a person who knew that his house was going to be burned to buy insurance to cover his loss. Other kinds of insurance coverage may include continuation of salary if a person becomes ill, or disability benefits if a person is unable to be fully rehabilitated once an illness has been incurred.

Indemnity versus Service Benefits

When Blue Cross was started in the 1930s, it provided a "service" benefit for hospital care, which meant that the price to the patient for the stay in the hospital (up to a maximum period) was reimbursed in full to the hospital. There were no cost-sharing provisions, deductibles, or coinsurance features for the patient. An indemnity benefit, which was offered by commercial insurance carriers, differed from a service benefit in that it reimbursed the patient, not the hospital, for medical costs the patient incurred. The amount of reimbursement was often a fixed dollar amount per hospital day or admission or a percentage of the bill. Naturally, the hospitals that had founded Blue

Cross preferred the service-benefit approach, since it meant that they would be reimbursed for all their services and there would be no incentive for the patient to shop around for the least expensive hospital. By providing coverage only for hospital care, Blue Cross made nonhospital services more costly to the patient; therefore, hospital use was encouraged when other settings could have been used to treat the patient. Further, the hospitals would incur lower collection costs if they could bill Blue Cross for all of their patients rather than collect from each patient. A more detailed discussion of the Blue Cross service benefit policy and a comparison between it and an indemnity policy is provided in Appendix 1 of this chapter.

THE THEORY OF DEMAND FOR HEALTH INSURANCE

The consumer's demand for health insurance represents the amount of insurance coverage that he or she is willing to buy at different prices (premiums) for health insurance. Additional insurance coverage will be purchased if the insurance premium (actually, the loading charge) declines; once the consumer has *some* insurance, the marginal benefit of increasing the comprehensiveness of the insurance declines with the more coverage that he or she has. When the marginal benefit to the consumer of additional coverage equals the cost of buying that insurance, then, other things being equal, the "appropriate" amount of insurance will have been purchased. Appropriateness, in the economic sense, is defined as occurring when the marginal benefit of additional insurance to the consumer equals the marginal cost of purchasing that increased coverage.

According to this definition, 100 percent coverage of all medical expenses would be demanded by the consumer only when insurance is sold at its pure premium; that is, no administrative cost is added. At positive administrative prices for insurance, the consumer would demand less than 100 percent coverage. This is because the marginal benefit of the last unit of insurance coverage would be purchased only if the price of that additional coverage to the consumer were small. Adding an administrative price to the pure premium would cause the total price of those last units to be greater than their marginal benefits. The consumer would purchase additional coverage only to the point where the benefit of additional coverage equaled the total price of additional coverage.

Keeping in mind that the appropriateness of the amount of insurance coverage consumers will buy will be related to their perception of the value of additional coverage compared with the additional cost of that coverage, the demand for health insurance will be examined under two conditions. In the first situation it is assumed that there is no "moral hazard." The demand for medical care is assumed to be completely price inelastic; that is, patients cannot affect the size of their loss once they are ill (1). The second situation considers the demand for insurance coverage when moral hazard does exist.

To understand the factors that affect the demand for health insurance, it is necessary to be familiar with the economic theory underlying the purchase of insurance. This discussion should clarify why people buy insurance for some risks and not for others. The economic theory of insurance is then used to predict the type of insurance expected to be most prevalent in the health field.[1]

Underlying the demand for insurance is the assumption that an individual wishes to maximize his or her utility, which is the usual assumption made in demand analysis. Since a person does not know whether they will be affected by an illness, consequently, a loss of wealth to pay for it, the individual who seeks to maximize his or her utility when subject to uncertain events seeks to maximize his or her *expected* utility. That is, the person can choose between two alternative courses of action:

1. He or she can purchase insurance and thereby incur a small loss in the form of the insurance premium, or
2. He or she can self-insure, which means facing the small possibility of a large loss in the event that the illness occurs, or the large possibility that the medical loss will not occur.

To determine whether consumers will purchase insurance for an unexpected medical event or self-insure and bear the risk themselves, it is necessary to compare courses 1 and 2 to determine which choice provides them with a higher level of utility.

The use of expected utility, as discussed by M. Friedman and L. Savage in their classic article "The Utility Analysis of Choices Involving Risk" (2), assumes that the consumer selects among alternative choices according to whether one choice is preferred to the others, and ranks these choices according to how much one choice is preferred over another (i.e., cardinal rankings). Although one can think of the utility function as having no unique origin or unit of measure, once some unit of measure and a point of origin are accepted, the utility function of an individual can be described for all levels of wealth. Further, for an individual to purchase insurance, he or she must believe that the marginal utility of wealth is decreasing; although the preference is for more wealth rather than less wealth, additional wealth has a lower marginal utility. The relationship between total utility and wealth is shown in Figure 6–2A; as will be shown, unless the utility function exhibits this relationship to wealth, the "rational" individual will not purchase insurance.

To illustrate the choices an individual has who is trying to decide whether or not to purchase health insurance, we will assume that if an illness occurs, it will cost $8,000. If the individual is currently at W_3, meaning that his or her wealth is $10,000, then if the event occurs, $8,000 must be paid out, thereby moving the individual to wealth position W_1. (The corresponding utility levels at W_3 and W_1 are U_3 and U_1, respectively.) Let us assume that the probability of the individual's requiring medical services costing $8,000 is .025—that is, 2½ percent. The "pure premium" of the insurance that would cover the actuarial value of the expected loss would therefore be .025 × $8,000 = $200.

The pure premium is a function of *both* the size of the expected loss ($8,000) and the probability of it occurring (.025) *for a large group of people* (the law of large numbers). If the person were to buy insurance priced at the actuarial value of the expected loss, he or she would pay $200, thereby reducing their wealth, with certainty, to point W_2 on Figure 6–2A, which represents $9,800. Let us further assume that as a result of

---

[1]Throughout this analysis, for the sake of simplicity, it is assumed that utility functions are independent, that is, the degree to which others have insurance to cover their medical loss does not affect an individual's desire to subsidize another person's purchase of insurance.

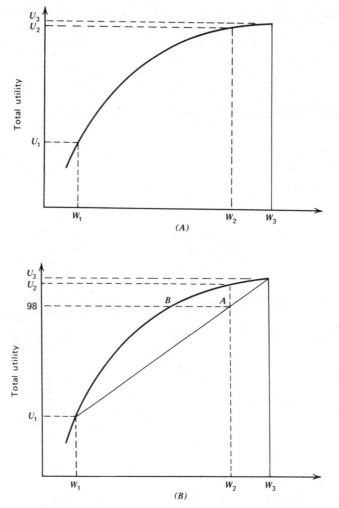

Figure 6-2. The relationship between total utility and wealth: *(A)* diminishing marginal utility with increased wealth, *(B)* expected utility.

purchasing insurance and decreasing one's wealth to $9,800, the individual is now at U_2, which is equivalent to being at a total utility level of 99, U_3 being 100 and U_1 being 20. The choices facing the individual therefore are:

a. To purchase insurance for $200 and move to a lower level of utility, 99, or

b. Not to purchase insurance and have a 2.5 percent chance that he or she will incur an $8,000 loss and thereby move to a utility level of 20 (U_1), which is associated with a wealth position of $2,000, or face a high probability of 97.5 (100–2.5 percent) that a loss will not be incurred and thereby remain at a wealth position of $10,000 with an associated utility level of 100.

To compare choices *a* and *b*, we must use expected utility. The expected utility of choice b is the weighted sum of the utilities of each outcome, with the weights being the probabilities of each outcome. Therefore, the expected utility of choice b is

$$P(U_1) + (1 - P)(U_3) = .025(20) + .975(100) = 98$$

Expected total utility is also a function of the expected loss ($8,000) and the probability of it occurring (.025), but for a single individual and, as a consequence, it is also a function of the shape of the individual's own utility function. To determine whether a person would buy health insurance, we compare the utility level of choice a, which represents purchasing insurance and thereby leaves the person at utility level $U = 99$, with the expected utility level of choice b, which represents not purchasing insurance and thereby results in an expected utility level $U = 98$. Since the utility level of choice a is greater than that of choice b, we predict that the person would purchase insurance. In this example it is assumed that the insurance is sold at the actuarially fair premium and that the utility function with respect to wealth is similar to the one described in Figure 6–2A—namely, diminishing marginal utility with respect to increased wealth.

The expected utility of choice b, $U = 98$, is shown in Figure 6–2B, by the straight line drawn on the utility curve extending from U_3, W_3, to U_1, W_1. The straight line represents expected utility for different probabilities that the illness will occur. The *lower* the probability that the event will occur, the closer the expected utility will be to the point farthest to the right on the utility curve. As the probability that the loss will occur increases, the expected utility value moves down to the left on the straight line, closer to the point represented by U_1 on the curve. In other words, if the loss is certain to occur, the individual will be at W_1 ($2,000) with a corresponding utility level of U_1 (= 20). Since the calculation of expected utility is based on the weighted sum of the probabilities of being at the different utility levels, as the probability of being at U_1 increases, the expected utility estimate declines in a linear fashion.

To show that expected utility declines linearly, the probability of the event occurring can be assumed to increase from .05, to .10, to .15, to .20. The expected utility of each of these events would then be as follows:

$$\begin{aligned} P(U_1) + (1 - P)(U_3) &= .05(20) + .95(100) = 96 \\ &= .10(20) + .90(100) = 92 \\ &= .15(20) + .85(100) = 88 \\ &= .20(20) + .80(100) = 84 \end{aligned}$$

Because the individual's actual utility curve (decreasing marginal utility with respect to wealth) is always above the expected utility line (constant marginal utility with respect to wealth), this individual will always buy insurance if it is sold at its actuarially fair value (its pure premium). However, insurance is never sold at its pure premium because there are administrative, claims processing, and marketing costs (loading costs). To determine whether or not an individual, as represented in Figure 6–2B, will buy insurance when there are these additional costs, the maximum amount above the pure premium he or she would be willing to pay for insurance must be calculated.

Referring back to Figure 6–2B, $W_3 - W_2$ represents the dollar amount of the pure premium for an $8,000 loss that has a 2.5 percent probability of occurring. Since the utility level with insurance is greater than the expected utility level (99 versus 98), the person purchasing insurance will be willing to pay an amount above the pure premium that makes the actual utility level *after* the additional payment equal to the expected utility level. When the actual utility level is equal to the expected utility level (at $U = 98$), the person will be indifferent as to whether he or she purchases insurance or self-insures. If an additional payment places the individual's actual utility level below his or her expected utility level, the person would be better off by self insuring; that is, the person would be willing to pay an amount above the pure premium as long as his expected utility is not greater than his actual utility.

This discussion is illustrated in Figure 6–2 B. Point A is the expected utility without insurance. If one draws a straight line from point A to where it crosses the actual utility curve, then at this point, B, a person's actual utility level and expected utility level are the same, $U = 98$. The distance from A to B on the wealth axis is the additional amount above the pure premium that a person would be willing to pay for that insurance. At every point along the expected utility line, which represents a different probability of the event's occurring, there is an additional amount above the pure premium that a person would be willing to pay for insurance. At points close to W_1, which represent a high probability that a person will incur a large enough loss to leave him or her at wealth position W_1, *a person would be willing to pay a smaller amount above the pure premium; the distance between the expected utility line and the actual utility curve, which would leave him or her at the same level of utility, is closer at that point.*

As shown in Figure 6–3 A, with an expected utility level at point E, the pure premium would be $W_3 - W_4$, which is a fairly large amount, since the probability of the loss's occurring is quite high. A person would be willing to pay an additional amount above the pure premium equal to the distance EF, since at point F expected utility is equal to actual utility. Any amount greater than EF would place the person at a lower point on his or her actual utility curve. Actual utility would then be less than the expected utility of not buying insurance. The amount above the pure premium, which is equal to the distance EF, is smaller than at another part of the graph, for example, CD. At point C a person is willing to pay an additional amount equal to CD, which would make the actual utility level indicated by D equal to the expected level indicated by C. CD is greater than EF because the probability of the loss's occurring is larger at point E. As the loss becomes almost certain to occur, the person can save for the event instead of paying the same amount (equal to the pure premium) to an insurance company *plus* an additional amount to cover other insurance company costs. In the case of near-certain events such as annual medical or dental checkups (probabilities approximately 1.0), it would be cheaper to self-insure. At large probabilities and at very small probabilities (very rare events) a person is willing to pay less over the pure premium than at other, more intermediate probabilities.

Another factor that influences how much over the pure premium the person is willing to pay for insurance is the magnitude of the expected loss. When the expected loss is relatively large, as shown in Figure 6–3 B, a person can lose $W_3 - W_1$ ($8,000) if the illness occurs and they do not have insurance. If, on the other hand, the loss is relatively small, as for a visit to the dentist for a filling, this loss will be represented by a smaller possible loss in wealth if it occurs, $W_3 - W_5$. The expected utility line for the large loss is AC; for the small loss it is AB. The distances $W_3 - W_1$ (expected utility line AC) and $W_3 - W_5$ (expected utility line AB) represent different-sized losses with the same probabilities of occurrence. The area between the actual utility curve and the expected utility line is much greater for the large loss than for the small one. Given

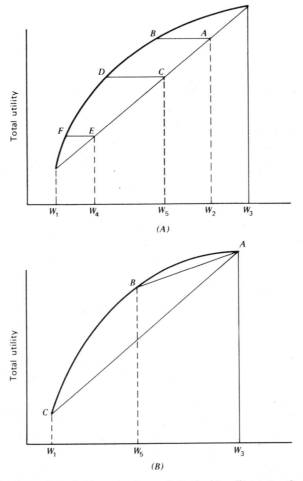

Figure 6–3. The amount above the pure premium an individual is willing to pay for health insurance: *(A)* according to different probabilites of the event occurring, *(B)* according to different magnitudes of the expected loss.

the same probability that either the large or the small loss will occur, a person is willing to pay a larger amount above the pure premium for the large loss than for the small one.

To determine the demand for health insurance, we must now combine the preceding discussion of risk aversion (the total utility curve of the individual that increases but at a decreasing rate), the probability that a loss will occur, the magnitude of that loss if it should occur, and information on the price of insurance—that is, the amount charged above the pure premium. To illustrate the price-quantity relationship of the demand for health insurance, reference is made to Figure 6–4.

The price of insurance along the vertical axis in Figure 6–4 is the amount *above* the pure premium that the person must pay for insurance; along the horizontal axis is the probability that the event will occur. The curved line starting at 0 probability of the event's occurring and ending at a probability of 1.0 (certainty) is the amount above

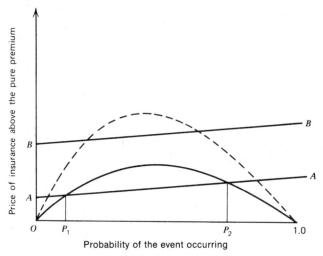

Figure 6-4. The relationship between price of insurance and quantity demanded.

the pure premium that the person is willing to pay for insurance. This area is taken from the previous figures and is merely the distance between the actual utility curve and the expected utility line. Since insurance is never sold at a price just equaling the pure premium (included are costs for marketing, administration, and claims process-ing), the price of insurance is represented by line AA in Figure 6–4. The reason it increases as the probability of the event's occurring increases is that there are greater administrative costs, such as record keeping and verification, when claims are more frequent (have a higher probability of occurring). Since line AA intersects the solid curved line representing the amount above the pure premium the person is willing to pay for insurance, the person will buy insurance for events that fall between P_1 and P_2. Between those two points the price the person has to pay for insurance is *less* than the amount he or she would be willing to pay, meaning that he or she would be better off (at a higher level of utility) if the insurance were purchased. The price of insurance is *greater* than the amount he or she is willing to pay for events that have either a very small probability of occurring (the area $0-P_1$) or a very high probability of occurring (to the right of P_2). Based upon Figure 6–4, we would predict that illnesses having both a very small probability of occurrence as well as those that have a high probabil-ity of occurrence (i.e., routine care) would be unlikely to be insured against by indi-viduals. If required to purchase insurance for these two events, an individual would be worse off, since the marginal benefits to be derived from that coverage would be smaller than the costs of insurance!

If the price of insurance were to rise to line BB, we would expect the individual represented by the solid curved line to self-insure—that is, to demand *less* insurance coverage. With a higher price of insurance, the new price will now *exceed* the addi-tional amount above the pure premium the individual is willing to pay. Regardless of the probability of the event's occurrence, the individual would be worse off if more had to be paid for insurance than he or she was willing to pay. Only if the magnitude of the loss, as shown by the dashed curved line, were greater than price line BB would the individual purchase insurance for that probable loss. Thus, as the price of insurance rises, the individual will be less likely to insure for certain events. This inverse relationship between the price of insurance and the quantity of insurance demanded is the demand schedule for insurance.

A person is also more likely to insure against events that have a greater magnitude of loss than against events with smaller possible losses. This aspect of the demand for health insurance can be seen with reference to the price of insurance (*BB*) in Figure 6–4 and the two curved lines representing different possible losses. Referring back to Figure 6–3, we saw that the amount above the pure premium that a person was willing to pay was less for small losses than for large losses, given the same probability of the event's occurring. One interesting implication of this relationship between the price of insurance and the size of the loss is that as the cost of medical care has risen, so has the size of the probable loss, and this by itself has resulted in an increase (a shift) in the demand for health insurance.

In summarizing this theory of the demand for health insurance, attention should be drawn to two areas: (a) the factors that affect the demand for health insurance, and (b) the welfare implications (Is the person better or worse off?) of requiring an individual to purchase health insurance against all types of medical illness, the routine as well as the low-cost services. The following factors would affect the demand for health insurance:

1. *How risk averse the individual is.* If he or she has a utility curve that is increasing but at a decreasing rate (i.e., diminishing marginal utility with respect to increased income), the individual is willing to pay an amount above the pure premium for insurance coverage.

2. *The probability of the event's occurring.* As shown in Figure 6–3, for those events that have a very low or a very high probability of occurring, a person is willing to pay less above the pure premium than for events that have a more intermediate probability of occurring.

3. *The magnitude of the loss.* The larger the magnitude of the loss, as in Figure 6–3, the greater will be the amount above the pure premium that the individual is willing to pay for insurance.

4. *The price of insurance.* The higher the price of insurance (the amount above the pure premium), the fewer will be the events the individual will insure against.[2]

5. *The income of the individual.* The size of a person's income and wealth will affect the amount above the pure premium they are willing to pay for health insurance. At both low and high incomes the marginal utility of income is either relatively high or low, so that such persons might prefer to self insure (3); the distance be-

---

[2]In a study using state-level cross-sectional data for fiscal year 1977, Roehrig estimated the elasticity of demand for health insurance with respect to the price of health insurance to be in the neighborhood of − 1.0. Demand was measured as the proportion of total private health care spending (hospital, physician, and dentist services) paid by Blue Cross-Blue Shield and other private health insurers. The price of insurance was taken to be proportional to the load factor (the premium/benefit ratio) and was corrected for the tax deductibility of health insurance using state-specific estimates of the marginal income tax rates (including social security taxes, federal income taxes, and state income taxes). The estimated elasticities with respect to income and the hospital semi-private room rate were small and not statistically significant while the elasticity with respect to the price of physician services was estimated to be -.60. Charles S. Roehrig, *The Impact of Technology on the Demand for Hospital and Medical Care,* Chapter 4, Final Report to the Division of Health Professions Analysis, HRA, Department of Health and Human Services, 1982, Contract HRA-232-80-0041 (Rockville, Md.: Human Resources Administration, 1982).

tween the expected and actual utility curve is less at high and low incomes than for intermediate income levels. High income has another, opposite, effect on the demand for health insurance because health insurance, as a fringe benefit, is not considered to be taxable income. The tax treatment of health insurance is discussed below.

An important factor that affects the price of insurance is whether the individual is part of a large group when purchasing insurance. Group policies are sold at substantially lower prices. In part the reduced price reflects lower administrative costs per individual; some of the administrative costs are handled by the group itself. Another reason for lower prices to group members is that there is less likelihood of adverse selection. Individuals seeking to purchase health insurance may be doing so because they believe they will be using such coverage in the near future. To guard against such self-selection and the possibly higher risks associated with it, the price of the policy will be higher to an individual than to a person who is part of a large group, where such adverse selection is less likely. The higher price of insurance to persons who are not part of a group leads to a smaller demand for health insurance.

The demand for health insurance is also affected by the tax treatment of health insurance premiums. This tax subsidy for the purchase of health insurance lowers the price of insurance to those in high-income groups. As incomes increase and people move into higher tax brackets, there is greater incentive for them to demand fringe benefits rather than increases in their cash incomes. Health insurance premiums paid by the employer are excluded from the taxable income of the employee (not just federal taxes, but state and social security taxes as well). This tax treatment of health insurance as a fringe benefit lowers its price and has led to a much greater demand for insurance than would have otherwise occurred. (See Appendix 2 for a graphical illustration of this issue.) It has been estimated that this tax incentive for the purchase of health insurance, in 1985, resulted in a loss of revenue to the government of between $30 and $40 billion a year (4). The tax treatment of health insurance coverage is, in effect, a subsidy for the purchase of health insurance and is greater for persons in higher income tax brackets. For example, a person in a 33 percent marginal tax bracket can purchase insurance, as an employee fringe benefit, at less than its pure premium. If the administrative cost of the insurance policy is approximately 10 percent, a person in a 33 percent tax bracket would be willing to purchase insurance with before-tax dollars since their tax subsidy exceeds the administrative cost of the insurance. [It has been estimated that the price elasticity of the tax subsidy with respect to insurance coverage is quite large, approximately -1.0 to -1.9 (5).] Thus an important reason for the increasing comprehensiveness of health insurance coverage for small claims ("first-dollar coverage") is that the premium for such losses is *less* than the actuarial value of such losses as the individual moves into higher and higher tax brackets. This government tax policy has stimulated the demand for health insurance and has increased its comprehensiveness.

A factor that has (until recently) affected the demand for health insurance through its effect on the size of the loss has been the method used for reimbursing the provider. Cost-based reimbursement and the use of service benefit policies removed any incentives that may have existed either for the patient to shop around or for the provider to provide care more efficiently. If the provider's costs are reimbursed in full, regardless of what other hospitals may charge, and if the patient is not required to pay any portion of the hospital's bill, as is the case under a service benefit policy, then any incentives for cost constraint on either the demander or the supplier have been removed. This method of provider reimbursement, preferred by hospitals and accepted by Blue Cross, increased hospital costs, increased the magnitude of the probable loss due to a hospital episode, and thereby resulted in a further *increase* in the demand for protection against such large losses. The greater the probable loss, the greater will be the demand for health insurance.

The demand for health insurance is thus affected by economic variables, price and income, the tastes of the individual toward risk aversion, and the size of the probable loss.

It is interesting to speculate on the welfare implications of this theory of demand for insurance. In attempting to maximize their utility, consumers will allocate their income so that the marginal benefit from each of the goods and services they consume equals the prices they must pay for those goods and services. If the price (which represents the marginal cost of producing those goods and services) exceeds the marginal benefits to them, they will be worse off by purchasing those goods and services. They can increase their utility by cutting back on those goods and services for which the marginal benefit is less than the price that must be paid and using the funds saved to purchase other goods and services whose marginal benefits (per dollar) are greater. In this manner they will achieve a higher level of utility than by any other allocation process. If, however, consumers are *forced* to purchase a good whose price is greater than its marginal benefit, they clearly end up worse off than before. Forcing consumers to pay a price for a good that is higher than its marginal benefit is a situation that can occur in the health field if all consumers are required to have complete comprehensive insurance coverage against all of their medical expenses.

As shown in Figure 6–4, there are two situations in which the price of insurance will exceed the amount above the pure premium that the consumer is willing to pay. The first is for medical losses that have either a very high or a very low probability of occurring. In Figure 6–4, the area to the right of P_2 represents medical losses that have a high probability of occurring; these routine medical expenses are for such purchases as physician office visits, a dental visit, and over-the-counter drugs. Comprehensive insurance coverage to include such routine medical expenses would necessitate a price, perhaps in the form of a tax on the consumer, that would have to exceed what they would be willing to pay above the actuarial value of those losses; requiring consumers to pay that price by law clearly leaves them worse off than if they could self-insure for those losses.

A second situation in which a consumer is made worse off by being required to purchase complete insurance coverage is where there are small medical losses. The price of insurance for that coverage (line *BB*) is greater than the amount above the pure premium (the solid curved line) the consumer would be willing to pay.

It might be argued that since the price of insurance is less than the aggregate amount consumers would be willing to pay in all situations, requiring insurance coverage for even those medical expenses that they would prefer not to insure against would, on an aggregate basis, still leave them better off with insurance than without. As long as the different forms of coverage are divisible and do not have to be sold together, consumers would be better off with *some* coverage than with either complete coverage or none at all. The welfare implication of mandatory insurance coverage that covers all medical losses, no matter how small or routine and expected they may be, is that some consumers will be worse off than if they had a choice and could self-insure in those situations.

AN APPLICATION OF THE THEORY OF THE DEMAND FOR HEALTH INSURANCE

The theory of the demand for health insurance can now be used to explain why we observe some people insuring against certain types of medical loss (e.g., hospital care) and not others (e.g., dental care). (When we later introduce the concept of moral hazard, we will see that although people may buy insurance for hospital services, they still may not insure against all hospital expenses, preferring to bear some of the costs themselves.) Also, since not everyone is a "risk averter" (their expected utility curve may be equal to or greater than their actual utility curve with respect to wealth), we would expect some people not to buy *any* health insurance. They would do so, not out of ignorance or irrationality, but because they are not risk averters (i.e., for the same reason that some people gamble). Before the price of health insurance was greatly reduced as a result of being widely available as a fringe benefit, a sizable percentage of the uninsured, 37 percent, according to a survey conducted in the mid-1950s, indicated that they felt they were just as well off without health insurance (6). The potential market for health insurance at that time was less than 100 percent of the population. As the price of medical care increased over time (i.e., the size of the potential loss became larger if an illness were to occur), and as personal income also increased, the demand for health insurance also grew. [In 1974, only 10 percent of the uninsured believed they were just as well off without health insurance; the percentage of persons believing this increased with higher incomes: 15 percent of those with incomes greater than $15,000 were in this category (7).] Thus, at any time, the potential market for health insurance depends on the various factors that affect the demand for health insurance.

To determine how well the foregoing model of demand for health insurance predicts the type of health insurance found in the population, we examine the purchase of insurance coverage by type of medical expense. Costs for hospitalization and for surgery would seem far more likely to qualify as high expected losses, with a relatively low probability of occurrence, than would medical losses such as physician visits, in the home or office, optometric services, drugs, and dental care, all of which involve relatively smaller medical expenses and are considered by families to be more routine and budgetable.

In examining older rather than more recent data (before the sizable effect on demand of the tax subsidy for health insurance), we find that the economic theory of demand for health insurance is able to explain the type of health insurance observed in the population quite well. Using data from a 1957–1958 household survey of the U.S. population, medical expenses by type of service were classified according to whether they had a high or a low probability of occurring and whether they had a high or a low potential loss if they did occur. Low probability of occurrence was arbitrarily defined by whether 20 percent of the population incurred an expense for that medical service during the past year; high potential loss was also arbitrarily defined by whether the average cost incurred by persons using that medical service was greater than $40. These data are shown in Table 6–1, together with the actual percentage of expenditures covered by insurance for each of the medical services examined.

According to the data, the prevalence of insurance was generally consistent with what the economic theory of demand for health insurance would lead us to expect. Those medical services that have a low probability of occurrence and a high expected

TABLE 6-1. Classification of Medical Services by Probability of Occurrence, Potential Loss, and Insurance Benefits, 1957-1958

Type of Medical Service	Probability of Occurrence	Magnitude of Expense	Percent of Expenditures Covered by Insurance	Expenditures on This Type of Service as a Percent of Total Medical Expenditures
Hospital care	Low	High	58	23
Physician charges for:				
Surgery	Low	High⎱	48	7
In-hospital visits	Low	High⎰		
Office visits	High	Low⎱	7	24
House calls	High	Low⎰		
Drugs and medicines	High	Low	1	20
Other medical services	Low	Low	1	8
Dental care	High	Low	—[a]	15

Sources: R. G. Rice, "Some Health Insurance Implications of the Economics of Uncertainty," unpublished paper presented before The American Public Health Association, October 6, 1964. Tables 1 and 2 based on data published in O. W. Anderson, P. Collete, and J. J. Feldman, *Changes in Family Medical Care Expenditures and Voluntary Health Insurance: A Five Year Resurvey* (Cambridge, Mass.: Harvard University Press, 1963).

[a]Less than one-half of 1 percent.

loss are more likely to be covered by insurance than are those expenses with either a high or a low probability of occurrence and low expected loss.

The cost of a medical event has greatly increased over time, which should be expected to result in an increase in the demand for insurance. Also contributing to an increase in demand was the growth in incomes and the rise in inflation throughout the 1960s and 1970s. As incomes and inflation increased, more employees preferred to receive additional income in the form of health insurance, which was not subject to personal income taxes. Thus, although the percentage of medical expenditures covered by insurance has greatly increased since the period covered by the data cited above, we would still expect to observe a difference in the distribution of medical expenses covered by health insurance. Those medical services having a lower probability of occurrence and a high potential loss are still more likely to have more of their expenses covered by insurance than are those services considered to be routine and/or with a relatively lower potential loss. The same relationship holds for more recent data as well. Table 6-2 shows the percent of bill paid for by insurance (for those over and under 65 years of age) by type of medical service, by probability of use, and by average cost per unit for 1977, the latest year for which such data were available. Where the probability of use is low and the expected cost is high, the percent of the bill paid for by insurance is highest. Aggregate data for 1985 also support this finding. Consumer out-of-pocket expenditures for short-term hospital care are approximately 9.3 percent of total hospital expenditures, with the remainder being paid for by private insurance and government programs. For physician services, approximately 26.3 percent of total expenditures are out of pocket; the out-of-pocket percentage is 63.4 percent for dental care, 69.3 percent for eyeglasses, and 76.1 percent for drugs (8).

TABLE 6-2. Classification of Medical Services by Probability of Occurrence, Potential Loss, and Insurance Benefits, 1977

Medical Service	Percent of Bill Paid by Insurance	Probability of Use	Average Cost/Unit
Hospital admission			
Persons under 65 years	.83	.14	$1,208.00
Persons 65 years and older	.91	.30	2,198.00
Physician visit (persons with at least one contact)			
Persons under 65 years	.44	.74	25.70
Persons 65 years and older	.52	.79	44.00
Dental visit	.24	.41	44.00
Vision aids (purchases or repair of glasses or contact lenses)	.16	.14	67.00
Drugs (person with at least one prescribed medicine)	.26	.58	6.20

SOURCES: Data obtained from NCHSR's *National Health Care Expenditure Study*, Data Preview Series; 1982: 8, 9, 11; 1983: 15, 16; U.S. Department of Health and Human Services, NMCES household data; United States, 1977.

In summary, the model of demand for health insurance suggests that a measure of the adequacy of health insurance should *not* be the percentage of aggregate medical expenses covered by health insurance, with anything less than 100 percent being considered inadequate. Instead, the adequacy of health coverage should be examined separately for each type of medical service. Even if everyone were a risk averter, we would not expect people to buy insurance for all of their medical expenses. The price of insurance (i.e., the amount above the pure premium) for some medical expenses would exceed the amount some people were willing to pay. Requiring everyone under such circumstances to purchase health insurance for *all* of their medical expenses would make people *worse off*, since the costs of the coverage for some expenses would exceed the benefits.

ADVERSE SELECTION

The earlier discussion of demand for health insurance assumed that the insured population was of the same risk group, that is, that they all had the same probability of incurring the illness. The pure premium was based on the average expected loss of that group. An insurance company, however, may not have as complete information as to an individual's risk group as does the individual. When this difference in information between the insurance company and the individual occurs, high-risk individuals are able to purchase insurance at a premium that is based on a lower-risk group. This situation is referred to as "adverse selection."

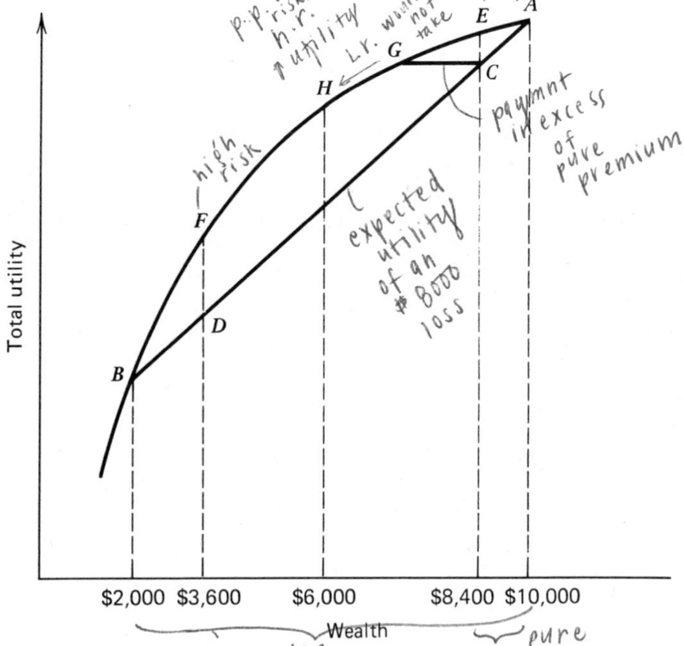

Figure 6–5. Adverse selection.

An insurance company may realize that there are population groups with differing levels of risk. However, if the insurance company is unable to distinguish between high and low risks, the insurance premium will reflect the average risk of the two groups. In this situation, the high-risk group will purchase insurance since a premium based on the average risk of the two groups is still lower than a premium based solely on their own risk group. Low-risk individuals may not purchase insurance since a premium based on the average of the two risk groups would be greater than their own risk-based premium. Adverse selection would result in a biased sample of those that purchase health insurance; predominately more higher-risk individuals would purchase insurance.

When adverse selection occurs, the insurance company loses money. To remain in business, the insurance company raises its premium to reflect the proportionately greater number of high-risk individuals. As the premium is increased, more low-risk individuals drop out.

The discussion above is illustrated in Figure 6–5. Assume the following: both high- and low-risk individuals have the same relationship between total utility and wealth; they each have $10,000; and if an illness occurs, the loss is $8,000. Low-risk individuals have only a .2 probability of incurring an illness, while high-risk individuals have a .8 probability. It is further assumed that there are an equal number of low- and high-risk individuals.

The pure premium for the low-risk group is $1,600 ($8,000 multiplied by .2) and a resulting wealth position of $8,400. For high-risk individuals the pure premium would be $6,400 ($8,000 multiplied by .8) and a resulting wealth position of $3,600.

The straight line *AB* shows the expected utility of an $8,000 loss occurring at different probabilities. If health insurance were sold at the pure premium to each risk group, both risk groups would be willing to purchase insurance. The low-risk individual would be at a higher utility level, *E*, which is greater than their expected utility, *C*. The low-risk individual would also be willing to pay distance *CG* in excess of the pure premium. (The expected utility of a high-risk individual is at *D*, which is less than their actual utility, *F*, when insurance is sold at the pure premium.)

If the insurance company cannot distinguish between high- and low-risk individuals, the pure premium will be based on the average risk of the two populations. The pure premium for everyone would then be $4,000 ($8,000 multiplied by .5). High-risk individuals would purchase the insurance because they would be at a higher utility level, *H* instead of *F*. Low-risk individuals, however, would not buy insurance since their utility level with insurance, *H*, would be lower than *G*, which is the maximum amount above the pure premium they would have been willing to pay.

A number of approaches are used by insurance companies to protect themselves against adverse selection. The insurance company may exclude coverage for preexisting conditions, which the individual may be aware of but not the insurance company. The insurance premium is reduced for persons who have been insured for a longer period than for those just purchasing insurance. Low-risk individuals may "signal" (i.e., provide information on their risk status) by their willingness to accept insurance policies that contain high deductibles and coinsurance.

THE DEMAND FOR HEALTH INSURANCE UNDER CONDITIONS OF MORAL HAZARD

We have shown that if the demand for medical care were completely price inelastic and therefore involved no moral hazard, people would still not demand completely comprehensive health insurance because of selling and transactions costs. In this section we introduce the concept of moral hazard in order to show that its existence would result in a demand for health insurance coverage that would cover less than 100 percent of a person's medical expenses (9).

If demand for medical care were inelastic with respect to price, the individual's demand curve in the event of illness would look like D_1 in Figure 6–6; that is, the individual would demand Q_1 units of medical care. In the case of moral hazard, it is possible for the patient to affect the size of his or her loss. If an individual became ill, the quantity of medical care that he or she would demand would depend, in part, on the price that had to be paid for that care. If insurance covered the entire cost of the illness episode, the individual represented by demand curve D_2 would demand Q_2 units of medical care. The presence of some elasticity in the individual's demand curve indicates that the individual will demand different quantities of medical care depending upon how much must be paid for that care. Since insurance lowers the price of medical care to individuals, they will consume more care than if they had to pay the entire price themselves. It is this behavior of individuals that is termed "moral hazard." To the individual consuming medical care under these circumstances, it is perfectly rational behavior—he or she is equating the marginal cost of purchasing that care with the marginal benefit of additional units. Since the marginal benefit of additional units of medical care decreases as the quantity of medical care consumed in-

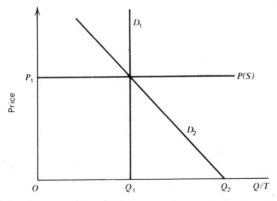

Figure 6–6. The demand for medical care under conditions of moral hazard.

creases, the individual will continue to consume additional units as long as the marginal benefit of those additional units exceeds their additional cost. Insurance coverage that reduces the price of care to zero under these circumstances results in an inefficient use of medical resources. Since the individual with insurance consumes medical care until the marginal benefits and marginal costs of the last units are equal, this will be at a point where the "true" marginal costs (the costs of *producing* those units) are greater than the marginal benefits. "Too much" medical care will be consumed, and the value of those additional units will be less than the costs of their production. This is illustrated in Figure 6–6 at the point where Q_2 units of medical care are consumed by an individual with 100 percent insurance coverage, with the costs of producing each unit indicated by the supply curve (S).

Another implication of the existence of moral hazard is that although individuals with insurance will consume Q_2 units of medical care if they become ill, they may be unwilling to purchase an insurance policy that provides such extensive coverage. As both consumers of medical care and purchasers of insurance, individuals are expected to consider the price involved in both cases: as consumers of medical services, greater utilization resulting from having insurance will result in their having to pay a higher premium for it. Instead of paying that higher premium, an individual may well prefer to self-insure or to purchase a less comprehensive insurance policy. For example, with reference to Figure 6–6, assume that an individual has both a .5 probability of not incurring any medical illness during the year, in which case his or her demand for medical care would be zero units, and a .5 probability of requiring medical care for an illness during that year. If the individual required medical care, with a corresponding demand curve of D_1, the individual would consume Q_1 units (which represents 100 units) at a cost of $10 per unit. The pure premium in this situation would be .5(0) + .5($1,000) = $500 per year. If, however, the individual's demand curve were D_2 (where Q_2 represents 200 units of medical care), the pure premium under these circumstances would be .5(0) + .5($2,000) = $1,000 per year.

These differences in premiums resulting from the price elasticity of the demand curve may be great enough for some individuals to prefer self-insurance, in which case the expected loss to them would be $500 per year [.5(0) + .5($1,000)]. They would consume Q_1 units of medical care if they became ill because, even though their demand curve may be represented by D_2, they would have to pay P_1 dollars per unit

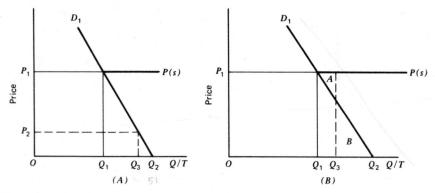

Figure 6-7. The effect of (A) coinsurance and (B) deductibles on the demand for medical care.

(which is the intersection of D_2 and S) and would consequently consume Q_1 units of care.

Individuals differ in their demands for medical care. If Figure 6-6 represents different demands for medical care, and one individual's demand is D_1 while the average demand among the rest of the population is D_2, then a premium for comprehensive insurance to the individual represented by demand curve D_1 would be based upon a utilization level indicated by Q_2, multiplied by a price of P_1. Under these circumstances an individual may well prefer self-insurance, which would mean a .5 probability (as in the previous case) of being ill and, if so, paying a price P_1 multiplied by Q_1 units of medical care. In both of these examples, *requiring* the individual to purchase comprehensive insurance that is the same as that which is purchased by the rest of the population will make the individual worse off (the marginal costs of the premium for the comprehensive coverage will exceed the marginal benefits of that insurance).

As a result of the effect of moral hazard on the use of medical care, several approaches have been suggested to limit utilization. One approach, which has not been very successful, was to rely on hospital utilization review committees. As long as hospitals were reimbursed for their costs, physicians were paid separately by Blue Shield, and the patient was not responsible for any part of the bill (under a service benefit policy), none of the participants had an incentive to use the utilization review committee to impose a cost on any of the other participants. Two other approaches which have been more successful are to introduce incentives on the part of either the physician or the patient. Under capitation-based payment systems, such as health maintenance organizations, the physician is likely to have an incentive (e.g., bonuses at the end of the year) if the organization's expenditures are less than their premium income. An incentive to the patient for reducing utilization would be provided if deductibles and coinsurance were part of the insurance package. Some persons, when purchasing insurance, might prefer intermediate choices between the extremes of comprehensive coverage or self-insurance. Deductibles and coinsurance enable consumers to bear some of the risk themselves and pay a smaller premium than if all their medical costs were covered by insurance.

In Figure 6-7A, the pure premium for comprehensive insurance would be represented by utilization level Q_2, multiplied by price P_1 (multiplied by the probability of .5). The cost of self-insurance would be P_1 multiplied by Q_1 (.5). The cost of an insurance policy with a coinsurance feature that lowered the price to the patient from P_1 to P_2 would cost $P_1 - P_2$ multiplied by a utilization level of Q_3 (.5). The pure premium for a policy with a coinsurance feature would be between the premiums of the other two alternatives. The availability of coinsurance would make insurance more attractive to some people who would prefer no insurance if their only other choice were comprehensive insurance.

In his article on the economics of moral hazard, Pauly also discusses the use of deductibles to reduce the costs of insurance premiums. Using only deductibles results either in the consumption of the same amount of care as in the case of no insurance, or conversely, in consumption of the same amount of care as in the situation of complete insurance coverage. This effect of deductibles on utilization is illustrated in Figure 6–7B. Without insurance, the individual represented by demand curve D_1 would, in the event of illness, consume Q_1 units of medical care; with complete insurance coverage the same individual would consume Q_2 units of medical care. If a deductible were instituted for the individual with complete coverage, then before the insurance would pay the medical costs, the individual would have to use and pay for Q_3 units of medical care at a cost of P_1 times Q_3. After that amount had been paid, the price of additional care (assuming no coinsurance feature) would be zero and he or she would consume Q_2 units of care. If the individual decides not to consume up to the deductible, which is P_1 times Q_3 units of medical care, he or she will merely act as though he or she has no insurance and use Q_1 units of care. Whether or not the individual will pay the deductible ($P_1 \times Q_3$) and then consume up to Q_2 units of medical care depends upon whether the excess amount that must be paid for the deductible, area A in Figure 6–7, which is above the individual's demand curve, is less than the "consumer surplus," represented by area B. The consumer surplus is the area under the demand curve that consumers would be willing to spend, but do not have to, since it would be at no cost if they first bought Q_3 units of care. If area B exceeds area A, consumers will then pay the deductible and consume Q_2 units of medical care.

Just as the effect on utilization of the coinsurance feature will depend upon the price elasticity of demand and the amount of the coinsurance, the effect the deductible has will also depend upon its size and the price elasticity of demand. In our discussion of deductibles and coinsurance, differences in income have been ignored; it is obvious that any copayment feature that is unrelated to income levels will have a more important effect on lower-income persons than on higher-income persons.

The existence of moral hazard thus has two effects. The price (premium) of health insurance is increased because utilization is increased when the consumer does not have to pay anything out of pocket (the moral hazard issue). Second, there is a decrease in the demand for health insurance when the insurance premium is increased, because of the previous increase in utilization.

The conclusion to be drawn from the discussion of the demand for health insurance, whether moral hazard is assumed to exist or not, is that even if all individuals were risk averters, insurance coverage for 100 percent of all of their medical expenses should not be required for all persons. When there are transactions costs for administering claims, and when people have different demands for medical care, no single insurance policy is best for everyone. Some persons will prefer to have only some type of medical expense covered; because of the existence of moral hazard, others will prefer to have some cost-sharing features.

SUMMARY AND CONCLUDING COMMENTS

The preceding discussion on the demand for health insurance offers an approach to answering the following questions: How much health insurance should the population have (i.e., what percent of total health expenditures should be covered by insurance), and what components of medical services should health insurance cover? The answers would indicate the degree to which the provision of health insurance in the population is economically efficient. Government intervention to increase or to change the type of health insurance in the population can then be evaluated in terms of whether such action moves the population closer to or further from what would be an optimal quantity and type of health insurance.[3]

To discuss the efficient amount and type of health insurance in the population, it is necessary to have criteria to evaluate what is efficient and what is inefficient in the purchase of health insurance. Assuming competition in the provision (supply) of health insurance, the price at which health insurance is sold will equal the marginal costs of providing it. In a competitive market, the suppliers will also respond to demands for different types of health insurance coverage and provide such coverage at a price that reflects the cost of producing it (these two assumptions are discussed in Chapter 8). The condition for economic efficiency on the demand side is that consumers purchase the type of and quantity of health insurance coverage to the point where its price equals the marginal benefit to them from additional insurance coverage. Since the demand curve indicates the marginal benefit to be derived from the purchase of health insurance, if the cost of additional insurance exceeds its marginal benefit, consumers will be better off purchasing less coverage. When the quantity of health insurance demanded is equal to the cost of providing that insurance, the individual will purchase the appropriate quantity; that is, the conditions of economic efficiency are met. At that point, the marginal cost of producing health insurance equals the marginal benefit to the consumer of that additional coverage.

The demand for health insurance was analyzed under two assumptions: first, that no moral hazard existed, in that the price of medical care did not affect its utilization or the quality of care demanded; and second, that moral hazard did exist, meaning that there is some price elasticity with respect to the demand for quantity and quality of medical care. In the first situation it was shown that individuals would *not* want to insure against all events. Insurance would be more likely for those medical services where the expected loss is greater and where the probability of the event's occurring is neither extremely high nor rare. Requiring insurance for all losses and all probabilities of their occurring, as well as for all individuals, would be economically inefficient; the cost of the insurance would exceed the marginal benefits to the consumer of additional coverage.

Based on this discussion, what percentage of the distribution of health expenditures should be covered by health insurance? The distribution of health expenditures is skewed, as show in Figure 6–1: many people have relatively small expenditures, a smaller percentage of the population have larger expenditures. We would expect the

---

[3]This discussion assumes no redistribution of medical services; when national health insurance proposals are discussed later, this assumption will be changed. Another assumption, which will subsequently be discussed, is that there are no externalities in the provision of personal medical services. Since redistribution of medical care to low-income persons may in fact have external effects, the efficient distribution of health insurance coverage may necessitate a different amount and type of insurance to low-income groups.

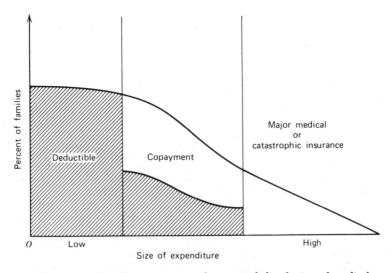

Figure 6-8. The effect of health insurance on the expected distribution of medical expenses among families.

large expenses with a low probability of occurrence to be covered by insurance, which suggests that the curve shown in Figure 6-1 should be modified. At a *minimum*, the tail of the distribution (relatively large expenditures for a small percentage of the families) should be covered by insurance, through major medical or catastrophic insurance, as shown in Figure 6-8.

When the demand for health insurance under conditions of moral hazard was discussed, it was shown that given the differences in preferences among people in their demands for medical care, it would be preferable to offer people more than an all-or-nothing choice. Some persons might prefer some insurance to either no insurance or complete coverage. What this suggests with regard to the distribution of medical expenditures is that the curve might be modified still further, as shown in Figure 6-8. Since the administrative costs of handling small claims are likely to exceed the amount above the pure premium that people that are willing to pay for relatively routine, smaller expenses, a deductible might be included for such expenses, as represented by the shaded portion of the curve in Figure 6-8.[4] Since there is moral hazard, people might prefer some copayment to reduce the size of their premium. Thus, a coinsurance feature would reduce the size of the medical expenses in the middle area. Insurance, in this instance, would cover less than 100 percent of medical expenditures (different components of the distribution of medical expenses would be covered at

---

[4]It has been claimed that deductibles and coinsurance provisions in health insurance will result in a decline in the demand for preventive services, which are lower-cost, more predictable medical services. Evidence of this alleged adverse effect is difficult to find. One can make the case that if preventive services have an effect on future medical demand, presumably insurance companies should be willing to subsidize the purchase of such services. Most, if not all, health insurance actually precludes such services from coverage. Similarly, HMOs and prepaid health plans have cut back on their use of preventive services, again presumably indicating that the costs of such services are greater than their potential savings. Thus if copayments actually reduce the demand for preventive care, it is not clear that increased demand for such services would have favorable cost/benefit ratios.

different percentages), and the premium for such insurance would be much lower than if it covered the entire distribution of medical expenses.

In discussing other factors affecting the demand for health insurance, the tax deductibility of premiums was mentioned; as incomes increase and people move into higher tax brackets, they have a greater incentive to purchase insurance against more, though smaller, medical expenses. The effect of the tax deductibility of health insurance premiums is a movement *away* from economic efficiency in the demand for health insurance. The "true" cost of health insurance has not been lowered, but its price to higher-income consumers has been. They will, therefore, be purchasing "too much" health insurance. The tax treatment of health insurance premiums has reduced the price of insurance against smaller, more predictable medical expenses to higher-income people to a point that may be *below* the actuarial value of those expenses. If the tax deductibility of health insurance premiums were no longer allowed, there would be less distortion in the purchase of health insurance, because the decision to purchase would more closely correspond to the cost of the insurance and the perceived marginal benefits to the consumer of that additional coverage. (The tax subsidy for the purchase of health insurance is discussed more technically in Appendix 2.)

An important question raised by the discussion of the demand for health insurance is which components of medical care should be covered by health insurance. When only one component of medical care, such as hospital services, is covered by insurance, the price of hospital care to the consumer relative to the prices of other forms of care has been distorted. The decision to use the different forms of care is based, in part, on the relative prices the patient must pay for such care. Inasmuch as these relative prices will not reflect the relative costs of care, moving toward greater economic efficiency in the use of medical care will require the patient to face prices proportional to the costs of such care. An example of insurance coverage that distorts the use of medical components by distorting the relative prices of medical care faced by the consumer is the Blue Cross service benefit policy. A service benefit policy provided very complete coverage for just hospital care, while it excluded nonhospital care; this led to an inefficient (more costly) form of treatment when services that could be performed on an outpatient basis were instead performed in a hospital. Blue Cross now provides coverage for nonhospital services.

Another aspect of the service benefit policy that leads to inefficiency, albeit in the production of hospital services, is that no incentive is provided to the patient to seek care in less expensive hospitals. Instead, the entire cost of a hospital episode is reimbursed (to the hospital) regardless of how costly that hospital is.

There are certain types of health insurance that do not distort the relative prices faced by the patient when seeking care. An example is indemnity insurance, which reimburses the patient a dollar amount. Patients and/or their physicians therefore have an incentive to minimize the cost of a medical treatment, and the relative prices of the different components of medical services will not be artificially distorted.

Another approach for achieving allocative efficiency in the use of medical services is the use of capitation payments (by or on behalf of patients) to an organization to cover the cost of medical services. Under these arrangements, a decisionmaker, generally a physician, prescribes that combination of services so that the relative costs of different medical services used by the patient equals their relative marginal benefits. Prepaid group practices and health maintenance organizations (discussed more completely later) are organizational arrangements whereby the patient is covered by a capitation payment system.

Finally, the method of provider reimbursement has affected economic efficiency in the demand for health insurance. Cost-based reimbursement of hospitals, which has recently ended, resulted in higher health care costs. These higher costs increased the size of the probable loss, thereby resulting in a greater demand for health insurance than if other, more-efficiency-oriented payment mechanisms had been used.

An important reason for understanding the demand for medical care, as well as the demand for health insurance, is to be able to determine whether or not the quantity (and quality) of medical care consumed is optimal. The optimal rate of output of medical care will be achieved when the price of that care (which is presumed to equal the costs of producing that care under a competitive system) is equal to the marginal benefit of that care. As has been shown, the type of insurance coverage that existed (service benefit coverage) and the tax treatment of health insurance premiums are two reasons why prices in medical care to consumers have been (and still are) distorted, thereby resulting in consumption of a nonoptimal amount of medical care.

To determine whether the price of medical care to the patient reflects the minimum cost of producing that care, it is necessary to turn to an analysis of the supply side of the medical care market.

APPENDIX 1: THE ALLOCATIVE INEFFICIENCY OF BLUE CROSS'S SERVICE BENEFIT POLICY

Blue Cross's service benefit policy provided complete coverage against hospital expenses, in a semiprivate room accommodation. A person with Blue Cross did not have to pay any of the charges for hospital care (up to a maximum number of days), but he or she had to pay the full price for any other forms of medical services, such as outpatient services or nursing home care, used in the treatment of that illness. Blue Cross's service benefit policy caused an "overuse" of hospital care relative to other medical components used in treatment. The consequence was a cost of treatment that was higher than if other, less costly, but equally efficacious forms of care were used.

The foregoing conclusion is illustrated in Figure 6–9. Assume that treatment for a medical illness can be achieved with varying amounts of hospital and/or physician services. This substitutability in the use of components for treatment is shown by the indifference curves in Figure 6–9. The shape of the indifference curve indicates the degree of substitutability among components, and it depends upon the particular illness and its seriousness. The budget constraint AB indicates the quantity of physician and hospital services that the patient can purchase without insurance; if they spent all their funds on physician services, they could purchase OA units of physician services; if they spent all their funds on hospital care, they could purchase OB units of hospital care; or they could purchase some combination of the two. The slope of the budget constraint indicates the relative prices of physician and hospital services. With no insurance, a patient with a particular illness and with budget constraint AB will consume OC units of physician services and OD units of hospital care. If the patient had indemnity insurance which reimbursed a given amount of money for medical care, then if the patient became ill, the budget constraint would shift out parallel and become JK. With indemnity insurance the patient could purchase more medical care than previously. The slope of the new budget constraint would remain the same; the relative prices of the components used in treatment would not change but the patient

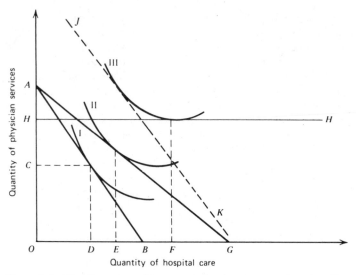

Figure 6-9. The allocative inefficiency of Blue Cross's service benefit policy.

could buy more of each, thereby moving to a higher indifference curve (III). The effect of indemnity insurance is similar to an increase in income when the patient is ill.

However, if the patient merely had hospitalization coverage with a coinsurance feature, the price of hospital care to the patient would be reduced, and the budget constraint would rotate to the right and become AG. The patient could now purchase more hospital care. The effect on the mix and quantity of components used when there is just insurance for hospital care and not for any of the other components is similar to the income and substitution effects of a price change. The patient will use relatively more hospital care, since the price of hospital care relative to out-of-hospital care has been reduced. This is the substitution effect. The income effect will be an increase in the use of both components, as long as they are normal goods.

If the patient were now to receive a service benefit policy, hospital care becomes essentially free, since there is no out-of-pocket cost to the patient. The substitution effect of this price reduction to the patient becomes even greater than in the previous case. Line HH is horizontal, to indicate that there is no price constraint on the purchase of additional units of hospital care. (It is lower than point A because, presumably, it would require more of the consumer's income to purchase the policy; hence less would be available to purchase physician services.) The individual, when ill, will use relatively more hospital care than in any of the previous cases. Because there is some disutility to being in the hospital, use of the hospital will not increase infinitely. Patients, through their physicians, will substitute hospital care for nonhospital services when these nonhospital services would be equally efficacious. In the case above, diagnostic testing would be free to the patient if performed in the hospital, whereas the full price would have to be paid if it were performed outside the hospital. We would therefore predict that such testing would be performed in a hospital.

The misallocation of resources resulting from a service benefit policy is shown as follows. The budget constraint JK, since it is tangent to indifference curve III, would make the patient as well off as would the service benefit policy; however, the combination of services used in the treatment represents the use of fewer resources. The slope of line *JK* represents the relative prices of hospital and physician services if the patient had an indemnity type of insurance or had to pay the full price of these services in the event that he or she did not have insurance. The relative prices of physician and hospital services are assumed to represent their relative marginal costs. The quantity of hospital care used in treatment with a service benefit policy is given by the point where indifference curve III is tangent to line *HH*. Since the patient is equally well off at any point along the same indifference curve, the least costly combination of services would be achieved by using the medical components according to their relative prices (as well as their relative benefits in treatment). The magnitude of misallocation is the difference between line *JK* and a line with the same slope intersecting the point of tangency between the indifference curve and line *HH*.

Although quality of hospital care is not shown in these diagrams, part of the increase in quantity of hospital care may be viewed as an increase in quality. Since the price of hospital care to the patient has been reduced to zero with a service benefit policy, the patient will also demand higher-quality hospital services, such as requesting the removal of an appendix in a teaching hospital when a smaller, less care-intensive community hospital would be equally satisfactory. This demand for increased quality of hospital services will result in an even greater misallocation of resources.

In this discussion, the allocative inefficiency resulting from insurance which provides coverage just for hospital care depends upon how much the price of hospital care is subsidized relative to the prices of other medical components (the most severe case being the Blue Cross service benefit policy), the degree of substitutability of hospital care for other forms of care, and the price elasticity of demand both for hospital utilization and for increased hospital quality.

The effects of a hospital service benefit policy have been threefold: one, the hospital has been used when other less expensive but equally effective forms of treatment could have been used, thereby raising the cost of producing medical care; and second, hospital use has increased to a point where the additional benefits to the patient of time spent in the hospital are very low. The real cost of resources to produce the additional care was greater than the price faced by the patient, thereby resulting in a situation where the marginal cost of producing the additional care *exceeded* the marginal value to the patient of increased use. Third, there has been a much greater demand for quality of hospital services on the part of patients and their physicians because the price of higher-quality services to the patients is zero and quality may be considered a normal good; therefore, they will demand increased quality to the point where the additional benefits derived from it equal the price to them. Since the price of higher-quality hospital services is zero, the amount of quality demanded will be greater than it otherwise would be; the cost of resources used in producing higher-quality care will, at the margin, exceed the additional benefits derived from it by the patients. These, then, are the three misallocative effects of different types of hospital insurance policies, with the greatest misallocation occurring in the case of a service benefit policy.

An approach that has been suggested for remedying these inefficiencies is to mandate the use of utilization review procedures. These review mechanisms attempt to reduce excess utilization instead of changing the distortion in the relative prices of care to the patient, which has brought these inefficiencies about in the first place. An alternative approach for correcting such inefficiencies, when it may not be desirable to reinstitute patient incentives, is to provide incentives to the *physician* to use the least costly mix of components. An example of such an incentive system (discussed more fully later) is the development of capitation plans for payment of medical services, such as health maintenance organizations.

APPENDIX 2: THE TAX ADVANTAGE OF HEALTH INSURANCE AS A FRINGE BENEFIT

Employees may receive increased income from their employer in either cash or as a fringe benefit in the form of health insurance. The cost to the employer of either choice is the same. To an employee in a high tax bracket, however, employer-purchased health insurance may be worth more than an equivalent payment in cash.

If an employee receives an income of $1,000 a week, then, as shown in Figure 6–10, the employee's budget line is $I_1 M_1$. If the employee spent his or her entire income on other goods and services, the employee could purchase quantity OI_1 of other goods and services each week. If she chose instead to purchase just health insurance with her weekly income, the employee could purchase a maximum of OM_1 quantity of health insurance each week. The slope of $I_1 M_1$ represents the relative prices of health insurance and all other goods and services. The combination of health insurance and other goods and services that the employee will actually purchase depends on the employee's tastes and preferences.

Assume that the employee receives a raise of $200 a week. If the employer gave the raise to the employee in cash, the employee's budget line would increase to $I_2 M_2$. In addition to being able to purchase more health insurance, the increased cash would enable the employee to purchase more of other goods and services.

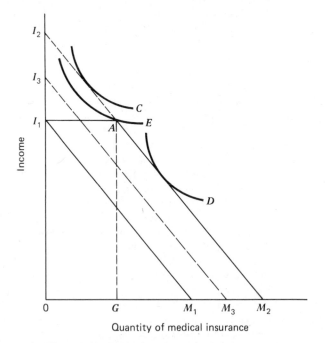

Figure 6–10. Fringe benefits versus money income.

If the employee has to pay income taxes (and social security taxes) on a cash raise, then the after-tax value of that cash raise is reduced and is shown by the budget line I_3M_3. The after-tax budget line would depend upon the employee's marginal tax bracket. The higher the marginal tax rate of the employee, the lower will be the new budget line.

If, instead of cash, the employer uses the money to purchase health insurance for the employee, which is not considered as taxable income, the employee's budget line changes to I_1AM_2. The budget line becomes horizontal from I_1 to A. The employee receives OG quantity of health insurance while retaining her current income. (The cash amount of the raise divided by the price of health insurance equals quantity OG.) Thus the employee receives OG quantity of health insurance and still has a budget line of I_1M_1. The employee can still purchase OI_1 of other goods and services (if she spent her entire income) or can purchase GM_2 of additional health insurance (for a total quantity of OM_2 if she spent her entire income on health insurance).

An employee who prefers more of other goods and services rather than additional health insurance would, with a cash raise, be on indifference curve C. An employee who prefers additional health insurance would move to indifference curve D after a cash raise. If the cash raise is then taxed so that the new after-tax income is budget line I_3M_3, those employees could no longer be on indifference curves C and D; they could only be on an indifference curve that is tangent to the budget line I_3M_3. With a fringe benefit, however, both employees could move to higher indifference curves. The employee preferring additional insurance can attain indifference curve D. Indifference curve C is still unattainable under fringe benefits; the highest indifference curve achievable by that employee is indifference curve E. However, E is still preferable to any indifference curve on budget line I_3M_3.

Employer-purchased health insurance is in the interest of the employees. As long as employees pay taxes on their cash income but not on employer-purchased health insurance, they have an incentive to receive additional income in the form of fringe benefits. The higher the employees' marginal tax bracket, the greater is their incentive for fringe benefits.

(There is also another reason why employees have an incentive for their employer to purchase health insurance rather than purchasing it themselves. Individual insurance coverage is more expensive than group coverage; there are lower administrative costs when a person is part of a group and there is less of a problem of adverse selection.)

With high marginal tax rates employees have an incentive to purchase more insurance than they would otherwise. Employees purchase more first-dollar coverage as well as new types of coverage, such as vision and dental benefits. In the last six years marginal tax rates have fallen from a top rate of 70 percent to 33 percent. The incentive to purchase additional coverage has therefore declined. If health insurance fringes were taxed at the same rate as cash income (or taxed above a certain amount), employees would demand less health insurance coverage.

APPENDIX 3: THE EFFECT ON THE INSURANCE PREMIUM OF EXTENDING COVERAGE TO INCLUDE ADDITIONAL BENEFITS

As insurance companies compete with one another, it becomes important for them to be able to provide a given set of benefits at the lowest possible cost. Since a treatment for an illness can be provided using a combination of settings (e.g., hospital, physician's office, and home care), insurance companies are experimenting with the effect on their premiums of adding less costly substitutes to their policies. This design of benefits offered by insurance companies has also been applicable to Blue Cross. As a consequence of its hospital service benefit policy, with its resulting "overutilization" of the hospital, Blue Cross has begun to broaden its coverage to include out-of-hospital care. The hoped-for effect of adding additional coverage is that substitution away from the hospital toward lower-cost substitutes will occur and the insurance premium can be reduced.

To determine whether or not adding coverage for a nonhospital benefit will reduce the total costs of care (i.e., the premium), the following information is needed:

1. the price elasticity of demand for the newly covered benefit;
2. the copayment factor for the new benefit;
3. the cross-elasticity of demand between hospitalization and the new benefits;
4. the cross-elasticity of demand between the new benefit and any complementary components of care; and
5. the relative prices of hospital care, the new benefit, and any other complementary components affected.

This information would be used in the following manner to determine whether adding a new insurance benefit would lower the insurance premium. Assuming that the demand for hospital care is as it appears in Figure 6–11A, then without any insurance, the patient would have to pay the full cost of a hospital episode if he or she became ill; the patient would have to pay PH_1, and according to his or her expected demand, would use QH_1 days of hospital care. The consumer's total expenditures for hospital care would be $(PH_1 \times QH_1)$. With an insurance policy that provided complete coverage for hospital care but not for substitutes to the hospital, such as the Blue Cross service benefit policy, the price of hospital care to the patient would become "zero," and the expected utilization in the event of illness would be QH_2. The total expenditure for hospital care in this case would be $(PH_1 \times QH_2)$.

Including in the insurance contract home health visits with a coinsurance feature will now result in a lower price to the patient, from PM_1 to PM_2, and an increase in utilization of home health visits, from QM_1 to QM_2, as shown in Figure 6–11B. The amount of the increase in home health visits will depend upon the price elasticity of demand for home health visits and the size of the coinsurance payment. The cost to the insurance company of covering home health visits is that part of the actual price that the insurance company will have to pay $(PM_1 - PM_2)$, multiplied by the number of home health visits, QM_2. (The patient would pay the remainder, $PM_2 \times QM_2$.)

If the new benefit acts as a partial substitute for hospital care, then with the reduction in the price of home health visits, patients (through their physicians) will demand less hospital care. How much less hospital care will be demanded will depend upon the cross-elasticity of demand between hospital utilization and the price of home health

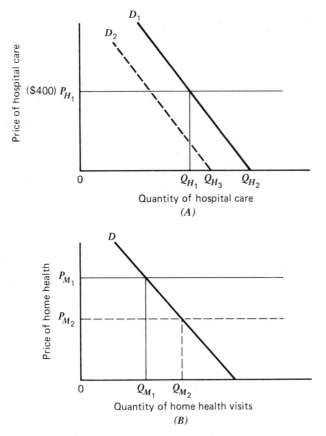

Figure 6-11. The effect on hospital utilization of insuring out-of-hospital services: *(A)* hospital utilization, *(B)* home health visits.

visits, which is equal to the percent change in hospital utilization divided by the percent change in the price of home health visits. This is shown in Figure 6–11A by a shift in the demand for hospital care to the left, indicated by demand curve D_2. Since the price of hospital care to the patient with his initial insurance policy has been assumed to be "zero," the new quantity demanded will be QH_3. The size of the shift in demand for hospital care will depend upon the magnitude of the cross-elasticity of demand and the size of the reduction in the price to the patient of the new benefit.

The savings in hospital expenditures to the insurance company of including coverage for a nonhospital service would be the difference in hospital utilization ($QH_2 - QH_3$), multiplied by the price of hospital care, PH_1. If the savings in hospital expenditures were greater than the cost to the insurance company of adding the new benefit, the total cost (the premium) would be reduced.

In actuality, other services might be affected by the provision of a new benefit (i.e., subsidizing home health visits). If there are medical services that are complementary to the use of home health visits, there will be an increase in use of these complementary services (a shift to the right in their demand curve). These additional costs may be borne by the patient rather than by the insurance company if the complementary service is not insured.

Following is a numerical example of a change in benefit design illustrating whether or not insuring a nonhospital service will reduce the total cost of an insurance premium. Let us assume the following values for each of the data required in our example:

1. Hospital utilization (QH_2) when home health visits are not covered by insurance is 800 patient days per 1,000 population.
2. The price of hospital care is $400 per day.
3. The price of a home health visit is $40.
4. Home health visits are 600 per 1,000 population.
5. The price elasticity of demand for home health visits is − 1.0 (a 10 percent decrease in price leads to a 10 percent increase in home health visits).
6. The cross-elasticity of demand between hospital patient days and the price of home health visits is + .2 (a 10 percent decrease in the price of a home health visit leads to a 2 percent decrease in hospital patient days).
7. After home health visits are included in the insurance coverage, the coinsurance rate is 20 percent; that is, the patient has to pay only 20 percent of the price of home health visits. (It is also assumed that the price of home health visits remains at its previous level.)

With this information we can now calculate the change in the cost of the premium as a result of including home health visits with a 20 percent coinsurance feature.

The total cost of the premium per 1,000 population before the new benefit is added to the coverage is

$$\frac{TC}{1,000} = P_{H1} \frac{Q_{H2}}{1,000}$$

$$\frac{\$320,000}{1,000} = \$400 \times \frac{800}{1,000}$$

or $320 per person. The total cost of the premium *after* home health visits are covered at a 20 percent coinsurance rate is

$$\frac{TC}{1,000} = P_{H1}\left(\frac{Q_{H3}}{1,000}\right) + .8P_{M1}\left(\frac{Q_{M2}}{1,000}\right)$$

which is

$$\frac{\$303,360}{1,000} = \$400\left(\frac{672}{1,000}\right) + .8(\$40)\left(\frac{1080}{1,000}\right)$$

or $303.36 per person.

The difference is computed as follows:

1. The increased expenditure on home health visits is

$$.8(\$40)\left(\frac{600}{1,000}\right)(1.8) = \frac{\$34,560}{1,000}$$

This is the percentage of the home health price paid by the insurance company (.8), multiplied by the price of home health visits ($40), multiplied by the number of home health visits per 1,000 population (600/1,000), multiplied by the percent increase in home health visits as a result of the 80 percent reduction in home health prices to the patient (a − 1.0 price elasticity multiplied by a 80 percent reduction in price).

2. Subtract the saving on decreased hospital utilization, which is

$$\$400\left(\frac{128}{1,000}\right) = \frac{\$51,200}{1,000}$$

This is the price of hospital care, multiplied by reduction in patient days as a result of a lower price of home health visits. (The cross-elasticity of + .2 when multiplied by a 80 percent reduction in the price of home health visits is equal to a 16 percent reduction in hospital utilization; this is then multiplied by 800/1,000.)

3. The net effect of the savings on hospital expenditures less the increased home health expenditures is

$$\frac{\$51,200}{1,000} - \frac{\$34,560}{1,000} = \frac{\$16,640}{1,000} \quad \text{or} \quad \$16.64 \text{ per person}$$

Given the data and assumptions used in this example, the effect of insuring home health visits would be a net decrease of $16.64 per person in the total cost of the premium ($303.36 versus $320 per person).

In the preceding example, insuring an out-of-hospital service would further reduce the insurance premium if the price of hospital care increased relatively faster than that of the nonhospital service, if the substitutability between the two services (cross-elasticity) increased, and if the price elasticity of demand for the nonhospital service were reduced.

Adding insurance coverage for an out-of-hospital service is more likely to reduce hospital utilization when this service is used *in conjunction with* hospital care in treatment of an illness episode. If home health visits are covered by insurance and are not used as part of the treatment for an illness, there may be a large increase in home health utilization without any consequent lowering of hospital utilization. A major medical policy, which covers all the medical services used in treatment (after a sizable deductible has been paid), is more likely to result in substitution away from the more costly components (10).

REFERENCES

1. The discussion in this section borrows heavily from an unpublished article by J. J. German, "A Note on the Economic Theory of Insurance with Implications for Health Insurance," mimeographed, January 1967; and the article by Dennis Lees and Robert Rice, "Uncertainty and the Welfare Economics of Medical Care: Comment," *American Economic Review*, March 1965. The comment by D. Lees and R. Rice (as well as the comment by M. Pauly in the next section of this chapter) were written in response to Kenneth J. Arrow, "Uncertainty and the Welfare Economics of Medical Care," *American Economic Review*, December 1963. Arrow claimed that the market for health insurance requires government intervention because there are gaps in consumer's health insurance coverage, and that this is evidence that the market is not producing certain services that consumers are willing to purchase. Lees and Rice argued that Arrow's claims are not evidence of market imperfections but rather are a result of transactions costs. For example, "the transactions cost to the individual of completing and filing applications and forms, paying premiums, keeping records, etc., as well as possible costs of obtaining information, may be of sufficient magnitude to make insurance policies against certain losses not worthwhile." Arrow replied that individuals who cannot take advantage of the economies of group health insurance will face too high a transactions cost (i.e., the price of insurance is greatly in excess of its pure premium) and thus may not purchase health insurance.

2. M. Friedman and L. Savage, "The Utility Analysis of Choices Involving Risk," *Journal of Political Economy*, 56(4), 1948: 279–304.

3. On this last point see the discussion by Jan Mossin, "Aspects of Rational Insurance Purchasing," *Journal of Political Economy*, July/August 1968.

4. Charles E. Phelps, "Large Scale Tax Reform: The Case of Employer Paid Health Insurance Premiums," Workshop Paper 20, Applied Economics Workshop, University of Rochester, Rochester, N.Y., September 1985. Several other studies have estimated the effect of the tax rate on insurance coverage. See, for example, Martin Holmer, "Tax Policy and the Demand for Health Insurance," *Journal of Health Economics*, 3, 1984: 203–221; and Amy K. Taylor and Gail R. Wilensky, "The Effect of Tax Policies on Expenditures for Private Health Insurance," in Jack Meyer, ed., *Market Reforms in Health Care* (Washington, D.C.: American Enterprise Institute, 1983), 163–184. The foregoing two studies estimate price elasticities of -.2 and less, which are lower than Phelps's estimates.

5. *Ibid.*

6. E. Friedson and J. Feldman, *Public Attitudes Toward Health Insurance*, Research Series 5 (New York: Health Information Foundation, 1958).

7. Based on unpublished data in the 1974 Health Interview Survey and published in *Catastrophic Health Insurance* (Washington, D.C.: Congressional Budget Office, Congress of the United States, January 1977), p. 58.

8. Daniel L. Waldo, Katherine R. Levit, and Helen Lazenby, "National Health Expenditures, 1985," *Health Care Financing Review*, 8(1), Fall 1986: p. 15, Table 3.

9. The discussion in this section is based on the article by Mark Pauly, "The Economics of Moral Hazard: Comment," *American Economic Review*, June 1968. In

Pauly's comment to Arrow's reply to Lees and Rice, he argues that even if there are certain economies in government provision of health insurance that would lower transactions costs, other costs may more than offset such possible savings. In addition to a loss of consumer choice, the existence of "moral hazard" would cause consumers to demand less insurance "at the premium its behavior as a purchaser of insurance and as a demander of medical care under insurance makes necessary." In other words, the existence of moral hazard would result in higher prices for insurance and, consequently, a decreased demand. The lack of complete health insurance coverage in the private market can also be explained by moral hazard, which would not be lessened even if government were somehow able to reduce the transactions costs of insurance to individuals.

10. The reader is referred to the following articles for a more complete discussion of the issues covered in this section: Mark V. Pauly, "Taxation, Health Insurance, and Market Failure in the Medical Economy," *Journal of Economic Literature*, 24(2), June 1986: 629–675. Mark V. Pauly, "A Measure of the Welfare Costs of Health Insurance," *Health Services Research*, Winter 1969, Karen Davis and Louise B. Russell, "The Substitution of Hospital Outpatient Care for Inpatient Care," *The Review of Economics and Statistics*, May 1972; and Martin S. Feldstein, "The Welfare Loss of Excess Health Insurance," *Journal of Political Economy*, March-April 1973.

CHAPTER 7

The Supply of Medical Care: An Overview

DETERMINANTS OF SUPPLY

Characteristics of Production Functions

Underlying the supply of any good or service is the production function. The production function describes the technical relation between the output of that good or service and the resources (or inputs) used to produce it. If the output were nursing care per patient, then included in the inputs would be the number of and type of nurses on the nursing unit. This technical relationship between nursing care per patient and the types of nurses may be expressed in the following general form:

$$Q_{npc} = f(\text{RNs, LPNs, ADs, UN})$$

where Q_{npc}, which represents quantity of nursing patient care, is functionally related to the number of registered nurses (RNs), licensed practical nurses (LPNs), nursing aides (ADs), and the type of nursing unit (UN).

Certain characteristics of medical production functions affect the cost and quantity of care provided. The relationship just stated between nursing care per patient and the type of nurses suggests that to some extent the various types of nurses are substitutable for one another in the production of nursing care. The substitutability is not one-to-one (i.e., one LPN cannot substitute for one RN). RNs presumably have more skills as a result of their additional training, and therefore LPNs can substitute for some or most, but perhaps not all, the tasks the RN performs. The degree of substitutability between different types of health workers is important to determine, since it provides information the decisionmaker needs if he or she is to minimize the costs of providing nursing care.

In the health field there are a number of legal restrictions on the tasks that various health professionals can perform. Even if a nurse is capable of performing certain tasks that are reserved solely for the physician, the nurse may not perform them because she would be violating the state practice acts. The effect of these legal restrictions is to limit the degree of substitutability in the production function. Thus, the decisionmaker is not legally able to combine the inputs at will; the law limits the extent to which inputs may be substituted in producing a given level of output. If legal restrictions prevent substitution from occurring when it would not result in a diminution of the quality of care, the legal restrictions have increased the cost of producing that care. The "costs" of restrictive practices, therefore, are the additional resources required to produce a given level of care at a given level of quality.

Another characteristic of the stated production function is that not all the inputs can be varied simultaneously at each point in time. At any time, the decisionmaker can vary the combination of nurses and their numbers on the nursing unit. To change the type of nursing unit itself, by enlarging it or improving it through greater use of monitoring mechanisms, would take longer. The "long run" is that period of time in which the administrator can vary not only the number and type of nurses but also the size and character of the nursing unit. The "short run" is that period of time in which the administrator can vary only the other inputs, not make changes in the nursing unit itself. Another example of the short versus the long run would be with regard to physician services. In the short run, an increase in physician services can be achieved by having the physician work longer hours or by hiring auxiliary workers. In the long run, medical schools may increase the number of physicians, which are the fixed input in the short run.

These distinctions between the long run and the short run are important for determining the least costly way of producing nursing and other types of medical care. If there is an increase in the demand for nursing care derived from an increased demand for medical and hospital care, the administrator can increase the number of nurses on the unit to provide more care. (The combination of nurses used to provide that increased care will depend upon which combination is least costly.) It might be much less costly if the nursing unit itself were changed; therefore, in the long run, all the inputs, including the nursing unit, will be changed to form a combination that will minimize the cost of providing that greater amount of nursing care. [Varying the size of the nursing unit is equivalent to moving along a long-run average cost curve (i.e., determining the effects of scale of the nursing unit on cost per unit of output).]

One further aspect of the production function is worth mentioning. Technical change has usually been defined as a greater output that is produced with the same or fewer inputs. In medical care, technical change has usually meant that illnesses that formerly could not be treated can now be cared for with a higher probability of a successful outcome. Such technical change, which is really a change in medical care output, usually results in increased rather than decreased use of inputs. An example of technical change that has led to a decrease in input use is the use of new drugs, which has decreased the use of more expensive institutional care. Thus, both types of technical change have occurred in medical care. It is important to hold the effects of such technical change constant when analyzing the production function for medical care.

Determining the Least-Cost Combination of Inputs

To determine the least costly combination of inputs to be used as output is increased, the following information is required. First, it is necessary to have some knowledge of the marginal increase in nursing care as each type of nursing personnel is increased. If the number of LPNs and ADs is held constant, the increase in patient care corresponding to an increase in the number of RNs is not constant; the law of variable proportions states that after some point the marginal product (contribution) of an additional RN will begin to decline. The same will be true for each of the other categories of nursing personnel. The marginal contribution to increased patient care for each type of input can be empirically determined, and both it and a second type of information are necessary if the decisionmaker is to minimize his or her costs of increasing patient care. The second type of information needed is the relative prices of the different inputs used in the production function. Even if an RN contributed one and a half times more than an LPN to patient care, increases in patient care should not necessarily be achieved through increases in the number of RNs. If RNs' wages were twice as great as those of LPNs, it would be less expensive to achieve an increase in nursing care by increasing LPNs rather than RNs, assuming no change in quality. The relative prices (wages) of different inputs, together with knowledge of the relative productivity of the inputs, will determine which combination of inputs to use for producing a given level of output or for meeting an increase in output.

To go from the production function to the supply schedule, it is necessary to combine information on the productivity of the inputs with information on their relative prices. Once prices are used in conjunction with the production function, we can describe the minimum-cost combination (i.e., relative prices and relative marginal products) for each level of output, which is the supply schedule or the amount of output that can be provided at different prices of that output. Supply schedules are rising because in order to provide a greater amount of output, the marginal productivity of inputs eventually declines and marginal costs rise, hence the costs of that additional output increase. Also, to increase the quantity of services, more resources must be drawn into production, and it is necessary to pay higher wages for these resources to bid them away from their current use. (The marginal cost curve shifts to the left.) In the long run, when all the inputs in the production function can be varied, the supply schedule will become more elastic (i.e., it will require less of an increase in cost to increase supply).

Certain assumptions implicit in the foregoing discussion should be made explicit, since they may not prevail, or perhaps are believed not to prevail, in medical markets. The first is the assumption of substitutability in the use of inputs to produce a given output. In the health field, a great deal of emphasis is placed on the use of ratios of skilled health manpower to the population. If there is substitution between skilled and other types of manpower to provide medical services, the use of such simple ratios (i.e., fixed coefficients of production) is inappropriate. Another assumption usually made with respect to production functions and supply schedules is that the different combinations of inputs that could be used to provide medical care are all technically efficient; that is, they are the minimum quantities necessary to produce a given level of service. It has been alleged that in certain sectors of the medical market too many inputs are used in producing a given service. It has also been alleged that the most economically efficient combinations of inputs are not used, because the input combinations that are used may be based upon the marginal productivities of the inputs without regard to their relative prices. The assumption that decisionmakers are desirous of minimizing the cost of producing medical services must be examined.

Goals and Incentives of Decisionmakers

Economic efficiency in production requires decisionmakers to use knowledge of the marginal productivity of their inputs and their relative prices to produce the output at minimum cost. In the health field decisionmakers may have goals other than cost minimization; further, the relative prices of the inputs used in production may be distorted. If there are government subsidies for certain inputs, such as hospital capital or educational programs for certain manpower categories, then the relative price of the subsidized input has been lowered and relatively more of it may be used in production because it is cheaper to the decisionmakers.

To the extent that the goals of the decisionmakers differ from cost minimization, and the provider payment mechanisms enable them to pursue these other goals (and to the extent that there are legal restrictions on the use of inputs), the supply curve of medical care will be less elastic. In other words, it will take larger price increases to produce an increase in services than it would if the objectives and constraints were similar to those of a competitive industry.

The example of the production function used above (nursing care), the information required to be able to minimize costs (marginal productivity and relative prices), and the assumptions underlying the behavior of the decisionmakers (a desire to minimize costs) can be applied equally well to other levels of the medical sector. The physician faces a production function in providing treatment for an illness of a particular diagnosis and of a given level of severity. The inputs in this instance would be the different institutional settings, such as a hospital, a physician's office, or a nursing home.

The concern with the production function at the aggregate level is usually discussed in terms of the organization for the delivery of medical care—namely, the combinations of institutional settings that are least expensive for producing patient care. To determine which delivery systems (combinations of inputs or institutional settings) in a production function to provide medical care are least expensive, we would need to have information pertaining to marginal productivities and the relative costs of the different institutional settings, and an understanding of the objectives of the decisionmakers who are responsible for combining these inputs to produce patient services.

EVALUATION OF ECONOMIC EFFCIENCY IN PRODUCTION

The concept of economic efficiency is relevant to both the demand and the supply side of an industry. When evaluating economic efficiency, we are concerned that the rate (and type) of output be "optimal." Economic efficiency in demand is related to economic efficiency in supply through prices. In discussing the demand for medical care, we saw that it is unlikely that economic efficiency, so defined, would occur in the output of medical care. The reason was that the price of medical care and of its various components is distorted as a result of existing insurance coverage, the tax deductibility of insurance premiums, and the incentives faced by the patient's physician, who may act not to minimize the patient's cost of treatment but rather to minimize the physician's own cost of providing that treatment and/or to maximize the net revenue garnered from the components used in treatment.

In our examination of the supply side of the medical care sector, we are also interested in the criterion of economic efficiency. If the various markets within the medical

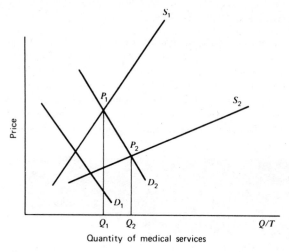

Figure 7-1. The effect of different supply elasticities on the price, quantity, and cost of national health insurance.

care sector are determined to be economically inefficient, the cost of medical care is higher than it should be. By examining the reasons for deviations from economic efficiency, we can make policy recommendations that would improve the efficiency of the market and inhibit the rapid rise in the cost of medical care. The "return" to greater economic efficiency in the production of medical care is the discounted present value of the possible cost savings. In an industry in which more than $400 billion is spent, and in which expenditures are rising at approximately 10 percent per year, a savings of even 1 to 2 percent would result in a return in excess of $50 billion.

The economic efficiency of the supply side of the medical care sector also has important policy implications. If the supply side of medical care is relatively inelastic, requiring relatively large price increases to bring forth an increase in medical care output (because the providers are not attempting to minimize their costs), this will influence the type of redistribution programs proposed on the demand side, specifically, the type of national health insurance programs that can be instituted. As shown in Figure 7-1, a relatively inelastic supply curve, represented by S_1, would, with an increase in demand from D_1 to D_2, result in a greater price rise and a smaller increase in services provided than if the supply of medical services were more elastic. A more elastic supply schedule would, for the same increase in demand, provide $Q_2 - Q_1$ more services at a smaller increase in price: P_2 rather than P_1. The total cost of the increase in demand would be $P_1 \times Q_1$ in the inelastic case versus $P_2 \times Q_2$ in the situation where supply is more elastic. In the latter case more of the increase in total expenditures would go for increased medical services, whereas in the former there would be more rapid price increases with a smaller increase in services. The cost of a national health insurance program would be greater and the availability of services diminished when supply is more inelastic; because of greater costs, the feasibility of instituting such a program, as well as its comprehensiveness, is reduced.

The economic efficiency of the supply side of medical care will influence decision-makers as to the type of national health insurance program that is developed, when it will be implemented, and what it will cover. There will also be redistributive effects among different population groups in society, depending upon the inelasticity of the supply of medical services. Greater inelasticity will mean greater increases in prices, wages, and incomes of the providers of medical services. The rest of the population will finance such increases from their own incomes and from taxes they pay to support demand-shift programs in medical care.

By analyzing the elasticity of the supply of medical services, it is possible to forecast more accurately the effect on prices and expenditures of demand-increasing programs and to evaluate the performance of the providers of medical care. If analysis reveals that the supply of medical services is determined solely by the nature of the production function for producing those services, and further, that the providers are attempting to minimize their costs, then very few changes will be possible to improve the performance of the industry. The increase in medical prices and the type of output being produced could not be altered without serious and harmful effects on the industry and the patients. If, however, the production function is artificially constrained by legal restrictions, and there are few incentives for the providers to minimize their costs of production, it would be possible to improve the performance of the medical sector.

In evaluating the performance of each of the medical markets, our first step will be to examine the market structure of each of the separate markets, beginning with the institutional settings in which care is provided, proceeding to the manpower markets, and ending with the education markets. Each medical market will be compared with a hypothetically competitive medical market. The competitive market is used as the yardstick for comparison, since it is inclusive of the conditions necessary for economic efficiency. The performance that might be expected under a competitive market will then be compared with what is observed in the particular medical market. Any divergence in performance between what is expected theoretically and what is observed will be analyzed in terms of differences in the structure and assumptions underlying the hypothetically competitive and actual markets. Public policy recommendations to improve the performance of the particular market studied will be made with reference to the differences in the structure and, consequently, the expected performance of the two markets.

Market performance can presumably be improved through alternative approaches: First, the actual market can be restructured to more closely approximate a competitive industry, wherein decisionmaking is decentralized and greater reliance is placed on competitive pressures to achieve the goal of economic efficiency. Alternatively, greater emphasis can be placed on regulation and centralized decisionmaking to achieve the desirable outcomes of a competitive market. Under either of these approaches there needs to be a comparable set of measures by which to evaluate the performance of each market. Unless there is some similarity between the desired outcome measures, differences between the advocates of increased regulation and the proponents of greater use of market pressures will be expressed in terms of value judgments rather than in more measurable terms reflecting the most efficient way to achieve a given outcome. In the health field, proposals for restructuring the delivery of medical services are often based more upon a general set of values that stop short of a clear definition of what the performance outcomes of the industry should be. If the health industry is evaluated using performance measures that are different from those traditionally used in evaluating economic efficiency, those measures should be clearly enunciated and the implicit values underlying them should also be clearly explained. The two approaches suggested for improving market performance—increased regulation versus greater reliance on market pressures—will also be examined. A theoretical analysis and empirical evidence will be provided to indicate what might be expected to occur under these different approaches toward improving market performance in medical care.

For each of the institutional and educational markets, we are interested in the following aspects of economic efficiency: (a) Is each "firm" (hospitals, physicians' offices, medical schools) minimizing its costs of production? (b) Is the number of firms in the industry the "right" number; that is, is each firm taking advantage of whatever economies of scale may exist? (c) Are the firms, and the industry as a whole, producing both a type and a quantity of output demanded by the consumers?

Taking each of the foregoing concerns in order, in a competitive industry, (a) each firm must be efficient, otherwise it will not be able to survive; (b) the number of firms in the industry is determined by two factors: first, the extent of economies of scale in production, that is, in the long run, each firm is operating at that plant size that is most efficient, namely, at the minimum point on the long-run average cost curve, and second, the importance of patient travel cost; and (c) the suppliers each respond in the short run to changes in demand (and in the long run through the entry of new firms). To what extent does this performance occur in each of the medical markets? For each of the institutional and educational markets an analysis will be made of firm efficiency, of system efficiency (which determines the number of firms), and of the supply response to changes in demand. To the extent that there are indications of inadequate performance in any particular industry, we will examine several of the assumptions that underlie a competitive industry: Is entry permitted into that industry by other firms, what are the goals and objectives of the suppliers, and what are the payment and incentive mechanisms in that industry? Major segments of the medical sector, such as hospitals and medical schools, are dominated by nonprofit firms. Do their objectives, which differ from those of traditional for-profit firms, lead to either desirable or undesirable differences in performance? Did previous cost-based reimbursement methods in certain medical markets have any effects on performance? What effects are new payment systems expected to have? Finally, what have been the effects on performance of barriers to entry into various medical markets that have been advanced on the grounds of consumer protection?

CHAPTER 8

The Market for Health Insurance: Its Performance and Structure

It is important to determine how efficiently each sector of the medical care market performs. If these separate submarkets do not perform efficiently, then there may be a legitimate role for public intervention to increase the efficiency of the marketplace. Government intervention to increase efficiency is different from, and should be kept separate from, government intervention to redistribute the output of the medical care market. A government policy that attempts to do both simultaneously, either through a government agency or comprehensive regulation, may do neither as well as separate policies directed toward either efficiency or equity.

Economic efficiency should be judged from both the demand side and the supply side of the market being examined. Economic efficiency with regard to supply usually means two things: that the number of firms in the market is the "right" number—that is, each firm operates at a minimum point on the long run average cost curve; and that each firm attempts to minimize its cost of production—that is, achieve internal efficiency. With respect to the demand side, adjudgment of economic efficiency is based on the "optimal" quantity (and varieties) of the product being produced. In discussing the performance of each of the markets being studied, we shall examine economic efficiency in demand as well as in supply. Hypotheses will be offered to explain possible divergence from economic efficiency, since any intervention to improve economic efficiency in this market should be consistent with the reasons for inadequate performance.

THE DEMAND SIDE OF THE HEALTH INSURANCE MARKET

The Market Demand for Health Insurance

The factors affecting the aggregate demand for health insurance, as discussed previously, are the price of insurance, the probability of loss, the magnitude of the loss if it occurs, the income of the consumer, and how risk averse the individual is. With increases in the price of medical care, the size of the potential loss increases, which in turn causes an increase (shift to the right) in the demand for health insurance. Increases in incomes lead to a greater demand for fringe benefits, which in turn also results in an increase in the demand for health insurance. (An increase in the aggregate demand for health insurance represents an increase in the percentage of the population with some insurance, an increase in the portion of the bill covered by insurance, as well as coverage for new benefits.) The price elasticity of the overall market demand for health insurance is considered to be approximately − 1; for each 1 percent increase in the price of insurance there will be a 1 percent decrease in the demand for insurance (1).

The Demand for Health Insurance Faced by the Individual Firm

Health insurance is provided primarily by Blue Cross and Blue Shield (BCBS) plans, which are nonprofit, and the commercial carriers, which are for-profit. A small but growing portion of the health insurance market consists of prepaid health plans, such as Kaiser Permanente. More recently, a number of larger companies have decided upon self-insurance as an alternative means of providing their employees with health insurance. Smaller companies are also considering this option, together with a reinsurance component, to protect themselves against catastrophic losses. Thus the increased aggregate demand for health insurance has expressed itself in increased demand for each of these competitive arrangements. Table 8–1 shows the increase in the population covered by hospital insurance both over time and by type of carrier.

What is of interest in this table is the changing market shares by type of insurance company. Since 1970, the share of the market held by commercial carriers has remained relatively stable at approximately 57 percent of the market. Blue Cross's share has declined over that period from 47 percent in 1970 to 40 percent in 1984. Independent plans, which include prepaid health plans, company self-insurance plans, and administrative service contracts only, have increased their share of the market from 5 percent in 1970 to almost 29 percent in 1984. Although the overall market demand for health insurance may not be very responsive to the price of insurance, that portion of the aggregate demand sold by each firm is much more price elastic. The simple reason is that although there are few substitutes for health insurance in general, there are good substitutes available for any one firm selling insurance. The demand curve facing each firm is more elastic than the aggregate demand for insurance; however, each firm is not a perfect substitute for every other firm. Each firm has some leeway in how it sets its price (i.e., determines its insurance premium). One of the factors that differentiate one firm from another is the type of benefits provided; not all firms offer the

TABLE 8-1. Enrollment of Persons with Hospital Expense Protection, 1950–1984

Year	Civilian Population	Net Number of Persons Insured (Thousands)		Commercial Insurance		Gross Number of Persons Insured (Thousands)			
		Total Number[a]	Percent of Population	Number	Percent of Total[b]	Blue Cross–Blue Shield		Independent Plans	
						Number	Percent of Total[b]	Number	Percent of Total[b]
1950	151,135	76,639	50.7	36,955	48.2	37,645	49.1	4,445	5.8
1955	164,588	101,400	61.6	53,480	52.7	48,924	48.2	6,545	6.5
1960	179,386	122,500	68.3	69,226	56.5	57,464	46.9	5,994	4.9
1965	193,223	138,671	71.8	77,642	56.0	63,662	45.9	6,984	5.0
1970	203,849	158,847	77.9	89,688	56.5	75,464	47.5	8,131	5.1
1975	214,931	178,180	82.4	99,547	55.9	85,762	48.1	13,145	7.4
1979	223,880	186,808	83.4	105,263	56.3	83,500	44.7	25,502c	13.7
1980	226,451	189,000	83.5	107,313	56.8	83,500	44.2	33,152c	17.5
1981	228,976	188,340	82.3	108,372	57.5	82,600	43.9	40,305c	21.4
1982	231,271	191,069	82.6	112,728	59.0	77,900	40.8	48,246c	25.3
1983	223,529	189,891	85.0	109,580	57.7	76,000	40.0	53,560c	28.2
1984	235,671	188,166	79.8	107,217	57.0	75,900	40.3	54,106c	28.8

SOURCES: *Source Book of Health Insurance Data; 1986 update* Washington, D.C.: Health Insurance Association of America, 1986); pp. 3–4; Blue Cross–Blue Shield statistics obtained from Arlene F. Flom, Information Services, 676 North St. Clair Street, Chicago, IL 60611; population figures come from Bureau of the Census, *Statistical Abstract of the United States, 1986*, 106th edition (Washington, D.C.: U.S. Department of Commerce, December 1985).

[a]Duplicate coverage (i.e., similar coverage by more than one insurer) has been eliminated in this column. No adjustment has been made for duplicate coverage in the other columns.

[b]Percentages of total, based on total net number of persons insured.

[c]Estimates.

same type of insurance coverage and they differ on the use and extent of copayments. The insurance carriers also differ as to whether the patient is reimbursed by the insurance company after he or she has reimbursed the health care provider, or whether the insurance company pays the provider directly. Insurance companies also have different reputations, and in markets where information on the relative performance of competing firms is not complete, people may be willing to pay a higher price for what they perceive to be a favorable reputation.

The "product," health insurance, differs both according to "real" characteristics, such as type of coverage, patient cost-sharing arrangements, and methods of payment of claims, as well as according to perceived differences in product, such as reputation for payment of claims. We would therefore expect to observe price differences between insurance firms in accordance with these product differences. If the prices of insurance differ between firms by a greater amount than what is justified by product difference, we would expect groups of insured persons to begin to switch their insurance coverage. Thus, insurance companies will compete among themselves for the insured population on the basis of price as well as in terms of product differences. If insured groups move between insurance firms according to differences in prices and products, the market will perform in an efficient manner. The "product" will be expected to change over time and also to conform more closely to the preferences of the insured group.[1] If additional firms selling insurance enter the industry, we would expect the resulting price competition to bring the price of insurance relatively close to the pure premium; that is, the cost of administration, claims processing, and marketing functions would be produced efficiently and there would be no excess profits in the industry. (The more price elastic the demand curve facing the individual firm, the closer the price will be to average costs and the less likelihood there will be of excess profits in the long run.) The efficient performance of this industry is not contingent upon each consumer's having perfect information regarding all the price and product differences among firms. The costs of acquiring such information are clearly too great for each individual; however, large groups such as unions would be expected to develop such expertise. Also, since approximately 85 percent of insurance is purchased by groups, it is the information acquired by these groups that brings about competition among insurance firms. (Because such information is costly to acquire, we might also expect the product and price differences to be more favorable to large groups that acquire it.)

The price of insurance that we have been referring to is the benefit/premium ratio, which is the percent of the total premium paid out in benefits to each insured group. If, for example, the premium for each member in a group were $1,000 per year and the utilization experience of that group resulted in an average payout of benefits equal to $900 per member per year, the benefit/premium ratio would be .9. The difference between benefits and total premiums goes to administration, claims processing, marketing, and profit for the insuring firm. When the benefit/premium ratio is close to 1.0, the group is "experience rated," which means that the premium reflects the expected experience of the group. The more the health insurance industry approximates a competitive industry, the closer we would expect the benefit/premium ratio to be 1.0. Where information is inadequate or where there are monopolies in the sale of

---

[1]Since there are such large differences in the costs of handling a group and an individual, we would expect that most individuals in a group would prefer to forgo the benefits of individually tailored policies to take advantage of the lower cost of a single group policy.

TABLE 8-2. Ratio of Benefit Expenditures to Premium Income, According to Type of Plan, 1955–1986

Year	All Plans	Blue Cross–Blue Shield			Commercial Insurance Companies			Independent Plans[a]
		Total	Blue Cross	Blue Shield	Total	Group Policies	Individual Policies	
1955	.805	.887	.915	.824	.725	.839	.530	.912
1960	.855	.921	.928	.904	.789	.904	.529	.965
1965	.874	.939	.953	.901	.819	.936	.547	.906
1970	.915	.958	.973	.922	.872	.958	.581	.962
1975	.927	.982	1.001	.939	.886	.984	.511	.867
1980	.928	.967	.973	.959	.888	.909	.645	.944
1981	.928	.966	.974	.952	.890	.891	.674	.956
1982	.919	.942	.949	.929	.892	.902	.648	.951
1983	.914	.920	.926	.911	.900	.903	.645	.952
1984	.889	.895	.899	.889	.872	.861	.650	.926
1985	– [b]	.904	.909	.899	– [b]	– [b]	– [b]	– [b]
1986	– [b]	.940[c]	.943[c]	.936[c]	– [b]	– [b]	– [b]	– [b]

SOURCES: This table was developed from data provided in Marjorie Smith Carroll and Ross H. Arnett, "Private Health Insurance Plans in 1978 and 1979: A Review of Coverage, Enrollment and Financial Experience," *Health Care Financing Review*, 3 September 1981: p. 75; figures after 1979 come from unpublished data from the Health Care Financing Administration, Blue Cross–Blue Shield data obtained from Arlene F. Flom, Information Services, BC/BS, 676 North St. Clair Street, Chicago, IL 60611.

[a] "Independent Plans" includes plans that offer health services on a prepaid basis, and self-insured health plans.
[b] Data not available.
[c] Estimate.

health insurance, there is greater divergence from 1.0 in the benefit/premium ratio. In a competitive industry we would expect groups to change insurance companies when their benefit/premium ratio surpasses the amount they are willing to pay for real or perceived product differences between firms. One indication of the performance of the industry would be the variation in benefit/premium ratios when size of group is held constant: the smaller the variation, the more efficient the market. (Because of economies of scale in administering different-sized groups, the larger the size of group, the closer the benefit/premium ratio would be to 1.0.) Not only would price reflect the minimum costs of producing the services of the insurance industry in a competitive market, but the choice of insurance packages would most closely approximate the preferences of the insured group.

To provide some indication of the competitiveness, hence performance, of the health insurance industry, it is important to examine the pricing of health insurance policies.

Table 8–2 shows the ratios of expenditures (benefits) to premiums by different types of insurance plans for the period 1955–1986. There are two points of interest in this table. First, the benefit/premium ratio for both the Blues and commercials have increased over time. The relative closeness of these ratios, both between the Blues and commercials and to a benefit/premium ratio of 1, suggests that this is a relatively price-competitive industry. [2] Second, the differences in the benefit/premium ratio between group and individual policies indicate the large savings to an individual from participating in a group plan.

A further indication of the price competitiveness of the insurance industry was the approach used by Blue Cross for many years to price its insurance coverage (community rating) and how market forces caused a change in that approach.

The Efficiency and Equity Aspects of Community Rating

When Blue Cross was started, premiums were based on the concept of community rating; that is, premiums were the same to all subscribers regardless of the experience of the group. (Blue Cross initially covered only hospitalization, which is still the dominant form of its coverage.) Aged persons, who would be expected to have much higher hospital use rates than younger persons, were charged the *same premium*.[3] The benefit/premium ratio for aged persons was, therefore, greater than 1.0; the benefits paid on their behalf exceeded the premiums they paid for insurance. Since the average benefit/premium ratio for all groups in a community rating system had to be close to 1.0, this meant that groups of low users of hospital services had benefit/premium ratios of much less than 1.0.

The effect of community rating, when the expected costs of groups differ, is that a subsidy is provided to high-use groups, financed by a "tax" on the lower-use groups (2). Any such "subsidy-tax" system can be evaluated on the basis of two economic criteria: first, its effect on efficiency—namely, does it affect the quantity of health insurance purchased?—and second, its equity—does such a redistribution scheme cause the higher-income subscribers of Blue Cross to subsidize the lower-income subscribers?

With regard to the efficiency aspects of community rating, low-user groups are typically low-risk groups. There is a certain amount above the pure premium that the individual is willing to pay for health insurance. Charging low-risk groups an amount above their pure premium much greater than the amount they would be charged if they were experience rated would result in fewer low-user groups' purchasing insurance. Such low-user groups might decide to self-insure rather than pay the Blue Cross community rate. Depending upon the price elasticity of demand for insurance, low-user groups would, under community rating, demand less insurance. Like an excise tax that is placed on some goods and services and hence distorts their relative prices, a community rate is a tax on the insurance premium of a low-risk person. The result of such a "tax" is a decreased demand for health insurance coverage. Changing from a community rating system to one based on experience rating should result in the low-risk group's purchasing more health insurance. For this reason a community rate is considered economically inefficient. (A similar inefficiency occurs when a monopolist charges a price for a service that exceeds its cost of production.) Community rating

---

[2]It may be argued that the increasing benefit/premium ratio is the result of more efficient methods of administration. Increased computerization of claims processing has undoubtedly occurred over the time period examined. However, unless there were competition between firms, these decreased administrative costs would not have been passed on to the subscribers; the benefit/premium ratio could have remained the same and the companies would instead have received larger profits. Competition forces these savings to be passed on in either lower premiums or greater benefits, thereby increasing the ratio.

[3]Even under community rating, however, premiums differed according to whether the individual was married or single and whether or not he or she belonged to a group.

does not permit the low-risk person to purchase insurance at its costs of production, which is its actuarial value plus administrative cost.

Perhaps the main reason for community rating, according to its advocates, was that it enabled persons who would otherwise not be able to afford health insurance to pay the premium. Without government subsidies, Blue Cross, in using community rating, acted as a welfare agency as it subsidized high-risk/low-income persons by taxing low-risk/higher-income persons.[4] The redistribution argument in favor of community rating offered by its proponents can be countered by the argument that community rating is an inefficient mechanism for redistributing medical care, and a mechanism that may not have had its desired effects.

Using risk as a basis for determining a subsidy for medical insurance involved the assumption that all high-risk people have lower incomes than those of low-risk people. This may be accurate on the average, but there are certainly high-risk aged persons who have higher incomes than those of low-risk younger persons. The direction of the subsidy, however, goes from the low risk to the high risk, regardless of their relative incomes. Further, the actual subsidy goes to the group that *uses* hospital services more, not necessarily to the group that has the highest risk of hospitalization. A study of Michigan Blue Cross revealed that the most heavily subsidized group were auto workers. The next most heavily subsidized group was comprised of health care professionals—physicians, nurses, and other hospital employees (3). These subsidized groups were *not* the lowest-income groups belonging to Michigan Blue Cross. (One possible reason for the auto workers' being subsidized in their purchase of Blue Cross is that they represent a large group with more market power than that of many of the other smaller groups that belong to Blue Cross.) What appears to have occurred in practice under community rating was that the subsidy-tax concept operated in reverse: higher-income persons were subsidized by lower-income persons.

If everyone agreed on the value judgment that subsidies should be provided to lower-income families to purchase health insurance, these values could be realized more efficiently through a system of direct subsidies to those families instead of authorizing Blue Cross to operate the subsidy-tax system. Blue Cross's goals do not include being the most efficient welfare agent. Instead, Blue Cross may attempt to increase its enrollment, and in so doing, it will allocate its taxes and subsidies according to a policy that will facilitate the greatest increase in its growth. This policy would be to charge lower premiums to groups whose demands are more elastic, such as large unions, and higher premiums to groups with less elastic demands, instead of matching the subsidy to income level.

The community rating concept used by Blue Cross was inefficient because it raised the price of health insurance to low-user groups, thereby decreasing their demand for health insurance. Their demand for health insurance was less than if they had been experience rated. Community rating was also an inefficient method of distributing subsidies for the purchase of health insurance.

Community rating, as a pricing system for health insurance, could not survive in a price competitive market. Unless community rating were legally mandated as the method for pricing premiums among all health insurance companies, competitive

---

[4]An additional reason suggested for community rating is that it is insurance with a longer time horizon. Since everyone grows old, the young (low-risk) who subsidize the aged eventually receive such a subsidy themselves. Still another reason offered is that the administrative costs for determining the necessary information to experience-rate each group may outweigh the possible savings to different groups receiving a lower premium.

forces would cause insurance premiums to become experience rated. If Blue Cross used community rating, a competitor could sell health insurance to lower-user groups at a price that approximated their expected experience rate. Assuming a comparable insurance product, low-user groups would be expected to switch their insurance coverage away from Blue Cross. As more lower-user groups left Blue Cross, the Blue Cross premium to the remaining subscribers would increase, in turn causing additional groups that were subsidizing others to change their insurance coverage. As long as the various groups purchasing health insurance attempt to maximize their health care benefits per dollar spent and if the groups had sufficient information on the different benefit packages, premiums charged by different companies, and performance of insurance companies in payment of claims, a community rated system would not be expected to survive in a competitive environment. Obviously, not every group has the necessary information or expertise to determine whether it should insure with a company other than Blue Cross. All it takes for the community rating concept to be changed, however, is for a few groups to decide to change their coverage. Some companies (or unions) have a sufficiently large number of employees to provide them with an incentive to develop the expertise and information on alternatives to Blue Cross. All purchasers in the market do not have to be informed for competition in health insurance to work. If only some of them have the necessary information and act on it, the effects of their behavior will be sufficient to produce a more competitive rate structure; price competition among the insurers will result in lower rates to the smaller, less-informed groups.

As expected, Blue Cross abandoned its community rating concept as competition from commercial insurance companies increased. This provides some evidence that competition in the health insurance market causes providers to respond to consumer demands. Some of the larger Blue Cross plans, less subject to competitive pressures, have not gone all the way to experience rating. They have what is called "merit rating," which is a modified experience rate that allows for some subsidies and taxes to different groups. It is doubtful, however, that these subsidies and taxes are based on the incomes of the group; they are more likely related to the size of the group and the likelihood of its switching to another insurance company.

Even legally mandating community rating among all insurance carriers would not be a workable system. The major health insurance benefit offered by Blue Cross under community rating was service benefit coverage for hospital care: Blue Cross paid each hospital on the basis of the hospital's own costs or charges; the patient was not responsible for any hospitalization costs and was entitled to a semiprivate accommodation while in the hospital. If subscribers have different preferences regarding the benefits for which they would like to purchase insurance and the amount of copayment desired (both of which determine their premium), it would be very difficult to maintain a series of community rates that would accommodate such preferences. Maintaining a community rate for the single set of benefits provided by Blue Cross, when subscribers differ in their utilization experience and in their preference for benefits and cost sharing, is highly inefficient. Diversity in consumer preferences can be dealt with most efficiently by a health insurance system that offers a variety of benefits, cost-sharing arrangements, and rate structures. If it is determined that certain groups have incomes that are inadequate to purchase a "minimum" level of health insurance, and if it is society's desire to provide them with at least a minimum level of health insurance, subsidies can be provided directly to those groups instead of mandating a similar insurance scheme for all persons that would be administered by a company that would use an internal subsidy and tax system.

THE SUPPLY SIDE OF THE HEALTH INSURANCE MARKET

Based on the discussion above, it appears that the demand side of the insurance market is quite competitive. The supply side is examined next to determine the efficiency with which health insurance is produced. Efficiency in production concerns both the number of firms selling health insurance, that is, the extent to which there are economies of scale among health insurance firms, and whether each firm is itself operating in the most efficient manner. The determination of economies of scale would indicate how many firms could compete in the sale of insurance and whether or not the insurance business is a "natural" monopoly; that is, can the functions performed by insurance companies be performed less expensively by just one firm? Following is a discussion of the evidence on economies of scale in the production of health insurance.

There are financial requirements for becoming a supplier of health insurance, such as minimum reserve requirements. These requirements, however, have not been sufficiently restrictive to prevent new firms from entering different regional markets. There are currently over 1,000 for-profit commercial health insurers and 85 Blue Cross and Blue Shield plans.

It is difficult to estimate empirically the extent of economies of scale among different health insurance carriers. Determining the reasons for differences in costs between companies for performing the administrative function requires the assumption that each company performs the same tasks and does them equally well. In fact, however, the administrative function varies among firms. The range of functions includes marketing and selling policies, processing applications and policies, maintaining the policy file, processing claims, reviewing claims, and paying claims. The variety of contracts offered, each entailing a different cost, and the extent to which the company has group or individual policies (it is more costly to handle individual policies) will also differ among firms; taxes may be included in the commercial companies' expenses but not in those of Blue Cross. It is difficult to compare the differences in costs, taking care to separate differences that are due to economies of scale from differences in efficiency and in functions performed.

One investigation that attempted to analyze the effect on administrative cost of differences in the size of health insurance carriers, while holding constant the effect of other factors, involved several separate studies. Using data from the early 1970s, Vogel and Blair examined economies of scale for commercial health insurance companies only, since their output mix (e.g., variety of contracts, percentage of nongroup policies, etc.) is so different from that of Blue Cross. The authors determined that economies of scale do exist and that the administrative cost ratio declines with increased size of operation (4). When economies of scale were investigated separately for Blue Cross and for Blue Shield (in their non-Medicare business), no economies of scale were found. The authors then included in their analysis BCBS plans that had merged. They observed lower administrative costs for these merged, larger firms. Based on these studies, the authors concluded that economies of scale do exist in the nonprofit sector, although the gains from such economies are offset by internal inefficiency ("x-inefficiency") because they are nonprofit firms (5).

In a follow-up study, Blair and Vogel undertook a "survivors" analysis to test for economies of scale among health insurers (6). In this type of analysis, firms are assigned to different categories according to their size. The growth of firms in each size category is studied over time. If substantial economies of scale exist, then firms in the largest size classes will grow rapidly at the expense of firms in the smaller size categories. Smaller firms will either have to expand their scale of operation (and/or merge) or they will be forced to leave the industry. The authors found that all but the smallest size categories expanded over the period 1958–1973. They concluded that economies of scale existed but that they were not as large as originally believed, since other size categories also grew.

Vogel and Blair also attempted to determine whether economies of scale exist in the administration of Medicare Part A (hospital claims payment). They found results opposite of what they expected. Administrative costs per claim increased with the size of the firm. The interpretation of this finding was that the method of Medicare reimbursement of intermediaries, which was cost-based, encouraged higher administrative costs (7). An experiment in the method of selecting Medicare Part B contractors provided an opportunity for determining the existence of economies of scale in this portion of the Medicare business. The government was permitted to award Medicare Part B contracts in selected areas on the basis of a competitive bid. Even though the administrative cost per claim had declined from $6.56 in 1971 to $2.62 in 1981 (in constant 1981 dollars), submitted bids were quite low relative to their historical cost and lower than carriers reimbursed on a cost basis (8). The author concludes that with respect to economies of scale, approximately 7 percent of the annual administrative cost of Part B could be saved if small firms were merged.

Fixed-price contracting, that is, providing a financial incentive to firms for performing the Medicare Part B intermediary function at their lowest cost, revealed that greater internal efficiency among the intermediaries is possible as well as determining that there are significant economies of scale in performing such functions. A similar experiment is being undertaken with regard to the intermediary functions for Part A of Medicare. It would appear that sizable savings to the government are possible if Medicare intermediaries were chosen and paid according to a competitive bid rather than the current cost-based payment system.

As determined from the studies above, there are substantial economies of scale in the insurance industry, and under appropriate incentives, firms can be internally efficient. There are, however, several aspects of the health insurance industry that not only distinguish it from other industries but also affect the degree of competition among firms.

Blue Cross and Blue Shield have received certain competitive advantages over commercial insurers that are believed to enable BCBS to achieve greater market shares than they would otherwise. One such advantage was that because Blue Cross plans are nonprofit, they received more favorable tax treatment than did commercial companies:

> Typically, the Blue Cross and Blue Shield plans pay no premium tax while the commercial insurers pay 2 percent or so. As a percentage of the insurance firms' costs, this 2 percent represents an enormous advantage for the Blues. For example, only 5 percent of Blue Cross premiums are kept to pay expenses. Thus, the typical tax advantage lowers Blue Cross costs by more than 30 percent. Blue Shield expenses are a larger percentage of premiums, but even for Blue Cross

and Blue Shield combined, only about 8 percent of premium income pays expenses, so that the premium tax break alone lowers costs by more than 20 percent.

Furthermore, many states exempt the Blues from other taxes that commercial insurers must pay, such as property taxes. Some states regulate the ratio of benefits to premiums for commercial insurance sold to individuals. This eliminates sales of certain types of commercial policies with high selling costs or administrative costs or both (9).[5]

Frech conducted an empirical study to determine the effect that the 2 percent tax advantage had on Blue Cross's market share. It was estimated that Blue Cross was able to increase its market share, on average, by 6.7 percent.

A more recent study, however, concludes that the premium tax advantages of the Blues is not that large. The authors find that eliminating the Blues' tax advantages would decrease their market share by only 1 percent (10).

In return for such favorable tax treatment, however, the Blues have been subject to greater regulation by the insurance commissioners in each state, who must approve their premium increases. Some states have limited the amount of premium increase that the Blues wanted to charge their nongroup enrollees. Some Blue Cross plans also have open enrollment periods. The regulation by insurance commissioners over the Blues' actions toward their nongroup enrollees is believed by the Blues to result in higher rates for their more competitive group business. To escape such regulation, a number of Blue Cross plans have become mutual insurance companies.

The Blues, however, lost their federal tax-exempt status under the tax reform legislation passed at the end of 1986. Over Blue Cross and Blue Shield objections, the need for additional federal revenues, and perhaps as a result of a Government Accounting Office (GAO) report, a change was made in the tax status of the Blues. The GAO report found that the pricing practices of the Blues were similar to those of the commercials, namely experience rating of large groups; there were few subsidies for high-risk individuals enrolling in the Blues; that the Blues had profit-making subsidiaries; that the open enrollment programs of the Blues varied (not all the plans had such programs and some placed restrictions on the medical benefits available during these open enrollment periods); and that "all these activities tend to reinforce the perception that the plans are similar to commercial companies" (11).

A second competitive advantage that the Blues have over the commercials (which they retain) is that the Blues do not compete with one another. Blue Cross is a loose federation of independently operating plans joined together by an interplan system for handling claims incurred in other areas. The national Blue Cross organization provides certain important functions, such as representing all Blue Cross plans in their relations with the federal government and testifying on legislation affecting the health

---

[5]In a study on *The Regulation of Health Insurance* (unpublished doctoral dissertation, Department of Economics, University of California, Santa Barbara, 1974), H. E. Frech states that "most states charge no premium taxes on Blue Cross while charging between .5 percent and 4.0 percent of premium for domestic and foreign (out of state) commercial insurers" (p. 59). In his empirical findings, Frech finds that "regulation of rates or prices of health insurance leads to a higher Blue Cross market share, more extensive insurance purchases and higher prices and quantities in the hospital market." He concludes: "An examination of the actual regulation of health insurance and of the legal status of Blue Cross hospital insurance plans, which are controlled by hospitals, shows that health insurance regulation provides competitive advantages for Blue Cross over commercial insurers" (p. xii).

insurance industry. Each Blue Cross and Blue Shield plan has a monopoly within its market over its type of service.[6] If one Blue Cross firm is more efficient and wishes to expand its market, it cannot enter another Blue Cross plan's area. (Should a Blue Cross plan try and do so, however, it may be able to do so in the current climate of the applicability of antitrust laws to the health field.) Each Blue Cross plan benefits by being the designated representative of Blue Cross's reputation and by being the only one to offer the Blue Cross insurance package to subscribers. Commercial companies, on the other hand, compete with one another as well as with Blue Cross.

The third, and perhaps most important, competitive advantage that Blue Cross has over the commercial insurers is that Blue Cross receives a discount compared with the charges that commercial companies pay to hospitals for the same care in the same institution. According to one study, the hospital discount averaged 14 percent for Blue Cross plans in 1979, with a range of 4 to 27 percent, as compared to only 4 percent for commercial insurers. The effect of this greater discount for the Blues resulted in an average increase in their market share of 7 percent (12).

Another important effect of the Blue Cross hospital discount is with regard to preferred provider organizations (PPOs). A PPO usually consists of one or more providers (e.g., hospitals or physicians) that offer to discount their services for an exclusive arrangement with a purchaser. Insurance companies and the Blues, in addition to providers themselves, may organize providers into PPOs and market them to employers. The subscriber to a PPO pays lower premiums or prices when they restrict their choice of provider to only those participating in the PPO. In those areas where Blue Cross receives a substantial hospital discount, a non-Blue Cross PPO has a competitive disadvantage. In an area where Blue Cross may be receiving a 20 percent hospital discount, an insurance company marketing a hospital PPO would have to negotiate a greater than 20 percent discount with its participating hospitals if it were to be able to convince its PPO subscribers to restrict their use of hospitals.

If one type of firm in a competitive market had a cost advantage, it could undercut the prices of other firms and drive them from the market. The cost advantage could provide the firm with a monopoly position. If this were to occur, the public would receive the benefits of that cost reduction in terms of lower prices. However, when Blue Cross plans with a cost advantage are analyzed, it appears that they have been able to increase their market shares but not to the extent thought possible by researchers investigating this issue. This finding has led researchers to develop several hypotheses as to how Blue Cross groups use their competitive advantage. Since the Blues are nonprofit organizations, there is the issue of what the Blues do with their increased market power. To whom do the competitive advantages of BCBS accrue? Are the consumers the beneficiaries, in terms of lower health care costs? Or, alternatively, are the beneficiaries the providers, hospitals and physicians, and the Blues themselves, in terms of higher salaries and internal "slack" within the organization?

Frech argues that since the Blues are nonprofit and their governing boards are often controlled by hospital and physician representatives, the Blues use their competitive

---

[6]Each Blue Cross plan was required to sign up 75 percent of the hospitals and beds in its area. M. Olson claims that "this requirement ensured that no Blue Cross plan could select only the most efficient hospitals in its area. Its effect was to reduce competitive pressures on less efficient hospitals." Mancur Olson, "Introduction" in Mancur Olson, ed., *A New Approach to the Economics of Health Care* (Washington, D.C.: American Enterprise Institute, 1981), p. 10.

advantages to benefit both the providers of care and those working for the Blues (13). For example, hospitals favor complete coverage for hospital care; such coverage increases the demand for hospitals and removes the patient's incentive to shop around. By having Blue Cross use their cost advantage to subsidize the sale of this type of coverage, hospitals benefit. Therefore, the Blues benefit the providers by offering their subscribers more complete insurance plans, such as paying a higher percentage of the hospital bill than commercial carriers and not having copayments or deductibles. With lower out-of-pocket costs, the subscribers will increase their demand for medical care. The consequence of this type of coverage is that providers are able to raise their prices and hospital costs increase faster than they would otherwise.

Because the Blues were controlled by the providers, it was in the interest of providers that the Blues had competitive cost advantages. When viewed in this manner, it was also in hospitals' interests to provide Blue Cross with a discount. Hospitals used the discount as a way of providing Blue Cross with a competitive advantage; the price of Blue Cross coverage was lowered relative to commercial insurance. Hospitals thereby benefited by assisting the expansion of a preferred (more expensive) type of hospital coverage. Weller distinguishes between discounts that are procompetitive (i.e., a firm is a tough bargainer and tries to get the lowest price possible from its suppliers) and discounts that are anticompetitive (i.e., a supplier gives a favored purchaser a preferential price). Based on the findings that Blue Cross plans were started and controlled by hospitals and that those Blue Cross plans with relatively high market shares are also in areas where hospital costs are relatively high, Weller concludes that the hospital discount can be explained more adequately in terms of anticompetitive behavior on the part of hospitals (14).

Anticompetitive measures have also been used by medical societies and physician-controlled Blue Shield plans to make it difficult for certain insurers to compete. Assume that Blue Shield plans do not have any cost advantages over other insurers. A commercial insurer could increase its market share by reducing its premium through the use of cost-saving measures such as copayments, preauthorization of services, utilization review, and preferred providers. To prevent the growth of such plans, medical societies have both boycotted and threatened to boycott patients with this type of insurance coverage. In this manner, providers have precluded certain types of coverage from being offered in the insurance market.[7]

---

[7]Goldberg and Greenberg describe how early (1930s–1940s) insurance companies in Oregon placed restraints on physician utilization. Preauthorization of services and monitoring of claims were used. When they were faced with competition, the insurance companies acted to lower their costs. Physicians accepted such constraints on their behavior since it was during the depression; physicians did not have as many patients and were not sure of their ability to collect from those they did have. Consumers benefited from the utilization review and the lower insurance premiums. The response to this situation by the medical societies in Oregon was twofold: first, to threaten expulsion from the medical society of physicians that participated in such insurance plans; second, the medical societies started their own insurance plans. These plans did not use aggressive utilization review procedures. With the growth of their own insurance plan, physicians were encouraged to boycott the other insurance plans. The effect of these policies was to increase the growth of the insurance plan sponsored by organized medicine and to cause a decline in the other insurance plans. To receive the participation of physicians, these other plans also had to become less aggressive in their cost containment efforts. Lawrence G. Goldberg and Warren Greenberg, "The Emergence of Physician-Sponsored Health Insurance: A Historical Perspective," in Warren Greenberg, ed., *Competition in the Health Care Sector* (Germantown, Md.: Aspen Systems Corporation, 1978).

The cost advantage of the Blues can also be used to benefit their management and employees. They can pay themselves higher salaries, work in more pleasant surroundings, and have a larger staff than necessary.

As a test of the hypotheses that the Blues use their competitive position to benefit both the providers of care and those working for the Blues, Frech and Ginsburg conducted an empirical study and found that Blue Cross plans with greater market power, namely those with a larger market share, offered more complete insurance coverage (15). Frech and Ginsburg also attempted to estimate the effect that increased market power has on the Blues' efficiency. Since Blue plans are nonprofit, it was hypothesized that the managers and employees also share in the Blues' competitive advantage. Frech and Ginsburg found that Blue Cross and Blue Shield plans with lower taxes, hence a competitive advantage, had higher administrative costs per enrollee (16).

Several studies, including a Federal Trade Commission investigation, have been conducted on Blue Shield plans to determine whether the regulatory advantages of such plans, which lower their costs relative to those of commercial insurers, benefit the physicians in control of the plan, Blue Shield plan administrators, or consumers by lowering the price of insurance and thereby increasing Blue Shield's market share.

Eisenstat and Kennedy hypothesized that greater physician control of Blue Shield plans should result in an increase in the efficiency of the plan; greater plan efficiency would result in more funds being available to increase reimbursement to the providers. In their empirical work, the authors found that for Blue Shield plans having a tax, hence competitive, advantage over commercial insurers, their administrative costs decreased as the percentage of physicians on the Blue Shield board increased. However, for those Blue Shield plans without a tax advantage, hence less market power, the composition of the board had no significant effect on the plan's administrative costs (17). The authors concluded that in markets where the Blues had a competitive advantage, the physicians were the beneficiaries and acted to reduce inefficient operations. Among plans that have no competitive advantage, market competition acts to reduce any plan inefficiency.

Sloan concluded that in physician-controlled Blue Shield plans, reimbursement levels and the number of services provided were greater than in those plans not controlled by physicians (18). Arnould and DeBrock found that in physician-controlled plans with cost advantages the benefits went to the physicians in the form of higher fees (19). Plan administrative costs and Blue Shield market share were lower in physician-controlled plans, thereby enabling the physicians to capture the benefits of the regulatory advantages for themselves. In non-physician-controlled plans, the authors found that at least some of the benefits went to the plan administrators.

Lynk, however, concludes that physician fees would not be increased in physician-controlled plans (20). He argues that if Blue Shield is acting in the physician's interest, it will set its maximum allowable charge equal to the median charge in the market area. If it were above the median charge, then physicians whose charges were below that level—the majority of physicians—would benefit by a reduction of the maximum allowable charge. The majority of physicians would benefit because they would receive the patients that shift away from those physicians with higher fees that are no longer fully reimbursed by Blue Shield. When the maximum allowable charge equals the median fee in the market area, a majority of physicians will be satisfied, and the market will be stable. Thus physician-controlled Blue Shield boards should result in lower, not higher, average levels of payment for insured procedures.[8] However, regardless of whether physician control of Blue Shield plans increases or decreases physician fees, the author agrees that physician control will be used to benefit the physicians.

CONCLUDING COMMENTS

Blue Cross was established by hospitals and grew at a rapid rate because it was able to see the vast potential demand for coverage of health care costs. The commercial insurance companies, entering the market after Blue Cross, also grew, because of their product and pricing innovations. They offered a benefit coverage (major medical insurance) that was different from that offered by Blue Cross, they offered indemnity payments rather than a service benefit policy to subscribers and providers, and they priced their premiums according to the experience of the group. Unless competition had been possible, it is unlikely that consumers would have been offered a greater choice in benefits, cost-sharing arrangements, and premiums to match their own experience.

The overall conclusion that appears to emerge from the studies described above is that the Blues have certain competitive advantages over the commercials. To the extent that individual Blue plans have been able to benefit from these advantages, they have been able to increase their market shares. As a result of their increased market power, the Blues have been able to sell more comprehensive health insurance, which has benefited the providers and led to increased health care costs. The Blues themselves have also benefited from these competitive advantages. The internal efficiency of the firm is affected by the objectives of the firm and the extent to which it is subject to competitive pressures. Their increased market power as a result of these cost advantages has enabled the Blues to have greater organizational slack than would have been possible in a competitive market. With regard to the studies of economies of scale, it appears that economies of scale do exist in the administrative function in health insurance companies. However, large Blue Cross and Blue Shield companies, which are less subject to competitive pressures, appear to have internal "slack," which more than offsets gains resulting from economies of scale. Therefore, if monopolies were created to administer any national health insurance scheme, either at a national or regional level, in order to take advantage of economies of scale, the lack of competitive pressures as a result of having a monopoly (such as allowing the Social Security Adminis-

---

[8]In a discussion on whether physician-controlled Blue Shield plans are anticompetitive, which was the subject of the Federal Trade Commission inquiry, Watts claims the results from both the Sloan and Lynk studies are inadequate on this point. Both studies focus on input prices (the fees paid to participating physicians), rather than on the policy premiums, which are more appropriate indicators of market competition. As long as there are no entry barriers, premiums for similar policies should be comparable. Thus the competitiveness of the insurance market cannot be determined by whether physician reimbursement levels are high or low. Carolyn A. Watts, "FTC Sings the Blues: A Comment," *Journal of Health Politics, Policy, and Law*, Fall 1980.

tration to perform this function) might cause administrative costs to be higher than if more firms competed against one another.[9]

Maintaining a competitive market structure for Blue Cross and commercial companies forces these companies to respond to consumer demands for different types of insurance coverage and to minimize their administrative costs. In such a situation, health insurance will be produced at the lowest cost and the type of services available will approximate the demands of the insured group. The incentives inherent in such competition are more effective for achieving economic efficiency in the demand and supply of health insurance than having one large firm administer a standard insurance policy for everyone. Innovations in benefit packages and in cost minimization are more likely to occur when there are strong competitive pressures than when firms, whether they are for-profit or nonprofit, are protected from such competition.

The benefits of increased competition in the insurance market appear to be passed on to the purchasers of insurance. As shown in Table 8-2, the benefit/premium ratio appears to average at approximately .9 over time. As insurance companies attempt to reduce their costs, such as by reducing hospital use, unless these cost savings were passed on to the purchasers, the benefit/premium ratio would get smaller and smaller. Since the ratio remains relatively constant, this suggests that insurance firms are competing away any savings that they are able to achieve.

Given the foregoing, admittedly brief description of the supply side of the health insurance market, what changes, if any, should be made? In the administration of health insurance under public programs (Medicare and Medicaid), it appears that cost-based reimbursement to intermediaries provides them with no incentives to perform their functions at minimum cost. Reimbursement of intermediaries might be changed to a competitive-bid basis; the performance of the intermediaries should be monitored to ensure that all administrative functions contracted for are carried out.

Individuals lack information on insurance benefits and on the performance of competing insurance companies. Further, it is costly for consumers to gather this information. This lack of information, however, is more severe for individuals who are not a part of groups. For the vast majority of the insured population who purchase their insurance through the workplace, assistance in their choice of insurance company is provided either by their employer or by their union. In an increasingly competitive insurance market where there are a greater number of choices facing the individual, along a number of product and price dimensions, it would be desirable if additional information on insurance products and premiums became more readily available.

Blue Cross and Blue Shield plans no longer enjoy a competitive federal tax advantage over commercial firms. A number of Blue Cross plans, however, still have a large cost advantage in the form of a hospital discount.

The health insurance industry is becoming very competitive. As shown in Table 8-1, although the population is slowly increasing, the percentage of the population

---

[9]Hsiao attempted to determine whether competitive pressures resulted in lower administrative costs. For the years 1971 and 1972, he compared the administrative costs under the Medicare program, which was administered by the Social Security Administration, with that of the Federal Employees Health Benefit Program (FEBP). The FEBP was administered by a consortium of private carriers, which included both profit and nonprofit firms. After adjusting for some differences in the functions performed in administration of the two programs, he found that administrative costs per claim were lower under the FEBP. Hsiao concluded that the greater efficiency of the private firms was due to the competition among those firms. William Hsiao, "Public Versus Private Administration of Health Insurance: A Study in Relative Economic Efficiency," *Inquiry*, 15, December 1978.

with hospital insurance is remaining relatively stable, at approximately 80 percent. The implication of this for health insurers is that it is becoming more difficult for them to increase their enrollments. Independent plans, such as prepaid, company self-insurance, and administrative services only, are experiencing the largest percentage growth, almost sixfold, from 5 to 29 percent since 1970. If the insurance carriers are to at least maintain their market shares, they will have to be competitive with respect to their premiums and their insurance products.

Continued large increases in their insurance premiums have made business firms aware of the impact this has on the firms' labor costs, and consequently on the prices of their goods and services. Labor leaders are also aware that merely to maintain the same health benefits, their members will have to forgo wage increases. It is therefore likely that the trend toward self-insurance by large companies and experimentation with prepaid health plans will continue to remain an important alternative to the traditional insurance coverage (21).

Both the commercials and the Blues are diversifying their insurance products. In addition to their traditional coverage, namely unlimited subscriber choice of hospital and physician provider, these companies are also forming their own prepaid health plans and PPOs for those subscribers who are willing to restrict their choice of provider in return for greater benefits and/or lower premiums.

Increased competition among health insurers is likely to have adverse effects upon hospitals. To keep their premiums competitive with other insurance companies, as well as with prepaid health plans, insurance companies will have to reduce their expenditures for hospital care. Hospital expenditures are a major portion of the insurance premium, representing 93 percent of Blue Cross expenditures (22). First, insurance companies are likely to place greater pressure on hospitals to hold down the rate of increase in hospital costs. Second, the insurers will attempt to reduce hospital utilization of their subscribers through stronger utilization review mechanisms and by insuring less costly substitutes for hospital care. The effect of these policies should be to reduce the portion of the insurance premium that is spent on hospitals.

Competitive pressures and the high portion of their premium represented by hospital expenditures provides Blue Cross with an incentive to control hospital expenditures. However, important to understanding the limited and generally ineffective approach used by Blue Cross in the past, namely, controls on increases in the number of beds, was the fact that Blue Cross was started, supported, and controlled by hospitals. Hospitals viewed Blue Cross as a means of increasing the demand for hospital care and of insuring payment to hospitals for their services. As such, it was not in the interests of hospitals to have Blue Cross provide any coverage to patients other than for hospitalization. Out-of-hospital coverage could serve only to decrease hospital utilization. Similarly, it was not in the interests of hospitals to have Blue Cross include any copayments such as coinsurance, because this would provide patients with an incentive to shop around for the least costly hospital. To compete with Blue Cross, commercial companies offered lower-priced coverage by including patient cost sharing and coverage for out-of-hospital care. Blue Cross, whose benefits were entirely for hospital care, could have kept its premiums from rising rapidly by introducing patient cost-sharing provisions, by monitoring hospital costs, or by decreasing hospital utilization. The first two approaches would have placed Blue Cross in an adversary position with the hospitals that controlled it. Therefore, the only other approach was to control hospital utilization indirectly by decreasing the availability of hospital beds in an area. Blue Cross was already committed to reimbursing hospitals for all of their beds, whether or not they were filled. If Blue Cross could prevent new hospitals from being built, it would not be in conflict with existing hospital administrators. Controls on hospital beds could limit total hospital utilization; because Blue Cross's premium consisted of a greater portion of hospital costs than did the premiums of commercial companies, Blue Cross's premium would be reduced by a proportionately greater amount.

Increased competitive pressures among insurance companies for insured groups has led Blue Cross to undertake more direct and effective cost control approaches, such as utilization review, out-of-hospital coverage, patient incentives, monitoring of hospitals costs, and preauthorization on admissions.

These intensified competitive pressures are changing Blue Cross's traditional relationship to hospitals. Blue Cross is developing a more adversarial relationship with hospitals in order to survive in this new environment.

REFERENCES

1. In a recent review article, Pauly concludes: "The results generally support the view that the impact of loading or loading proxies on insurance purchases is significantly negative. The actual numerical estimates of the elasticity of insurance with respect to the loading 'price,' however, vary considerably, ranging from about − 0.2 . . . to numbers greater than unity . . . ." Mark V. Pauly, "Taxation, Health Insurance, and Market Failure in the Medical Economy," *Journal of Economic Literature*, 24, June 1986: p. 644.

2. For a more extensive discussion of community rating, see Pauly, "The Welfare Economics of Community Rating," *Journal of Risk and Insurance*, September 1979.

3. *Health Care Insurance Regulation Program: An Assessment of Effectiveness*, Executive Office of the Governor, Lewis Cass Building, Lansing, Mich., March 1973, p. 11.

4. Ronald J. Vogel and Roger D. Blair, *Health Insurance Administrative Costs*, Social Security Administration, Office of Research and Statistics Paper 21, October 1975, p. 56.

5. *Ibid.*, p. 63.

6. Roger D. Blair and Ronald J. Vogel, "A Survivor Analysis of Commercial Insurers," *Journal of Business*, 51, July 1978.

7. Ronald J. Vogel and Roger D. Blair, *Journal of Business*, October 1975: 92–93. Also, in another study of the performance of Medicare (Part A) processing costs, H. E. Frech found lower cost per dollar processed, lower average processing time (in days), and fewer errors per $1,000 processed in for-profit as compared to not-for-profit firms. H. E. Frech III, "The Property Rights Theory of the Firm: Empirical Results from a Natural Experiment," *Journal of Political Economy*, February 1976.

8. Stephen T. Mennemeyer, "Effects of Competition on Medicare Administrative Costs," *Journal of Health Economics*, 3(2), August 1984: 137–154.

9. H. E. Frech III, "Blue Cross, Blue Shield, and Health Care Costs: A Review of the Economic Evidence," in Mark V. Pauly, ed., *National Insurance: What Now,*

What Later, What Never? (Washington, D.C.: American Enterprise Institute, 1980), 251–252.

10. Killard Adamache and Frank Sloan, "Competition Between Non-Profit and For-Profit Health Insurers," <i>Journal of Health Economics</i>, 2(3), December 1983: 225–243.

11. <i>Health Insurance: Comparing Blue Cross and Blue Shield Plans with Commercial Insurers</i>, Report to the Chairman, Subcommittee on Health, Committee on Ways and Means, House of Representatives (Washington, D.C.: U.S. General Accounting Office, July 1986), p. 20.

12. Adamache and Sloan, <i>op. cit.</i>

13. Frech, "Blue Cross, Blue Shield, and Health Care Costs."

14. Charles D. Weller, "On 'FTC Sings the Blues' and Its Respondents," <i>Journal of Health Politics, Policy and Law</i>, Summer 1982.

15. H. E. Frech III and Paul Ginsburg, "Competition Among Health Insurers," in Warren Greenburg, ed., <i>Competition in the Health Care Sector: Past, Present, and Future</i> (Germantown, Md.: Aspen Systems Corporation, 1978).

16. <i>Ibid.</i>

17. David Eisenstat and Thomas Kennedy, "Control and Behavior of Non-Profit Firms: The Case of Blue Shield," <i>Southern Economic Journal</i>, 48, July 1981.

18. Frank A. Sloan, "Physicians and Blue Shield: A Study of the Effects of Physician Control on Blue Shield Reimbursements," in <i>Conference Proceedings, Issues in Physician Reimbursement</i> (Washington, D.C.: Health Care Financing Administration, Department of Health and Human Services, 1980).

19. Richard J. Arnould and Lawrence M. DeBrock, "The Effect of Provider Control of Blue Shield Plans on Health Care Markets," <i>Economic Inquiry</i>, 23(3), July 1985: 449–474.

20. William J. Lynk, "Regulatory Control of the Membership of Corporate Boards of Directors: The Blue Shield Case," <i>Journal of Law and Economics</i>, April 1981.

21. For a more complete discussion on the self-insurance option, see Richard Egdahl and Diana Chapman Walsh, eds., <i>Containing Health Benefits Costs: The Self-Insurance Option</i>, Springer Series on Industry and Health Care 6 (New York: Springer-Verlag, 1979).

22. Marjorie Smith Carroll and Ross H. Arnett, "Private Health Insurance Plans in 1978 and 1979: A Review of Coverage, Enrollment, and Financial Experience," <i>Health Care Financing Review</i>, 3, September 1981: p. 79.

CHAPTER 9

The Physician Services Market

INTRODUCTION AND OVERVIEW

Physician services may be provided using different combinations of physicians and other health manpower. Physicians may undertake to perform all of their tasks themselves or they may delegate varying amounts of those tasks to their auxiliaries. With a greater degree of task delegation, physicians will be able to increase their productivity and provide a greater variety of services than do physicians who use fewer auxiliaries. The extent to which physicians delegate their tasks will affect not only the quantity and type of physician services available but also their cost. In evaluating how well the supply side of the physician services market performs, an examination will be made to determine whether physician services could be produced at lower cost and whether a greater variety of services could be provided than is currently the case.

Even if it were determined that physician services are produced at minimum cost, the prices at which they are sold might be greatly in excess of their costs. If such a situation were to exist, fewer physician services would be purchased than if their prices were lower and closer to the costs of production. Thus, another measure of how well the market for physician services performs is the relationship of prices to costs in that market; because it is often difficult to measure costs directly, this price–cost relationship may be inferred through the method by which physician prices are determined. In relatively competitive markets, prices will approximate costs; in monopolistic markets, the seller's price may greatly exceed the cost of providing that service. If, after an examination of the physician services market, it is determined that a greater quantity (and variety) of physician services, at lower prices, is possible in this market, policies to achieve such an outcome will be proposed.

The emphasis of this chapter is on the efficiency with which physician services are provided rather than on the efficiency with which medical treatments, of which physician services are an important component, are produced and priced. In a subsequent chapter we discuss the broader issues, which have important ramifications for the physician services market itself. To delineate further the subject area included in this

172

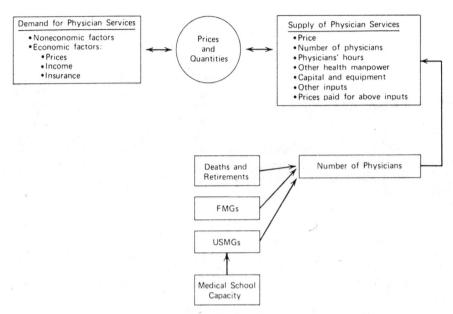

Figure 9-1. The market for physician services.

chapter, it should be noted that the determination of the optimal number of physicians in the labor market is excluded; the market for medical education is also discussed in a separate chapter. Although these markets are closely related to the market for physician services, the rationale for discussing these subjects and the pricing and provision of physician services separately is that the determinants of the number of physicians are not identical to the factors that determine the quantity of physician services or how they are priced. The interrelationship between these two markets, the determinants of supply and demand in each market, and the different types of public policies that influence these separate markets are more easily visualized with reference to Figure 9-1.

The demand for physician services is determined by factors such as those discussed previously. There are noneconomic factors, such as need and cultural-demographic factors; the economic factors are the patient's income, the price the patient must pay for physician services (as well as the price of substitute and complementary services), the type and comprehensiveness of insurance coverage, and any time costs that are involved in the purchase and use of physician services. The supply of physician services is affected by the price received for physician services and by the cost of producing those services, which depends upon input productivities and input prices. These are affected by the number of physicians, the amount of hours they work, their use of auxiliaries, the capital and equipment available, and other inputs and expenses necessary to the provision of physician services, such as malpractice coverage.

The price of physician services, as shown in Figure 9-1, is determined by the interaction of both supply and demand factors; in turn, price influences patient demand and the amount of services providers are willing to provide. How the physician services market differs from the traditional demand and supply models is also discussed.

On the supply side of the market, the number of physicians combined with other inputs determines the available supply of such services. In the short run, all of the inputs except physicians can be varied. Physician hours, which can also be varied, are determined by the labor–leisure trade-off; what happens to the physician's hours of work as both the price received per hour of work and his or her income increases? Namely, do physicians reduce their hours of work as their prices increase? The long run is that period of time in which there can be an increase in the number of physicians. Changes in the number of physicians result from deaths and retirements, immigration of foreign-trained medical graduates and physicians, and increases in the number of U.S.-trained medical graduates (USMGs). The number of USMGs is determined by the demand for and supply of medical education. The demand for a medical education is influenced by a number of factors, among which is the relative rate of return to such an education; as shown in Figure 9–1, the price and quantity determined in the physician services market (which is equivalent to gross physician income) is a component of that rate of return.

Government policies have intervened at several points in the physician markets. With respect to the demand for services, Medicare and Medicaid have served to stimulate the demand for services among specific population groups. Further, the imposition of federal price controls between 1971 and 1974 controlled the annual percent increase in physician fees. In addition to the direct effects of these two programs, there were also indirect consequences: persons not subsidized by Medicare and Medicaid faced higher prices for physician services; controls on physician prices affected the quantity of those services, the hours physicians were willing to work, and the time patients had to wait to receive such services.

Government policies on the supply side have been directed at increasing the number of physicians by providing subsidies for both the construction of new medical schools and for existing schools to increase their enrollments. Loans and scholarships have also been provided (through the medical schools) to medical students, which influences their demand for a medical education. The government has affected the inflow of foreign-trained medical graduates and physicians by its immigration policies. Of more direct effect on the supply of physician services has been legislation at a state level that places limits on who can practice medicine and defines the tasks that may be performed by various categories of health manpower.

As shown in Figure 9–1, medical education is an important determinant of the number of physicians and, consequently, the supply of physicians' services. Separate chapters are devoted to an analysis of both the physician manpower and medical education markets, to include the development of their structural characteristics, their consequent effect on performance, and the relevant public policies within each market.[1] In this chapter the performance of the physician services market is evaluated to determine whether physician services are produced in the least costly manner and whether the prices charged for such services are related to their costs of production. A better understanding of costs and the determination of prices in this market will en-

---

[1]Quality-assurance mechanisms are placed, primarily, on medical inputs, such as on the training requirements for physicians, and not on the services provided. The development of such "process" quality measures has had important effects on the structure of health manpower and health education markets. Alternative approaches to achieving quality assurance, and their effect on performance, are therefore discussed in chapters dealing with the manpower and education markets.

hance our ability to predict physician prices and expenditures. The consequences of public policy in this market should also be more easily anticipated.

As a basis for evaluating the performance of the market for physician services, observed measures of performance will be compared with what might be expected to occur in a hypothetical competitive market. The reasons for any possible divergence between the observed and hypothetical outcomes will then be analyzed. Policies to improve the performance of the physician services market will be suggested based on the structural characteristics of a competitive market that give rise to desired outcomes.

OBSERVED PERFORMANCE IN THE PHYSICIAN SERVICES MARKET

Variations in Physician Fees

In a competitive market, prices for similar services would be expected to vary within a relatively narrow range. Prices are unlikely to be identical even for seemingly comparable services, for several reasons: some patients may prefer particular physicians because of real or perceived quality differentials; patients may incur less waiting time when seeing certain physicians and therefore be willing to pay higher physician fees; and there are always search costs involved in finding a particular physician. Since it is costly to gather information on different physicians, some patients who place a high value on their time will do less search and be willing to take a chance on paying higher prices. In fact, identical prices in a market such as physician services would be more indicative of collusion or price fixing than of competition. If prices for specified services diverge too greatly, however, some patients will be willing to shift to other providers. As the price differential increases, it will eventually exceed the value the patient places on particular providers and on perceived quality differences. Although prices for the same physician services are unlikely to be exactly the same, they would be expected to vary only within a narrow range.

Physician fees for the same procedure have shown substantial variation, both between geographical areas and within an area. For example, in 1984, the average physician fee for an initial limited office visit, new patient, varied between $31 and $53 between two counties in Florida; for a normal delivery, the fees varied from $775 to $1,450 (1). In 1985, cardiologists in Montgomery County, Maryland, charged between $100 and $300 for a stress test; 22 percent of the physicians in that county charged $1,200 to $1,499 for a transurethal resection of the prostate, while 25 percent of the physicians charged more than $2,000; and surgeons in the Baltimore area charged between $450 and $1,030 for a hernia repair (2).

The range in fees within a locality is usually smaller than the range between cities. Variations in prices are reduced as patients seek lower prices. Even in competitive markets, search costs, time costs, and quality differentials among physicians would be expected to result in price differences. But it is questionable whether these factors can explain the relatively large price differences for similar services within an area or a city. Also contributing to price variation, particularly between cities and regions of the country, are differences in wage rates and in costs of living. However, even when physician fees are adjusted for differences in costs between cities, fees for similar surgical procedures are still almost twice as great between cities. Based on these data, it would appear that the range in fees for similar services is greater than would be expected in a competitive market.

Increases in Physician Fees

In a competitive system the level at which physician fees are established over time is determined by the cost of providing the service. One would expect increased prices to occur in the short run to ration demand; in the long run, however, one would expect increased prices to reflect the costs of the output provided. When the actual trend in physician fees is examined, it appears that fees have increased more rapidly than the costs of providing physician services. As shown in Table 9-1, physician fees have generally risen more rapidly than either the Consumer Price Index (CPI) (all items less medical care) or the All Services component of the Consumer Price Index. Prior to 1965, physician fees rose faster than the CPI. When Medicare and Medicaid were passed in 1966, physician fees increased at an even faster annual rate. In 1966 and 1967, the CPI increased by 3.0 percent and 2.4 percent, respectively. In those same years, physician fees increased by 5.8 and 7.1 percent, which was more than twice the annual rate of increase in physician fees for the previous five years. Price controls were imposed on the U.S. economy in mid-1971 and remained in effect for the medical care sector until April 1974. During that period, physician fees increased at a little over 3 percent per year. After the removal of price controls, physician fees rose sharply, from 3.3 percent in 1973 to 9.2 percent in 1974, reaching 12.3 percent in 1975. In 1976, physician fees rose twice as fast as the CPI and their annual rate of increase remained above the CPI for the next several years. In 1979 and 1980, however, the CPI increased more rapidly than physician fees. Between 1981 and the present time, physician fees have been increasing faster than the CPI.

It is possible that the more rapid increase in physician fees in recent years is the result, in part, of measurement error. As more of the physician's fee is paid by insurance companies and government, a smaller portion of the patient population pays the physician's usual and customary fee, which is what is collected as part of the CPI. The CPI does not take into consideration what the physician actually receives. Medicare, Medicaid, and Blue Shield do not pay the physician's billed fee; fee screens are used and the physician's fee is often reimbursed at a lower amount. Thus only a small portion of the physician's patients may be paying the fee measured by the CPI.

Expenditures on physician services have continued to increase over time, even when adjusted for population change, as shown in Table 9-2. After the passage of Medicare and Medicaid, physician expenditures increased rapidly. The imposition of price control in the medical sector between 1971 and 1974 slowed the rate of increase in expenditures; however, immediately following the removal of those controls in 1974, physician expenditures increased sharply, reaching 17.5 percent in 1975. After several years of high annual increases in the late 1970s and early 1980s, the rate of increase diminished. However, it should be kept in mind that the rate of inflation in the economy has decreased, thus even though the rate of increase in physician expenditures has decreased, it is still much higher than the increase in the CPI. The more recent annual increases in physician expenditures appear to be, in large part, a result of price increases rather than increases in physician visits. The population has in-

TABLE 9-1. Annual Rate of Change in the CPI and in Physician
Fees, 1955–1987

Year	CPI All Services Less Medical Care	CPI All Items Less Medical Care	CPI Physician Fees
1955–1960	2.0	3.5	3.3
1960–1965	1.2	1.8	2.8
1966	3.0	3.4	5.8
1967	2.4	3.7	7.1
1968	4.1	4.9	5.6
1969	5.4	6.8	6.9
1970	5.8	8.3	7.5
1971	4.1	5.3	6.9
1972	3.3	3.8	3.1
1973	6.4	4.3	3.3
1974	11.1	9.2	9.2
1975	8.9	9.1	12.3
1976	5.5	7.9	11.3
1977	6.2	7.3	9.3
1978	7.6	8.6	8.3
1979	11.4	11.2	9.2
1980	13.6	15.9	11.7
1981	10.3	13.4	11.0
1982	5.9	8.7	9.4
1983	2.9	2.9	7.7
1984	4.1	5.2	7.0
1985[a]	3.4	5.1	5.2
1986	3.7	5.1	6.8
1987	1.0	3.9	8.1

SOURCE: Bureau of Labor Statistics, *CPI Detailed Report*, various issues.

Note: The rates of change are based on the change in the annual average of each index listed in the Table. The All Urban Consumer Index is used for 1978–1987. Prior to 1978 the only available index was for urban wage earners and clerical workers.

[a]Data are from February CPI Detailed Report and therefore measures change from February 1984 to February 1985.

creased at less than 1 percent per year and the number of visits per patient has remained relatively steady; thus the major portion of the increase in expenditures must be attributed to increases in physician prices.[2]

An important change that has been occurring over time with regard to payment for physician services is the increasing role of third-party payors. As shown in Table 9-2, direct consumer payment has declined from 61.4 percent of total physician expendi-

---

[2]It is also possible that there has been an important change in the definition of a visit in the last several years. For example, an increase in the number of services per visit would be reflected in a higher price per visit but not as an increase in the number of visits. If there has been a large increase in the number of services per visit, it must be determined whether these additional services were in fact demanded by patients or whether it is a means whereby physicians can increase their revenues.

TABLE 9-2. Total Expenditures on Physicians' Services by Source of Funds, 1950–1985

Calendar Year	Physician Expenditures (Billions)	Annual Increase in Total Expenditures (%)	Per Capita Physician Expenditures	Distribution of Physician Expenditures (%)				
				Total	Direct Payment	Third-Party Payment		
						Total	Private Insurance	Public Insurance
1950	$ 2.7	—	$ 17.76	100	83.2	16.8	11.4	5.2
1955	3.7	6.5	21.91	100	69.8	30.2	23.2	6.7
1960	5.7	9.0	30.92	100	65.4	34.6	28.0	6.4
1965	8.5	8.3	42.82	100	61.4	38.6	31.7	6.9
1970	14.3	11.0	68.74	100	45.1	54.9	33.9	20.9
1971	15.9	11.2	75.35	100	44.9	55.1	33.3	21.7
1972	17.2	8.2	80.36	100	42.4	57.6	34.8	22.8
1973	19.1	11.1	88.45	100	41.8	58.2	34.9	23.2
1974	21.2	11.0	97.60	100	37.9	62.1	37.0	25.0
1975	24.9	17.5	113.38	100	36.2	63.8	37.6	26.2
1976	27.6	10.8	124.17	100	31.5	64.9	39.1	25.8
1977	31.9	15.6	142.05	100	35.7	64.3	39.0	25.2
1978	35.8	12.2	158.03	100	36.6	63.4	37.7	25.7
1979	40.7	13.7	177.65	100	37.7	62.3	36.1	26.2
1980	46.6	14.5	201.18	100	37.3	62.7	36.3	26.4
1981	54.8	17.6	230[a]	100	29.7	70.3	42.8	27.4
1982	61.8	12.8	257[a]	100	28.7	71.3	43.8	27.4
1983	69.0	11.7	282[a]	100	27.7	72.3	44.0	28.3
1984	75.4	9.3	307[a]	100	27.8	72.2	44.4	27.8
1985	82.8	9.8	335.36	100	26.3	73.7	44.4	29.3

SOURCES: Robert M. Gibson and Daniel R. Waldo, "National Health Expenditures, 1980," *Health Care Financing Review*, 3, 1981: 32–35, Table 3; 40, Table 5. Daniel R. Waldo, Katherine R. Louit, and Helen Lazenby, "National Health Expenditures, 1985," *Health Care Financing Review*, 8, 1985: 14, Table 2; 15, Table 3.

[a]Figures have been rounded off.

TABLE 9-3. Number of Physician Visits per Person per Year and Number of
Visits per Physician per Week

Calendar Year	Number of Visits per Person per Year	Number of Visits per M.D. per Week	Number of Visits per M.D. per Week[a]
1958–1959	4.7	—	—
1963–1964	4.5	—	—
1966–1967	4.3	124.1	—
1968	4.2	—	—
1969	4.3	126.9	—
1970	4.6	132.5	—
1971	4.9	135.8	—
1972	5.0	—	—
1973	5.0	137.7	—
1974	4.9	125.8	—
1975	5.1	126.5	139.2
1976	4.9	128.5	137.2
1977	4.8	—	—
1978	4.8	130.6	136.3
1979	4.7	122.7	129.6
1980	4.8	—	—
1981	4.6	—	—
1982	5.2	—	130.9
1983	5.1	—	125.3
1984	5.1	—	120.4
1985	5.3	—	118.4

SOURCES: The data for the number of visits per person per year came from the National Center for Health Statistics, "Current Estimates of Health Interview Surveys," *Vital and Health Statistics*, Series 10 (Washington, D.C.: Department of Health, Education and Welfare, various years); and Marcus Goldstein, *Income of Physicians, Osteopaths, and Dentists from 1965–1969*, (Washington, D.C.: Department of Health, Education and Welfare Publication 155A, 73-1182, 1972), p. 49. The data for the number of visits per M.D. per week came from Marcus Goldstein, *op. cit.*, p. 48; David Goldfarb, ed., *Profile of Medical Practice, 1981* (Monroe, Wis: American Medical Association, 1981), p. 156, Table 14; Martin Gonzalez and David Emmons, eds., *Socioeconomic Characteristics of Medical Practice, 1986* (Chicago: American Medical Association, 1986), p. 56, Table 13.

[a]Data in this column are based on information from physicians in all specialties, excluding psychiatry, radiology, anesthesiology, and pathology. The column to the left differs because it includes these specialties.

tures in 1965 to 26.3 percent in 1985. The rise in government as a payor of physician services has increased from less than 7 percent to almost 30 percent over that period. Physicians have become more reliant not only on third parties but are more affected by government payment methods.

Table 9–3 shows the trend in visits per person, which started increasing at the start of the price control program in 1971 and has remained relatively constant, except for a slight increase in recent years. Also of interest in Table 9–3 is the trend in weekly visits per physician, which has been falling since 1975. A possible explanation for this decline in visits per physician is the limited increase in patient demand (relatively constant over the last several years) and the increasing supply of physicians (see Table 13–2) to compete for that limited demand.

When physician fees were increasing faster than the costs of providing those services and visits per physician were also increasing, physician incomes would also be expected to increase rapidly. This is apparently what occurred after Medicare and Medicaid were passed. Between 1965 and 1975, physician incomes increased by more than 100 percent, which was a more rapid rate of increase than that of dentists, lawyers, and most likely, any other profession. Except for psychiatry, the annual rate of increase in physician incomes exceeded that of the CPI. However, since the mid-1970s, the incomes of primary care physicians have not kept up with the rate of inflation. As shown in Table 9–4, since 1975, "real" incomes of primary care physicians have fallen.

The data on physician fees, visits per physician, and physician real income appear to be consistent with each other in showing that a change occurred in the physician services market in the late 1970s.[3]

The Production of Physician Services at Minimum Cost

If physician services were produced in a competitive market, cost-minimizing behavior would result in physicians hiring the optimal number and mix of auxiliaries, and the size of the physician's practice would be determined by the extent of economies of scale in providing services.

As a first step in determining whether physicians are minimizing the cost of providing their services, it is necessary to estimate a production function for physician services. Estimates of the productivity of each of the inputs used in producing physician services and the extent of economies of scale can then be made. An important problem in specifying and estimating a production function is the definition and measurement of outputs and inputs. Unless outputs and inputs are measured accurately, the results of the studies will be questionable.

The output—physician services—consists of examinations, treatment, tests, history taking as well as health education, record keeping, and patient billing. Detailed information on the quantity and mix of each of the services provided in a physician's office is generally unavailable. Empirical studies must therefore use proxy measures for physician services. One often-used proxy for the output of a physician's practice is the weekly number of office visits. When office visits are used, it is implicitly assumed that quality differences, if any, will not bias the results of the study. In physician productivity studies it is also generally assumed that the mix of patient visits among different

---

[3]Also indicative of this change in the physician market during the late 1970s is the changing geographic distribution of physicians. With the increase in the supply of physicians during the 1970s, there has been an increase in the number of physicians locating in small communities. "The percentage of small cities and towns with specialists grew appreciably during the period 1970 to 1979. In general, the specialties that grew the most (in percentage terms) also moved in the largest numbers into previously unserved towns" (p. 2392). This diffusion of physicians into smaller communities is contrary to the views of those who believe that physicians can create their own demand so as to locate where they prefer. Instead, these changes in the geographic distribution of physicians are believed to be the result of competitive market forces. As the supply of physicians continues to increase, these trends in location patterns of physicians should continue during the 1980s. Joseph P. Newhouse, Albert P. Williams, Bruce Bennett, and Williams B. Schwartz, "Where Have All the Doctors Gone?" *Journal of the American Medical Association*, May 7, 1982. See also William B. Schwartz, Joseph P. Newhouse, Bruce Bennett, and Albert P. Williams, "The Changing Geographic Distribution of Board-Certified Physicians," *New England Journal of Medicine*, October 30, 1980.

TABLE 9-4. Average Pretax Net Income from Medical Practice by Specialty, Selected Years

Specialty	1965	1970	1975	1980[a]	1985	Annual Percent Growth 1965–1975	Annual Percent Growth 1975–1985
General practice	$23,000	$33,900	$45,400	$ 67,100	$ 77,900	7.0	5.5
Internal medicine	27,800	40,300	57,000	80,700	101,000	7.4	5.9
Surgery	34,300	50,700	68,200	107,300	155,400	7.1	8.6
Pediatrics	24,500	34,800	44,300	62,800	77,100	6.1	5.7
OB/gyn.	29,700	47,100	63,300	101,300	122,700	7.9	6.8
Psychiatry	30,600	39,900	44,800	66,600	88,600	3.9	7.1
Anesthesiology	31,900	39,400	57,100	105,000	140,200	6.0	9.4
Radiology	43,000	—	75,200	—	150,800	5.7	7.2
All specialties	—	41,800	56,400	107,500	113,200	—	7.2
CPI all items	94.5	116.3	161.2	247.0	319.1	5.5	7.1

SOURCES: Zachary Dyckman, *Study of Physicians' Income in the Pre-Medicare Period-1965*, United States Department of Health, Education, and Welfare, Social Security Administration (Washington, D.C.: U.S. Government Printing Office, 1976), p. 10. David Goldfarb, "Trends in Physicians Incomes, Expenses and Fees: 1970–1980," in David Goldfarb, ed., *Profile of Medical Practice* (Monroe, Wis.: American Medical Association, 1981), p. 114, Table 1. *Socioeconomic Characteristics of Medical Practice* (American Medical Association, 1986), p. 106, Table 39.

Note: In 1981 the American Medical Association changed its methodology for calculating physician incomes from its Periodic Surveys of Physicians to its Socioeconomic Monitoring System Core Surveys. Therefore, there may be slight differences between the post-1981 data and the pre-1981 data.

[a] 1980 figures have been interpolated from 1979 and 1981 figures.

181

TABLE 9-5. Estimated Optimal Levels of Aide Input at Various Weekly Salaries and Net Proceeds per Visit (Solo General Practitioners)

Net Proceeds Per Visit	Weekly Cost Per Aide		
	$70	$100	$160
$ 5	3.7	3.2	1.6
7	4.0	3.7	2.9
10	4.2	4.0	3.5

Source: Uwe Reinhardt. Reprinted with permission from *Physician Productivity and the Demand for Health Manpower* (Cambridge, Mass.: Ballinger, 1974), p. 184, Table 6-14.

physician practices is similar.[4] Over time, however, there have been important changes in the physician output mix. For example, there has been a large increase in the proportion of all physician services performed by specialists. Further, since the 1930s there has been a large decline in the number of home visits, with a corresponding increase in the number of office and hospital visits and telephone consultations. For example, between 1930 and 1965, home visits declined from 45 percent of total outpatient visits to only 4 percent. Since the time spent by a physician on an office visit is approximately half that of a home visit, this change in output mix over time contributed to a large increase in physician productivity (3).

Another output proxy used is annual gross patient billings. Although this measure may reflect differences in quality and service mix among practices, it contains a serious problem in that higher patient billings may not reflect differences in output but may result from higher prices being charged for similar services.

The measurement of manpower inputs in production function studies is also troublesome. In addition to quality differences among manpower of a given type, which affect their relative productivities, the categories of health manpower employed in physicians' offices vary. Physician extenders, such as physician assistants and pediatric nurse practitioners, are the closest substitutes for the physician and are more productive than are allied health workers (e.g., registered nurses), medical technicians (e.g., x-ray and lab technicians), and nonmedical assistants (e.g., clerical and administrative persons). Productivity estimates of auxiliaries are likely to fall within a wide range and thereby bias the results unless these different manpower categories are measured separately.

A number of studies have attempted to estimate the optimal use of inputs and the extent of economies of scale in physician practices. Based on his studies, Uwe Reinhardt concluded that the average solo physician could profitably employ twice as many auxiliaries as he or she currently does. Employing four rather than two auxiliaries, which is the current average, would result in a 25 percent increase in the number of patient visits per physician (4). As shown in Table 9-5, Reinhardt has calculated the optimal number of aides for a solo physician to hire based on the price received per visit and the weekly wage of the aide. Based on estimates of the marginal productivity of aides, the table indicates that the employment of aides should increase as the price of the visit increases; as the cost of the aide increases, the optimal number of aides decreases.

[4]If physician practices are being compared and some of these practices have different specialists or use a greater number of auxiliaries, the output mix and the productivity estimates may be systematically biased.

TABLE 9-6. Average Weekly Patient Visits, Practice Hours, and Number of Aides per Physician

Practice Mode	Average Weekly Patient Visits	Average Number of Practice Hours	Average Number of Aides Per Physician
Solo	183	60	1.81
Group	213	64	2.12
Group as percent of solo	116	107	117

Source: Uwe Reinhardt, "A Production Function for Physician Services," *The Review of Economics and Statistics* (February 1972): 60.

Other studies on the productivity of aides have reached similar conclusions. Kehrer and Zaretsky concluded that a doubling of allied health personnel in physicians' offices would result in a 20–25 percent increase in total patient visits per physician (5). These authors also found that internal medicine and general practice were more likely to be able to absorb additional auxiliaries. Kimbell and Lorant also found in their study that additional aides would add significantly to the productivity of physicians (6).

Golladay, Smith, and Miller used activity analysis to develop a normative model of how a primary care practice should be organized (7). Their procedure consisted of enumerating 263 tasks in eight major categories of activity that fully describe a typical primary care practice. Five medical school students then acted as observers in a sample of primary care practices for two-week periods and collected data on the frequency with which tasks were performed and who performed them. From this they developed a model of optimal input mix at given levels of output. They estimated that introduction of a physician assistant (PA) increases physician productivity by 49–74 percent. That is, a physician usually producing 147 office visits per week may increase that number up to 265 visits per week simply by hiring a PA.

With regard to economies of scale in physicians' practices, Reinhardt concluded that physicians in groups generate between 4.5 and 5.1 percent more patient visits and about 5.6 percent more patient billings than do those in solo practice. These results suggest that there are slight economies of scale in the production of physician services. Reinhardt also found that productivity of physicians increased with group size because of greater manpower substitution in groups (8).

As shown in Table 9-6, taken from Reinhardt's study, the average number of weekly patient visits for GPs in groups was 16 percent higher than for solo GPs. But the group practitioners also seemed to work more hours per week and employ more aides per physician; therefore, mode of practice accounted for about a 5 percent increase in patient visits.

In 1978 a large survey was undertaken of group practices (9). This comprehensive examination of group practice examined such subjects as workload of physicians, physician incentives, size and specialty of group, and method of payment for the group's services (i.e., fee for service or prepayment). The study also investigated the extent of economies of scale, however, because solo practice was excluded from the study, the findings are limited on this point. When groups of different sizes were analyzed, it was found that there was a negative effect of group size on the physician's hourly patient load; the larger the group, the lower the physician's hourly patient load. The researchers, however, did find that surgical workloads were higher in groups than were estimates derived from another study that examined all persons performing surgery. An interesting finding was with respect to the use of nonphysician inputs. In a comparison between prepaid and fee-for-service groups, it was found that prepaid groups employed approximately 28 percent more support staff and that expenditures on support staff were approximately 40 percent higher. Again, since solo practices were not included, productivity comparisons could not be made.

In another study, Frech and Ginsburg tried to determine optimal size of practice by conducting a "survivor test" (10). This technique, developed by Stigler (11), assumes that over time market competition will produce an optimal size distribution of medical practices. Until the optimum is reached, the fastest growing size is identified as the most efficient. By use of this type of analysis, Frech and Ginsburg, using data for the period 1965–1969, conclude that solo practice is very inefficient, and very small practices (3–7 physicians) and very large practices (greater than 26 physicians) are most efficient. Hence they conclude that there are economies of scale in the production of physician services.

In a follow-up study, Marder and Zuckerman examined changes in the size distribution of medical practices for three periods, 1965–1969, 1969–1975, and 1975–1980 (12). The authors conclude that in the period up to 1975 solo practices were less efficient; in the more recent period studied, 1975–1980, large groups were considered efficient whereas small and medium-sized practices were not. The authors believe that in the latter period the medical marketplace had changed.

The findings on economies of scale in physician practices appear to be confirmed by more recent data indicating that more physicians are joining group practices. In 1969, 21.7 percent of physicians were in group practice; by 1975, this had increased to 31.6 percent. There was little change between 1975 and 1980; however, between 1980 and 1984 there was a dramatic increase, the percent of physicians practicing in group practices increased from 32.8 to 44.3 percent. The fastest-growing form of group practice was the single specialty form of practice, increasing from 10.9 to 18.9 percent of physicians between 1980 and 1984. These data are shown in Table 9–7.

The recent growth in group practice is also indicated by the number of group practices over time. Again, the largest growth occurred in the single specialty groups, which experienced a 73 percent increase between 1980 and 1984. As shown in Table 9–8, there has also been an increase in the average size of each form of group practice, with the multispecialty form of practice having the largest number of members, 26.6 compared to 5.8 in single-specialty groups.

There thus appears to have occurred an important change in the structure of the physician services industry over time. The image of the typical physician being in solo practice is no longer the case. Almost half of all physicians are part of a larger economic entity, and the average size of these firms is increasing. This change in the structure of the industry will have important implications for competition in the physician services market.

There are several reasons for the recent changes in physicians' type of practice. The market for medical care has become more competitive since 1980; therefore, physicians have more of an incentive to minimize their costs by taking advantage of economies of scale. Economies exist not only in internal management but also in marketing and advertising. Large groups are more likely to be able to market their services directly to employers and to health maintenance organizations. Large groups that serve a large patient population are able to have greater leverage over hospitals that want

TABLE 9-7. Distribution of Office-Based Physicians by Group Affiliation, Selected Years, 1969–1984

Type of Practice	Number of Physicians				Percent of Physicians According to Type of Practice			
	1969	1975	1980	1984	1969	1975	1980	1984
Total office-based physicians (nonfederal)[a]	184,355	211,776	269,001	316,757	100	100	100	100
Individual practice	144,262	144,934	180,711	176,365	78.3	68.4	67.2	55.7
Group practice	40,093	66,842	88,290	140,392[b]	21.7	31.6	32.8	44.3[c]
Single-specialty group practice	13,053	23,572	29,456	59,917	7.1	11.1	10.9	18.9
Multispecialty group practice	24,349	39,311	54,122	69,371	13.2	18.6	20.1	21.9
Family or general group practice	2,691	3,959	4,712	9,839	1.5	1.9	1.8	3.1

sources: National Center for Health Statistics, *Health, United States, 1986*, DHHS Publication (PHS) 87-1232, Public Health Service (Washington, D.C.: U.S. Government Printing Office, December 1986), p. 163. J. N. Hung and G. A. Roeback *Distribution of Physicians, Hospitals, and Hospital Beds in the United States, 1969*, Vol. 2, Metropolitan Areas Center for Health Services Research and Development (Chicago: American Medical Association, 1970). Penny L. Havlicek, *Medical Groups in the United States, 1984* (Chicago: American Medical Association, 1985), pp. 4–16.

[a]"Total office-based physicians" includes all patient care physicians except residents, interns, and full-time hospital staff. In 1984 there were 316,757 office-based physicians, which excluded 69,506 residents and interns and 28,651 full-time hospital staff who provided patient care.

[b]This figure, representing physician positions, was obtained by asking groups for their number of members. Since physicians may practice in more than one group, the actual number of group physicians would tend to be smaller than this estimate.

[c]Total number of group practice is larger than the summation of the specialty breakdowns because there were 1,265 physician positions in groups whose specialty composition was unknown.

TABLE 9-8. Number and Average Size of Physician Groups, Selected Years, 1969–1984

Type of Practice	Number of Group Practices				Average Size of Physician Group			
	1969	1975	1980	1984	1969	1975	1980	1984
Total group practice	6,371	8,483	10,762	15,485[a]	6.3	7.9	8.2	9.1
Single-specialty group practice	3,169	4,601	6,156	10,635	4.1	5.1	4.8	5.8
Multispecialty group practice	2,418	2,976	3,552	2,781	10.1	13.2	15.2	26.6
Family or general group practice	784	906	1,054	1,770	3.5	4.4	4.5	5.7

SOURCE: Penny L. Havlicek, *Medical Groups in the United States, 1984* (Chicago: American Medical Association, 1985), pp. 4–16.

[a] "Total group practice" is larger than summation of specialty breakdown because this figure includes 299 groups whose specialty composition was unknown.

their patient referrals; such groups are able to negotiate joint ventures with the hospital and investment by the hospital in the group's equipment needs. Physicians within large multispecialty groups are also able to refer to other physicians within that group. In a more competitive environment, large groups are not only able to bid for contracts but also offer greater quality assurance to purchasers. Large group practices have a reputation for strong peer review procedures; poor quality of care by a colleague or a lawsuit places all the group's assets at risk.

In the past, generally up until 1980, physician practices were smaller in size than the data suggested was optimal. Yet physician practices were able to survive and even prosper. This evidence is inconsistent with cost-minimizing behavior in a competitive market.

Physician fees, expenditures, and income could not have increased as rapidly as they had until the late 1970s if the physician services market were competitive. The rapid rise in physician fees could not be explained by increases in physician expenses; nor could differences in costs provide the explanation for the large differences in prices between locations for the same service. A competitive model of physician pricing, which relies on differences in costs to explain differences in prices, did not appear consistent with observed data.

DETERMINATION OF PHYSICIAN PRICES

A Monopoly Model of Physician Pricing

When a competitive model, which relies on costs to explain the level of prices, is not able to explain changes in prices and quantities in a market, then a monopoly framework is used to explain the phenomenon observed. To show where monopoly elements are likely to have their impact, the probable effects of an increase in demand are analyzed. With an increase in demand for physician services, prices would increase as existing providers ration the increased demand. As profits increase, an increase in supply would also be expected; with an increase in supply, prices would begin to fall (what would actually be observed is that prices would not rise as rapidly as demand

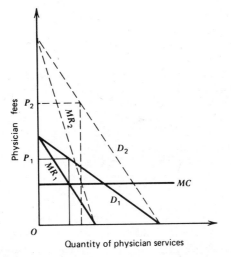

Figure 9-2. The impact of insurance on physician fees.

continues to increase). An increase in supply of physician services would be expected from two sources. In the short run, existing physicians can increase their productivity by hiring more auxiliaries and/or by increasing their own hours of work. In the long run, additional physicians would be trained and would enter the practice of medicine. Entry barriers are one possible source of monopoly power. A discussion of the long-run supply of physicians and whether or not there are barriers to entry in that market is reserved for Chapter 14. In the short run, however, the number of practicing physicians is sufficiently large that if physicians were to increase their productivity to the level that is technically feasible, the increased supply of services would inhibit the rise in physician prices. Physicians, however, are not likely to encourage unlimited increases in physician productivity. If physicians were allowed to expand the size of their practices to whatever size is technically feasible, the increased capacity for providing medical services might exceed the increased demand for such services. In that event, competitive pressures on physicians could increase, which would adversely affect their incomes. Thus, under a monopoly model of physician pricing, only gradual increases in productivity would be expected as demands for physician services increased; the purpose would be to ensure that increased supply would not outstrip increases in demand. The mechanism whereby productivity increases are limited is the state practice acts. Such acts, which are usually proposed to the state legislature and controlled in their implementation by the medical profession, specify the tasks that different professionals can perform and often the number of physician assistants that can be hired. The consequence of such supply-restricting behavior would be a greater increase in physician fees than would otherwise occur.

The application of a monopoly model to explain physician pricing behavior would not necessarily end with an explanation of restrictions on increased supplies of physician services. Physician prices in excess of costs can occur even though there may be no increases in demand. A decrease in the price elasticity of demand for physician services would be expected to result in an increase in physician fees. This effect on physician fees of a less elastic demand curve for physician services is shown in Figure 9-2. The initial demand and marginal revenue curves are D_1 and MR_1. The physician's marginal cost curve is MC, which, for simplicity, is assumed to be constant. The resulting price is P_1. With increased insurance coverage for physician services, the demand for physician services becomes less elastic, shifting from D_1 to D_2. The marginal revenue curve also shifts rightward. Thus, even though marginal costs have not changed, the intersection of the steeper MR_2 with MC results in a higher price, P_2, on the demand curve. Economic theory would therefore suggest that a second possible explanation for the rapid increase in physician fees has been a change in the price elasticity of demand for physician services.[5] Evidence to test this hypothesis is examined next.

The method of reimbursement preferred by physicians is fee for service, according to their "usual, customary, and reasonable" (UCR) fees. Such a pricing strategy enables the physician to set what he or she believes is the profit-maximizing price. With the growth in private insurance for physician services, the amount the patient had to pay out of pocket for such services was reduced; however, patients were still responsible for the major portion of their bill. It was not until 1966, when Medicare and Medicaid were passed, that third-party payors, private insurance and government, became the predominant payors of physicians' services. As shown in Table 9–2, public payments for physician services increased from 6.9 percent in 1965 to 29.3 percent in 1985. Together with private insurance, all third-party payors now pay 73.7 percent of total physician expenditures. When physician fees are adjusted both for inflation and by the decline in the out-of-pocket price as a result of third-party coverage, the physician fee, *in constant dollars faced by the average patient,* has actually declined since 1950 (13). As the patients' responsibility for payment of physician fees declined and physicians charged third-party payors according to their UCR fee, physician fees increased rapidly. As more of a physician's fees were reimbursed by a third party, the constraints holding down physician fees were removed (14).

Insurance coverage for payment of physician fees has not been uniform among all physician specialties. The hospital-based specialties, such as radiology and anesthesiology, have the largest percent of their revenues (approximately 80 percent) covered by third-party payors; surgeons also received a majority of their revenues from third-party payors. The decline in the patient's sensitivity to prices lowers the price elasticity of demand; rapidly increasing prices would be expected in such a situation. Those specialties of medicine that require less use of the hospital, such as pediatrics and psychiatry, have the smallest percent of their revenues covered by third-party payors. Not surprisingly, members of those specialties with the largest percent of their revenues paid by third-party payors also have the highest incomes. The usual market constraints, such as patients' seeking lower prices, began to disappear as more of the physicians' fees were reimbursed by third-party payors. As a consequence, third party-payors began to place limits on physicians' fees. Medicare, Medicaid, and some

---

[5]One explanation for rising physician fees has been the rapid increases in malpractice premiums. Malpractice premiums, however, are a fixed cost; they do not vary according to the number of deliveries or the number of surgical procedures performed. If a physician sets a profit-maximizing price (i.e., marginal revenue equal to marginal cost), changes in fixed cost should not have any effect on the physician's price. If physicians were able to pass on increases in their fixed costs, it is unlikely that they would spend their time in marches on their respective state capitols seeking legislative relief. Only in the long run in a competitive industry would increased fixed costs result in higher consumer prices. Since there is evidence that physicians were receiving above-normal rates of return during this period (Chapter 13), the long-run explanation is not applicable. Increased malpractice premiums may be used as a reason for increasing prices by physicians even though the more accurate explanation was a lessening price elasticity of the patient's demand curve; higher costs are a more palatable explanation than increased ability to pay.

third-party payors each place different limits on how much physician fees are permitted to increase.

When patients are uninformed about the prices charged by physicians, it is costly for them to seek out this information. Physicians about whom the patient has little knowledge are poor substitutes for the patient's own physician. The poorer the substitute the other physicians are for a patient's own physician, the less elastic the individual physician's demand curve will be. It is for these reasons that the medical profession has opposed advertising among physicians. State medical societies had prohibitions against advertising as part of their code of ethics; if physicians were found guilty of such "unethical" behavior, they could be subject to severe sanctions. Prohibitions against advertising were also included in state medical practice acts. In 1975, the Federal Trade Commission (FTC) charged the American Medical Association, the Connecticut State Medical Association, and the New Haven County Medical Association with attempting to prevent their members from advertising, engaging in price competition, and other competitive practices. The finding by the FTC administrative law judge that the AMA and two medical societies had attempted to limit competition among physicians was upheld by the FTC commissioners, the Court of Appeals, and in 1982, by a tie vote, the Supreme Court. The less information available to patients on physicians' prices, their qualifications, and their availability, the more likely it is that variations in fees (for comparable services) will persist; it becomes too costly, in terms of a patient's time, to search for lower fees and for the type of physician that he or she prefers. With little or no information available on physicians' fees and services and as more of the physicians' charges are covered by private insurance or public payments, the potential savings to the patient from searching for a lower fee declines. A more complete discussion of the effect on prices of advertising, together with a review of empirical evidence, will be found in Chapter 12.

The Target-Income Hypothesis

The uncertainty that patients have regarding their medical needs and their reduced sensitivity to physician prices have given rise to the idea that physicians can both induce their own demand and set their own prices. It has been suggested by some economists that the extent of the demand the physician will "create" and the price that will be established are based upon what target income the physician desires (15). The target-income hypothesis of physician pricing suggests that with an increase in the number of physicians, physicians will increase both their prices and their demand to provide themselves with a target income. The target income is said to be determined by the local income distribution, particularly with respect to the incomes of other physicians and professionals, such as dentists and lawyers, in the area. The prediction of the target-income hypothesis—namely, that an increase in the supply of physicians will result in *higher* prices and/or greater demand—is contrary to traditional economic theory, which suggests that increased supplies will lead to *lower* prices.

Figure 9-3 shows the effect on physician fees of an increase in the number of physicians using traditional economic theory as well as the target-income hypothesis. If market demand and supply were originally D_0 and quantity S_0, respectively, equilibrium will be at price P_0 and quantity Q_0. An increase in the number of physicians in an area would shift supply to the right, to S_1, which would, under traditional economic theory, result in a *lower* equilibrium price, P_1. Under the target-income hy-

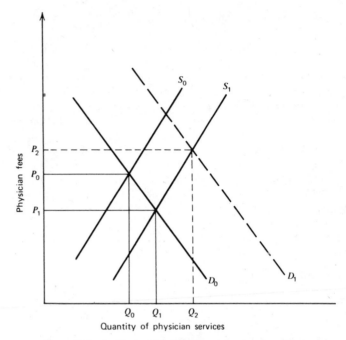

Figure 9-3. An illustration of the target-income hypothesis.

pothesis, with an increase in the number of physicians in the community, physicians induce an increase in their demand to D_1. The effect is an increase rather than a decrease in physician fees.

The major evidence upon which the target-income hypothesis is based is the finding that physician/population ratios are positively related to physician fees, after adjusting for other variables.[6] Critics of the target-income hypothesis find fault with both the logic and the empirical work on which it is based. For example, why should the target income vary among physicians? Further, how does the physician decide on the trade-off between increased fees and increased visits to achieve the target income? The empirical finding of a positive association between physician fees and physician/population ratios is believed to be a result of not adjusting adequately for changes in patient time and quality of a physician visit. As the number of physicians in an area increases, there are decreased travel and waiting times to see physicians; this would result in an increase in patient demand as the patient's time costs are lowered. Similarly, as the quality aspects of a physician visit are increased, as measured by the amount of physician time per visit and the length of the visit, the patient would be willing to pay a higher price for a physician visit. For example, after adjusting for physician characteristics and physician time spent with the patient, Wilensky and Rossiter found that the physician/population ratio had no impact on three separate types of fees, for three different types of physician output (16).

---

[6]Robert Evans concludes that "the market for physicians' services is not self-equilibrating in the usual sense, that price does not serve primarily to balance supply and demand [but that] the primary role of price is instead as an input to supplier incomes, which are not themselves the product of explicit maximizing behavior, but rather of target-seeking through the manipulation of several control variables" [Evans (15), p. 173].

As it becomes possible to adjust physician prices more adequately for such differences, particularly quality and amenity differences among physicians, it should be possible to determine a negative relationship between physician fees and physician/population ratios, which is what would be predicted using traditional economic theory. However, in his study on the effect of increased number of surgeons on operations, V. Fuchs argues that time costs are likely to be less relevant when it comes to in-hospital operations, "because the psychic costs of surgery and the time costs of hospitalization are likely to be large relative to the time costs of search, travel and waiting." Fuchs finds that a 10 percent increase in the surgeon/population ratio results in a 3 percent increase in per capita utilization. Also, opposite to what would be expected using traditional economic analysis, he finds that prices are increased in this situation of induced demand. Thus, although the average surgeon's workload decreased by 7 percent, income per surgeon declined by a smaller amount. The extent of demand inducement, even among surgeons, is, however, limited, since "the average number of operations per surgeon . . . is far below the level that surgeons consider a full workload . . . and below the quantity that surgeons would be willing and able to perform at the going price" (17).

In an article on this subject, Pauly and Satterthwaite examine the situation among primary care physicians, where the patient's insurance coverage is less than for surgeons and therefore price incentives still exist (18). They attempt to explain the observed relationship between an increase in the number of physicians and fees and a decline in consumer information. In choosing a physician, consumers depend on the recommendations of others rather than shopping, as they typically do in other markets. When there are few physicians in an area, each physician's reputation is known throughout the community. Consumers are likely to know people who have gone to each physician. However, when there are a large number of physicians in a metropolitan area, the consumer's knowledge of each physician's reputation is less. There is also less information on each physician's qualifications and prices. An increase in the number of physicians in an area therefore increases the consumer's difficulty in finding out about each physician. As this occurs, the consumer becomes less price sensitive and the physician's demand curve becomes less elastic. Physicians (or firms in monopolistically competitive markets) will then raise their prices.

While the foregoing model and the target-income hypothesis both predict that an increase in the number of physicians in an area leads to an increase in physician fees, the theories differ in their concepts of physician and consumer behavior. In the target-income theory there is a trade-off between a physician's income and diagnostic accuracy. Physicians are believed to be able to manipulate demand by reducing the accuracy of information they provide to their patients. There is presumably a limit to the extent to which physicians can create demand since they incur a psychic cost from demand manipulation. At some point this disutility to the physician exceeds the value of the additional income they earn. In the Pauly and Satterthwaite model, it is the increased cost of search to consumers as the number of physicians increase that results in higher fees. It has little to do with physicians manipulating demand.

The policy implications of these theories differ. Providing consumers with comparative information on physicians will enhance their ability to select among physicians. As physicians are viewed as better substitutes for one another, their elasticity of demand increases; consequently, fees should be reduced.

In reply to critics of the target-income hypothesis, Uwe Reinhardt suggests that physicians may also increase their revenues by prescribing additional ancillary services rather than by increasing their own time. Increased laboratory tests and x-rays may be prescribed by physicians in the belief that quality of care is increased and that the possibility of a malpractice suit is reduced. Reinhardt observed that in West Germany, where the physician/population ratio has increased rapidly in the last decade, the incomes of physicians have not decreased; rather, they have continued to increase. Reinhardt believes that increases in fees accounted for only a small part of the growth in physicians' incomes. The bulk of the increase has come from increased delivery of minor medical, x-ray, and diagnostic procedures per patient treated. German physicians have shifted away from time-consuming procedures toward laboratory and diagnostic procedures. There was a 90 percent increase in x-rays between 1965 and 1974 per patient treated by a physician as more and more physicians in private practice equipped their offices with technical equipment or joined with colleagues in the establishment of profit-making, physician-owned laboratory co-ops (19).

As insurance coverage for physician and ancillary services becomes more widespread, it becomes relatively easy for the physician to increase fees and to prescribe more ancillary services. If the patient perceives that there is some benefit from such tests, no matter how small, and the price to the patient is zero because of insurance, an increase in ancillary services would be expected. Such behavior is also consistent with physicians maximizing their incomes.

If the target-income hypothesis of physician pricing behavior is correct, there are important implications for public policy. With the recent increase in the number of physicians as a result of federal subsidies to medical schools, physician fees would be expected to rise even faster than in the past, as more physicians attempt to attain their target income. Increased expenditures on physician services (with doubtful effects on health status) will not be the only cost to society of such pricing behavior. It has also been claimed that each physician generates between $200,000 and $300,000 in other medical expenses each year. Thus, with an increase in the number of physicians, expenditures on physician and medical services would be expected to increase rapidly. The policy prescription for inhibiting these price and expenditure increases is likely to be the establishment of arbitrary limits on expenditures for physician services and on the number of physicians, as opposed to inducing increases in the supply of physician services. However, before such regulatory approaches are implemented in the physician services market, it should be clear whether or not this market responds to traditional economic incentives. Although there appears to be evidence of some demand inducement among certain groups of specialized physicians, there appears to be sufficient doubt about the extent of such a phenomenon to suggest caution in the use of this hypothesis as a rationale for certain types of public policy.

PROPOSED CHANGES IN THE PHYSICIAN SERVICES MARKET

The divergence between what was observed in the physician services market and what would have been expected if this market were relatively competitive included a wide range in prices for similar procedures, both between and within cities, that appear to be greater than differences in costs between those locations; a more rapid increase in prices for physician services than in the costs of performing those services; and a more costly mix of manpower (relatively high physician/auxiliary ratios) for providing physician services than was technically or economically feasible. It was hypothesized that these differences from what might be expected if the market were competitive were a result of a lack of information on which patients can base their choice of physicians; uncertainty by patients as to their medical needs and treatment requirements; reduced patient incentives for being concerned with physician prices because of increasing third-party payment for physician services; and reimbursement of physician services under private insurance and government programs on a fee-for-service basis according to the physician's usual, customary, and reasonable fee.

However, as mentioned previously, the market for physicians' services has been changing; it is becoming more competitive. Third-party payors, such as Medicare, Medicaid, and Blue Shield, place limits on the amounts they pay physicians; physicians that participate in HMOs and PPOs negotiate their fees with these organizations. Physicians are responding to these new market arrangements; they are joining groups, the size of physician groups is increasing, and groups are using nonphysician support staff to increase the physician's productivity. Due to a lack of data, it is difficult to track these trends in physician productivity as competitive pressures have increased.

As the physicians' services market continues to adapt to the new competitive environment, it is expected that trends toward greater efficiency in the provision of physician services will continue. There are likely to be smaller variations in physicians' fees to large purchasers of physicians' services; however, private-pay patients are likely to continue to observe such variations because of a lack of information. Although advertising is now permitted, the purchase of physician services is based on a number of factors in addition to price; it is still difficult for patients to gather information on these other dimensions of the physician's service.

Two types of public policy proposals are discussed. The first relates to methods of increasing efficiency in the market for physician services; the second involves analysis of current and proposed methods of payment for physicians' services under Medicare.

Increased Efficiency in the Provision of Physician Services

Recent court rulings that the antitrust laws are applicable to health care should serve to stimulate competition and provide incentives for efficiency. To ensure that physicians are able to combine resources so as to minimize their costs, it is necessary that any additional restrictions, unrelated to quality, be reduced. The degree to which physicians can delegate tasks and use physician extenders in their practices is often limited on grounds generally unrelated to issues of quality. In many states, medical licensing boards retain control over the introduction and use of such personnel. To produce physician services at minimum cost, it is first necessary to be able to *legally* employ the quantity of health manpower that is desired and to be able to delegate such tasks to them as they are trained to perform. Any restrictions limiting the physician's use of such persons should be removed; continuing to hold the physician responsible for maintaining quality should provide the same assurance as today that quality is not diminished.

The number of tasks that any physician will delegate will depend, in part, on the size of the physician's practice. In small practices, physicians might prefer an auxiliary to undertake a variety of tasks; in larger practices there would presumably be a greater division of labor. Delegating tasks to be performed according to which profession is licensed to perform those tasks, as is the case today, rather than on the basis of training and experience can only raise the costs of providing physician services.

One way to increase efficiency in the provision of physician services would be to have the person who is both qualified and has the least amount of training perform any given task. This would be similar to a competitive market in which the price for a given service approximates the least costly method of producing that service. An incentive for moving in this direction would be reimbursing physician fees at a level equivalent to the level of reimbursement for the individual with the lowest level of training who can perform the particular task (20). If the time of a lesser-skilled individual—a nurse or physician assistant, for example—can be substituted for a physician's time, the allocation of resources is improved. In the short run, the physician's time is freed for more complex tasks; in the longer run, if lesser-trained manpower takes over some of the tasks now performed by physicians, a smaller supply of physicians will be needed. An important feature of a system designed to promote delegation is that it would provide greater financial rewards to physicians who delegate tasks than to those who do not. Under a fee-for-service reimbursement system, this would occur if the same payment were made for a particular task regardless of whether it was performed by a physician or an aide (assuming the quality to be the same in each case). (This would also occur automatically under a capitation system of payment, since physicians or groups of physicians who delegated tasks efficiently would be able to treat a larger number of patients and would end up with more net revenue after covering practice expenses.)[7]

Reimbursement for physician services according to the task performed rather than the level of training of the person performing it might also affect the specialty distribution of physicians. If a particular procedure can be performed equally well by a family practitioner, a surgeon should not receive a higher fee for performing it. If surgeons are not as busy as they would like to be, and they use their excess time performing services that nonsurgeons can perform equally well, reimbursing surgeons at a higher rate will provide them with a higher income than they would otherwise have. Applying the same principle of reimbursement to performing anesthesia services should result either in more procedures being performed by nurse anesthetists or in anesthesiologists receiving lower incomes.[8] All physicians do not base their decisions as to which specialty to enter solely on financial considerations; however, for some physicians, income differentials do play a more important role, and in this manner changes in the specialty distribution can occur.

---

[7]The relationship between the salary method of payment and task delegation is not very clear. Since a salaried physician is rewarded financially for the time spent working, but not necessarily for the efficient use of that time, salary payment does not inherently promote efficient task delegation. A salaried physician might conceivably go too far in either direction—overusing a staff of auxiliaries in order to minimize his or her own work effort, or refusing to make full use of a staff because the physician finds personally caring for a small number of patients to be more satisfying than supervising the care of a larger number. This is not to suggest that a salaried physician will never use auxiliaries efficiently, but without a strong financial incentive, efficient task delegation would have to be promoted by educating physicians as to what style of practice is efficient, and by monitoring their performance in some way to determine how well they approach the standard.

[8]For hospitals to increase their use of nurse anesthetists, an incentive should be provided, such as allowing the hospital to bill for those services as would a physician.

Physician Payment under Medicare

Physician Assignment under Medicare

The concept of a participating physician under Part B of Medicare has changed. When Medicare started, and until 1984, participating physicians had the option of accepting or rejecting assignment for payment of a beneficiary's claim. If the physician accepted assignment, he or she accepted as full payment the amount that Medicare reimbursed; in addition, the patient was responsible for a 20 percent copayment, which had to be paid directly to the physician. When the physician did not accept assignment, the patient was responsible not only for the copayment but also for the difference between what Medicare reimbursed and what the physician charged. The beneficiary also had the increased burden of submitting the claim for payment before being reimbursed by Medicare for 80 percent of the physician's reasonable charge. A physician was able to accept or reject assignment on a claim basis; that is, for the same Medicare-eligible patient, the physician could accept assignment for one claim while rejecting assignment for another claim.

When physicians did not accept assignment, Medicare beneficiaries had an increased financial liability for their medical care. Particularly for the low-income aged, increased copayments result in a decrease in use of physician services. The aged's access to medical care becomes more restricted.

In 1969 the physician assignment rate (assigned claims as a percent of total claims) was 61.5 percent. By 1977, the net assignment rate had declined to a low of 50.5 percent. By 1979 the assignment rate started rising and reached a high in 1985 of 68.5 percent and then declined to 63.4 percent in 1986. The increase from 1984 to 1985, which was in part the result of a change in the definition of a participating physician (discussed below), was the largest one-year increase, from 59.0 to 68.5 (21).

The assignment rate varies both according to region of the country and by physician specialty. South Dakota had the lowest percent of services assigned, 17.0 percent, while Rhode Island had the highest, 87 percent (as of 1982) (22). When assignment rates are examined by physician specialties, podiatrists and pathologists had the highest percent of services assigned, 65.0 and 64.8 percent, respectively, while internists had the lowest, 44.4 percent. One factor that appears to be important in determining whether a physician accepts assignment is the size of a beneficiary's total charges.

> "For persons with annual charges under $100, only 38.2 percent were assigned. For persons with annual charges of $2,500 or more, 60.8 percent of the charges were assigned" (23).

Assignment by physicians in these circumstances may be a means of minimizing the risk of nonpayment. Surgeons, who have larger total charges, would therefore be more likely to accept assignment than would primary care physicians.

If Medicare is to be effective in increasing access by its beneficiaries, it is important that the physician assignment rate be high. The following is an analysis of the effect that economic factors, including Medicare reimbursement rates, have on physician assignment. For purposes of this analysis it is assumed that a physician has the following types of patients: private-pay patients, which includes those with private insurance as well as Medicare nonassigned patients; Medicare-assigned patients; and Medicaid patients. It is further assumed that the physician's fee is highest for the

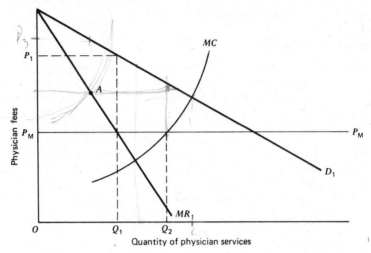

Figure 9-4. Physician decision whether to accept Medicare assignment.

private-pay patients, lower for Medicare-assigned patients, and lowest for Medicaid patients. To maximize his or her income, the physician will serve patients paying the highest fees before serving other patients. How many patients in each category will be served by the physician will depend on the size of those markets and the physician's marginal cost schedule.

The Medicare assignment problem can be described with reference to Figure 9-4 (24). The demand curve for physician services is D_1. The marginal revenue curve associated with that demand curve is MR_1. The downward-sloping demand curve assumes that physicians have some monopoly power. For private pay patients the physician is a "price setter." The Medicare price is a horizontal line at P_M. The physician is thus a "price taker" in the Medicare (and Medicaid) markets. The physician will start by serving the private market. If the physician's marginal cost curve (MC) intersects the downward sloping MR curve at a point above P_M, such as A, this will determine the quantity of physician services to be produced and the price charged (the price charged will be that point on the demand curve directly above point A, which is where MR = MC). A physician in such a situation would not serve any Medicare-assigned patients. If, however, the physician's MC curve intersected MR at a point below the Medicare price (P_M), the physician would serve that number of private patients given by the intersection of MR and P_M (shown by Q_1). The physician would also serve Medicare-assigned patients up to the point where MC equals P_M. As shown in Figure 9-4, the physician would serve OQ_1 private patients and Q_1Q_2 Medicare-assigned patients. The marginal revenue of both private pay and Medicare patients would be equal at that point. The price for private patients would be P_1, while the Medicare price would be P_M. The physician's MR curve is changed so that it becomes MR up to the point of intersection with P_M and then it is horizontal (P_M). (In this example the physician would not serve Medicaid patients, assuming that Medicaid pays a price less than P_M.) A physician would enter the Medicaid market if the number of both private and Medicare patients is relatively small so that the physician's MC curve intersects the Medicaid price, which would be horizontal, as is the Medicare price, but presumably at a lower level.)

Several important factors affect the physician's assignment rate. These may be classified as demand factors, supply factors, and Medicare policies. For example, if there is an increase in incomes or private insurance so that the private demand for physicians' services increases, the demand and MR curves would shift to the right. If MC is unchanged, then MC would intersect MR at a point to the right of Q_1. The physician would serve more private patients and fewer assigned patients. The reverse would occur if there were a decrease in private demand. A change in the factors affecting the physician's MC curve, such as increased wages for personnel working in the physician's office, would also affect the assignment rate. With an increase in MC, the new MC curve would intersect P_M to the left of Q_2. There would thus be a decrease in the acceptance of assigned patients. Similarly, a decrease in MC should result in an increase in assignment. Medicare policies also have an effect on assignment. An increase in Medicare's price would raise P_M. The higher P_M would intersect the MR curve at a point to the left and higher than the previous point. Assuming that the higher P_M intersected MR at point A, there would be a decrease in private-pay patients served (as well as an increase in their price) and an increase in the number of assigned patients. Other Medicare policies may have an effect on P_M without explicitly changing it. For example, if Medicare makes it more (less) difficult for physicians to collect their fees for assigned patients, such as by delaying (speeding up) payment, this would be similar to a decrease (increase) in Medicare's net price. The consequence would be an increase (decrease) in the number of private patients served and a decrease (increase) in the number of assigned patients.

The factors affecting assignment rates noted above suggest alternative policies that may be used to increase assignment. Medicare reimbursement rates can be increased, physicians accepting assignment could be reimbursed faster, and policies to lower the physician's MC curve could be instituted. Each of these policies would increase assignment. The costs of these policies would, however, vary greatly. Another alternative, in addition to the above, is to eliminate the physician's option of participating in Medicare on a claim-by-claim basis. Physicians would face an all-or-nothing choice of either accepting assignment for all their Medicare patients or not participating in Medicare. Undoubtedly, a number of physicians would decide not to participate. However, Medicare patients represent a significant portion of the total practice of many physicians.

Recent legislation has affected the physician assignment rate. In 1984 the Deficit Reduction Act was passed, which made several changes in the way the assignment option works. In 1984, Medicare physician fees were frozen for 15 months and the definition of a participating physician was changed so that a physician must accept assignment for all of his or her Medicare patients and for all services. A nonparticipating physician could still accept assignment on a claim-by-claim basis. The incentive for physicians to participate was that their fees would be increased at the end of the freeze. The result was a large increase in the assignment rate, 5.3 percentage points, in the year when this change took effect (25). The increasing supply of physicians, the growing competition among physicians for patients, and the promise of increased fees led many physicians, offered such an all-or-nothing choice, to decide that it was in their economic interest to accept assignment.

Alternative Methods of Physician Payment Under Medicare

Alternative proposals are being examined for payment of physicians under Medicare. The impetus for changes in physician reimbursement comes from two sources. The first, and by far the most important, is the federal government, which is interested in reducing expenditures under Part B of Medicare, which is funded out of general revenues. Lowering the rate of increase in physician expenditures (under Medicare) would contribute toward resolving an important political problem—that of reducing the federal budget deficit. The government is, however, reluctant to achieve this objective by having a large number of physicians drop their Medicare participation. The second impetus for change comes from various physician specialties, third-party payors, and a number of academicians who believe that the current fee-for-service system is inequitable and inefficient.

These two constituencies for change, the federal government and those favoring increased efficiency and equity, are not necessarily allies. Unless a new system also achieved the federal objective, it is unlikely that it would be adopted. Or if adopted, a new system would then have superimposed on it the federal objective, thereby making it unlikely that the efficiency and equity goals would be achievable over time. Thus any new physician payment system should be judged according to the twin criteria of reducing the rate of increase in federal physician payments (while not lowering physician participation) and increased efficiency and equity.

To understand the direction of federal policy with respect to physician payment, it is important to understand the goals of government, the likely responses by the private sector, and the eventual responses by the government if it is to be able to achieve its objective.

Federal Objectives. Seventy-five percent of Medicare Part B expenditures are financed out of the federal government's general tax revenues. The remaining 25 percent is paid for by premium contributions from the aged to that program. Federal contributions under Part B now represent one of our larger federal programs; they have risen from $1.6 billion in 1970 to $7.9 billion in 1980 to $17.1 billion in 1985. These expenditures are expected to reach $25 billion by 1990. Any reduction in this expenditure increase will contribute toward reducing the federal budget deficit.

Several alternative approaches are being explored to reduce these federal expenditures. Each approach imposes a cost on some constituency. The aged currently pay a deductible and copayment for their use of physician services. One proposal would have the aged pay larger copayments or deductibles. It has also been proposed that the aged pay a larger fraction of the Part B premium, from 25 to 35 percent. The consequence of either of these proposals would be to increase the financial burden on the elderly. Unless these increased costs to the elderly make allowance for differences in the elderly's income, the consequences could be particularly severe on low-income elderly. Proposals to shift a greater portion of the Part B costs to the elderly must contend with their political implications. The elderly have a high voting participation, associations representing their interests are quite active, and members of congress run for reelection every two years. Thus while some increase in contribution from the elderly, such as an increase in their premium contribution, may occur, the federal government's concern with rising Medicare expenditures is unlikely to be resolved by shifting all the costs to the elderly.

Another approach that has been suggested for reducing expenditures for physician services under Medicare is to delay the date of Medicare eligibility. While changing eligibility requirements would decrease the rate of increase in projected physician expenditures over the long run, it would offer little savings over the next several years— and it is over the next several years that spending reductions must be achieved.

An alternative to reducing federal expenditures is to increase payroll or general taxes or to impose a specific tax, such as an excise tax on alcohol or cigarettes. Such taxes would be a substitute for current federal expenditures on physician services. However, any proposal to increase tax revenues would have to be viewed as part of an overall approach to reduce the federal deficit and the Health Insurance Trust Fund.

In the past, as a means of reducing the rise in its expenditures, the federal government reduced provider fees. This approach was used during the Economic Stabilization Program in the early 1970s; it was also the basis of the Medicare Economic Index.

A constraint on the federal government's behavior in designing any physician payment system is that a sufficient number of physicians must participate under that system. No matter how attractive the payment system may be to the elderly, if physicians will not participate, access to care by the elderly will decline and Congress will be forced to make changes. Physician threat of nonparticipation, however, may have been a more important lever used by physicians in the past than currently. The increased supply of physicians has lessened physician influence in this regard.

The Efficiency and Equity of the Current Physician Payment System. Fee for service results in inefficiencies for three reasons. First, the physician has an incentive to perform more services. The physician's revenue will be greater the greater the number of services performed. Second, the mix of services performed is not necessarily the most desirable. Some services are priced much higher than other services in relation to their cost or their value. Those services having a higher relative "profit" provide physicians with an incentive to perform a greater number of services. For example, procedures are more amply rewarded than are cognitive services. A smaller percent of general/ family practitioners adopt new procedures each year (19 percent) than other physician specialties, (e.g., 62 percent of radiologists adopted one or more new procedures in 1982) (26). Thus the adoption of new, more remunerative, procedures is associated with the specialty status of physicians.

Third, as procedures become routine and their costs fall with experience and volume, the fee for performing that procedure should also decline. However, this has not been occurring. For example, the fee for coronary artery bypass surgery was initially established when the procedure required a great amount of a surgeon's time. As the surgeon's experience with this procedure increased and it became possible to delegate various aspects of the care for this procedure (e.g., pre- and post-care), the price for the procedure should have fallen, but it did not. B. Roe estimated that by performing fewer than three such procedures a week (requiring approximately 2–4 hours per procedure) cardiac surgeons could have earned at least $350,000 in 1979 (27).

These inefficiencies have been a result of third-party coverage and freezes in fee schedules over time. Services that are included under third party coverage have increased faster than other services. Also, as a result of various limits on fee increases, such as the Medicare Economic Index, fees are no longer flexible. Past relationships among fees for various services have been frozen. There is little economic justification for current relationships among fees.

In addition, when fees are frozen, physicians may subdivide their services (fractionalization) so that charges are submitted for each of the components of those services. Some physicians may also increase the volume of services, such as tests, in order to increase their revenues. Past attempts to limit increases in physician expenditures through limits on physician fee increases have not been very successful (28).

Inequities occur because, under UCR, new physicians within the same specialty are able to charge higher fees than are older, established physicians in an area. Further, there are large differences in fees for the same service between regions, unrelated to differences in cost of living. Also, fees charged by physicians for the same service vary depending upon the physician's specialty. For example, for three common types of visits, undefined by time or content (e.g., minimal follow-up office visit), specialist reimbursement averaged 22–53 percent greater than for nonspecialists (29).

These inefficiencies and resulting inequities in physician fees cause differences in physician incomes, choice of specialty, and practice location. To correct these inefficiencies and resulting inequities, there is the belief that the fee structure should be overhauled.

The following is a discussion of different methods that have been proposed to change physician payment under Medicare (30). Each of the proposals will be examined in terms of how well they meet the twin objectives of limiting the rise in federal payments for physician services and the desire to correct the inefficiencies and inequities in physician payment.

A. Modified Fee Schedules: Relative Value Scales

A fee schedule based upon a relative value scale consists of two parts. First, relative values or weights are assigned to all services and procedures. Second, a multiplier is applied to those relative values so as to translate them into dollars or fees. For example, if the multiplier is $50 and a procedure has a weight or a relative value of 2.5, the fee for that procedure will be $125.

The multiplier used to generate fees for the various services and procedures is likely to be the result of political negotiation between the government and physicians. If the government sets the multiplier too low, physician fees and expenditures will be reduced, but physician participation will also be reduced. Conceptually, it is possible to establish a multiplier based upon an estimate of what physician incomes should be. It is unlikely, however, that this task would be left solely to researchers and economists. It would be the outcome of a negotiation process.

The major advantage of relative value scales is the belief that it would be a more equitable and efficient system than current fee schedules. Based on several studies that have calculated relative values, fees for cognitive services would be increased while fees for technical procedures would be decreased. Primary care physicians would gain at the expense of procedure-oriented specialists.

The disadvantage to the government of a relative value scale is that it will not limit the rise in Medicare physician expenditures. To achieve this federal objective, the government will have to impose a limit on the annual percent increase in physician fees as well as an overall expenditure limit.

The federal government would have to require that a limit be placed on the annual increase in physician fees, similar to the current Medicare Economic Index. However, as with the current system, this limit on the annual increase in fees is unlikely to control the rise in total physician expenditures. Under a fee-for-service payment system, in which relative values are used, there is still an incentive for physicians to increase their revenues by increasing the volume of services provided, prescribing increased numbers of tests, and charging for services having a higher relative value. Each of these methods to increase income have been used when limits were previously placed on physician fee increases (e.g., the Economic Stabilization Program in the early 1970s and in various Blue Shield plans). To be effective in limiting the total annual increase in physician expenditures, the federal government would then have to place a limit on the annual total amount spent for physician services. An expenditure limit is likely to be imposed in the following manner. The multiplier used to translate the relative values into fees would be adjusted downward. In this way an increased volume of services can be contained within the expenditure limit by multiplying the relative value of each service by a smaller amount. In essence, fees are reduced so that when they are multiplied by a larger number of services, the total expenditure remains constant.

An expenditure limit has important implications for physicians. Once such a limit is announced, physicians might be concerned that if they do not prescribe more tests, upgrade the services they charge for, and increase their volume of services, other physicians will, thereby leaving less revenue available to themselves.

To provide physicians with an incentive to participate in the Medicare program, the federal government is likely to offer a new relative value scale only to participating physicians. Much of the current attention with respect to relative value scales is concerned with its construction. Since the main purpose of a relative value scale is to correct the inefficiencies and inequities of current fee schedules, the following principles need to be followed (31). First, there should be one price for each service regardless of the training and background of the person performing that service. Second, fees should be proportional to the costs of performing each service, so as not to bias the mix of services. Third, the costs of providing the service should be based upon the most efficient method (i.e., lowest level of training required) rather than on averages of costs or charges.

Several methods for constructing a relative value scale are possible; the simplest approach is to base the relative values according to the relative differences of current fees or charges. The advantage of this approach is that data are readily available. This approach can be useful if it is desired to eliminate wide variations in fees for the same service as well as regional differences in fees. The disadvantage is that the current structure of fees, with all its inefficiencies and inequities, is preserved.

A modification of the method described above is to use professional and/or political judgment to structure the relative weights. The extreme of this approach is to rely only on negotiation to establish relative weights.

Another method for developing relative values is to use a Delphi or "consensus" approach. Panels of professionals decide what the relative values should be for different services and procedures.

Developing relative values based upon the cost of performing the service has been proposed by Hsiao and Stason (32). The basic underlying concept is that in a competitive economic market, the price of a service will, in the long run, reflect the cost of producing that service. Given the interest expressed in the cost-based approach, a brief discussion is provided.

The cost-based approach to determining relative values is complex, requires a great deal of analysis and data, must be continually updated, and involves a number of assumptions which, if different, could change the outcomes.

There are four cost components used by Hsiao and Stason to construct their relative value scale:

- The physician's time
- The complexity of the service, to allow for differences in skill and effort required
- Opportunity cost, so that physicians with different training times can earn the same rate of return
- Overhead expenses of the practice, such as malpractice insurance, office payroll, and depreciation on equipment, which vary across specialties

Involved in the calculation of each of these "resource costs" are a number of assumptions. For example, the calculation of the physician's time assumes that a certain amount of time is spent by the surgeon before and after the operation and for each day thereafter, what the average length of time is for the various tasks that the physician performs, and that these times are normally distributed.

When estimating the complexity of the task, two methods were used: personal interviews, and a modified Delphi technique in which each physician was able to compare his or her own estimate to the average of physicians within that specialty. A high degree of correlation was found between complexity and time, each of which are separate resource costs. However, complexity is assumed to be separate from the amount of time when each is used as a resource cost.

One assumption used in calculating opportunity cost was that the years required for training in a specialty are the minimum necessary. It was also implicitly assumed that each specialty is equally desirable. If this is not the case, then to achieve equilibrium across specialties, differences in rates of return would have to exist. Further assumptions were made regarding the lengths of working careers across specialties, residency salaries, hours worked per week, and an interest rate to discount future earnings.

With respect to overhead expenses, it was implicitly assumed that there were no economies of scale in certain specialties; that is, certain specialties were not more likely than others to belong to groups. It was further assumed that equipment and payroll costs were on average appropriate for that particular specialty.

Hsiao and Stason performed a very useful service in trying to calculate a relative value scale based on resource costs. In doing so they had to specify their data requirements and assumptions. Although it is always possible to be critical of any empirical study, especially one so innovative, one concern with this approach is that a great amount of data would be required to update the results continually. If such an approach were used to allocate physician payments, technological changes, as well as changes in equipment and time required to perform a task, would have to be studied continually. Malpractice premiums, residents' salaries, physician incomes, and office expenses are changing continually.[9]

---

[9]A second concern is somewhat technical. The opportunity costs of physician training would be a resource cost when comparing costs across specialties. It is not clear, however, why different opportunity costs are needed if different specialties were performing the same service. According to economic theory (and the principles referred to earlier), the costs for performing a given service (of given quality) should be the same regardless of who performs it. If physicians of different specialties perform the same service (perhaps because some specialties are

A possible concern to primary care physicians is whether relative value scales would be used to limit the tasks that are being performed by such physicians. Some family practitioners have enlarged their scope of practice. It is possible that specialists who feel threatened by this increased role of the family practitioner may try and deny reimbursement for the relative values that specialists believe to be within their scope of practice.

Researchers at the Urban Institute concluded that of the different approaches that could be used to determine relative values (i.e., using charges, developing a cost function as proposed by Hsiao and Stason, relying on professional consensus, or some modification of these methods), the charge based and consensus methods were most practicable (33).

Establishing and updating the basic fee around which the other fees will be related will determine the incomes of primary care physicians; the relative incomes of the various specialties will then be determined by their fee schedules relative to the fees of primary care physicians.

B. Inclusion of Physician Services In DRG Payments

1. All Hospital DRGs and All Physicians' Services

Achieving the federal objective of limiting the rise in total physician expenditures suggests that emphasis first be placed on those areas where the magnitude and growth in physician expenditures have been highest. Physician inpatient hospital services account for 60 percent of Medicare physician payments (34). Over the period 1968–1975, the annual rate of growth in Medicare-allowed charges was 9.3 percent when the place of service was the hospital, as compared to 3.4 percent when the place of service was the physician's office (35).

Thus an alternative to the fee schedule is to broaden the unit of payment. Under a broader unit of payment, such as an illness episode, physicians would no longer have an incentive to prescribe additional tests or services. In fact, the incentive is reversed. A payment for a given illness provides the physician with an incentive to do less, since the payment is the same.

Hospitals did not have the option, as physicians did, to accept assignment on a claim basis. Hospitals must accept Medicare assignment. Mandatory hospital assignment makes it possible for the government to include in that assignment more providers related to the hospitalization of a Medicare patient. Physician specialties that perform most of their service in the hospital would find it difficult not to participate in the assignment for a hospitalized patient.

By including more providers in a DRG payment,[10] the government reduces the ability of the provider to bill for additional services and is able to reduce payments to providers whose fees or costs are above the average, both within a locality as well as

---

not busy enough) and those specialties are paid different amounts, based on differences in opportunity costs, this would be economically inefficient. The opportunity costs of physician training should only be used when specialists are performing services specific to their specialty. If relative value scales are not to perpetuate the inefficiencies and inequities of the current payment system, fees for the same service should be the same regardless of who performs it. The fee should reflect the lowest cost of providing that service.

[10]DRGs are diagnostic related groupings, which is the basis of Medicare payment for hospitals. Under DRGs, hospitals are paid a single amount for a Medicare patient according to the patient's DRG classification. This subject is discussed more completely in Chapter 11.

among localities. By controlling the annual rate of increase in the broader DRG payment, the government is also able to limit the rise in Medicare expenditures.

There are several problems, however, with including all physician services as part of the DRG payment. For some diagnoses it is difficult to define when the particular hospital episode starts and ends. Medical DRGs may require a great deal of physician time after (and even before) a patient is discharged from the hospital. To include all of these physician services in a single DRG payment would be both difficult to calculate as well as cause problems of access for Medicare patients with chronic problems. The average amount of physician services both before and after a hospitalization would have to be measured. Adjustments would have to be made for the patient's age and health condition. One could envision problems with coding, as a physician may decide to rehospitalize a patient, under a different DRG category, to continue being reimbursed for a patient requiring extensive treatment. Alternatively, patients requiring extensive treatment after a hospitalization might be referred to another physician.

According to recent research on this subject, the authors concluded that including all physicians in a hospital DRG system is not feasible for medical admissions (36).

A separate issue, but equally important, relates to who should receive the payment. A single DRG payment that included hospital and physician services could be paid either to the hospital, the physician, or split between the hospital and the medical staff.

Both physicians and hospitals would be concerned about who receives the payment. If the physician component went to the medical staff, they would have to decide how to allocate it to the various physicians involved (e.g., the attending physician, the surgeon, and the hospital-based physicians). Under any such arrangement the members of the medical staff would become intimately concerned with the charges of their colleagues.

2. Physician Services for Surgical DRGs

Although it does not seem feasible to include in a single payment physician services for all DRGs, it might be possible to do so just for surgical DRGs. Defining the beginning and the end of a surgical DRG is less complicated. It would also be simpler to exclude the attending physician's charges from the single DRG payment. The attending physician's charges are likely to be a small fraction of the overall charge for a surgical DRG and the costs of including these physicians would probably outweigh any savings.

The issue of which group would receive the payment would again be politically sensitive. To the extent that the payment goes to one group, either to the physicians or to the hospital, there is greater incentive to minimize the costs of care provided by the other group. Physicians would be more concerned with the costs of hospital care if they had to reimburse the hospital for the hospital's portion of the DRG. Similarly, the hospital would consider ways to reduce physician costs if they were to reimburse the physicians. If the physician portion went to the medical staff, there would be negotiation over the charges among the surgeon and hospital based physicians over each one's contribution.

3. Including Only Hospital-Based Physicians in a Single DRG Payment

Another alternative is to include fewer physicians-namely just the hospital-based physicians, anesthesiologist, radiologist, and pathologist-in a single surgical DRG payment. A disadvantage of this approach is that by excluding surgeons, the wide variation in surgeons' fees for similar procedures would not be reduced. The appropriateness of surgeons' fees would have to be handled according to a relative value scale. Hospital-based physicians are clearly different from other physicians in that they do not compete for patients. There is also ample precedent for hospitals negotiating payment with hospital-based physicians. A single surgical DRG payment that included hospital-based physicians would merely be an extension of exclusive contracts.

C. Establishing Preferred Provider Organizations (PPOs) Under Medicare

Medicare is such a large purchaser of physician and hospital services that it could use its market power to reduce the price it pays for these services. Medicare's purchasing power is particularly large in certain markets (e.g., Florida) and for certain procedures (e.g., cataracts). Especially where there is a surplus of physicians, Medicare can establish a bidding arrangement for certain services, as is done by some states under Medicaid. Some services lend themselves more easily than others to a bidding procedure. For example, surgical procedures are more easily defined than medical treatments. Further, within surgical procedures, the physician's time required and their costs are likely to be within a smaller range, hence more predictable, for those performed in an outpatient rather than in a hospital setting (e.g., cataracts). Medicare, through its intermediaries, could take bids from specialists in various localities.

D. Capitation Payment for Physician, Ancillary, and Referral Services

The federal government has already approved the concept of capitation under Medicare, but with regard to annual hospital and medical expenditures. The Medicare Voucher, which is the combination of Parts A and B of Medicare, is available to Medicare enrollees as part of an HMO. A capitation system for physician services, likely to include ancillary services as well as referrals could be separate from the Medicare Voucher. Such a payment system might work as follows. Medicare would announce that it is willing to allow participating physicians a choice as to how they wish to be paid under Medicare. They may choose, for example, a relative value scale or they could be paid according to a capitated basis; the amount of the capitation payment would equal 95 percent of the average area per capita cost (AAPCC) of a Medicare eligible person, categorized by age, and so on. The AAPCC would include physician services, ancillary services, and those of referral specialists. [In addition, physicians might be paid fees for unusual services (e.g., deliveries).] The amount of the savings that can be kept by the physician at the end of the year (or the fraction of losses they would be responsible for) would have to be determined and could be changed over time. There would also have to be an annual percent increase in the AAPCC each year to allow for inflation. Presumably, if the annual percent increase in the AAPCC is too small, then over time fewer physicians would choose to participate.

Several advantages accrue to the government from a physician capitation payment system. As the payment unit is broadened, it becomes easier for the government to monitor and to forecast its expenditures. The incentive for some physicians to increase volume or to unbundle services is diminished. An incentive has been given to the physician to decrease the use of tests and the charges for those tests, and to be concerned with referrals and the charges of referral specialists. The government would save money by paying only 95 percent of the AAPCC and it might be able to have a lower annual rate of increase in the AAPCC if physicians are able to reduce the use of ancillary and referral services.

The advantages of a capitated system to physicians is that they can increase their own incomes by decreasing expenditures on ancillary services and on referrals. The physician is not only the decisionmaker, but bears the fiscal responsibility of those decisions.

Unfortunately, there are a number of potential problems with a capitation method as described above. Would physicians be required to place all their Medicare patients on capitation, or could they select some, as is done under assignment? If physicians could pick and choose, there is the problem of preferred risk selection. Some physicians might recommend capitation only to those patients requiring relatively few services. Such a system could end up costing the government more money than previously. (The same problem can occur under the Medicare Voucher system.) Preferred risk selection would not be a problem if capitation were an all-or-nothing choice to the physician. Similarly, adverse selection could occur. Only those patients requiring large amounts of services might sign up for the capitated system. Capitation payments reflecting the patient's health status would have to be developed if patients and physicians could decide who should be capitated.

Another potential problem is whether a physician would be required to have a minimum number of patients on capitation. If too few of a physician's patients are capitated, some may have very high needs for services and for use of referral specialists. For a physician with a large number of capitated patients, a high variation in use among a few patients would represent a smaller fraction of the physician's total payments and would be offset by patients who have relatively little use.

Since the incentive under a capitation system is the opposite of the fee-for-service system, there will be a concern that some physicians might provide too few services. A monitoring system to guard against this would be difficult to develop and implement. A mechanism would have to be available to permit patients to transfer to other physicians if they are dissatisfied; a similar mechanism might be developed for physicians.

If a capitated system were to be adopted, permitting a fee-for-service system to coexist alongside a capitated system would provide patients and physicians with a mechanism to express their dissatisfaction with either system. Too great an exit by either group would be an immediate indication of problems with one of the systems.

E. Paying Physicians to be Case Managers

The case manager approach is an intermediate step between the fee-for-service system and capitation. It offers the advantages of both systems without some of their disadvantages. As case managers, primary care physicians would be paid several dollars a month for each Medicare patient that the physician regularly treats. This payment is in addition to the amount that the physician charges on a fee-for-service basis. (Thus the case manager method could also incorporate a relative value scale.) In return for this monthly payment, the physician is expected to make appropriate use of ancillary services and the services of referral specialists.

The physician becomes a gatekeeper, a designated provider who can be held responsible for the patient's care. The patient cannot go to other providers on his or her own. The monthly per capita payment is expected to provide the physician with an incentive to be concerned with the costs of other services and perhaps even with hospital admissions. The physician is not placed at great risk, since there is no immediate cost to the physician if the physician's behavior is not changed.

The savings to the government from a case manager system presumably come from the difference between the additional monthly payment and less use of other services. The physician case manager may even be inclined to act as an informed purchaser and refer patients to less costly specialists and providers of ancillary services, as well as to use fewer such services.

There are some concerns, however, with a case manager approach to physician payment. The physician's incentive is expected to be related to the amount of risk (personal loss or gain). Since the physician's risk is minimal under such a system, it is questionable how strong the physician's incentive will be.

To be able to evaluate physicians as case managers, patients would have to agree to remain with one provider for a given period of time. Patients might have to be provided with an incentive to do so. If the incentive is financial, such as reducing the deductible required under Medicare, this may lead to increased utilization, hence higher government expenditures. There is also the issue of adverse selection and preferred risk groups, as discussed previously. Another issue, also discussed above, is whether there should be a minimum number of patients to be signed up for each physician designated as a case manager.

Whether or not physician behavior is changed and the government saves money would have to be determined empirically. An approach similar to the area average per capita cost used for the capitation method could be developed. Similarly, data on hospital use rates could be calculated to determine whether case managers have lower hospitalization rates for their Medicare patients. Physicians not performing well on these measures could be denied case manager status in subsequent periods.

It is important to recognize that any change in physician payment will have redistributive effects. If the federal government pays physicians less, there will be a corresponding gain either to tax payors or to beneficiaries of other government programs. If some physicians benefit as a result of a new payment system, it will come at the expense of reduced incomes of other physicians or from other health care providers. Any federal attempt at redistribution, which would be the consequence of a change in physician payment, is ultimately settled in the political arena. Successful attempts at redistribution are usually characterized by widespread diffusion of the costs to be borne by those financing it and by a lack of clarity as to who is actually financing it.

Relative value scales are of topical interest. They address the issues of inequity among physicians but not necessarily the inefficiency of the current fee-for-service payment system. Because such a system is clear in its redistributive effects among physicians, the relative value scale is likely to be determined by negotiation among the interested parties.

To meet the federal objectives, however, relative value scales would eventually have to include mandatory participation, limits on expenditure increases, and an expenditure cap, since the incentive to prescribe more services and tests has not been eliminated.

The federal government does not need to rely on a single-payment method. Changes in payment systems could be implemented according to which provide the greatest savings rather than one that necessarily covers all physicians. These different payment systems could also be introduced at different times. The advantage of a variety of payment methods is that it will allow both patients and physicians to move into those systems that are most preferable.

Physician payment systems are likely to evolve over the next several years. Allowing patients and physicians to have the flexibility of different options will provide information on how each of these systems performs.

CONCLUDING COMMENTS

What is the economic outlook for the physician services market? If one believes that physicians can create their own demand, then an increasing supply of physicians suggests more rapidly rising physicians' fees and expenditures in the years ahead. In such a scenario market forces will not be able to prevent an increasing share of our resources from being devoted to physician services.

Alternatively, certain trends in this market suggest that market forces do operate. In the years ahead these market forces are likely to become stronger and to inhibit rapid increases in fees and expenditures. First, the FTC's victory over the American Medical Association, permitting advertising, should result in increased information to consumers about physicians' fees, qualifications, accessibility, and so forth. The consumer's cost of search should be lowered as physicians begin advertising. Second, the increase in the number of physicians should continue through the 1990s. Physicians will strive to increase their workloads to maintain their real incomes.

Visits per physician have been declining. Thus incentives have been created for increased competition among physicians for patients and referrals and the applicability of the antitrust laws will ensure that anticompetitive behavior does not prevent such competition from occurring. Thus whether advertising and the increasing supply of physicians result in price competition depends on the insurance sector.

Medicare has already placed limits on how much the physician will be reimbursed. Physician fees under Medicaid are typically set below Medicare levels. Although these two large payors act as a constraint on physician fee increases, their success depends on what happens in the private sector. Private insurance does not reimburse all physician services at a uniformly high level. For some physician services the amount paid out of pocket by the patient is much larger than for other types of services. Thus an important constraint on the increase in physician fees is the limited coverage for certain types of services. Also, when the patient is responsible for the full amount above the physician's allowable charge, as in the case of Medicare patients and those privately insured patients whose physicians do not take assignment, price incentives are reintroduced into the market. In the current market, price incentives exist and serve to limit fee increases. This is particularly the case for those physician services where there is little or no insurance coverage and for those insured patients who are responsible for all or a large part of the fee above a certain limit.

Another important market force affecting the physician services market is increased competition among health insurers. Insurers compete according to premiums as well as other factors. If an insurance company merely reimburses the physician in full regardless of the size of the fee, the insurance company's premiums will increase sharply. As premiums increase, two things will occur. There will be a decrease in demand for such coverage, and new insurance companies enter the market. (One such entrant might be a company offering its employees their own self-insurance plan.) As long as some purchasers are willing to buy less comprehensive insurance (i.e., deductibles, copayments, and perhaps restrictions on which physicians they can use), insurance companies will respond to these demands. The remaining insurance companies will suffer losses in their market shares. With the increase in the supply of physicians, there should be a sufficient number of physicians willing to participate under more restrictive agreements, at lower fee levels, and become "preferred providers." To maintain their market shares, the other insurance companies will be forced to hold down their premiums. This might be accomplished by setting more stringent fee schedules (if the insurance company offers a service benefit policy) and/or increased patient copayments. Whether physicians participate in different insurance programs will depend, in part, on what their competitors—other physicians—are willing to do.

The slow growth in the size of the population, the increased supply of physicians, the ability of physicians to advertise, a market where the patient is still responsible for a sizable portion of the bill, and (even if there were 100 percent insurance coverage) competition among health insurers should serve to stimulate market forces so that price competition begins to play its traditional role in the physician services market.

REFERENCES

1. "Statistical Briefs," *Journal of Medical Practice Management*, 1(4), 1986: 225.

2. Based on a list compiled by the Maryland Attorney General's office and reported in *Business and Health*, 4(6), April 1987: 60.

3. Uwe E. Reinhardt, *Physician Productivity and the Demand for Health Manpower* (Cambridge, Mass.: Ballinger, 1975), p. 82.

4. Uwe Reinhardt, "A Production Function for Physician Services," *Review of Economics and Statistics*, February 1972: 63.

5. B. Kehrer and H. Zaretsky, "A Preliminary Analysis of Allied Health Personnel in Primary Medical Practice," Working Paper, Center for Health Services Research and Development (Chicago: American Medical Association, 1972), p. 95.

6. L. Kimbell and J. Lorant, "Production Functions for Physicians' Services," Working Paper submitted by Human Resources Research Center to Economic Analysis Branch under Contract 110–70–354 (Rockville, Md.: Health Services and Mental Health Administration, Department of Health, Education, and Welfare, 1972).

7. Kenneth R. Smith, Marriene Miller, and Frederick L. Golladay, "An Analysis of the Optimal Use of Inputs in Production of Medical Services," *Journal of Human Resources*, 7, Spring 1972: 208–224.

8. Uwe Reinhardt, "A Production Function for Physician Services."

9. Philip J. Held and Uwe Reinhardt, eds., *Final Report: Analysis of Economic Performance in Medical Group Practices* (Princeton, N.J.: Mathematica Policy Research, 1979), p. 440. See also, Philip Held and Uwe Reinhardt, "Prepaid Medical Practice: A Summary of Recent Findings from a Survey of Group Practices in the United States," *Group Health Journal*, 1(2), Summer 1980: 4–15.

10. H. E. Frech III and P. Ginsburg, "Optimal Scale in Medical Practice: A Survivor Analysis," *Journal of Business*, January 1974.

11. George J. Stigler, "The Economics of Scale," *Journal of Law and Economics*, 1, 1958: 54–71.

12. William D. Marder and Stephen Zuckerman, "Competition and Medical Groups: A Survivor Analysis," *Journal of Health Economics*, 4(2), June 1985: 167–176.

13. James R. Cantwell, "Copayment and Consumer Search: Increasing Competition in Medicare and Other Insured Markets," *Health Care Financing Review*, December 1981.

14. Several researchers have investigated the hypothesis that physicians raise their UCR fees in the expectation that third-party payors, such as Blue Shield, will raise the physician's fee in a future time period. When Blue Shield updates its fee schedules, the physician's fee is higher and Blue Shield pays, for a given percentile, a higher prevailing fee. Whether such a policy increases the physician's net revenues depends upon the proportion of their patients that are covered by third-party payors, the higher fee, and the effect of the increased copayment on the physician's patients. The following study concludes that the UCR system encourages excessive price increases. Donald E. Yett, William Der, Richard Ernst, and Joel W. Hay, "Fee-Screen Reimbursement and Physician Fee Inflation," *Journal of Human Resources*, 20(2), 1985.

15. Examples of empirical studies lending support to the target-income hypothesis are Martin S. Feldstein, "The Rising Price of Physicians' Services," *Review of Economics and Statistics*, 52, May 1970: 121–133; and Robert G. Evans, "Supplier Induced Demand: Some Empirical Evidence and Implications," in Mark Perlman, ed., *The Economics of Health and Medical Care* (New York: Halstead Press, 1974), 162–173. For an excellent review of the target-income hypothesis and a reply to its critics, see Uwe E. Reinhardt, "Comment on 'Competition Among Physicians' by Frank Sloan and Roger Feldman," in Warren Greenberg, ed., *Competition in the Health Care Sector: Past, Present, and Future*, Proceedings of a Conference, sponsored by the Bureau of Economics, Federal Trade Commission, March 1978 (Germantown, Md.: Aspen Systems Corporation, 1978).

16. Gail R. Wilensky and Louis F. Rossiter, "Physician-Induced Demand for Medical Care," *Milbank Memorial Fund Quarterly*, 61(2), 1983: 252.

17. Victor R. Fuchs, "The Supply of Surgeons and the Demand for Operations," *Journal of Human Resources*, 13, Supplement, 1978: 35–36, 38.

18. Mark V. Pauly and Mark A. Satterthwaite, "The Pricing of Primary Care Physicians' Services: A Test of the Role of Consumer Information," *Bell Journal of Economics*, Autumn 1981.

19. Uwe Reinhardt, "Proposed Changes in the Organization of Health Care Delivery: An Overview and Critique," *Milbank Memorial Fund Quarterly*, 51, Spring 1973: 169–222.

20. This concept is discussed more completely in S. O. Schweitzer and J.O. Record, "Third Party Payments for New Health Professionals: An Alternative to Fractional Reimbursement in Outpatient Care," *Public Health Reports*, 92 November-December 1977: 518–526.

21. Alma McMillan, James Lubitz, and Marilyn Newton, "Trends in Physician Assignment Rates for Medicare Services, 1968–85," *Health Care Financing Review*, 7(2), Winter 1985: 62.

22. *Ibid.* p. 65.

23. Thomas P. Ferry, Marian Gornick, Marilyn Newton, and Carl Hackerman, "Physician Charges Under Medicare: Assignment Rates and Beneficiary Responsibility," *Health Care Financing Review*, Winter 1980: 57.

24. The discussion in this section is based on Lynn Paringer, "Medicare Assignment Rates of Physicians: Their Responses to Changes in Reimbursement Policy," *Health Care Financing Review*, Winter 1980. See also Donald E. Yett, William Der, Richard L. Ernst, and Joel Hay, "Blue Shield Plan Physician Participation," *Health Care Financing Review*, Spring 1981; Frank Sloan, Janet Mitchell, and Jerry Cromwell, "Physician Participation in State Medicaid Programs," *Journal of Human Resources*, 13, Supplement, 1978; and Frank Sloan and Bruce Steinwald, "Physician Participation in Health Insurance Plans: Evidence on Blue Shield," *Journal of Human Resources*, Spring 1978. The articles above also contain empirical estimates for the different factors affecting physician participation rates.

25. McMillan et al., *op. cit.* p. 63.

26. Special Committee on Aging, U. S. Senate,*Medicare: Paying the Physician–History, Issues and Options* (Washington, D.C.: U.S. Government Printing Office, March 1984), p. 8.

27. B. Roe, "The UCR Boondoggle: A Death Knell for Private Practice?" *New England Journal of Medicine*, 305, 1981: 41–45.

28. John Holahan and William Scanlon, *Price Controls, Physician Fees, and Physician Incomes from Medicare and Medicaid* (Washington, D.C.: Urban Institute, April 1978).

29. Special Committee on Aging, *op.cit.* p. 23.

30. There are a number of recent papers discussing physician payment proposals. Among these are *Physician Reimbursement Under Medicare: Options for Change* (Washington, D.C.: Congressional Budget Office, April 1986); Sandra Christensen, *Effects of Selected Fee Schedule Options on Physicians' Medicare Receipts*, mimeographed (Washington, D.C.: Congressional Budget Office, Congress of the United States, 1987); and *Medicare Physician Payment: An Agenda for Reform*, (Washington D.C.: Physician Payment Review Commission, March 1, 1987). In the Spring 1986 issue of *Medical Care Review*, 43(1), the following articles are devoted to physician payment: Kathryn Langwell and Lyle Nelson, "Physician Payment Systems: A Review of History, Alternatives and Evidence;" Frank Sloan and Joel Hay, "Medicare Pricing Mechanisms for Physician Services: An Overview of Alternative Approaches;" Mark Pauly and Kathryn Langwell, "Physician Payment Reform: Who Shall be Paid?"; and Gail Wilensky and Louis Rossiter, "Alternative Units of Payment for Physician Services: An Overview of the Issues."

31. Uwe E. Reinhardt, "Alternative Methods of Reimbursing Non-institutional Providers of Health Services," in *Controls on Health Care*, Proceedings of a Conference, January 7–9, 1974 (Washington, D.C.: National Academy of Sciences, 1975).

32. William C. Hsiao and William B. Stason, "Toward Developing a Relative Value Scale for Medical and Surgical Services," *Health Care Financing Review*, Fall 1979: 23–37.

33. *Alternative Methods for Developing a Relative Value Scale of Physician Fees*, (Washington, D.C.: Urban Institute, 1984).
34. Special Committee on Aging, *op.cit.* p. 28.
35. Ira Burney et al., "Medicare and Medicaid Physician Payment Incentives," *Health Care Financing Review*, 1, Summer 1979.
36. Janet Mitchell and J. Cromwell, *Methods of Describing Physician Services Billed and Rendered*, unpublished (Chestnut Hill, Mass.: Health Economics Research, 1984).

CHAPTER 10

The Market for Hospital Services

BACKGROUND

The most important institutional setting to be analyzed is that of hospitals. In 1985, hospital expenditures totaled more than $166 billion, or 44 percent of personal health care expenditures. Hospital expenditures constitute the largest single health care expenditure category and are rising at a rate of 7 percent per year, which is a higher annual rate than the Consumer Price Index (1). The hospital is also the most expensive setting on a per unit of service basis, and it has been both the object and the beneficiary of much federal and state legislation. A great deal more emphasis is therefore devoted to hospitals than to the other institutional settings.

Hospitals are classified according to the major type of service delivered, length of stay, and control or ownership. A short-term hospital is one in which its patients, on average, have lengths of stay of less than 30 days. Hospitals with lengths of stay in excess of 30 days are referred to as long-term hospitals. Of the 6,872 hospitals listed by the American Hospital Association, 6,339 are classified as short-term hospitals. The major types of services by which short-term hospitals are classified are general, psychiatric, and tuberculosis and other respiratory diseases. The general hospital is the predominant type of hospital; 5,938 hospitals have this service classification. Hospital control or ownership can be categorized as either governmental (i.e., federal, state, and local), nonprofit (i.e., voluntary or community), or for-profit.

Psychiatric, tuberculosis, and long-term hospitals have generally been public institutions, for welfare reasons and because of externalities, such as the contagiousness of tuberculosis, which led the state to provide care for such persons so as to protect the rest of the population. The demand for such public institutions, however, has been declining. From 1955 to 1985, the average daily census in tuberculosis hospitals declined 98 percent, 78 percent in psychiatric hospitals, and 61 percent in long-term hospitals. The decline in demand for tuberculosis hospitals has been the result of improved environmental conditions, widespread testing and earlier discovery, and improved treatment techniques. New treatment techniques for mental illness, specifically drug and shock therapy, have changed the demand for incarceration in a psychiatric hospital to a demand for qualified personnel, facilities for treatment, and a shorter length of stay. Short-term general hospitals have also developed substitute facilities in the form of psychiatric units; these, together with community mental health centers, provide services that have left only the poor, the senile, and the incurable to the care of mental hospitals, which provide care of a different quality at much lower cost. The decline in demand for long-term hospitals is partly attributable to the development of substitute facilities (i.e., nursing homes), along with increased patient incomes and public insurance to pay for such care.

The demand for care in short-term general and other special hospitals during this period (1955–1985), however, increased 54 percent in its average daily census. The rapid increase in demand for these facilities has been the result of changes in medical technology as well as various economic and demographic factors.

The analysis of the market for hospital services emphasizes the performance of the short-term general hospital, and within that type of hospital, the voluntary, nonprofit institution. The predominant form of control and organization of the short-term general hospital is nongovernmental and nonprofit; these hospitals number 3,262. State and local governmental are next in predominance, numbering 1,597; then come the for-profit (investor-owned) hospitals, with 774; and finally, federal hospitals, 305. When one examines the data in Table 10–1 on admissions and the number of beds, the voluntary nonprofit short-term general hospital is even more predominant as the major institution involved in the delivery of hospital services. These institutions have more than half of the short-term general beds, admit 68 percent of the patients, and employ more than 67 percent of all hospital employees.

The same table reveals that the large majority of short-term general hospitals have fewer than 200 beds, with one-third of the voluntary hospitals having fewer than 100 beds. From Table 10–2, which shows the distribution of Community hospitals by bed size, it is clear that the average size of hospitals has been increasing over time. The number of hospitals in the smaller bed size categories has been declining while the number of hospitals in the larger bed size categories has been increasing. This change has occurred through the expansion of the smaller hospitals. The growth in the size of hospitals was greater in the period 1965–1975 than in the more recent period. In 1975–1985, part of the decrease in the number of small hospitals has been a result of their closure rather than increases in their size.

The changes occurring in the market for short-term general hospitals is shown more vividly in Table 10–3. The period from 1965 to 1975 was one of growth. Medicare and Medicaid started in 1966 and coverage for hospital care became quite extensive. From 1975 to 1985, particularly in the last several years, cost constraints began to be imposed on hospitals and the industry grew at a less rapid pace. There was a slight expansion in the number of hospitals in the former period and then a reversal in the latter period. While there was little change in the number of hospitals, growth occurred in the number of beds, both in total and per hospital. The 27 percent increase in beds during 1965–1975 was in response to the 26 percent increase in admissions during this period. In the 1975–1985 period, admissions no longer increased and in fact have been declining in the last several years. The decline in admissions in the latter period together with the faster decrease in length of stay resulted in a sharp drop in hospital occupancy in the period 1975–1985. An indication of the changing role of the hospital is the rapid increase in hospital outpatient visits. An increasing portion of hospital revenues are from provision of ambulatory services. As discussed below, changing re-

TABLE 10-1. Selected Data on U.S. Hospitals, 1985

Type of Hospital	Number of Hospitals	Beds	Admissions	Percent Distribution of Admissions	Percent Occupancy
Short term				
General	5,938	1,069,960	35,039,278	100	65.5
State and Local government				
6–99 beds	1,092	55,154	1,497,230	4.3	46.7
100–199 beds	273	38,129	1,163,472	3.3	62.1
200–499 beds	174	53,295	1,976,109	5.6	68.9
500 + beds	58	41,560	1,393,013	4.0	76.5
Voluntary				
6–99 beds	1,101	62,857	1,847,921	5.3	50.2
100–199 beds	823	118,298	3,981,056	11.4	61.9
200–499 beds	1,085	342,403	12,157,054	34.7	68.6
500 + beds	253	173,405	5,890,217	16.8	74.1
Investor-owned				
6–99 beds	351	21,122	649,578	1.9	44.9
100–199 beds	276	38,440	1,200,384	3.4	51.0
200–299 beds	104	24,647	801,620	2.3	56.7
300 + beds	43	17,008	520,115	1.5	58.6
Federal	305	83,642	1,961,479	5.6	74.3
Long term[a]	533	206,046	536,817	—	86.9

SOURCE: *Hospital Statistics*, 1965, 1976, and 1986 editions, copyright 1965, 1976, and 1986 by the American Hospital Association.

[a]Includes general, psychiatric, tuberculosis and other respiratory diseases, and all others.

imbursement methods have given hospitals an incentive to provide more services outside the hospital. The increase in the CPI is shown to dramatize the percent increases in expense per hospital admission and per patient day that has occurred over time. While the CPI almost doubled (97.7) between 1975 and 1985, expense per patient day increased by 243 percent. Not all of this increase was an increase in price for the same patient day; increased technology and a different patient mix are indicated by the large, continuing increases in personnel per patient day over the period 1965–1985.

Trends in Hospital Cost Inflation

The difficulty of measuring hospital output is well recognized. To discuss cost trends, we must focus on the cost of some unit. The units most commonly chosen for cost comparisons are patient days and admissions (i.e., cases). Neither one is a homogeneous unit; there have been many changes in both the type of patient treated and in the patient's outcome over time. These changes in the nature of the average patient day or the average case have important effects on costs. Further, major payors of hospital care are also probably more interested in total hospital expense per capita than in expense per patient day or per admission, since their total payouts depend on total hospital expenses for the population covered. However expense per capita is also subject to

TABLE 10-2. Distribution of Community Hospitals, by
Size, 1965, 1975, and 1985

	1965	1975	1985	Percent Change 1965–1975	1975–1985
Total community hospitals	5,736	5,875	5,732	2.4	– 2.4
Bedsize category					
6–24	562	299	208	– 46.8	– 30.4
25–49	1,445	1,155	982	– 20.1	– 15.0
50–99	1,482	1,481	1,399	– .1	– 5.5
100–199	1,108	1,363	1,407	23.0	3.2
200–299	541	678	739	25.3	9.0
300–399	306	378	439	23.5	16.1
400–499	129	230	239	78.3	3.9
500 or more	163	291	319	78.5	9.6

SOURCE: *Hospital Statistics*, 1965, 1976, and 1986 editions, copyright 1965, 1976, and 1986 by the American Hospital Association.

measurement problems; for example, if more of the treatment is shifted outside the hospital, expenditures in these other settings may increase while hospital expenses decline. Although these measures are far from perfect, they are useful for providing an overall impression of what has been occurring.

Table 10–4 presents some basic statistics on several commonly cited measures of hospital costs since 1950. The first of these measures is the Consumer Price Index (CPI) so that the rise in hospital expenses can be compared to what has been happening in the rest of the economy. Next is the hospital semiprivate room charge, which is a component of the CPI. It is a measure of changes over time in the basic daily room rate, without inclusion of charges for ancillary services.

The other measures in Table 10–4 are all based on data collected by the American Hospital Association (AHA) in its annual survey of hospitals. The figures reported in the table are for nonfederal short-term general and other special hospitals. The first three of these measures—expense per patient day, expense per adjusted patient day, and expense per admission—are often cited as measures of hospital prices or unit costs. Expenses per patient day are merely total hospital expenses divided by total inpatient days. Since total expenses include those for outpatient care, expense per patient day gives a somewhat misleading picture of the average cost of a day of hospital care. Therefore, the AHA calculates an adjusted expense per patient day by converting the number of outpatient visits according to the ratio of the average revenue per outpatient visit to the average revenue per inpatient day. This adjustment has been criticized as arbitrary, since the revenue ratio may not reflect the ratio of the costs of outpatient visits to inpatient days. (An expense per adjusted admission figure can also be calculated that adjusts the number of admissions for outpatient volume in a manner similar to that in which patient days are adjusted in the expense per adjusted patient day calculation.)

The last two measures in Table 10–4 represent the hospitals' total expenses. The first is in per capita terms (dividing by the U.S. civilian population) and the second is

TABLE 10-3. Selected Characteristics of Community Hospitals, 1965-1985

	1965	1975	1985	Percent Change	
				1965–1975	1975–1985
Number of hospitals	5,736	5,875	5,732	2.4	-2.4
Total beds (thousands)	741	942	1,001	27.1	6.3
Average number of beds per hospital	129	160	175	24.0	9.4
Total admissions (thousands)	26,463	33,435	33,449	26.3	0.0
Average daily census (thousands)	563	706	649	25.4	8.1
Average length of stay (days)	7.8	7.7	7.1	-1.3	-7.8
Percent occupancy	76.0	75.0	64.8	-1.3	-13.6
Surgical operations (thousands)	13,100	16,664	20,113	27.2	20.7
Births (thousands)[a]	3,413	2,999	3,521	-12.1	17.4
Outpatient visits (thousands)[b]	92,631	190,672	218,716	105.8	14.7
Adjusted expenses per inpatient stay (dollars)	—	$1,030	$3,245	—	215.0
Adjusted expenses per inpatient day (dollars)	$40.6	$134	$460	230.0	243.3
Full-time equivalent personnel per 100 adjusted census	224	300	386	33.9	28.7
Consumer Price Index	94.5	161.2	318.7	70.6	97.7

SOURCE: *Hospital Statistics*, 1965, 1976, and 1986 editions, copyright 1965, 1976, and 1986 by the American Hospital Association.

217

TABLE 10-4. Measures of Hospital Costs and Percentage Rates of Increase, 1950–1985

Calendar Year	Annual Percent Increase				Expense per Admission		Expense per Capita		Total Expenses	
	CPI All Items	CPI Semiprivate Room Charge	Expense per Patient Day	Expense per Adjusted Patient Day[a]	Dollars	Annual Percent Increase	Dollars	Annual Percent Increase	Millions of Dollars	Annual Percent Increase
1950	—	—	—	—	$ 127.23	—	$ 14.06	—	$ 2,120	—
1955	2.2	6.9	8.1	—	179.79	7.1	21.07	8.4	3,434	10.1
1960	2.0	6.3	6.8	—	244.54	6.4	31.53	8.4	5,617	10.3
1965	1.3	5.8	6.6	—	345.65	7.1	47.73	8.7	9,147	10.3
1966	2.9	10.0	8.3	7.6	382.05	10.5	53.12	11.3	10,276	12.3
1967	2.9	19.8	12.3	13.3	447.64	17.2	61.87	16.5	12,081	17.6
1968	4.2	13.6	13.5	12.8	519.21	16.0	71.84	16.1	14,162	16.4
1969	5.4	13.4	14.1	15.2	587.99	13.2	83.42	16.1	16,613	17.3
1970	5.9	12.4	15.7	14.7	668.67	13.7	96.97	16.2	19,560	17.7
1971	4.3	12.2	13.9	13.2	743.15	11.1	109.67	13.1	22,400	14.5
1972	3.3	6.6	14.0	13.4	830.13	11.7	123.75	12.8	25,549	14.1
1973	6.2	4.7	9.0	7.6	897.20	8.1	136.94	10.7	28,496	11.5
1974	10.9	10.7	11.6	11.2	994.17	11.1	156.19	14.1	32,751	14.9
1975	9.1	17.2	18.3	17.6	1,166.80	17.4	184.97	18.4	39,110	19.4
1976	5.8	13.8	14.0	14.4	1,324.28	13.5	206.61	11.7	45,402	16.1
1977	6.5	11.5	13.9	13.8	1,508.81	13.2	237.65	13.0	51,832	14.2
1978	7.6	11.0	12.1	11.9	1,687.58	11.9	264.62	11.3	58,348	12.6
1979	11.5	11.4	12.0	11.3	1,882.37	11.5	296.79	12.2	66,184	13.4
1980	13.5	13.1	13.3	13.3	2,126.36	13.0	341.18	15.0	76,970	16.3
1981	10.2	14.8	16.0	16.2	2,486.41	16.9	398.21	16.7	90,739	17.9
1982	6.0	15.7	16.0	13.1	2,884.90	16.0	456.70	14.7	105,094	15.8
1983	3.0	11.3	11.7	12.7	3,221.79	11.7	502.11	9.9	116,632	11.0
1984	3.4	8.2	13.4	11.4	3,509.74	8.9	527.10	5.0	123,550	5.9
1985	3.6	5.5	14.3	12.1	3,901.38	11.2	552.90	4.9	130,700	5.8

SOURCES: *Hospital Statistics*, 1965, 1976, and 1986 editions, copyright 1965, 1976, and 1986 by the American Hospital Association, p. 3; for Data on CPI and civilian population, *Social Security Bulletin*, 48(11) November 1985: 55–59.

[a]Adjusted expense per patient day is calculated by converting the number of outpatient visits into patient days according to the ratio of the average revenue per outpatient visit to the average revenue per inpatient day. These data are not available prior to 1963.

merely total hospital expenses. These measures make no attempt to separate quantity from price changes.

Although each of the cost measures in Table 10–4 is somewhat different from the others, all show similar patterns of increase over time. The trends in these measures of hospital costs suggest the following:

1. The phenomenon of rapidly rising hospital costs is not new. Throughout the 1950s, hospital costs rose 6 to 9 percent annually, depending on which measure one examines. Hospital cost increases were 5 to 6 percent per year greater than the all-items CPI.

2. A marked speedup in the rate of increase in hospital costs occurred after 1966. Although rates of cost increase from 1960 to 1965 remained about what they had been in the 1950s, the rates of increase in all measures of hospital costs in Table 10–4 accelerated in 1966, and even more markedly in 1967. This acceleration is also evident when costs are measured in relation to the rest of the economy.

   Concern over rising hospital costs heightened considerably after 1966. The annual rate of increase was greater and the more rapid increases produced a tremendous growth in the total number of dollars involved—each percentage increase in costs amounts to a much larger number of dollars than it did in the 1950s. Cost increases also became more visible after 1966; a larger share of hospital expenditures were financed by the government. The Medicare program, under which the federal government finances hospital care for the aged, was initiated in mid-1966. The striking association between this event and the acceleration in hospital costs strongly suggests a cause-and-effect relationship.

3. The increase in hospital costs abated during the period 1972–1974. The annual rate of increase in hospital expenditures was smaller as a result of the price controls imposed by the Economic Stabilization Program (ESP) in 1971 (2). The controls were removed from the rest of the economy in 1972 and from the health industry in April 1974. After removal of the controls, expenditures increased very rapidly and then returned to their more familiar post-1966 rates of increase.

4. Although the rate of inflation (CPI) increased during the late 1970s, the rise in hospital expenses remained constant. One possible reason for this constant annual rate of change was the threat effect of federal hospital controls and the subsequent voluntary effort (VE) started by hospitals to slow down the rate of increase. The Carter administration proposed cost controls on hospitals. Fearing the imposition of these controls, hospitals started the VE as a means of showing the Congress that the industry did not need federal controls. A voluntary effort, however, can never be very effective for very long. When the Reagan administration began, hospital and medical associations believed that President Reagan would be opposed to federal controls. To limit its growing budgetary commitment under Medicare and Medicaid, however, the Reagan administration introduced price controls on hospitals (DRGs) in October 1983.

5. The economy went into a recession in 1981 and the rate of inflation also declined. The rise in total hospital expenses and expenses per capita also began to moderate. As the economy began to recover, the rate of increase in total hospital expenses and expenses per capita kept falling. The annual rise in these measures were at their lowest rate in over 30 years. Starting in 1983, changes had occurred in the hospital

sector; annual rates of increase in total and per capita hospital expenditures were lower than previous annual increases and also lower in relation to the CPI.

The descriptive data above illustrate the changes that have been occurring in this market. The short-term general hospital has increased in size and in the volume of services delivered; it has changed its product, and in turn there have been very large increases in the cost of its output. The large sums of money being expended in this market, and the continuing rapid increases in its costs, make it important to determine the efficiency with which it performs.

THEORIES OF HOSPITAL COST INFLATION

Wage-Push (or Catching-Up) Hypotheses

The theory that the upward push of wages is an important force behind the overall increase in costs has been prevalent in the hospital literature for some time. This wage-push theory has intuitive appeal for several reasons. Since the hospital industry is labor intensive, changes in average wage levels affect a large portion of total costs. Historically, hospital workers are believed to have been underpaid relative to other workers, and therefore relatively rapid increases in hospital wages are explained as a catching-up with wages in other industries. Further, changes in labor productivity in the hospital industry are thought to lag behind that of most other industries. As hospitals match wage increases granted in other industries in the absence of an offsetting rise in productivity, the net effect is rising hospital costs.

Labor expenses represented 60 percent of total hospital expenses in the period 1965–1970. This has steadily declined to where labor expenses are now (1985) approximately 55 percent of total hospital expenses. The average hospital employee's wage has risen much more rapidly than the number of employees per patient day. From 1965 to 1970, average wages increased 7.7 percent per year while the number of employees per patient day increased 3.4 percent. In 1970–1975, 1975–1980, and 1980–1985 wages rose an average of 10.3, 9.3, and 9.8 percent per year, respectively. Over those same three time periods, the number of employees per patient day increased 2.4, 2.3, and 2.9 percent per year (3).

Rising wages have by no means been the only contributor to hospital cost increases since 1965. The use of nonlabor inputs has actually increased faster than labor expenses. Nonetheless, average wages in hospitals have increased relative to the wages of all private nonagricultural workers throughout the post-1950 period, with the exception of 1971–1974. This phenomenon and the catching-up hypothesis deserve further investigation.

Martin Feldstein has used data collected by the Bureau of Labor Statistics to investigate whether hospital employees were underpaid relative to other workers in the past, and how the situation changed between 1957 and 1972 (4). For types of workers also employed in substantial numbers outside the hospital industry, such as clerical workers and housekeepers, he compared wages of hospital workers with those of non-hospital workers in several metropolitan areas for which data were available. He found that in 1957 hospital employees did, in fact, receive lower wages—the differential was more than 20 percent in a number of jobs and locations. However, by 1964 hospital personnel were often paid more than nonhospital personnel of the same type. In spite of this, hospital workers from 1969 to 1972 continued to make greater wage gains than those of other industry workers.

By comparing the rates of wage increase of different types of hospital workers during the period 1962–1972, Feldstein also found that percentage increases in the wages of more highly skilled hospital personnel, such as professional nurses and technical workers (administrative workers were not included in the BLS surveys), were at least as great as those of less skilled personnel. Wage gains were not disproportionately large among the lowest-paid workers. Using a different data base and methodology, Victor Fuchs essentially corroborated Feldstein's findings. He, too, found evidence of catching up during the 1960s and concluded that "health workers, starting at a relatively low wage level in 1954, has risen by 1969 to a point of almost parity with other industries" (5). Hospital workers, in particular, were found to have made larger gains than health workers in general. In fact, by 1969, registered nurses in hospitals earned on the average 13 percent *more* than other workers of the same sex, color, age, and schooling.

These findings by Feldstein and Fuchs reveal that hospital workers were generally paid less in the past than workers in other industries with similar functions or apparently similar qualifications, and that hospital workers made substantial relative gains in the 1960s. The catching-up hypothesis does not indicate why these differentials existed to begin with, or why wages of hospital workers increased more rapidly in the 1960s. If hospitals had traditionally been able to obtain sufficient manpower while paying relatively low wages, why were they no longer able to do so? The catching-up hypothesis also does not explain why hospital wages continued to increase more rapidly than wages in other industries—except during the period of the ESP—even though Feldstein and Fuchs both suggest that they had essentially caught up by 1969.

Another problem with the catching-up hypothesis is that it does not explain why hospitals increased their use of labor and nonlabor inputs per patient day so rapidly. It seems clear that a large portion of the increases in hospital costs per patient day have been due to increases in input use. Thus the reasons for increased input use need to be explained if the process of hospital cost inflation is to be understood.

It might be argued that increased input intensity was a result of a change in the type of hospital care demanded. For example, an increase in the number of older people in the population would require a more intensive type of hospital care than that required for younger persons. However, despite the fact that the average age of the population has increased, it seems unlikely that changes in the population mix have been responsible for a very large portion of the increase in input use in hospitals. An index of demographic structure in which the proportions of the population in each of 16 age, sex, and color classes were weighted by hospital admission rates in 1963–1964 changed less than 1 percent between 1950 and 1968 (6). A similar index using six age classes and 1970 admission rates as weights increased about 4.5 percent from 1960 to 1974 (7). The increases would be slightly larger if patient day rates were used as weights, since average length of stay also increases with age, as do admission rates. Patient days and admissions, however, increased more than 20 percent on a per capita basis between 1960 and 1974; this is greater than would be expected on the basis of changes in the structure of the population. Further, given such large increases in utilization, it is difficult to see how small changes in the age structure of the population could have led to much larger increases in the use of inputs per patient day.

A further problem with the catching-up hypothesis as a theory of hospital cost inflation is that it does not provide an explanation for the rapid adoption of medical technology, which has frequently been suggested as an explanation for rising hospital costs. Medical technology made possible the treatment of illnesses previously considered untreatable, and provided new and presumably higher-quality treatments for other conditions—often at much higher costs than the methods it replaced. The diffusion of entirely new technologies does not account for a large portion of the tremendous increase in hospital input use. Instead, these increases can be explained by increases in more intensive use of basic ancillary services (laboratory tests, x-rays) and efforts to improve hospital ambience. These findings are borne out by Anne Scitovsky and Nelda McCall's study, which found large increases in the average number of laboratory tests for such relatively straightforward cases as appendicitis and maternity care (8). Further, the upward trend in hospital personnel per patient day did not support the hypothesis that increases in input use was primarily the result of the application of new technologies; hiring was not disproportionately greater among highly skilled personnel.

It appears that the increase in input use was not simply the result of entirely new technologies but the result of more hospitals adopting existing technologies or using them more intensively. For example, use of intensive care and coronary care units has grown since the late 1950s until, by 1974, it accounted for 4–5 percent of the short-term general hospitals' beds (9). An intensive care unit might employ over six persons per bed compared with an overall average of 2.5 employees per bed in 1975. Although to some extent the high costs in these units reflect the use of equipment unavailable 25 years ago, such high costs are also related to the very intensive use of technologies that have been available for a long time.

Much of the increase in input use has apparently come about separate from important technological developments. Perhaps such general increases in the intensity of care are economically justifiable; perhaps their marginal benefits in terms of improved health outcomes and greater patient comfort exceed their marginal costs, or perhaps they do not. Were there underlying reasons for the rapid introduction of new technologies? What influenced their rate of diffusion? Does the supplanting of one technique for treating an illness by another always represent a choice based on a cost-benefit comparison of the alternatives? An alternative theory of hospital cost inflation might provide a more satisfactory explanation of the adoption of existing and new technologies by hospitals.

A Demand-Pull Model of Hospital Cost Inflation

Economists have generally rejected the notion that hospital cost inflation can be fully or even largely explained by exogenous increases in input prices, changes in the population distribution, and increases in medical technology. Although economists do not agree on a precise theory or model of hospital cost inflation, they generally agree that the growth of third-party payment of hospital care (payment for care by some party other than the person receiving it) has drastically changed the financial constraints under which hospitals operate.

The percentage of hospital revenues coming from private insurance, government, and direct consumer payments changed over time. In 1950, 50 percent of hospital revenues were paid for directly by consumers. By 1985, about 10 cents of every dollar received by short-term general hospitals came directly from consumers. Through the 1950s and early 1960s, the growth of private insurance was responsible for the shift away from direct consumer payment, but since then the government's role as a third-party payor has grown relative both to consumer and private insurance. From 1965 to 1985, the government portion of total hospital expenditures increased from 39 to 54 percent, primarily because of the introduction of Medicare and Medicaid (see Table 3–1).

Rapid increases in the price of a product, coupled with small increases in the quantity consumed, suggest an obvious explanation: demand increasing along a relatively inelastic supply curve. The growth of demand pulls up prices as consumers bid for the available supply. (Upward shifts in supply along a fixed demand curve could produce rapid price increases, but even if demand were quite inelastic, some decrease in quantity consumed would be expected.) It therefore appears that the combination of rapidly increasing costs per patient day and per admission and slight increases in hospital utilization is a result of demand increasing more rapidly than supply: hence the demand-pull hypothesis. Although one can suggest several possible reasons why the demand for hospital care might increase, the most plausible is the spread of third-party coverage.

The experience following the introduction of Medicare in mid-1966 is consistent with a view that hospital utilization responds to changes in net price brought about by third-party coverage. At that time, insurance coverage for the elderly improved dramatically, while that of the rest of the population remained essentially unchanged. Survey data indicate that between the period July 1965-June 1966 and the year 1968, hospital admission rates decreased for every group except the elderly, for whom admission rates increased approximately 25 percent (10).

The early effects of Medicare on hospital use are illustrated in a study by John Rafferty (11). Rafferty examined changes in case mix and length of stay for the 65-and-over and the under-65 groups that took place between the 18 months before and the 18 months after the introduction of Medicare. He found that the case mix became more severe and the (case-mix-adjusted) lengths of stay shorter for the under-65 population, while case mix remained about the same and length of stay increased for the over-65 group.

These findings are consistent with the following hypothesis, as depicted in Figure 10–1. The total demand for hospital care can be divided into demand by the under-65 group and demand by the 65-and-over group. The older group received a substantial subsidy with the introduction of Medicare, thereby shifting its demand curve from D_2 to D'_2, while demand by the younger group remained essentially unchanged. The total demand curve thus shifted up, increasing equilibrium price (particularly if the supply of admissions was relatively inelastic). As price rose, some demand was choked off, and the net effect was an increase in admissions for the 65-and-over group and a decrease for the younger group. One would expect the elimination of the least serious admissions in the under-65 group and a shortening of length of stay within case types. Rafferty's case-mix and length-of-stay findings suggest that they did act in just this way. While case mix apparently did not change much for the elderly, stays for given case types were lengthened, and the latter phenomenon is consistent with the notion that demand for hospital care increases as net price falls.

An examination of the evidence on hospital utilization before and after Medicare makes a demand-pull model of hospital cost inflation seem plausible. The model is not complete, however, unless it explains why hospitals have responded to demand increases as they have.

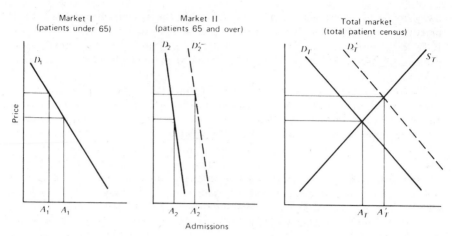

Figure 10-1. The effects of Medicare on hospital use, by age group. (John Rafferty, "Enfranchisement and Rationing Effects of Medicare on Discretionary Hospital Use." Reprinted with permission from *Health Services Research* 10(1) (Spring 1975):52. Copyright 1976 by the Hospital Research and Educational Trust, 840 N. Lake Shore Drive, Chicago, IL 60611).

Hospitals improved their financial positions after the introduction of Medicare, leading to a substantial increase in their net-income-to-total-income ratios (12). One study indicated that depreciation and interest expenses increased, on average, 29.5 percent per year from 1966 through 1968. It appears that hospitals had changed their accounting methods to obtain greater reimbursements from Medicare and other cost payors (13). Evidence of this kind of behavior seems to suggest that in increasing their costs so rapidly after Medicare was introduced, hospitals were not passively reacting to factors entirely beyond their control (i.e., the catching-up hypothesis). Rather, hospitals were taking advantage of loosened financial constraints to accumulate funds to pursue their own objectives.

DETERMINANTS OF HOSPITAL PERFORMANCE

To understand and to be able to evaluate the performance of the hospital industry, it is important to examine three aspects of this sector. The first are the incentives faced by hospitals based on the method by which hospitals are reimbursed. After the introduction of Medicare, the aged represented approximately 40 percent of hospitals' patient days. The federal government reimbursed hospitals for their costs of providing services to the aged. The method used was the "ratio of charges to charges to cost." The hospital's charges to Medicare patients as a portion of its charges to all patients was the ratio of the hospital's total costs that would be reimbursed by the government. As the proportion of Medicare charges increased, so did the portion of the hospital's costs that would be paid for by the government. During this period, insurance coverage of the nonaged also increased. As shown in Table 3-2, out-of-pocket payments by patients for hospital care decreased so that patients were, on average, responsible for less than 10 percent of their hospital expenditures. Patient sensitivity to hospital charges diminished. Other third-party payors of hospital care, such as Blue Cross, also paid hospitals according to their costs. The effect of these payment methods and the lack of patient sensitivity to hospital charges was to lessen hospitals' concern with the costs of their care.

In the early 1980s, purchaser concern with the costs of hospital care increased. Insurance companies and the federal government moved away from cost-based payment to fixed-price systems. As the payment system changed, so did the incentives facing hospitals.

The second determinant of hospital performance are the objectives of hospital decisionmakers. The industry is predominately nonprofit. Given the evolution of different payment systems, how was the nonprofit system expected to respond to these different payment incentives? The objectives of the nonprofit hospital and their likely effects on hospital performance are discussed below.

The third factor affecting hospital performance is the nature of hospital costs. The extent to which there are economies of scale in the provision of hospital services is an important determinant of the number of hospitals in a given market. (Another determinant of the number of hospitals is that of legal and regulatory restraints.) The market structure of hospitals can be classified as being competitive or monopolistic depending upon the number of competitors in a market. In a price-competitive market, the extent of economies of scale determines the number of firms in a market. The degree to which an industry is competitive or monopolistic will determine the type of competition among firms as well as the performance of that industry. Thus a separate section is devoted to empirical studies on hospital costs.

Finally, based upon the payment systems and incentives faced by hospitals, the objectives of the decisionmakers, and the structure of the industry, this chapter concludes with a discussion of hospital performance over time. The importance of these determinants of hospital performance varies depending upon the payment system. For example, in a price-competitive market, hospital objectives become less important than under a cost based payment system. Similarly, the nature of competition and the importance of economies of scale in determining the number of competitors will also depend upon the payment system. Thus the performance of the hospital industry will be examined as it has moved from a cost-based system to a fixed-price and more price-competitive system. To enhance our understanding of hospital performance, in the next section we discuss the objectives and incentives of hospital decisionmakers.

THEORIES OF HOSPITAL BEHAVIOR

In a competitive system, the simple assumption that firms will attempt to maximize their profits makes it possible to predict what a firm's supply response will be to changes in demand and/or changes in its input prices. With entry into the industry permitted, we would expect firms to minimize their costs and expect prices to reflect the costs of production; there would be no internal cross-subsidization of patients or of users of different services. If prices are not related to costs, new firms will enter the market and sell the service at a lower price. Because of the assumption of profit maximization and entry, we would expect prices to equal costs (in the long run); the different mix of services provided would reflect what people are willing to pay for those services, which in turn is a reflection of their full costs. The firms competing would all attempt to minimize their costs, and investment decisions would be based on profitability (i.e., demand and cost conditions).

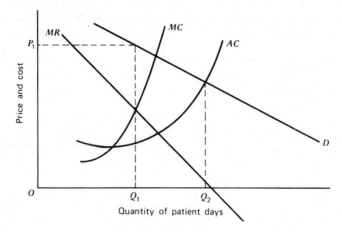

Figure 10-2. Price and output policies of a profit-maximizing hospital.

Since hospitals are predominantly nonprofit, what does this difference in owner-ship imply for the performance of the hospital industry? Does it, as some persons have alleged, result in lower costs of production, since the hospital does not have to earn a profit and pay dividends? Or are the incentives faced by the decisionmakers of the nonprofit hospital such that nonprofit hospitals have poorer performance? We need to develop a model of the nonprofit hospital to explain the observed performance of the hospital sector, to predict future performance, and to evaluate whether changes should be made. If changes are to be proposed, it is important to be able to predict how hospitals will respond to them, and for this we need to understand what moti-vates the behavior of hospital decisionmakers.

A number of theories have been developed to explain hospital behavior (14). These theories will be examined and their predictions summarized. The predictions will be tested by examining their consistency in relation to observed data. The most consistent theories will be examined with respect to their implications for hospital performance and for proposed changes in that performance.

A Profit-Maximizing Model of Hospital Behavior

To begin with our simplest model of hospital behavior, let us examine how a for-profit hospital would determine its price, output, and investment policy. This will pave the way for varying the assumption of for-profit behavior on the part of the hospital. Hos-pitals are assumed to have a downward-sloping demand curve; since each hospital has a somewhat differentiated product in that not all of its physicians have staff appoint-ments at the other hospitals, its mix of services may also differ, as would its location and reputation. To maximize profits, the hospital would select that price on the de-mand curve where its marginal cost curve intersects the marginal revenue curve; this is shown in Figure 10-2. The profit-maximizing price and output would be P_1 and Q_1, respectively, and the amount of profit would be the difference between P_1 and the average-cost curve at that price, multiplied by Q_1.

Further, since the hospital is a multiproduct firm with different payors, it can in-crease its profits by practicing price discrimination; it will price-discriminate accord-ing to the price elasticity of demand for each class of patient and type of service. The hospital's room rate is believed to be more elastic than the demand for ancillary services because patients and/or their physicians may decide to substitute out-of-hospital care or care in a different hospital if the room rate is higher in comparison. Once the patient has been hospitalized, ancillary services are complements to the use of the room, and fewer substitutes are available for those ancillary services. The charges for ancillary services are also generally a small portion of the room charge. Thus the demand for ancillary services is believed to be relatively price inelastic. If the hospital is interested in maximizing its profits, it will charge higher prices (relative to costs) for those services and that class of patients whose demands are less price elastic.

This simple model of profit-maximizing behavior predicts that hospitals will increase their prices if demand either increases or becomes less elastic, or if the prices of their inputs increase. This behavioral model also predicts that hospitals will attempt to minimize their costs of operation. If hospitals make a profit, then, under this model, they will reinvest those profits on the basis of which investments offer the highest rate of return. Examples of the types of investments they could undertake would be additions to bed capacity, if their occupancy rates were rising, cost-saving technology, or additional facilities and services. New facilities and services could be profitable in their own right or could serve to attract a greater number of physicians to the hospital's staff, thereby indirectly increasing the demand for the hospital's beds. An important aspect of this model is that the hospital would determine its prices as would a profit maximizer, minimize its costs (since higher costs represent forgone profits), and invest only in projects that offer a profitable return.

If there were free entry into the hospital market, excess profits would not exist in the long run. The performance of the industry would be similar to that of a monopolistically competitive industry; along with price competition and competition for physicians, hospitals would attempt to differentiate themselves from other hospitals. The prices of their services and classes of patients would, in the long run, reflect their respective average costs. If there were entry barriers, excess profits could exist in the long run, as prices exceeded average costs.

How well does this model reflect observed hospital behavior? With regard to hospital pricing policies, there is evidence that hospitals set price according to their price elasticity of demand. Prices have been much greater than average costs for those services believed to be less price elastic (ancillary services), but closer to average costs for those services believed to be more price elastic (room rates and delivery room) (15). For example, obstetric patients have the time to compare prices among hospitals.

Until the 1980s, observed hospital behavior diverged from the profit-maximizing model with regard to the assumptions of cost minimization and the profitability of investments. Hospitals invested in facilities and services that were known in advance to result in substantial losses; cross subsidies were provided to certain facilities and services to offset their losses rather than closing them. However, the main problem with the profit-maximizing model of the hospital is that it excludes any important role for the physician. According to this model, the only role for physicians is a passive one, to increase demand for the hospital. The model assumes that the hospital will attempt to keep adding physicians to its staff, whereas in the past the medical staff tightly controlled staff appointments and sought to limit rather than expand physician staff appointments.

There also appear to have been barriers to entry or other "peculiar" aspects to the hospital market, since previously hospitals were able to survive even though they did not minimize their costs and were able to undertake and maintain services that resulted in losses.

Another behavioral model posits that hospitals act as if they wanted to maximize their output or revenues. According to this model, hospitals attempt to maximize their profits in the short run (by setting prices and output to maximize profits) and invest either in additional capacity, cost-saving technology, or facilities and services that result in the largest increases in their output. Hospitals would still minimize their costs and maximize profits, since to do otherwise is to forgo revenue, which could be used to increase output. With reference to Figure 10-2, an output maximizer would increase output to Q_2, which would represent the point on the demand curve where average cost equals price. This does not mean that for every service or class of patients price equals average cost, but it does in the aggregate. This model is similar to the previous model both in its predictions and in its lack of consistency with observed data.

Utility-Maximizing Models of Hospital Behavior

The next set of models incorporate some of the observed inconsistencies of the previous models. The first of these models suggest that managers of nonprofit hospitals have objectives other than just profit (which they cannot keep or share) or being the administrator of the largest hospital. The decisionmakers are assumed to have a utility function that includes some measure of the quality of the institution as well as its size. The quality of a hospital is not a well-defined variable; quality may include the type of facilities and services offered in the institution, the quality of its medical staff and the specialists on that staff, as well as the caliber of its labor inputs. Under this "quality-quantity" behavioral model, the hospital will still seek to maximize its profits in the short run through its pricing strategy, but it will then attempt to invest that profit either in increased quantity—increased capacity, cost-saving technology, or facilities and services that result in an increase in quantity of patients—or in prestige/quality investments. Because quantity and quality are to some extent substitutable for one another in the utility function, the manager will have to make a trade-off according to the marginal increase in utility resulting from increased quality or from increased quantity.

The effect of adding quality to the hospital's objective is to cause an increase in hospital costs. This change in costs as a result of increased quality is shown as Figure 10–3. To start, assume that the hospital is operating on average-cost curve AC_1. Since it cannot keep any profits, its long-run price and output will be P_1 and Q_1, respectively. If the hospital invests in increased quality, this results in an increase in its costs; the average-cost curve rises to AC_2, but the increased quality also results in an increase in the hospital's demand, shifting its demand to D_2. The increase in demand may occur as a result of attracting additional physicians to the hospital. After some point, increased expenditures for quality will result in small or negligible increases in demand; at this point the additional cost of increased quality may exceed the additional revenue resulting from the small increments in demand. Additions to quality beyond that point continue to raise the average-cost curve to AC_3 but do not result in further shifts in demand. Since funds that are used to increase quality could be used to increase quantity by adding to capacity, the manager has to determine the relative weights to be placed on the quantity-quality trade-off.

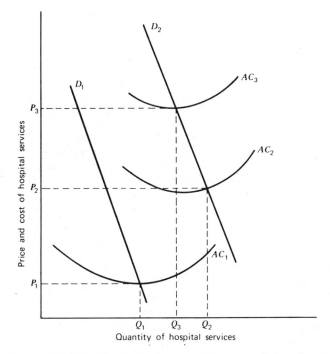

Figure 10-3. The effect on hospital costs of increases in hospital quality.

The consequences for economic efficiency of a utility model of a hospital attempting to maximize both quantity and quality is that the price of hospital care will be higher than if quality were not continually increased. Continued increases in quality without increased demand will shift the average-cost curve higher, possibly decreasing quantity and raising price. Further, hospitals will be producing a higher-quality product than consumers might be willing to pay for. Such a behavioral model could be accurate only if there were either some barriers to entry, such that lower-cost, lower-quality hospitals could not enter the market, or if consumers had an elastic demand with respect to hospital quality and the price of their care were subsidized. With entry and price competition, consumers would select that combination of price and quality that corresponded to what they were willing to pay for rather than to the quality-quantity preferences of the hospital administrator. Quality in such a case would increase in response to consumer demands for quality. If, on the other hand, barriers to entry existed or consumers did not have to pay the full price for hospital care, higher levels of quality could exist in the hospital market and would be determined by the preferences of hospital decisionmakers.

How consistent has the quantity-quality model been with observed behavior? This model still implies a profit-maximizing pricing strategy and cost-minimizing behavior since the forgone revenues could have been used to increase quality or quantity. It does explain why hospitals might make unprofitable investments or maintain unprofitable services, as long as these services add prestige to the institution. This model also suggests that a hospital will invest in new technology as soon as it becomes available, not necessarily because of its effect on demand, but because of its effect on the perceived image of the hospital. The quantity-quality model also suggests that hospitals with such objectives will be against the entry of for-profit hospitals into their communities. The nonprofit hospitals would be using internal cross-subsidization of their services to pay for the prestige services, which are money losers. For-profit hospitals, which do not have a prestige objective and do not have to resort to cross-subsidization of services, would not have to price their services as high as those of nonprofit hospitals. The for-profits attempt to compete with the nonprofits by lowering the price of the "profitable" services in comparison with the prices charged by the nonprofits. The nonprofits have claimed that these money-losing services are essential to meeting the needs of the community and that the for-profit hospitals are "skimming the cream" by not offering such services.[1] Others claim that the money-losing services are duplicative in the community and should not be offered by multiple hospitals.

The number of hospitals with open heart surgery facilities and their utilization has been cited as an example of this duplication. In 1961, 327 facilities reported having such facilities. The percentage breakdown of hospitals with specified cases per year is: 11 percent had *no* cases, 30 percent had 1–9 cases, 36 percent had 10–49 cases, 17 percent had 50 or more cases, and 6 percent were unknown. This survey of hospitals with open heart surgery facilities was repeated in 1969 with similar findings (16). It is difficult to believe that the quality of open heart surgery is the same regardless of the frequency of the surgery performed. To test this hypothesis, a study was conducted of the frequency with which different types of surgery were performed and the resulting mortality rates. In their analysis, the investigators controlled for other factors that might affect mortality, such as the patient's age, sex, and health status. It was found that for complicated types of surgery, the greater the volume of surgery performed, the lower the surgical mortality rates (17).

Although it provides additional explanations on the quality side, this model still has some drawbacks—namely, the expectation of cost-minimizing behavior, the lack of a clearly defined role for physicians in the decisionmaking process, and the failure to incorporate physician objectives.

The quantity-quality model has been modified to address one of these failings by including a "slack" variable in the manager's utility function. Hospital administrators, according to this utility model, are also interested in working in a pleasant environment, as defined by such amenities as thick rugs and higher wages for employees to minimize conflict. This broader utility function of the hospital administrator predicts that hospitals will still price to maximize profits, and then will spend those profits to achieve some combination of quantity, quality, and slack. Again, the survival of hospitals that act in such a manner depends upon a situation of strong barriers to entry, or one where patients are responsible for paying even less of their hospital costs than under the previous models. If entry exists and patients are responsible for payment of their hospitalization expenses (or the hospital faces fixed prices for its products), hospitals will have to compete on the basis partly of price as well as of their differentiated product. With the inclusion of slack in the manager's utility function, prices will be even higher than under the previous models. Such a model therefore assumes that patients (and/or the purchasers of hospital care) have become relatively indifferent to the

---

[1]"Skimming" by proprietaries has been investigated in a number of studies. One such study is Carson W. Bays, "Case-Mix Differences Between Nonprofit and For-Profit Hospitals," *Inquiry*, March 1977. In his conclusion Bays raises the appropriate question: "[W]hy is the pricing structure of nonprofits such that for-profits find it profitable to produce only certain types of care[?]" (p. 21).

prices charged or that few substitutes are available. Under these circumstances, hospitals would compete with one another, but the competition would be to see which hospitals could become the most prestigious, while providing the administrative staff with a pleasant working environment. There would be a great deal of duplication within the industry, as well as excess capacity, high costs, and rapidly rising prices to finance the described behavior.

The foregoing models of hospital behavior, although they apparently explain some observed data in the real world, do not explain other phenomena. For example, why are hospitals nonprofit? If it is because it is immoral to profit from sickness, why can people profit from hunger and the need for shelter? Also, these models attribute a passive role to physicians. Hospitals, under these models, attempt to attract more physicians to their staffs, yet physicians, according to our observations, attempt to limit additions to their staffs. The decisionmakers in the foregoing models appear to be hospital administrators or an undefined group, but in reality physicians have had a great deal of control over the hospital, its pricing policies, and investment behavior. The next model of hospital behavior attempts to rectify these weaknesses.

A Physician-Control Model of Hospital Behavior

The physician is the manager of the patient's illness, with responsibility for deciding upon the components to be used in providing treatment. As someone with a stake in what inputs are used, the physician might also be expected to combine the treatment inputs in such a manner so as to increase his or her own income and/or productivity. This view of the consumer's demand for medical care is based on the assumption that the total price of medical care is the relevant price to the consumer, not the individual price of specific inputs such as hospital care. (This assumption was more appropriate before there was such widespread insurance for hospital care and may again be more relevant currently.) If the consumer is more concerned with the total price of the treatment than with the price of its separate parts, more of the total price would be left for the physician the less the patient has to pay for any one component, such as hospital care. Conversely, "the greater the supply price of the inputs, the smaller the return to the producer of a given quantity of the final product" (18). That the total price of medical care is the relevant price to the consumer can be illustrated with reference to Figure 10-2. If two inputs are used in providing a medical treatment–hospital and physician services–then, given the patient's demand for medical care and an average-cost curve which represents the cost of hospital care, the difference between the price charged the patient and the amount that goes to pay the hospital is available to the physician. The physician acts as a contractor, retaining the amount left over after all the other inputs have been paid.[2]

This profit-maximizing model of the physician can be used to explain a number of apparent anomalies in the health field. The medical staff of a hospital is assumed to control the hospital under this model; it is further assumed that the decisions undertaken by the hospital represent the objectives of the staff physicians. If the demand for medical care were to increase, it would be in the physicians' interest that it be met by

---

[2]Such profit-maximizing behavior on the part of the physician is not necessarily inconsistent with the physician's acting in the patient's economic interest as well. If hospital care is free to the patient (because of insurance coverage), while the patient must pay the full price for use of other components, it may be in both the patient's and the physician's interest to hospitalize the patient.

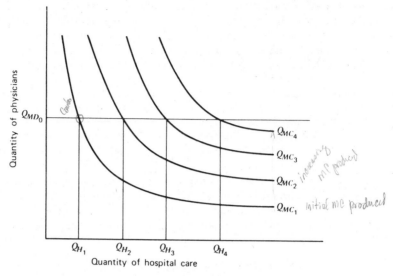

Figure 10–4. A production function for medical care.

an increase in hospital capacity, which would increase the physicians' productivity, rather than by an increase in the number of physicians. For example, with reference to Figure 10–4, physician and hospital services are two inputs in a production function. With an increase in the demand for medical care, the increased output, represented by the highest isoquant, can be produced with different quantities of either physician or hospital services. At the initial amount of medical care being produced, isoquant Q_{MC1}, the combination of physicians and hospital care is Q_{MD0} and Q_{H1}, respectively. As the quantity of medical care to be provided increases to isoquant Q_{MC4}, the number of physicians and the amount of hospital care can be increased in the same proportions as previously. However, it will be more in keeping with the interests of the physician if their number remains the same while the amount of hospital care is increased. With the same number of physicians, Q_{H4} of hospital care will be required. Since the quantity of medical care produced is greater, even though the number of physicians has remained unchanged, the marginal productivity of the physician has increased; correspondingly, the marginal productivity of the hospital has fallen. This is similar to the law of variable proportions, in which output is increased by increasing the use of one input while holding constant the quantity of another input; the marginal productivity of the variable input—in this case the hospital—will eventually decline. The higher the physician's productivity, the greater will be his or her income.

This model suggests that physicians would favor increases in the hospital's capacity to provide additional services; increases in the hospital's capacity to handle more physician services as demand increases, such as increasing the number of interns and residents, who provide physician services for which the physician can charge the patient; additional facilities and services, such as an excess of operating rooms and obstetric facilities, so the physician does not have to wait or be inconvenienced; and facilities and services that are available in other community hospitals so that the physician does not have to refer a patient to another hospital and physician, thereby risking the loss of a fee. The staff physicians who do not have staff appointments at other hospitals would thereby favor hospital investment, even though it may be duplicative for the community, because it increases their productivity and income. Physicians would also prefer some hospital slack, enabling them to economize on their own time.

The effect of physician control over hospital investment policies is to cause technical inefficiency in production; too many inputs are used relative to the physician input in meeting increased demands for medical care. The price to the physician for these other inputs is zero, particularly if they are paid in full by some third-party payor or the government. Before a large percentage of the population had coverage for hospitalization, the physician would be expected to be more concerned with the hospital's costs, since the higher those costs, the lower would be the payment available to the physician. In larger hospitals, however, the effect on any one physician's income of inefficient behavior on the part of the hospital would be small. Only in smaller hospitals, with correspondingly fewer physicians, would physicians be expected to be concerned with the efficiency of the hospital's operation. As insurance coverage for hospital care became more widespread, however, and as payment to hospitals was based on the hospital's costs, regardless of what they were, increases in hospital prices became less of a concern to the physician. As the price of hospital care to the patient became smaller, physicians were able to increase their charges to the patient and were unconcerned with the effect on costs of the hospital's investment and efficiency behavior.

The physician-control model also provides some explanation of hospital pricing behavior. The physician would prefer that the hospital assign relatively low prices to services that are complementary to the physician's services, in which case we might expect (prior to the widespread availability of hospital insurance) to find hospital charges for the operating room priced at or below cost. Similarly, obstetricians would prefer the same type of pricing policy for the hospital's delivery room. As insurance coverage increased, physicians would be expected to favor hospital profit-maximizing pricing policies (when they did not conflict with their own pricing strategies), since such prices would result in greater hospital profits, which could then be invested internally according to physician preferences. Physicians might also want their hospital to have an outpatient department and to provide preventive care services, which might at first appear to compete with the physicians. The outpatient department, however, is a convenient way of avoiding the financial risk of caring for low-income patients and allows physicians to allocate more of their time to higher-income patients. Physicians are also relieved of providing emergency services, thereby allowing them more time for more remunerative services or for leisure. The same explanations can be offered for having the hospital provide preventive care, in that the physician's time is freed for acute services, which offer a higher return per unit of time.

An interesting aspect of the physician-control model is that it offers an explanation of why hospitals are nonprofit. If physicians were in fact the real decisionmakers in the hospital, hospitals are nonprofit because this form of control was more profitable for their physicians. The advantages to physicians of nonprofit hospitals are several. First, a nonprofit hospital could not sell medical services directly to the patient; consumers could not buy all their medical care from the hospital because they first had to go to a physician if they required hospitalization, thereby increasing the demand for physicians. Medical societies ensured that hospitals would not be able to compete with physicians by having the various states enact legislation prohibiting the corporate practice of medicine. Under such legislation, only physicians could practice medicine, not organizations operated by nonphysicians. Second, when physicians were concerned with the total price of care, they preferred that hospital services be sold at marginal cost. If hospitals were for-profit, hospitals would want to increase their profit by setting price above marginal cost (setting marginal cost equal to marginal revenue). If hospitals were able to do so, less of the total price would be available to the physician.

Nonprofit status would be preferable to a for-profit hospital owned by the physicians themselves. When hospitals are nonprofit, the hospital can receive relief from payment of taxes, become the recipients of philanthropic contributions (which are tax deductible), accept volunteers, who provide services at no charge, and receive substantial government subsidies, such as from the Hill-Burton program. In addition, the physicians could receive the assistance of interns and residents, for whom they do not have to pay salaries, and receive the benefit of their services. The effect of these various subsidies is to cause hospital costs to be lower than they would be otherwise.

If physicians are concerned with the total price of care that the patient pays, they would favor subsidies to their inputs of production. If physicians were to own (or use) a for-profit hospital, inputs would have to be paid their market price. By having hospital inputs subsidized, it is relatively cheaper to expand those inputs when there is an increase in demand for medical care. Further, if the physicians own the hospital, then the larger that hospital becomes, and the greater the number of physicians associated with it (or who share in its ownership), the less incentive each physician has to be concerned with the hospital's costs because the effect of any savings (or profit) on any one physician is so small. The advantages of for-profit ownership decline as the size of hospital and the number of physicians increase (19). Another advantage to the physician is that the nonprofit hospital can only use surplus funds internally. Hospitals would have to use a criterion other than profitability for the investment of their funds. In lieu of profitability, the hospital (the board of trustees and the managers) would settle upon prestige as a goal, which would also be consistent with the investment objectives of the hospital's staff physicians. The institution would be more willing to invest in duplicative services and facilities than if it were accountable to stockholders.

One additional advantage that accrues to the physicians of a nonprofit hospital is that they retain stronger control over the hospital's decisionmaking. In the past, medical societies have been viewed as being similar to a physicians' cartel. As such, it is useful to examine the method that the cartel had to control the amount of output produced by each of its members. The individual producer in a cartel always has an incentive to increase output, since the costs of doing so are less than the cartel's profit-maximizing price. Unless the cartel can prevent its members from expanding their output, the monopoly price will fall. Since there are so many physicians, it is relatively costly to monitor the output of individual physicians in their offices (although the cartel can limit the use of inputs contributing to increased production, i.e., which personnel can undertake different tasks). It was far easier to limit the number of hospital beds per physician, which also acted as a constraint on the physician's productivity. By controlling the number of hospital beds, the medical society was able to limit competition among physicians for patients. Limiting the number of hospital beds, however, makes them a scarce resource. If physicians were to bid for these scarce inputs, it would transfer income from the physician to the hospital. To retain these monopoly profits for themselves, the physicians in control of the hospital used a form of nonprice rationing, either seniority or some other standard, to distribute the scarce hospital privileges among themselves (20).

To sum up the physician-control model, before the mid-1960s, when hospital insurance was not widespread and major medical insurance was more prevalent, physicians would have been expected to minimize the cost of all the medical inputs used in providing a medical treatment. Patients were concerned about the total price of medical care and physicians would be able to receive the difference between the cost of the inputs and the total price of medical care charged to the patient. As hospital coverage became more extensive and hospitals were reimbursed for their costs, physicians no longer had to be concerned with the cost of hospital care. Physician payment was separated from payment for hospital services and physicians were neither financially responsible nor accountable for their decisions. There were no constraints on how the physician used the hospital or influenced its investment decisions. Planning efforts to reduce duplication of hospital facilities failed because they were contrary to both the physicians' and the hospital's interests. Then starting in the early 1980s, with the applicability of the antitrust laws to the health field, the growth of HMOs, payment of hospitals according to fixed prices, and the concern by business with reducing the rise in their health insurance premiums, the incentives of the pre-Medicare period reappeared. Once again, physicians have incentives to minimize the cost of producing medical treatments. With the decline in the monopoly power of physicians and the emergence of market competition among insurance companies and producers of medical services, pressure is being placed on physicians to minimize the cost of producing medical services.

One implication of the physician-control model is that as the supply of physicians increases at a more rapid rate than in the past, less care will be provided in the hospital and more of it will be provided in the physician's office. Refer back to Figure 10–4, where it was shown that physician and hospital inputs are somewhat substitutable for each other. Again, if payments of medical care are based on the total price of that care (e.g., a capitation payment per individual), the physician can retain more of those funds if less is paid to the hospital. Physicians will begin substituting more of their own input in the provision of medical care. (This assumes, however, that the total amount to be spent for medical care per patient is limited and what gets spent on other inputs is no longer available to the physician.) Unless reimbursement policies consider the various incentive effects of physicians, their effect may not only be different from but opposite that which was intended.

Concluding Comments

An examination of the behavioral objectives of hospitals was undertaken because of the effects on economic efficiency of different hospital objectives. Within the hospital, three groups are generally considered to be important in the determination of the hospital's objectives: the trustees, the administrators, and the medical staff. The behavioral models analyzed assume that one of the groups is dominant in the decisionmaking process (21). Several of the hospital and physician-control models provide consistent explanations of hospital decisionmaking. Because the determination of prices and investment in duplicative facilities are predicted by several models, it is difficult to distinguish between them. Assuming that either the utility-maximizing model or the physician-control model is the more accurate representation of hospital behavior, what are the effects of these objectives on hospital efficiency?

In an era of extensive third-party reimbursement and cost-based payment of hospitals, the incentives facing the decisionmakers are such that the output mix of the hospital industry is unlikely to be optimal. There is likely to be a bias toward higher "quality," meaning more facilities and services, greater capital intensity, and a tendency to introduce new technology before its benefits have been fully evaluated. The quantity-quality output mix of the hospital is likely to be different from what patients would be willing to pay for if they were to bear a greater share of the costs of hospitalization and had greater choice in this selection. As a result of the hospitals' desire to enhance prestige or the physicians' desire to enhance their income by increasing their productivity, there is also likely to be unnecessary duplication of facilities and services; that is, to the extent that there are economies of scale in certain services, more institutions are likely to be operating at higher costs than necessary because of low use of facilities. There will be system inefficiency, meaning that there are too many firms (facilities and services) operating in the industry. There is also likely to be firm inefficiency because of the desire for slack in the manager's utility function (and because the return to each physician declines, the larger the institution). When a large percentage of the population is covered by hospital insurance, with payment models based on each hospital's costs, it is less important for the hospital managers to minimize their costs of operation. Finally, there are redistributive effects (both as a result of the methods used to set hospital prices, such as internal cross-subsidization, and the taxes that are raised to pay for the increase in hospital expenditures) in that income is being redistributed from taxpayers to persons working directly and indirectly in the hospital sector.

As payment systems change and as hospitals face different incentives, the effects on performance are more related to the incentives than to the ownership or control of the hospital. Under a price-competitive system with entry, each of the behavioral models of the hospital would hypothesize that the decisionmakers will price so as to maximize profits and act to minimize their costs. How the "profits" are paid out, however, will differ according to the hospital's ownership and control.

Further, in more recent years, the group having control over the hospital has been changing. The supply of physicians, relative to hospitals, has been increasing. As their relative scarcities have been changing, so have their relative market power. Physicians need hospitals to practice and hospitals have found it relatively easier to attract physicians. With the new competitive environment and elimination of many legal restrictions, control by physicians over hospital decisionmaking has diminished.

DETERMINANTS OF MARKET STRUCTURE

The Extent of Economies of Scale in Hospitals

An important determinant of the degree of competition among hospitals is the extent of economies of scale in relation to the size of the market. With economies of scale, the larger the output of the firm, the lower will be its average costs. With price competition, firms with higher costs will not be able to survive. For a given size of market, more firms will be able to exist as the gains from being a facility size that is least costly occur at small levels of production. The larger the size of the plant required to achieve the minimum costs of production, the fewer the number of firms that will be able to compete. An important reason for wanting to determine the extent of economies of scale, therefore, is to ascertain whether hospitals are a "natural" monopoly, whereby only very large hospitals are able to achieve the most efficient scale of operation. Or, are hospitals similar to most other industries in that the gains from large-scale production can be achieved in institutions that are small enough to permit many firms to survive in an urban area? Hospitals have been referred to as public utilities, necessitating public utility regulation. An analysis of the extent of economies of scale in hospitals would indicate whether such public utility status is justified on economic grounds.

Several other factors are also important in determining whether hospitals could, theoretically, be a competitive industry. The first is the importance of the patients' distance from the hospital. Patients might be willing to go to a smaller, more expensive hospital if the value of their travel cost and time more than offset the lower costs of going to a larger hospital farther away. The total price of hospitalization is the relevant price to the patient, not just the hospital portion of that price. (The importance of travel cost varies with the particular service being demanded, as, for example, whether it is emergency or elective care.)

A second factor affecting the market structure of hospitals is whether there are barriers to entry. Regulatory controls on entry could provide hospitals with monopoly power. Similar to entry controls have been quasi-controls, such as the refusal of an insurance company (e.g., Blue Cross) to pay for hospital care in certain types of institutions (e.g., for-profit hospitals).

A third factor influencing the degree of competition among hospitals is the role of the physician. Patients do not generally purchase hospital care directly; their physician has a staff appointment at certain hospitals, and patients must generally enter the hospital where their physician practices. In this situation, competition among hospitals would still exist, but instead of competing for patients directly, hospitals would compete for physicians and, indirectly, for their patients. If physicians faced appropriate incentives and acted as their patient's agent, thereby minimizing their patients' costs of treatment, the effect of hospitals' competition for physicians would be similar to competition for patients.

Determination of economies of scale in the production of hospital services has also been useful for two other reasons. The finding of economies of scale together with the observation that hospitals are not taking advantage of such scale economies (excluding reasons such as patient travel costs) may indicate that hospitals are inefficient. The same output could be produced at lower cost if it were produced in fewer but larger institutions. Second, inefficiency in the production of hospital services is an indication that public policy may be appropriate. One type of policy is to regulate the number and size of health facilities. Knowledge of economies of scale could then be used for planning such facilities (22). Hospital planning has been proposed as a way of efficiently allocating resources for producing hospital care. If economic efficiency in production is to be achieved through planning, hospital planners will require the same information regarding economies of scale, travel costs, and other costs used in a competitive system to achieve economic efficiency. The concept of regionalization (where there are different levels of hospital facilities, the largest ones serve the population of a region and the smallest serve a community) is based on the belief that there are economies of scale in certain hospital services and that the extent of these economies varies with the particular hospital service. Thus the information that would indicate whether hospitals can be competitive would also be important for planning those services if planning were used as an alternative to competition to achieve an efficient production of hospital care.

Knowledge of the extent of economies of scale in hospital services is also necessary when regulation attempts to achieve an optimum allocation of resources through the setting of payment systems. Under rate regulation, one method for determining which hospitals should be permitted to maintain or add specified facilities and services is to establish a reimbursement rate that is related to the minimum average cost of providing the specified service. Hospitals able to take advantage of economies of scale in producing that service would be able to cover their costs and would thereby be able to offer that particular service.

Thus, for the purpose of understanding the structure of the hospital industry, its efficiency, and for purposes of hospital planning and rate regulation, it is important to determine the extent of economies of scale in the provision of hospital services. How the information on hospital costs can be used specifically for each of these purposes is discussed in subsequent sections.

Empirical Findings on the Extent of Economies of Scale in Hospital Services

The theoretical relationship between hospital cost and size is U-shaped. As the size of the facility (and its production) is increased, average cost per unit should decrease, reach a minimum, and then increase. The reasons for this expected relationship are several: with a larger facility there can be greater specialization of labor; further, with the emphasis on licensure as a means of assuring competent personnel in the health field and the consequent limited flexibility in delegation of tasks, licensed and specialized personnel can be used more fully in a larger institution than in a smaller one. Specialized equipment and facilities can also be used to their capacity in larger institutions. Finally, larger institutions are more likely to be able to take advantage of quantity discounts in purchasing than are smaller institutions.[3] Offsetting these advantages is the greater proportion of time and effort required to coordinate and control work in large organizations. In general, for sufficiently small outputs, efficiency increases with size, because the advantages that accrue from the use of specialized labor and equipment far outweigh the increased cost of management. As size increases, however, the reduction in per unit cost afforded by greater and greater specialization begins to decline and is eventually outweighted by increased costs of coordination and control. Other things being equal, average hospital costs thus may be expected to decline initially and then rise as size is increased, as shown by the U-shaped curve in Figure 10–5. How rapidly these gains and losses from scale of operation occur is what determines the shape of the long-run average cost curve.

The theoretical relationship is not easily determined, however. Hospitals are not homogeneous in size or other characteristics. Hospitals are multiproduct firms. In addition to producing inpatient services, which differ in their quality, the type of patient treated, and the severity of the particular case, hospitals also produce outpatient services, education, training, research, and community services. Hospitals also differ in the amenities they provide. There are further differences among hospitals, such as in the prices they must pay for their labor and nonlabor inputs as well as in hospital efficiency. A difficulty with studies that have attempted to estimate the effect of size on average cost has been to measure adequately and then to hold constant all the other factors that affect hospital costs, while estimating the net effect of size alone. The consequence of not being able to hold these other factors constant is that the relationship between size and costs is likely to be biased.

---

[3]To some extent small hospitals may circumvent the various diseconomies associated with their size by purchasing services from outside firms.

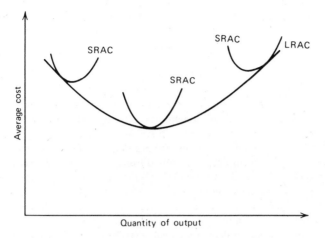

Figure 10–5. The relationship between hospital size and average cost.

For example, if economies of scale exist in larger hospitals, which usually treat patients who are more seriously ill, then unless differences in the type of patient are accounted for, it may seem that the observed relationship between cost and size is that larger hospitals have *higher* per unit costs. The result of failing to hold constant differences in costs between hospitals that are a result of factors other than size (such as seriousness of illness) may be seen in Figure 10–6. The hospital represented by the short-run average-cost curve at point C may be on a lower long-run average cost curve than hospital B or A because it may provide fewer services. If one were to observe raw data on average cost and size, one might observe data points that represent the relationship between hospitals D and A. It would appear that hospital D, which is smaller, has lower costs than hospital A, and that average costs increase as the size of the hospital is similarly increased. If adjustments are made for the differences between these two hospitals—namely, the reason they are on different average cost-curves—it

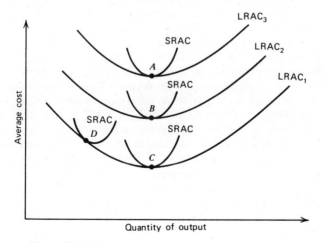

Figure 10–6. Variations in average cost between hospitals.

can be observed that for the product hospital A is producing (on long-run average-cost curve $LRAC_3$), it is producing its output in the least costly facility (it is operating in a facility that is at the minimum point on its long-run average cost curve). Hospital D, however, is not only producing a different product (one that is less costly to produce than the one produced by hospital A), but it is also in a facility that is not least costly; it is at point D rather than point C.

Investigators who have attempted to estimate the extent of economies of scale in hospitals have differed in their approaches used to control for these other factors affecting hospital costs (23). Early studies on hospital costs tended to use more aggregated data; subsequent studies have used more detailed data, particularly on their patient population. For example, to measure differences in the hospitals' product, various investigators have used the number of facilities and services, others have grouped hospitals by comparable facilities and services, while still others have classified facilities and services according to whether they are basic, quality-enhancing, complex, or community services. Investigators have also included patient case-mix measures—that is, the proportion of a hospital's patients classified into various diagnostic categories (24). In an attempt to include a quality variable, some investigators have included a measure of the use of hospital inputs or even some measure of the hospital's costs as a proxy for quality. More recent measures of quality that have been used are the probability that a patient will be turned away or a patient's expected waiting time (25). There are still severe data problems involved in adequately controlling for all the variations in hospital output. There are, in addition, the difficulties of measuring the non-patient care outputs of the hospital, such as teaching programs (and the impact that interns and residents have on hospital costs), outpatient services (which may share facilities and equipment with inpatient services in the hospital), and so on.

All the studies on hospital costs have also found it difficult to adjust for differences in hospital efficiency, making it difficult to separate the effects of efficiency on costs from the effects of differences in hospital size. Additional technical problems include the difficulty of adjusting for differences in prices paid by hospitals for their factor inputs that are unrelated to differences in hospital size. Since larger hospitals are located in large urban areas, where wage rates are often higher, it must be determined how much of the larger hospitals' higher wage costs are paid for the same type of hospital worker as elsewhere and how much for more highly skilled workers.

An important limitation of most previous hospital cost studies is the failure to adjust hospital costs for differences among hospitals in the contributions of physicians to the hospitals' output (26). Hospitals differ in their employment of staff physicians. In hospitals without salaried physicians, the physician charges the patient separately for services rendered. Hospitals that employ physicians will have higher costs than hospitals that do not, although there may be no differences in their output. Interns and residents also provide patient care; their costs are included in the costs of those hospitals that have such educational programs, although their (or the patient's physician's) contribution to hospital output is not included in hospitals that do not have such programs. The foregoing are some of the conceptual and data problems involved in estimating the net effect of hospital size on cost.

The empirical approach used to derive the effect of size on cost, while controlling for other differences between hospitals, is to use some form of multivariate analysis. The general form of such an equation is

$$AC = f(B, S, C, Q, V, P, E, D, O)$$

where AC = dependent variable, usually average cost per admission
      f = functional relationship, connoting the dependence of AC on the variables on the right-hand side of the equation
     B = measure of hospital size, usually measured in terms of number of beds
     S = hospital's service capability, usually measured by some enumeration of facilities and services in the hospital
     C = measure of patient case mix, measured by the proportion of patients in a given number of disease classifications
     Q = measure of quality, inadequately measured to date (if included at all) by a variable such as inputs per patient (e.g., lab tests)
     V = severity of illness within a patient disease classification, possibly measured (inadequately) by the number of surgical procedures
     P = adjustment for differences between hospitals for wages and other factor prices that are unrelated to hospital size
     E = differences in hospital efficiency that are unrelated to hospital size
     D = educational programs (e.g., number of interns and residents, affiliations with a medical school and a nursing school, as well as representing research and other training programs)
     O = other variables, such as the physicians' contribution and other hospital outputs, such as outpatient visits

Once the model has been specified in this manner and reasonable proxies have been developed for the various theoretical variables, data are collected on either a time-series or cross-sectional basis, or some combination of the two. That is, yearly data are collected on each of the listed variables for each hospital in a state, a region, or the country as a whole. [The assumption is that each data point for a hospital represents a given-sized facility (i.e., a short-run average-cost curve), which can then be used to trace out a long-run average-cost curve.] The advantage of using a cross-sectional analysis rather than a time-series approach (which would be yearly data from one or more hospitals over a long period) is that technology, medical practice, and illnesses can generally be assumed to be constant for a given period for each of the hospitals in the study. Other problems with conducting a time-series study are that data may be unavailable for long periods or accounting methods may have changed. There may also have been changes in the hospital's management and efficiency over time.

The method used to estimate the effect on cost of each of the factors above is multiple regression analysis. This method provides measures of the effects that each variable has on average cost, the significance of that variable, and the variation in average cost that is explained by all the variables in the equation. To determine whether there are economies of scale, the output measure is allowed to be curvilinear; that is, either the variables are transformed into logarithms or a squared term is included for the output measure.[4]

---

[4]For example, if the net effect of beds on average cost per admission is $-.04$ BEDS $+ .0001$ BEDS^2, then the size of hospital with lowest average costs is determined by taking the partial derivative of AC with respect to BEDS, setting it equal to zero, and solving for BEDS.

$$\frac{\partial AC}{\partial BEDS} = -.04 + .0002 \text{ BEDS} = 0$$
$$+ .0002 \text{ BEDS} = +.04$$
$$\text{BEDS} = 200$$

Average costs per admission would be at a minimum in hospitals with 200 beds.

The foregoing discussion of statistical estimation has been cursory. The interested reader who wishes to pursue it further is referred to several of the review articles that have been written on hospital costs; students with a background in econometrics are referred to the studies themselves, examples of which are referenced in the review articles.

The following is a brief summary of the findings on economies of scale. Because of the conceptual and data limitations in conducting such studies, it is difficult to be precise with regard to exact estimates for the effect of any of the theoretical variables on hospital costs. Economists studying hospital costs disagree as to whether the various studies have been able to hold constant all the other factors affecting hospital costs. Some general findings, however, do appear among the various studies. First, there appear to be slight economies of scale: hospitals with approximately 200–300 beds appear to have the lowest average costs. The shape of this average-cost curve is shallow; that is, it does not fall sharply, nor is the minimum point much below that of hospitals on the ends of the curve.

Although difficult to determine empirically, hospitals may also be subject to economies of scope, that is, hospitals with greater service capability may be subject to larger economies of scale. The reason for economies of scope is that it may be less expensive to produce several services jointly than it is to produce each separately. Services that have an interrelationship with one another may have lower costs when they are produced together within the hospital. The implication of the above is that services which are subject to economies of scope are more likely to be provided regionally or in larger markets.

Finding economies of scale (or not) for the hospital as a whole is insufficient for policy, planning, reimbursement, or any other purpose. For example, there are presumably large economies of scale in laundry operation; such information would be useful for a make-or-buy decision. Can a hospital produce its own laundry services more cheaply than it can buy such services from another hospital or from a centralized laundry service? The same analysis can be undertaken for other services within a hospital. For highly specialized services, such as lithotripters, the extent of economies of scale can be used to indicate how many such services can be offered in a given area. Which hospitals should be the ones to offer such services is a separate question, determined by the hospitals themselves in a market-competitive situation or by a regulatory agency when planning is used. Information on economies of scale by service can be used by a regulatory agency to set reimbursement levels, and then any hospital able to provide the service at that price can do so.

Another finding based on studies of economies of scale is that the mix of patients in the hospital is an important determinant of hospital costs: in some cases, case mix explains more than 50 percent of the variation in average costs between hospitals. The implication of this finding is that with prospective reimbursement for hospital payment, accurate measurement of the hospitals' patient mix and the complexity of the cases is important in establishing a hospital's prospective rate.

Studies that have attempted to estimate the effect on hospital costs of physician input have found that both the number and specialty mix of physicians have a significant effect on costs (27).

The finding of slight economies of scale suggests that many hospitals could exist in a community, possibly competing with one another. Since hospitals appear to add services in a very predictable way as they grow, "basic" hospital services are not subject to large economies of scale. [There are also probably good substitutes available for most of these services in a nonhospital setting (e.g., the physician's office).] In a large community there is little reason why there should not be multiple hospitals, although it is unlikely that each of the hospitals in the community would have all of the same specialized facilities. There would thus tend to be a less competitive market in a particular area as far as more highly specialized services such as open heart surgery are concerned. The demand for such highly specialized services is generally not of an emergency nature; the relevant market is likely to be at a state or even a regional level. Even for these services, it is unlikely that a case can be made for treating them as a natural monopoly.

Concluding Comments

The structure of the hospital market has changed over time. Until the late 1970s, hospitals were predominately nonprofit, independent institutions, generally competing in local markets, and providing inpatient services. The trend now is for hospitals to be part of a larger organization, a multihospital system, and to become vertically integrated, that is, provide an entire range of services, such as ambulatory services, inpatient care, home and nursing care, and operate retirement centers. One reason for the change in the structure of the hospital market has been the increasing importance of economies of scale and economies of scope.

Hospitals are becoming more concentrated; they have been affiliating with one another and forming what is referred to as "multihospital systems." The types of multihospital systems vary widely. In some systems, the hospital affiliation agreements are relatively weak. The hospital and its medical staff are able to retain their decision-making authority. The reasons usually given for weak forms of affiliation are the hospital being able to take advantage of economies of scale, such as in joint purchasing arrangements. At the other extreme, in terms of affiliation agreements, are hospitals that are completely merged into the larger organization; the institution loses its autonomy. The reasons for this type of arrangement are usually to take advantage of large economies of scale, such as lower interest charges on bond issues, improved cash management, lower malpractice premiums—each of which require the institution to be more tightly integrated with the other hospitals in the system, and because of the need for financial survival. Hospitals facing declining occupancy rates and more stringent reimbursement policies are more willing to give up their autonomy to survive.

In 1986, as shown in Table 10–5, 2,031 facilities belonged to 164 multihospital systems. These systems had a total of 355,859 beds, which represented approximately 33 percent of the total nonfederal short-term general beds. The trend toward hospital affiliations has increased in the last several years. Within the investor-owned systems, there has been a 21 percent growth in the number of units per system between 1981 and 1986. The fastest growth in the investor-owned group was in the number of managed beds, which increased 134 percent over that period (28). The growth in managed beds has also been the fastest-growing category for each of the other types of systems as well. As independent hospitals experience financial difficulties, they are more willing, in the current competitive environment, to turn to large systems to manage their institutions. Some members of the hospital industry believe that during the coming decade the unaffiliated community hospital will be the exception rather than the rule.

Hospital cost studies have examined the effects on costs of the size of an individual hospital. As such, these studies have generally neglected the effect on cost of hospitals

TABLE 10-5. Characteristics of Multihospital Systems, 1986

Type of System[a]	Total Number of Units in System	Total Number of Beds in System	Number of Beds per System	Number of Beds per Unit	Beds per System Owned or Leased	Beds per System Managed
Investor-owned (26)	967	140,289	5,395.7	145.1	3,939.1	2,705.2
Secular nonprofit (67)	442	71,790	1,071.5	162.4	989.5	338.6
Catholic (37)	358	85,035	2,298.2	237.5	2,220.6	339.5
Other religious (20)	158	35,837	1,791.9	226.8	1,535.8	393.9
Public (14)	106	22,908	1,636.3	216.1	1,636.3	—
Total (164)	2,031	355,859	2,169.9	175.2	1,870.7	844.0

SOURCE: "Multi-hospital Systems Survey," *Modern Health Care*, June 5, 1987, p. 52. Reprinted with permission from *Modern Healthcare* magazine. Copyright Crain Communications, Inc., 740 N. Rush Street, Chicago, IL 60611.
[a]Number of systems reporting in parentheses.

being part of larger organizations. Multihospital systems have been able to receive lower interest costs and greater access to the capital markets; purchasing discounts on supplies are also available to larger organizations. There are also economies in marketing a large organization as compared to a separate facility.

The role of the hospital and its product line have also been undergoing changes. In addition to horizontal integration, hospitals are becoming vertically integrated. For example, as a means of increasing referrals to their institution, hospitals have branched out into ambulatory care clinics, forming joint ventures with their medical staffs for certain patient activities, and developing retirement centers. These services act as feeder systems to the hospital. Similarly, hospitals are moving into substitute product lines. Rather than losing the revenues from outpatient surgery centers, hospitals are providing these services themselves. The same is occurring with regard to HMOs. Hospitals are participating and even forming their own HMOs so as to receive the admissions from HMO patients. Changes in the reimbursement system are also moving hospitals into complementary product lines. Under a fixed-price reimbursement system, hospitals now have the incentive to discharge Medicare patients sooner. By discharging patients to other institutional settings, such as nursing homes and home care, however, the hospital can receive additional reimbursement for care in these settings.

Multihospital systems choose their hospitals so as to increase their market share within a region; they also try to have a large teaching hospital which would be the referral center for their member hospitals within that region. By vertically integrating into related products, the multihospital system is then able to approach employers and offer a complete product line with broad geographic coverage. The next step in the process of vertical integration will be for the multihospital system to bear some risk, that is, offer insurance coverage to employers in their area.

The structure of the hospital industry is undergoing dramatic changes; hospitals are becoming part of larger systems and in turn becoming vertically integrated. The size of the organization is therefore increasing and competition is likely to be between larger organizations rather than between individual hospitals.

EFFECT OF MARKET STRUCTURE ON PERFORMANCE

Based on the evidence of economies of scale, competition can exist among hospitals in many market areas. Normally, competitive markets are expected to have desirable consequences; producers will choose the least cost size of facility, the firm will minimize its costs of production, and the price of the product will equal its marginal cost. These outcomes of a competitive market occur when there is price competition among firms. Firms may also compete on other grounds, but unless there is also price competition, purchasers will have no incentive to seek out those firms with the lowest prices. During the mid-1960s and 1970s, competition among hospitals occurred, but, it was not price competition. Medicare and Medicaid removed the incentive of the aged and the poor to be concerned with the price of hospital care. Also, the widespread existence of private health insurance, such as Blue Cross, removed any concerns over hospital prices by those with private insurance. Reimbursement by third party-payors, government, and private insurers on a cost basis also removed any incentives that hospitals may have had to be concerned with their costs.

Competition among hospitals during this period occurred without the usual constraints, that is, purchasers or hospitals having to make a choice and limited in their choices by prices and a budget. The nonprofit organizational form of the hospital also meant that any surpluses could not be retained by the hospital or its personnel. As the concern over prices was removed from patients and as budget constraints were removed from hospitals, nonprice competition among hospitals intensified.

The physician played a decisive role during this period. As the patient's agent, the physician determined the hospital to which the patient was admitted. Therefore hospitals competed for physicians. (In a physician control model of the hospital the outcome of nonprice competition would be similar.) The physician, under a cost based payment system to hospitals, can serve both the patient and hospital without any conflict (29). Providing additional benefits to the patient, as long as they have a positive effect, also provides additional payments to the hospital.

A number of studies have examined the effect of competition among hospitals during this period of cost-based hospital payment (30). The hypothesis of these studies was that hospitals in more competitive areas were likely to have higher costs than those of hospitals in less competitive areas, such as hospitals located in rural communities. When hospitals were monopolistic, they had less need to compete for physicians; there were fewer alternative hospitals available to physicians. In highly competitive markets, hospitals engaged in nonprice competition to have physicians join their staffs. The nonprice competition increased operating costs, resulted in the more rapid introduction of technology, and led to duplication of facilities and services. When physicians are viewed as the hospital decisionmakers, additional hospital expenditures in a competitive market enables physicians to increase their productivity and to increase their market share relative to other physicians.

Several of the studies have used the Standard Metropolitan Statistical Area (SMSA), a Census Bureau definition, as the geographical area for examining hospital competition; counties have also been used. Within the SMSA, some investigators have classified areas as more or less competitive based on the number of hospitals in that area; others have used the Herfindahl index (HI), which is the measure of concentration used by the Department of Justice in its merger guidelines.[5] The advantage of this index is that it is sensitive to both the number of firms and to their relative sizes (e.g., percent of total admissions). The higher the HI, the less competitive the market. Thus the index will be more monopolistic if a few firms have a high market share than if there were many firms, each with a small share. (The index is also used to indicate whether a merger between firms in the market is likely to lessen competition. If the merger raises the index to above 1,400, the merger is likely to be investigated on grounds of antitrust.)

A number of other factors affecting hospital costs in competitive and monopolistic areas, such as patient case mix, were included in the analyses so as to hold their effects constant.

---

[5]The Herfindahl Index is calculated by summing the squared market shares of each firm in the market. For example, if there are five hospitals in an area and each has the same market share, 20 percent, then the HI is

$$20^2 + 20^2 + 20^2 + 20^2 + 20^2 = 2,000$$

If the five firms had unequal market shares, the HI would be

$$40^2 + 30^2 + 10^2 + 10^2 + 10^2 = 2,800$$

Hospital ownership was also a variable included in these studies to determine whether for-profit and nonprofit hospitals differ in their competitive effects. For-profit hospitals, although they represent a small portion of all hospitals, have greatly increased their growth. According to a physician control theory of hospitals, for-profit hospitals would be expected to act differently than nonprofits since they have to earn a rate of return for their investors. Have such hospitals been able to increase their growth because they are more efficient than nonprofit hospitals? What effect have they had once they enter a market? Do they engage in cream skimming whereby they serve less severely ill patients or do not provide certain high-cost services? For-profit hospital chains have also had greater access to the capital markets since their larger revenues and assets make them better risks than independent community hospitals.

The evidence on for-profit hospitals is somewhat surprising. There is no significant difference between for-profit and nonprofit hospitals in their costs per admission, adjusted for case mix. However, for-profit hospitals are more profitable and their charges are higher, particularly for ancillary services. Their higher profits are apparently a result of higher prices rather than greater operating efficiency (31). One possible hypothesis to explain why for-profits have higher prices and are more profitable is that they have entered markets where the population is growing rapidly (e.g., the south and southwest), where there is less competition, where there are fewer entry restrictions, and where demand is less price elastic (or they profit maximize and nonprofits do not).

The empirical findings of several studies of hospital behavior, under a cost-based payment system, are that hospital costs are higher in competitive markets than in more monopolistic hospital markets. Economic theory suggests that in a price-competitive market, the greater the number of firms, the lower the price. However, given the limited degree of price competition among hospitals in the late 1960s and 1970s, competition occurred on a nonprice basis. Hospitals competed for physicians by offering additional facilities, the latest in technology, and increased staffing. The consequence was higher costs and duplication of expensive technology and facilities. Quality was also presumably higher, although it is difficult to measure (32).

In addition to the rapid increases in hospital costs, the performance of the hospital industry has been criticized on other grounds, namely, the large variations in costs among similar hospitals and extensive duplication of costly facilities and services. On numerous occasions, several hospitals in a community have been equipped with the same facility, even though one or two such facilities would easily accommodate the community's need.

Critics often cite the example of open heart surgery when making this argument. In 1969, 23 percent of all hospitals with facilities for open heart surgery performed less than one surgery per month, and 71 percent performed less than one per week (33). Radiation therapy would also seem to be excessively duplicated. A study of radiation therapy in New Hampshire, Massachusetts, and Rhode Island revealed that 20 of 67 hospitals equipped to provide radiation therapy in 1969 were providing 93 percent of all treatments. The authors concluded that five major centers might be adequate to accommodate all the needs for radiation therapy in the three states without seriously inconveniencing patients (34).

This kind of criticism might apply even to maternity care. Survey data collected by the American Hospital Association indicate that on average, newborn occupancy is only about 40 percent of the rate hospitals are equipped to handle (35). Teh-wei Hu has estimated a cost function for maternity care, based on data from 30 nonprofit hospitals in Pennsylvania (36). He found that most hospitals were operating at much smaller outputs than those associated with minimum average costs. His estimated cost function indicated a minimum-average-cost point of 1,616 deliveries per year, while the average annual number of actual deliveries in the sample hospitals was just under 1,000.

Large annual increases in hospital costs, wide variations in per unit costs among apparently similar hospitals, and the existence of underutilized facilities and services have been used as indications of extensive inefficiency in the hospital industry. The equivalent output could have been produced with fewer resources if they were used more efficiently. Cost-increasing changes in hospital resource use have improved the quality of care; for example, the adoption of new medical technology, increases in nurse/patient ratios, and even adding a new facility to a community's already underutilized facilities provides some quality improvement. Still, it is important to ask whether improvements in quality have always justified their high marginal costs. Previous methods of financing hospital care have not provided strong incentives for consumers, doctors, or the hospitals themselves to weigh the true costs of resource allocation decision for hospital care. Thus, even decisions that improve the quality of hospital care may often reflect less than optimal industry performance.

REFERENCES

1. Daniel Waldo, Katherine Levit, and Helen Lazenby, "National Health Expenditures, 1985," *Health Care Financing Review*, 8(1), Fall 1986: 14.
2. For descriptions of the controls as they applied to hospitals, see Stuart Altman and Joseph Eichenholz, "Control of Hospital Costs Under the Economic Stabilization Program," *Federal Register*, 39, January 23, 1974: 2693–2700; Richard Berman, "The Economic Stabilization Program of the United States: August 1971-April 1974," *World Hospitals*, 12, 1976; Paul Ginsburg, "Inflation and the Economic Stabilization Program," in Michael Zubkoff, ed., *Health: A Victim or Cause of Inflation?* (New York: PRODIST, 1976), pp. 31–51.
3. *Hospital Statistics* (Chicago: American Hospital Association, 1986), p. 3.
4. Martin Feldstein, *The Rising Cost of Hospital Care*, Chapter 5 (Washington, D.C.: Information Resources Press, 1971); and M. Feldstein and Amy Taylor, "The Rapid Rise of Hospital Costs," in Martin Feldstein, ed., *Hospital Costs and Health Insurance* (Cambridge, Mass.: Harvard University Press, 1981), pp. 19–56.
5. Victor Fuchs, "The Earnings of Allied Health Personnel—Are Health Workers Underpaid," *Explorations in Economic Research*, 3, Summer 1976: 408–431.
6. Martin Feldstein, "Hospital Cost Inflation: A Study of Non-profit Price Dynamics," *American Economic Review*, 61, December 1971: 861.
7. Calculated from data in National Center for Health Statistics, "Hospital Discharges and Length of Stay: Short-Stay Hospitals, United States—1972," *Vital and Health Statistics*, 10 (107), September 1976.
8. Anne Scitovsky and Nelda McCall, "Changes in the Costs of Treatment of Selected Illnesses 1951-1964-1971," Health Policy Discussion Paper, University of California School of Medicine, San Francisco, September 1975.

9. The information on intensive care units is taken from Louise Russell, "The Diffusion of New Hospital Technologies," *International Journal of Health Services*, 6(4), 1976: 557–580.

10. National Center for Health Statistics, *"Hospital Discharges and Lengths of Stay—1972"* (Washington, D.C.: U.S. Government Printing Office, 1972).

11. John Rafferty, "Enfranchisement and Rationing Effects of Medicare on Discretionary Hospital Use," *Health Services Research*, Spring 1975: 51–62.

12. See Paul J. Feldstein and Saul Waldman, "Financial Position of Hospitals in the Early Medicare Period," *Social Security Bulletin*, 31, October 1968: 18–23.

13. See Karen Davis, "Hospital Costs and the Medicare Program," *Social Security Bulletin*, 36, August 1973: 18–36.

14. The following is a representative list of articles dealing with hospital objectives. K. Davis, "Economic Theories of Behavior in Nonprofit Private Hospitals," *Economic and Business Bulletin*, Temple University, Winter 1972; M. S. Feldstein, "Hospital Cost Inflation: A Study of Non-profit Price Dynamics," *American Economic Review*, December 1971; P. Jacobs, "A Survey of Economic Models of Hospitals," *Inquiry*, June 1974; M. L. Lee, "A Conspicuous Production Theory of Hospital Behavior," *Southern Economic Journal*, July 1971; J. P. Newhouse, "Toward a Theory of Non-profit Institutions: An Economic Model of a Hospital," *American Economic Review*, March 1970; M. V. Pauly and M. Redisch, "The Not-for-Profit Hospital as a Physicians' Cooperative," *American Economic Review*, March 1973. M. Goldfarb, M. Hornbrook, and J. Rafferty, "Behavior of the Multiproduct Firm: A Model of the Nonprofit Hospital System," *Medical Care*, 18, February 1980: 185–201; and M. V. Pauly, "Nonprofit Firms in Medical Markets," *American Economic Review*, Papers and Proceedings, 77(2), May 1987: 257–262.

15. Patricia M. Danzon, "Hospital 'Profits': The Effects of Reimbursement Policies," *Journal of Health Economics*, 1(1), May 1982: 46.

16. F. C. Spencer and B. Eiseman, "The Occasional Open-Heart Surgeon," *Circulation*, February 1965: 161–162; and Roger D. Platt, "Letter to the Editor," *New England Journal of Medicine*, June 17, 1971: 1386–1387.

17. Harold Luft, John Bunker, and Alain Enthoven, "Should Operations Be Regionalized," *New England Journal of Medicine*, 301, December 20, 1979. See also Ann B. Flood, W. Richard Scott, and Wayne Ewy, "Does Practice Make Perfect? Part I: The Relation Between Hospital Volume and Outcomes for Selected Diagnostic Categories; Part II: The Relation Between Hospital Volume and Outcomes and Other Hospital Characteristics," *Medical Care*, 22(2) February 1984.

18. Robert Rice, "Analysis of the Hospital as an Economic Organism," *Modern Hospital*, April 1966: 91.

19. For a more complete discussion of this point see R. Rosett, "Proprietary Hospitals in the United States," in M. Perlman, ed., *The Economics of Health and Medical Care* (New York: Wiley, 1974).

20. For a more complete discussion of this hospital control mechanism by physicians see S. Shalit, "A Doctor-Hospital Cartel Theory," *Journal of Business*, January 1977.

21. Harris conceptualizes the hospital as two separate firms: a medical staff, which is the demand division, and the administration, which is the supply division. Each of these separate entities are believed to have their own managers, objectives, pricing strategies, and constraints. Jeffrey E. Harris, "The Internal Organization of Hospitals: Some Economic Implications," *Bell Journal of Economics*, 8, Autumn 1977.

22. For a discussion of the economics of health facilities planning and an illustration with respect to obstetric facilities, see Millard F. Long and Paul J. Feldstein, "The Economics of Hospital Systems: Peak Loads and Regional Coordination," *American Economic Review*, May 1967.

23. There have been a large number of hospital cost studies. The following contain reviews of these studies at different points in time. Judith R. Lave, "A Review of the Methods Used to Study Hospital Costs," *Inquiry*, 3(2) 1966: 57–81; Judith K. Mann and Donald E. Yett, "The Analysis of Hospital Costs: A Review Article," *Journal of Business*, 41, April 1968: 191–202; Thomas R. Hefty, "Returns to Scale in Hospitals: A Critical Review of Recent Research," *Health Services Research*, 4, Winter 1969: 269–280; S. E. Berki, *Hospital Economics* (Lexington, Mass.: Lexington Books, 1972); Martin S. Feldstein, "Econometric Studies of Health Economics," in M. Intriligator and D. Kendrick, eds., *Frontiers of Quantitative Economics* (Amsterdam: North Holland, 1974); Judith R. Lave and Lester B. Lave, "Hospital Cost Functions," in George Chacko, ed., *Health Handbook 1976* North (Amsterdam: Holland, 1980); T. G. Cowing, A. G. Holtmann, and S. Powers, "Hospital Cost Analysis: A Survey and Evaluation of Recent Studies," in R. Scheffler and L. Rossiter, eds., *Advances in Health Economics and Health Services*, Vol. 4 JAI Press, (Greenwich, Conn.: 1983).

24. For a comprehensive review of the hospital case-mix literature, see Mark C. Hornbrook, "Hospital Case Mix: Its Definition, Measurement and Use; Part I. The Conceptual Framework," *Medical Care Review*, 30(1), Spring 1982; and "Hospital Case Mix: Its Definition, Measurement and Use, Part II: Review of Alternative Measures," *Medical Care Review*, 39(2), Summer 1982.

25. Paul L. Joskow, "The Effects of Competition and Regulation on Hospital Bed Supply and the Reservation Quality of the Hospital," *Bell Journal of Economics*, Autumn 1980: 421–447.

26. Mark V. Pauly, "Medical Staff Characteristics and Hospital Costs," *Journal of Human Resources*, 13, Supplement, 1978.

27. For a recent article on the effect of physicians on hospital costs, see Gail A. Jensen and Michael A. Morrisey, "Medical Staff Specialty Mix and Hospital Production," *Journal of Health Economics*, 5(3), September 1986: 253–276.

28. "Multi-hospital Systems Survey," *Modern Health Care*, June 5, 1987 52.

29. Randall P. Ellis and Thomas G. McGuire, "Provider Behavior Under Prospective Reimbursement," *Journal of Health Economics*, 5(2), June 1986. Rather than examining the financial effect on the physician of their decisions, Ellis and McGuire view the physician as a decisionmaker who trades off benefits to the patient against the benefits to the hospital when making a treatment decision.

30. Richard J. Arnould and Lawrence M. DeBrock, "Competition and Market Failure in the Hospital Industry: A Review of the Evidence," *Medical Care Review*, 43(2), Fall 1986; Harold S. Luft et al., "Hospital Behavior in a Local Market Con-

text," *Medical Care Review*, 43(2), Fall 1986; Harold S. Luft et al., "The Role of Specialized Clinical Services in Competition Among Hospitals," *Inquiry*, 23(1) Spring 1986; Monica Noether, *Competition Among Hospitals* (Washington, D.C.: Federal Trade Commission, 1987); James Robinson and Harold Luft, "The Impact of Hospital Market Structure on Patient Volume, Average Length of Stay, and the Cost of Care," *Journal of Health Economics*, December 4, 1985; David Salkever, "Competition Among Hospitals," in W. Greenberg, ed., *Competition in the Health Sector: Past, Present and Future*, (Washington, D.C.: Federal Trade Commission, 1978); George Wilson and Joseph Jadlow, "Competition, Profit Incentives and Technical Efficiency in the Provision of Nuclear Medicine Services," *Bell Journal of Economics*, Autumn 1982.

31. J. Michael Watt et al., "The Comparative Economic Performance of Investor-Owned Chains and Not-for-Profit Hospitals", *New England Journal of Medicine*, 314(2) January 9, 1986; Edmund R. Becker and Frank A. Sloan, "Hospital Ownership and Performance," *Economic Inquiry*, 23, 1985; Bradford H. Gray, ed., *For-Profit Enterprise in Health Care*, (Washington, D.C.: National Academy Press, 1986).

32. Hospitals in more competitive areas were found to have a greater likelihood of having a bed available, which is one measure of quality, than hospitals in less competitive markets. Joskow *op. cit.*.

33. Roger Platt, "Utilization of Facilities for Heart Surgery," *New England Journal of Medicine*, 284, June 17, 1971: 1386–1387.

34. Bernard Bloom, Osler Peterson, and Samuel Martin, "Radiation Therapy in New Hampshire, Massachusetts, and Rhode Island," *New England Journal of Medicine*, 286, January 27, 1972: 189–194. It should be noted that when examining cost data from a small number of the hospitals with radiation therapy facilities, the authors found that costs per patient and per treatment were generally higher in the hospitals which performed a large volume of treatments. This is explained in part by the fact that the major radiation therapy centers treat a more complex mix of cases.

35. James Hauge and Dale Matthews, "Hospital Indicators," *Hospitals*, 51, February 16, 1977: 51–54.

36. Teh-wei Hu, "Hospital Costs and Pricing Behavior: The Maternity Ward," *Inquiry 8*, December 1971: 19–26.

CHAPTER 11

Relying on Regulation to Improve Hospital Performance

INTRODUCTION

Throughout the late 1960s and 1970s the hospital sector appeared to be performing inadequately. There was excessive duplication of expensive facilities and services, rapid inflation of hospital costs, wide variations in costs for similar services between hospitals, and the failure to substitute care in less costly settings for hospital care when medically possible. The following reasons for the industry's poor performance were cited: a service benefit health insurance policy that both removed any incentive for patients to reduce their hospitalization costs and that reimbursed the hospital on the basis of its costs; the physician's freedom from fiscal responsibility for the method of patient treatment selected; and the incentives and goals of the hospital physicians and administrative staff to undertake those pricing and investment policies that are to their advantage instead of those that would minimize the community's cost of medical care.

One approach that was proposed for improving the performance of the hospital sector, and actually implemented to a certain degree starting in the mid-1970s, was regulation. The regulatory approach places greater reliance on the use of controls over capital investment and hospital price setting through centralized decisionmaking. Under this approach, local and state health planning agencies, through their control over capital expenditure programs, determined which hospitals were permitted to enter certain markets and which hospitals should be permitted to offer certain hospital services.

The alternative policy approach for improving hospital performance is to rely on market forces to provide hospital decisionmakers with the appropriate incentives. Advocates of market competition favored elimination of many restrictions that prevailed in the medical sector preventing decisionmakers from minimizing their costs of care,

252

engaging in price competition, and forming new delivery systems to compete with the traditional form of medical practice.

It has been difficult to develop a clear dialogue in the health field between these alternative approaches to improving performance in the medical sector. Differences in opinion occur over the appropriateness of goals, such as what the measures of performance for the hospital system should be, and also over the consumer's ability to choose the appropriate quantity and quality of health care; rarely is the debate simply over which approach—regulation or competition—can achieve a more efficient allocation of medical resources and provide adequate consumer protection. However, unless the debate is clarified so that everyone is debating the same issues, it will remain impossible to separate value differences from differences in methods designed to achieve a given set of values most efficiently.

Some evidence has now been accumulated on the effects of regulation and competition on hospital performance. The following chapters review these two approaches to improving performance in the medical sector. The first chapter discusses the likelihood that planning will improve performance. The experience of regulation in other industries is examined, and based on that experience, the likely consequences of increased regulation in the health field are discussed; empirical studies on the effects of regulation are also reviewed. The next chapter examines the movement toward greater reliance on market forces to achieve improved performance. Although the competition movement is still young, the chapter describes the structural changes in the medical sector that have been occurring and empirical evidence as to its effects.

THE THEORY AND PRACTICE OF REGULATION

The Presumed Objectives of Regulation in the Medical Sector

Proponents of health sector regulation cite different reasons in support of their position. A review of these arguments will help us to determine whether regulation can achieve the various objectives that have been assigned to it, and it will develop a basis for contrasting regulatory and nonregulatory approaches by which regulatory proponents' goals can be achieved.

One set of reasons used to justify increased regulation focuses on inefficiencies in medical care demand. Patients are not knowledgeable as to the type of treatment an illness requires; they have neither the information upon which to choose different providers nor the ability to evaluate their competence. Because the costs of incompetent providers can be large, and may be impossible to rectify in some cases, consumers need the protection that regulation will afford. Another rationalization for regulation with respect to demand is that the type of insurance coverage available provides consumers with no incentive to select lower-cost providers; in fact, as patients pay a small portion of their medical expenses, their incentive is to select the highest-cost providers in the hopes of receiving high-quality care. The patient thereby also has an incentive to overutilize medical services. Certain persons favoring regulation prefer that professional medical judgment be substituted for consumer judgment in determining medical service use. Such persons would favor using professionally determined need as the determinant of utilization rather than the consumer's willingness to pay, even assuming that the consumer has the means to choose and can afford the medical care chosen.

A second set of reasons used to justify increased medical sector regulation addresses supply inefficiency. The natural-monopoly argument (that large economies of scale exist in the provision of services) is rarely made, except for rural areas and for highly specialized services. The most frequent reasons given for supply regulation are the duplication of expensive services which are subject to economies of scale, the excess of beds in communities, and the lack of provider incentives to be efficient.

A third reason offered for regulation is the need to hold down the large increases in governmental expenditures on medical care. States, as well as the federal government, are attempting to restrain the amounts they spend on medical care for the indigent and the aged. The main concern of these governmental entities is not so much efficiency as it is the total dollar amount, which is rapidly increasing each year. Unless the states and the federal government can contain these expenditures, they will either have to raise taxes or be unable to finance existing or new programs; both alternatives are politically unpalatable to elected administrations.

The last reasons used to justify regulation and planning are that without central planning, some persons would not have access to medical care, and scarce medical resources would be inequitably distributed. The proponents of this argument claim that reliance on market forces alone to allocate medical care would leave people living in rural or ghetto areas without access to care; who would be willing to serve them?

These reasons for favoring regulation and planning are not exhaustive, but they include the major concerns of the proponents. Demand inefficiencies, particularly the consumer-protection argument, are often used to justify regulation that requires licensure and erects barriers to entry into the profession. Utilization review procedures are also suggested, albeit by a different set of regulation proponents, to improve certain inefficiencies on the demand side. The regulations most often proposed for controlling supply inefficiencies are certificate of need (CON), rate regulation, and other centralized approaches to the allocation of resources. Rate regulation and expenditure limits are usually suggested as methods for containing the total increase in government funds spent on medical care. Certificate of need, which centralizes control over capital expenditures in a planning agency, is also considered by some persons to be a useful means to this end.

For dealing with the equity and maldistribution problem, national health insurance, controls on the location decision of all providers and professionals, rate regulation, and certificate of need are proposed. National health insurance and control over location decisions are fairly obvious approaches when judged by their intended effects, but the latter two methods may not be. Rate regulation would be used to set prices at a higher level for some services or patients so as to provide a subsidy for other services or persons. CON legislation would prevent the elimination of services or facilities from certain unprofitable regions and would also suggest which regions should be permitted to expand their facilities and services.

As can be seen from the foregoing discussion, the objectives to be achieved by regulation and planning in the medical care field are multiple. It is not possible, nor is it desirable, to compare market competition in the delivery of medical services with that of regulation as a means of achieving all of the above mentioned objectives. Greater reliance on competitive forces alone will not increase the amount of funds available to improve the poor's access to medical care. Neither will it necessarily improve the distribution of medical resources. Provider competition will not alleviate the concerns of those persons who believe medical care use should be based on professional judgment alone. It is thus inappropriate to fault a market approach to medical services delivery because it fails to meet the objectives sought by the different proponents of regulation. A fairer comparison would be carried out goal by goal. For example, if increased access to medical care is favored, a government subsidy is required. Given a government subsidy, it is then appropriate to ask which of the two approaches would achieve the goal of increased access more efficiently. If economic efficiency in supply is a desirable objective, which of the alternative approaches is more likely to achieve that objective? However, the two approaches cannot be comparatively applied to determine whether professional judgment should dictate medical services use. The desire of regulation proponents to base decisions affecting use on professional judgment involves a value judgment and, as such, substitutes a criterion other than economic efficiency in consumption as the objective. It is thus not possible to compare the two approaches with respect to achieving this goal. A market approach would come closer to achieving economic efficiency on the demand side; professional judgment is a negation of the criteria of economic efficiency in the use of medical services. Therefore, the two approaches cannot be compared.

Thus, in delineating the area in which the two approaches can be compared, we will not address inefficiencies in demand because the basis for comparison would not be acceptable to both sides. We shall also omit, at this point, issues dealing with welfare, equity, or distribution, since we will return to this subject when we discuss medical care financing. At that time, we will discuss alternative approaches to financing medical care, the different values involved, and the different approaches that may be used to deliver that care. The remaining area in which market competition and regulation can be compared is the achievement of economic efficiency in the supply or delivery of medical services. Thus, regardless of what we hold to be the appropriate criteria for evaluating efficiency in demand or for determining how much medical care should be redistributed and to whom, it is still possible to compare the regulatory and market approaches with respect to the supply side of the medical care market.

With this background on the general objectives of medical sector regulation, and with the specific objective of contrasting a market and regulatory approach to achieving efficiency in the provision of medical services, we turn now to an examination of the regulatory approach and its likely consequences.

The Performance of Regulatory Agencies Outside the Health Sector

To gain a better understanding of regulatory behavior in the health sector, it is instructive first to examine the performance of regulatory agencies in nonhealth sectors. To this end, we discuss behavioral models of regulatory agencies and, based upon these models, develop different hypotheses to predict the regulated industry's performance. The behavioral model of the regulatory agency that most closely approximates the regulated industry's actual performance is then selected as the most accurate behavioral model. The model selected is then applied to the health field, and its implications and predictive potential for hospitals are discussed.

The first model of regulatory agency behavior, referred to as the traditional or "public interest" view, assumes that such agencies were established to protect the consumer from the abuses of big business (natural monopolies) and to provide consumer protection in those cases where consumers were unable to judge the quality of the product or service they were purchasing. Under this traditional view of regulation, the regulatory agency, acting in the consumer's interest, should cause the prices of the goods and services produced by the regulated industries to be lower than they would be without such legislation. In this view, the profits of regulated industries would also be expected to be lower than they would be if such regulations did not exist. To protect the public interest, the regulatory agency would exercise tight controls over the regulated industry's prices and profits. Such a comprehensive set of regulatory controls is often referred to as public utility regulation.

Dissatisfaction arose, however, with this traditional view of regulation. It was asked: If public utility regulation was established to protect the consumer from being charged monopoly prices by such natural monopolies as railroads, telephone, and utility companies, why were such competitive industries as trucking, airlines, and taxicabs also regulated? Competitive industries were selectively regulated, a fact that the traditional model could not explain: Why was there such extensive regulation of what could be considered a competitive industry?

Another source of dissatisfaction with the traditional view of regulation is the fact that if the regulatory agency's intention was to lower the regulated industry's prices and profits, why would other firms desire to enter the markets served by regulated firms? There should be no reason for unregulated firms to want to compete in regulated markets. Yet in every regulated industry, the regulatory agency strictly limits the entry of unregulated firms into the regulated market. These two dissatisfactions with the traditional view of regulation—namely, the extension of regulation to include industries that could be competitive, and the persistent desire by unregulated firms to enter regulated markets—resulted in the development of an alternative model of the behavior of regulatory agencies.

The view of regulatory agency behavior that directly opposes the traditional view is known as the economic theory of regulation (1). According to this theory, regulatory agencies and their policies are developed for the express purpose of monopolizing the industry. Under the traditional view, the agency regulated the monopolistic firms to achieve the outcome that would occur in a competitive industry. The economic theory of regulation, however, hypothesizes that regulation enables what is or would be a competitive industry to act as though it were in fact a monopoly. The impetus for regulation, or for the capture of the regulatory agency by the industry it is meant to regulate, comes from the industry's desire to use the regulatory process as a vehicle for charging higher prices, restricting its output, raising its profits, and protecting itself from possible competitors.

The economic theory of regulation and legislation suggests that government policies and legislative outcomes can best be understood within a traditional economic framework. Namely, regulation is demanded by groups because of the benefits it confers and is supplied by legislators. The market price equilibrating the demand and supply of regulation is political support. Groups demanding regulatory benefits are willing to pay a price for those benefits, such as providing votes, campaign contributions, and volunteer time. The purpose of regulation under this theory is to use the power of government to transfer wealth from those with little political power to those with more. The suppliers of regulatory benefits, who are ultimately elected officials, require political support to maximize their reelection probabilities (their goal). In attempting to maximize political support, the suppliers of regulation are presumed to calculate the amount of political support gained as a result of providing benefits to one group compared to the political support they would lose by those opposed. Legislators delegate some of their authority since it becomes too costly to legislate constantly each aspect of regulatory behavior. The legislature's preference is to delegate to regulatory agencies rather than the courts. The courts are more insulated from political control since their tenure is for fixed terms and their budgets are less subject to legislative approval.

The success of a group in receiving regulatory benefits depends, not only on whether they are able to recognize what is in their self-interest, but on whether they can organize themselves, provide the necessary political support to those who will supply the regulation, and on whether there is organized opposition to their proposals. Special-interest groups are said to have a "concentrated" interest in regulation; regulation can have a major impact on their livelihood. It is in their economic interest to be informed on regulations affecting their members and to promote those interests actively. The members of such groups are also likely to be more informed as to the positions taken by their legislators at election time. It is for these reasons that Downs concluded: "Democratic governments tend to favor producers more than consumers in their actions" (2).

To minimize opposition, the costs of providing regulatory benefits to a particular group are spread over a large number of people. Consumers are said to have a "diffuse" interest in the outcome of regulation, since the increased prices they have to pay as a result of favorable regulation to an industry have a small effect on the consumer's overall budget. Although these costs are relatively small to those who bear them, in the aggregate these losses may be quite large. Given the diffuse nature of the costs of regulation, it is not in the interest of those bearing the costs to become involved in the regulatory process. If consumers were to organize other consumers, gather the necessary information to refute the information provided by the regulated industry, and to become an adversary in the agency's proceedings, the costs of doing so would exceed the diffuse costs imposed on them by the regulation. Thus because the high information and transactions costs generally exceed the benefits (in terms of defeating the regulation) to an individual, the public generally does not have much input into the regulatory process. The exclusion of the public from most regulatory decisionmaking is particularly true for legislation that is neither publicized nor obvious in its redistributive effects (3). To the regulated industry, which has a concentrated interest, such lobbying efforts before the legislature, its subcommittees, and before the regulatory agency are both worthwhile and necessary.

The economic theory of regulation provides an explanation of why industries that would otherwise be competitive demand regulation. Industries that are highly concentrated, that is, that consist of a few large firms, would be more likely to act as a cartel if it were not for the antitrust laws. It is less costly for a few firms to reach an agreement on price and output and to monitor whether each firm abides by their agreement. However, the costs of cartelizing an industry that consists of many small firms are relatively large. These costs consist of coordinating agreements among the many firms as to the price and output quotas to be established for each firm. It is also costly to monitor the firms to ensure that they do not cheat on the agreement. If they do, sanctions must be imposed. Once a price is established that is higher than the price that would prevail under competition, each firm has an incentive to charge a slightly lower price, thereby increasing its own output, hence profit. However, if this cheating becomes widespread, the higher price will fall back to the competitive price. Because organizational and enforcement costs are higher for firms in a competitive industry, it is unlikely that they could privately cartelize an industry. To receive the benefits of a cartel, firms in competitive industries must seek regulation. Only through regulation can the industry price be established above the competitive price, firms prevented from lowering that price to increase their sales, and new firms prevented from entering the industry.

The economic theory of regulation applies to diverse groups that have a concentrated interest in regulation, such as small businesses, labor unions, dairy farmers, and the professions. Unless they were protected by regulation, these groups could not receive the benefits of a cartelized industry. Thus the economic theory of regulation can resolve the two dissatisfactions with the traditional view of regulation. Normally competitive industries demand regulation to provide themselves with the benefits of monopoly power. Unregulated firms continually attempt to enter regulated markets because the prices established by the regulatory agency are higher than those which would prevail in a competitive situation.

At times the economic theory of regulation is similar in its predictions to the "capture" theory; that is, the regulated industry captures the regulatory agency so as to use the regulatory power to its own benefit. However, the economic theory of regulation is a more satisfactory theory than the capture theory since it provides greater explanatory power in more diverse situations. Groups other than the regulated firms, such as competing industries and labor unions, may also have a concentrated interest in the regulatory outcomes. For example, in the health field the government and large businesses have developed a concentrated interest in health care cost containment since increased health costs have such a large impact on the federal budget and on employees' insurance premiums. Since the economic theory of regulation views the regulator as attempting to maximize political support, regulatory benefits will be shared when there are competing groups, each with a concentrated interest. The division of those benefits, however, is unlikely to be equal.

Legislators, particularly the legislative sub-committee having jurisdiction over an industry, control the regulatory agency's appropriation. Thus the regulatory agency is expected to follow the direction set forth by the subcommittee; the regulatory agency is therefore assumed to have similar goals as the oversight committee. The bureaucrats responsible for the regulatory agency may, in addition, have their own goals, such as to increase the size and authority of their agency, thereby justifying higher salaries. To be able to increase its budget, the agency must receive support from the legislative subcommittee having control over its jurisdiction. To receive this support, the agency will act, as would the legislators, namely, to maximize political support from the agency's decisions. To achieve its own goals, as well as those of the legislators, the agency will attempt to minimize opposition to its decisions; the agency will consider the concerns, and attempt to reach a compromise, among all those with a concentrated interest that appear before it. The concentrated interests likely to appear before the agency are the regulated industry, their unions, and other organized interest groups, such as a competitive industry, that might provide vocal opposition to the agency's decisions. When the major interest group concerned with the regulatory agency's decisions is the regulated industry, this model would be similar in its predictions to those of the capture theory. When several divergent interest groups are affected by the agency's decision, the agency will arrive at compromise decisions, which minimize further opposition to the agency and forestall any appeal. Under this theory of agency behavior, when the regulated industry is the main interest group affected by the agency's decision, the agency will produce a decision that is approximate to what the regulated industry desires. As the number of competing interest groups increases, the agency will attempt to minimize its costs by reaching a compromise with the competing groups.

In this view, the regulatory agency will attempt to measure its performance according to fairly obvious indicators. Failure to perform well on these measures could result in opposition to the agency's plans for its budget, its size, and the extent of its legislative authority. Unfortunately, the success indicators will be those that are the most obvious, not necessarily the most important. There are always trade-offs between different measures of performance; however, the agency's decision will be biased toward the more obvious measures of success, neglecting the less obvious costs inherent in those choices.

These different theories of regulation, the traditional view and the economic theory, provide different hypotheses to explain the performance of the regulated industry. Under the traditional view of regulation, the regulated industry would be expected to have lower prices than if regulation did not exist. The regulatory agency would also be expected to eliminate inefficiencies inherent in monopolistic markets. Under the economic theory of regulation, the regulatory agency will enable the different firms in the industry to act as a cartel, thereby raising prices, restricting output, and providing regulated firms with higher profits than if regulation did not exist. When there are competing interest groups, compromises result, and no single group does as well as it would if it were the only group with a concentrated interest.

To date, the empirical evidence indicates that prices of comparable goods and services are *higher* in regulated than in nonregulated industries.[1] For example, airlines that flew intrastate only, such as between San Francisco and Los Angeles, were not subject to regulation by the Civil Aeronautics Board (CAB) and were 32 to 47 percent lower in price than airlines that flew comparable distances but were regulated by the CAB (4). Motor carriers that carried agricultural products, and were thereby exempt from Interstate Commerce Commission (ICC) regulation, had rates 41 to 58 percent lower than those charged by carriers subject to ICC regulation (5). "Pipeline tariffs in regulated interstate markets are not only higher than in the unregulated intrastate markets, but apparently in some cases even somewhat higher than an unconstrained monopolist would charge" (6).

The production of electricity, which is generally considered to be characteristic of a natural monopoly, is an interesting illustration of regulators' behavior. In earlier years, not all states regulated the prices at which electricity was sold. Since industrial users of electricity are fewer than residential users and are organized to press their interests, they should be able to exert more influence over the regulatory agency to act on their behalf in the setting of electricity rates. Under the economic theory of regulation, we would therefore expect industrial users in regulated states to receive more

---

[1]There is one exception. Natural gas prices are lower in regulated than in nonregulated competitive markets. The reason for this apparent anomaly is that the buyer of natural gas is the pipeline industry, which is itself regulated by the Federal Power Commission (FPC). The FPC set the price of natural gas lower than the cost of newly discovered natural gas. This pricing policy by the FPC to benefit the regulated pipelines has not been without certain consequences. Newly discovered natural gas has been sold on an intrastate basis, where it is not subject to FPC regulation. This reduction in natural gas in interstate commerce has resulted in shortages in those states relying on interstate pipelines. Paul MacAvoy, "The Regulation-Induced Shortage of Natural Gas," *Journal of Law and Economics*, April 1971. Such shortages were very noticeable during the winter of 1977, when factories, schools, and even residential homes could not receive an adequate supply. Since the price and availability of natural gas is higher in those states where it is sold on an intrastate basis, industry has begun to move to those states to ensure themselves of an adequate supply, albeit at higher prices.

favorable electricity rates than residential users. The price of electricity to industrial and residential users would be expected to differ to reflect actual differences in costs between the two user groups. Therefore, the ratio of the residential to the industrial price of electricity was compared between states that regulate such prices and states that do not. In the two time periods studied, the relative price of electricity was higher for residential users than for industrial users in the regulated states. Thus the data support the hypothesis that regulation was used to the advantage of the more organized interest group and to the disadvantage of residential users (7).

	1917	1937
Regulated states	1.616	2.459
Unregulated states	1.445	2.047

The fact that the regulatory agency restricts entry into regulated industries adds further weight to the evidence that prices are higher in such industries. If regulated prices were comparable to those that would prevail in a competitive industry, other firms should not find it profitable to enter the regulated market. Yet for all regulated markets an important function of the regulatory agency is to limit entry. This behavior of the regulatory agency is consistent with the hypothesis that the industry seeks regulation so as to establish a cartel. To maintain a high price for its member firms' products, the cartel must ensure that production does not exceed the level of output that would be demanded at the cartel's price. To limit the rate of output in the cartelized industry, the cartel must limit the industry's capacity to produce that output; otherwise, firms would find it profitable to increase their output by undercutting the cartel's price.

Regulatory agencies apparently undertake those functions that would normally be assigned to managers of the cartel. To protect its monopoly price, the cartel must limit productive capacity in two ways: First, the regulatory agency must prohibit entry by new firms. For example, since its inception, the CAB had not permitted the establishment of any new trunkline air carrier; entry by existing air carriers into markets served by other air carriers was strictly limited. Second, a well-controlled cartel will attempt to ensure that no excess capacity exists among its current members, lest they be encouraged to produce more than the cartel desires. When cartelization initially occurs in an industry, the industry's output has to be reduced, since the output demanded at the higher monopoly price will be less than it was previously. To ensure that member firms in the cartel do not increase their output, which would undercut and bring pressure on the monopoly price, the cartel must remove the excess capacity that exists among its members, which was appropriate to their previously larger output. As the cartel becomes solidly entrenched, it will be strict in granting permission to its members to expand their capacity so that increased production does not place pressure on the cartel's artificially maintained price. To date, most regulated industries have not been able to assign specific quotas to each regulated firm in each particular market. The consequence of this excess capacity has been intense nonprice competition among the regulated firms to increase their market shares. For example, it has been estimated "that at any given time 40 percent of the trucks on the road are running empty because of government regulations that prevent them from carrying cargo on return trips after making deliveries" (8).

The body of evidence on prices in regulated industries thus appears to support the economic theory of regulation and to contradict the traditional view that regulation will lower prices. The empirical evidence, however, indicates that rates of return in regulated industries are not as high as in nonregulated industries; further, the prices of common stocks of regulated industries has generally not risen as fast as the stock of nonregulated firms (9).

There are a number of reasons why profitability in some regulated industries is lower than expected. These reasons have to do with nonprice competition, prices are set above costs and excess capacity among firms exists, and the existence of multiple groups having a concentrated interest. For example, establishing a regulated price greater than that which would prevail in a competitive market causes competition to occur on aspects other than price, thereby raising the industry's costs and diminishing the profitability of the regulated prices. Nonprice competition also benefits the producers of these other services (10). The excess capacity caused by CAB regulation benefited the aircraft manufacturers, airline employees, and suppliers of airline services.

Following is a brief discussion of why profitability is reduced in some regulated industries.

Cross-Subsidization of Services

As a political support maximizer, the regulator allocates the benefits of regulation to competing interest groups. Although regulated firms are permitted to charge monopoly prices in some markets, when there are competing concentrated interests they are required to use some of those profits to serve these other interests; for example, an industry might be required to subsidize a certain set of organized customers by charging prices below the costs of providing the service. Using the profitable markets to subsidize unprofitable markets has been referred to as "taxation by regulation" (11). Regulatory agencies are thus able to bypass state and federal legislatures, whose function it is to levy taxes, by imposing what are in effect taxes on the goods and services of the industries they regulate. Using the taxes to subsidize certain customers expands the size of the regulated industry. For example, the Civil Aeronautics Board set airline prices that greatly exceeded costs in markets such as New York and Miami, and then required the airlines serving those markets to serve less-profitable cities as well. Passengers flying between New York and Miami paid a monopoly price for that service, part of which was used to subsidize passengers flying between smaller towns, markets for which the airlines might otherwise have discontinued service or sharply raised the price. As a result of this cross-subsidization, overall rates of return to the regulated industry were lower than they might otherwise have been.

The benefits of cross-subsidization are several: influential legislators are able to provide subsidized services to their constituents; the regulated industry is able to enlarge its investment through expansion, thereby increasing absolute profit by earning a fair return on the total investment (including the resources used to service less-profitable areas); other groups with a concentrated interest willing to provide political support receive net benefits; and the regulators themselves are able to justify increases in their agency's size and influence. The opponents of this hidden tax are the unorganized users of the service in the monopoly-priced markets.

There is little justification for an indirect tax-subsidy system. Regulatory agencies are not provided with legislative authority to redistribute income among the various users of regulated services, and it is unlikely that the redistribution that occurs is from higher- to lower-income groups. The use of monopoly pricing in one area to generate subsidies to increase use in other areas also results in an inefficient allocation of resources, as too many resources flow into the regulated sector from unregulated sectors in the economy. It has also been suggested that if these subsidies were removed, the communities losing subsidized services would suffer little, as substitute services would expand and replace those lost. If airline service to small communities by the major carriers decreased, other forms of transportation, such as commuter airlines and buses, would take its place (12).

Regulation-Induced Inefficiencies

Under regulation, price competition is eliminated by the establishment of minimum prices, but other forms of competition are permitted, leading to higher costs. Regulated firms compete among themselves in markets where monopoly prices are established by offering additional services to consumers. In the airline industry, airlines competed on such nonprice aspects as amenities, newer equipment, larger and faster planes, and frequency of schedules. The costs of nonprice competition generally exceed the value that consumers place on such services. (After deregulation of the airlines, consumers were provided with greater choice between lower or higher air fares for different types of services; a number of consumers preferred to pay lower prices for air travel and take "no frills" flights or have certain restrictions placed on their tickets, such as cancellation penalties.) Nonprice competition among regulated firms results in excess capacity and an increase in costs of operation. To ensure that the airlines did not use up all of their profits in nonprice competition (depleting funds to subsidize airline service to less profitable areas), the regulatory agency placed limits on the various aspects of nonprice competition. Thus the regulatory agency becomes involved in determining what amenities can be offered to airline passengers. The agency governing international air travel (IATA) was forced to define an open-faced sandwich. More and more regulation must be developed to cover services provided to customers as new forms of nonprice competition are generated by the competing regulated firms. The consequences of nonprice competition are an increase in the regulated industry's costs, the creation of excess capacity, and a resource cost that exceeds the value that consumers place on such nonprice competition.

Another consequence of regulation that results in higher costs for regulated industries is the removal of incentives for efficient operation. If the price of the regulated service is set high enough to cover the costs of even the highest-cost firm, and if all firms in the industry are able to earn a minimum rate of return, management has little incentive to be efficient. A more efficient firm cannot keep its savings, because any excess profit will be used to cross-subsidize other services. It is not surprising, therefore, that the caliber of management in regulated firms is lower than in nonregulated industries. The potential rewards for management creativity and efficiency in regulated industries are relatively small.

Regulatory agencies' methods for calculating a regulated firm's rate of return result in certain perverse incentives. The amount of profit allowed in some regulated industries is based on costs incurred, while in other regulated industries it may be based on the size of the firm's investment. In the former case, it is in the regulated firm's interest to increase its costs (hence increase its profits) or to undertake larger investments than necessary. The telephone company's profit increased when it built larger, more elaborate, and longer-lasting buildings.

The method regulatory agencies used to protect regulated firms from potential competition also increased the costs of providing a service in regulated industries. As mentioned earlier, prices in the regulated industry are set high enough to permit the firms with the highest costs to survive. If, for example, a lower-cost method of production is developed as a result of technological change, the regulatory agency will prevent the new, lower-cost industry from driving the regulated, higher-cost producers out of the market in the following ways. First, the regulatory agency will include the new, lower-cost industry (which can become a substitute for the regulated firms) within its regulatory authority. Second, the price of the service will be set high enough to permit the regulated firms to survive and compete (on a nonprice basis) with the lower-cost firms. For example, the ICC initially regulated railroads presumably because they were a monopoly. As trucks, a lower-cost substitute, were developed, the ICC regulated them to prevent this new industry from capturing large segments of the markets served by railroads. Barges and other water carriers were brought under ICC regulation in 1940 because of their competition with railroads (13). Rather than allowing the prices of goods shipped in various markets to reflect the costs of shipping, the ICC set minimum rates for goods shipped in interstate commerce that were not reflective of the least-costly method of shipping. Trucking, which could have been a competitive industry, was regulated to prevent railroads from losing some of their markets to lower-cost shippers.

The consequences of extending regulatory authority to include lower-cost producers is that consumers pay prices higher than if competition existed among the different industries and the price reflected the production cost of the lowest-cost industry. As long as the regulated industry and its unions continue to provide political support, the survival of the industry, even though it may be higher-cost and contain inefficient firms, becomes an objective of regulatory agencies.

Regulatory Response to Technological Change

Another reason for higher costs in regulated industries is the regulatory agencies' response to technological change developed outside the regulated industry. Technological innovations may result in new substitute services or similar services that consumers would be willing to purchase at a lower cost. To prevent the regulated industry from losing its market share and possibly going out of existence, the agency attempts to retard the introduction of technological innovations. For example, the FCC delayed giving its permission to a firm other than AT&T to put up a domestic communications satellite; the FCC restricted the development of cable television, which would threaten the monopoly of UHF television stations in large cities. The introduction of new technology is stalled because the firms that would profit from it are not those that are regulated.

Technological change is introduced very slowly in regulated industries because such change could have an adverse impact on the regulatory agency itself. To minimize criticism of its performance, an agency is unlikely to undertake actions that have a chance of failure. Since the effects of innovation cannot be entirely foreseen, an agency would prefer to delay, permitting a change until the benefits of the innovation are obvious to all or until the benefits are greatly in excess of the possible costs, according to the agency's determination. The agency's assessment of the possible benefits and costs of innovation is likely to differ from that of consumers, who might be willing to purchase such services were they available on the market. To avoid criticism, the agency is likely to use the most obvious measures of benefits and costs; the less obvious or hidden costs and benefits will be assigned less weight in the agency's deliberations.

In reviewing the empirical evidence on the behavior of regulation in other industries, it appears that the traditional view of regulation, whereby agencies act in the public interest and cause prices to be lower, is an inaccurate description of reality. It appears that a more accurate model is the economic theory of regulation; legislators and the regulatory agency act so as to maximize their political support. When there is only one group with a concentrated interest and willing to provide political support, that group will receive the benefits of regulation. When there are competing interest groups, each providing political support, compromises are reached and the benefits of regulation are shared. As has been shown, the consequence of allocating benefits according to provision of political support is that the prices of goods and services in the regulated industry will be higher than if the industry were not regulated. Cross-subsidization of services, inefficiency, a decline in the quality of management, and competition in the areas of amenities and extra services can also be expected in a regulated industry, together with the resulting higher costs. The agency will also impose entry barriers on technologically innovative firms and extend its regulatory authority to include lower-cost substitute providers to protect the regulated firms. The scope of regulation increases as the regulatory agency seeks to cover all the gaps that arise from nonprice competition and from the threat of new firms. Finally, as the scope of its authority and the number of competing interest groups served increases, the regulatory agency will, to protect its own interests, resort to using obvious measures of its success. Not only will obvious success measures minimize criticism of the agency's performance, but they will also result in the agency's failure to consider trade-offs and other costs that may be involved in its decision, possibly resulting in a shift of those costs to consumers.

The Probable Consequences of Regulation of Hospital Capital Investment

Although it is possible that the consequences of hospital regulation will differ from the regulatory experience of other industries, it is unlikely in the light of the evidence already presented. Hospitals have a great stake in any regulatory process affecting them. Their interests are concentrated, whereas, until the 1980s, those of consumers and other purchasers concerned about the rapid increase in hospital costs were diffuse. As long as hospitals were the only ones with a concentrated interest, we would expect hospital regulatory agencies to be favorably disposed to the hospital's interests; in fact, we would expect any hospital regulatory agency to protect the hospitals under its jurisdiction. Contrary to the traditional view of regulation, when hospitals were the only or major group with a concentrated interest, we would expect hospital prices to continue their upward rise; we would also expect to observe cross-subsidization of services and patients within the hospital. Both the regulatory agency and the hospitals themselves would favor expanding the number of services offered by hospitals. Monopoly pricing of certain hospital services, such as ancillary services, would continue under regulation; the regulatory agency would not become involved in an adversary relationship with the hospitals by requiring them to set prices equal to costs for each hospital service. Since price competition among hospitals was virtually nonexistent until the 1980s, nonprice competition to attract customers, namely physicians, would continue in the form of investment in facilities, services, and other inducements. The regulatory agency, on hospitals' behalf, would inhibit innovations in the delivery of medical care that decrease hospital utilization, regardless of its potential cost savings to customers; such innovations would potentially decrease hospital revenues and threaten the survival of some protected hospitals. Similarly, entry into the industry would be sharply curtailed lest a new hospital demonstrate greater efficiency, lower its costs, and render existing hospitals' capacity excessive.

The foregoing scenario of the likely consequences of hospital regulation (when hospitals were the only group with a concentrated interest in regulation) would not have obviated any of the reasons for proposing hospital regulation in the first place. The rapid increases in hospital costs, duplication of facilities and services, excess hospital capacity, and the lack of incentives to substitute less costly care when medically possible were the result of hospital payment systems, namely cost-based reimbursement, and the form of insurance coverage, resulting in a lack of incentives by hospitals, patients, and physicians, who were the decisionmakers in the use of the hospital and yet did not have the financial responsibility for those decisions. The experience with regulation in other industries would have suggested that as long as hospitals were the major group with a concentrated interest in hospital expenditures, the problems above would not have been resolved through the regulatory process.

A Review of Efforts to Control Hospital Investment

Regulation to control hospital costs has changed over time. The following discussion reviews the history of regulations designed to control hospital investment. These planning regulations culminated in the enactment of both state and federal certificate-of-need (CON) laws. As a result of such laws, hospitals had to secure the approval of planning agencies at several levels of government for all new hospital investment (exceeding a minimum dollar amount, such as $100,000). CON legislation was the natural extension of previous efforts to make the expansion of the health care system more "rational."

Hospital planning at the federal level started with the Hospital Survey and Construction Act (Hill-Burton) in 1946 (14). Federal funds were provided to each state for construction of new beds and for modernization according to a formula based on population and per capita income. To receive funds, a hospital (or a prospective hospital) had to obtain the approval of the Hill-Burton agency in its state. The criteria used by the state Hill-Burton agencies for the allocation of funds were relatively simple and considered data only on the number of beds, the population, and the population density in the area. It is difficult to identify the method used by Hill-Burton agencies to allocate Hill-Burton funds for modernization, which eventually became the major use of Hill-Burton funds. To receive these funds, each state had to produce a state plan for its hospital beds, but there is little evidence that such state plans were anything more than inventories of beds and facilities. Under the Hill-Burton program, many small hospitals were started in rural areas that previously did not have a hospital. The Hill-Burton program had the political support of the American Hospital Association and the continued endorsement of Congress for 25 years, since each state received a share of the federal funds for hospitals. Hill-Burton was responsible for starting many new hospitals, but only in areas where they would not compete with existing hospitals. After several years, the program changed its emphasis to modernizing existing hospitals rather than providing new hospital beds. Hospitals that did not receive Hill-Burton funds were still able to finance new beds from other sources. However, Hill-Burton did little, if anything, to coordinate hospital investment; perhaps for this reason, hospitals have considered it a success.

The next major development in hospital planning came with the development of voluntary planning agencies. In the mid-1960s Congress passed the Comprehensive Health Planning Act. Health planning agencies were set up locally within a state and coordinated by a state-level agency, but they could only attempt to improve hospital planning in a voluntary manner, as they did not have any authority to approve or disapprove hospital investment. When their effectiveness was evaluated, it was determined that planned and unplanned areas had the same amount of unnecessary duplication of facilities and services; also, planned areas experienced a larger percentage increase in their beds, a larger percentage decrease in proprietary hospitals in their area, and no difference in the rate of increase in hospital costs per patient (15). It appears that voluntary hospital planning had no significant effect on hospital costs or investment. Individual hospitals had little incentive to cooperate in hospital planning because it would have frustrated the achievement of their prestige goals. Perhaps as a means of ensuring that planning agencies did not obstruct hospital goals, but instead directed their efforts against potential entrants to the market, planning agencies were made dependent upon hospital contributions for part of their budgets (16).

By the mid-1970s several developments resulted in sufficient pressure for a new and stronger planning law to be passed. Hospital costs continued to rise rapidly since the passage of Medicare and Medicaid in 1966. Third-party payors, whose premiums were affected by these cost increases, and state and federal governments, whose expenditures under these programs were rising much more rapidly than expected, wanted to contain the increase in hospital expenditures. A stronger planning law was proposed as a solution to the problem of hospital costs. Blue Cross saw capital controls as a way of holding down hospital costs without becoming an adversary of the major hospitals in an area, whose interests Blue Cross served. Hospital associations had by this time also favored stronger controls through planning.

It is interesting to speculate on why hospitals, and their associations, favored constraints on their capital expenditures. By the mid-1970s, a high percentage of the population had insurance coverage for hospital care, and the demand for hospital care was no longer expected to increase as it had in the past. Further, all hospitals in an area were not equal. Some were already prestigious; they had a favored competitive position vis-à-vis other hospitals. Continued competition among hospitals presented a threat to the large hospital with many facilities and services and with a large number of staff physicians to keep its beds filled. The larger hospital's interest lay in strengthening local planning efforts to restrict further hospital investment. It was also in the interests of all the hospitals to keep potential competitors out of the industry. With the leveling off of the increases in demand for hospital care, combined with hospitals' fears that more drastic cost-containing measures would be proposed, and hospitals' desire to retain their favored competitive position, the time was ripe for hospitals to institute local hospital cartels.

The hypothesis above is supported in a study by Wendling and Werner (17). The authors attempted to explain the passage of state CON laws. The period 1968–1973 was selected for analysis; 22 states passed CON legislation, 16 states defeated such legislation, and 11 states did not undertake any action. (A change occurred in 1974 which made the years since then less appropriate for analysis. In 1974 the National Health Planning and Resources Development Act, was passed which provided incentives and penalties to encourage states to adopt CON.)

The traditional or public interest view of CON is that states passed it to control the increase in hospital expenditures, as measured by the percentage change in hospital expenditures per patient day for the six-year period preceding state action on CON. The economic theory of regulation suggests that hospitals favored passage of CON in those states in which there was greater competition among hospitals, as measured by the occupancy rate in the state for the preceding six years. An increase in competition would lower hospital revenues and make it more difficult for hospitals to expand. Several other variables were also included in the analysis. A measure of industry concentration was used to measure the costs of organizing hospitals to seek regulation. It was also hypothesized that CON was more likely in those states where there was greater competition among the political parties, hence a greater need for political support by the parties; a variable measuring this factor was also included.

The results of the statistical analysis were as expected. There was a greater likelihood of CON passage in those states having lower occupancy rates. The percent change in hospital expenditures per patient day was not related to the passage of state CON laws. Thus where the competitive threat was high (low occupancy rates) and hospitals were highly concentrated, the probability of CON in a state was .76. (The probability of defeat under these conditions was .13.) At the other extreme—hospitals facing little competitive threat and low concentration—the probability of CON in a state was .18; the probability of defeat, since it would be against the hospitals' interests, was .55.

The results of this study support the economic theory of regulation. The probability of CON in a state was highest when the potential benefit to hospitals was greatest and the costs of achieving it were relatively low. This study also suggests that CON was unlikely to have an impact on hospital expenditures because cost containment was not the real purpose of the legislation.

Federal legislation was passed in 1974 providing planning agencies with greater authority over hospital capital expenditures. Hospitals were required to receive planning agency approval for expansion and for investment in new facilities and services. The method proposed for dealing with rising hospital costs was to establish controls on hospital beds and on investment in new facilities and services.

Certificate-of-need legislation was a very conservative approach to containing the rise in hospital costs (18). CON legislation assumed that no changes were required in the method of hospital reimbursement and provided no new incentives to change patient or physician behavior. It is not surprising, therefore, that CON turned out to be unsuccessful in controlling hospital expenditures, which was the problem it was intended to redress. To control the increase in hospital costs, additional regulation was proposed. As each set of regulations failed to achieve the desired social goals, stronger regulations were proposed to do the job.

The Consequences of CON Legislation

Based upon the economic theory of regulation, it is possible to hypothesize how CON legislation would have performed in controlling hospital costs and to then test those hypotheses against actual studies. Based on evidence from other regulated industries, we would expect that unless (or until) competing interest groups develop, hospital planning agencies will use their legislative authority to protect the hospitals they are supposed to regulate; the agencies will prevent entry by competitors into markets served by existing hospitals and preclude innovations that might threaten existing hospitals' revenues.

Entry by potential competitors threatens existing hospitals for two reasons: first, a competitor might decrease existing hospitals' market share; and second, a competitor could undercut a hospital's monopoly pricing practices, which generate revenue for cross-subsidization. Cross-subsidization in hospital care occurs in several ways: profitable services, such as ancillary services, are used to subsidize unprofitable prestige facilities and services for which demand may be insufficient; some patients subsidize other patients who are more severely ill; and patients with commercial insurance subsidize Medicaid patients. Price discrimination is practiced by hospitals by type of service, type of patient, and type of third-party payor. A new hospital could, therefore, threaten these elaborate cross-subsidy schemes by failing to offer certain unprofitable services and by choosing not to admit severely ill patients, which would enable them to charge lower prices to more price sensitive purchasers. In the health field such pricing practices are referred to as cream skimming. The incentives for new firms to undercut the monopoly prices set by hospitals on certain services are the same as those that existed when airlines were regulated; new firms are willing to make less profit on services where the price is much greater than cost. The reason for agency and firm opposition to cream skimming is also similar: if monopoly profits are not made on certain services, patients, and third-party payors, funds would not be available for other uses. In effect, the regulated firm would have to reduce its size.

The objection to cream skimming in health care is based on the claim that unless some patients are subsidized, they will not be served. These consequences are more severe than a reduction in airline services to a community. Opposition to cream skimming is based on the premise that hospitals provide significant amounts of charity care. It is further claimed that the elimination of cross subsidies, funded by monopoly pricing on other services, would result in a reduction in needed hospital facilities and services. Hospital expenditures that can be attributed to philanthropy were estimated to be less than 1.5 percent of total hospital expenditures in 1970 (19). The argument that hospitals need to charge monopoly prices to provide charity services is difficult to justify. It has also never been proven that the funds generated by monopoly pricing are used to subsidize those patients who have lower incomes. Many poor patients may not enter the hospital at all or they may go to municipal hospitals. Further, the higher prices charged to patients who are less severely ill are reflected in higher insurance premiums, which fall on lower-income consumers as well.

The argument that without price discrimination a hospital would be forced to discontinue needed facilities and services is also complex. If a facility is costly because it is subject to economies of scale, all hospitals in a community should not necessarily have this facility. If such a facility is the only one in the community or if more than one hospital should have it, why should not its costs be reimbursable as part of the hospital costs of those patients requiring its use? The use of costly facilities and services, as well as of hospital care itself, is an insurable risk. Insurance policies that include major medical or catastrophic coverage (rather than those policies that provide front-end, shallow benefits) would reimburse the hospitals for use of such services. If patients cannot afford to pay for such services, the argument becomes similar to the charity argument. The extent of this occurrence should be determined and a separate subsidy should be provided to low-income patients to pay for their expected hospital expenses (i.e., their insurance coverage can be subsidized). It is likely, however, that the charity argument is not the major justification, nor even an important one, for hospitals' desire to maintain facilities and services that would have to be discontinued if subsidies for their operation could not be provided. It is more likely that hospitals used internal cross-subsidization to bolster prestige services and/or to increase the attending medical staff's productivity than to maintain facilities and services the community considered necessary.

The second argument against permitting entry of a new institution into an area currently served by hospitals is that entry will merely create excess hospital capacity, which the community will end up paying for through increases in insurance premiums. However, the costs of excess capacity will be passed on in the form of higher insurance premiums only if hospitals are reimbursed on a cost basis. As hospitals are reimbursed similar to other industries, the consumer would not bear the costs of hospitals that go into bankruptcy. The hospitals and its backers would bear those risks. Hospital proponents might claim that before hospitals go bankrupt they would fill those excess beds with patients who did not have to be there by extending lengths of stay as well as admitting additional patients. They implicitly threaten that unless existing hospitals are protected, they will knowingly fill their beds with patients who do not have to be there and the community will end up paying more for its hospital care. This "demand inducement" argument becomes less credible under a fixed price per admission system.

With a stable or declining demand for hospital care in a community, the only requirements for new beds will be replacement of existing ones. It is highly unlikely that a regulatory agency will refuse an existing hospital the right to replace its facilities and instead award that license to a new organization. CON agencies are likely to guarantee the survival of existing hospitals and preclude entry by new competitors, particularly at a time when bed needs in most communities appear to be satisfied. It is interesting to examine evidence of the use of CON legislation to restrict entry. For example, in Kansas City, Missouri, the decision of the planning agency was overturned by the courts on the following grounds:

"The areawide agency had denied the application of Extendicare, Inc., a proprietary institution. The court found that Mid-American CHP had approved all applications by not-for-profit institutions but had denied that of the only investor-owned organization in circumstances that the court described as 'arbitrary, capricious, and unreasonable to the extent of being tantamount to fraud'" (20).

The movement toward a fixed-price payment system is a more direct method than entry controls for preventing excess capacity. If a hospital could not compete with a potential competitor at a given reimbursement rate, the community would not have to pay for the excess capacity or the unnecessary services. A hospital with excess capacity, in a service subject to economies of scale, would either have to merge or close that facility if it could not cover all its costs at the fixed payment rate. Under such an alternative, the organization and its employees would bear the costs of duplication or inefficiency.

Competition is a threat to the survival and goals of existing hospitals, while barriers to entry guarantee the hospitals' survival. Entry barriers do not solve the problem of rapidly increasing hospital costs, which was their initial rationalization. Thus regulation proponents have to propose additional controls, rate regulation, to solve the problem of rising costs.

Another consequence of establishing a cartel over hospital capital investment is hypothesized to be a delay in the introduction of innovation by outside firms and the extension of the cartel's authority over lower-cost producers. Existing members of the cartel would introduce technological innovation themselves if it resulted in increased prestige for the institution or increased productivity for the hospitals' physicians. The members of the cartel would not be expected to approve of innovational changes in the delivery of medical care that would decrease their revenues. Railroads were protected from competition with trucks when the ICC extended its authority over such low-cost substitutes, thereby regulating their entry and prices to be charged. The health planning agency's treatment of innovation would be expected to be similar. If health planning agencies are viewed as protectors of the hospitals they are meant to regulate, we would predict that the agencies would want to inhibit the development of any substitute source of care that would decrease the revenues of existing hospitals. Once again, such action would probably be justified as an attempt to prevent substitutes from decreasing the demand for existing hospitals, thereby creating excess capacity. Again the threat would be made that the community would have to pay for this excess capacity through its third-party payors. If, on the other hand, planning agencies are viewed as attempting to minimize the cost of medical care to the community, they should be seeking to encourage lower-cost substitutes whenever possible. Any excess hospital capacity that results should then be eliminated by the planning agency or not be paid for by third-party payors.

Evidence of delayed innovation in the delivery of medical services supports the hypothesis that CON agencies tend to be more concerned with protecting existing hospitals than with encouraging lower-cost substitutes. A majority of CON laws included under their authority freestanding outpatient surgicenters and health maintenance organizations (21). There was little, if any, justification for placing these organizations under CON; these organizations did not have excess capacity, their services were not reimbursed on a cost-plus basis, their incentives or goals are not the same as those of the hospitals, and their costs were not a cause for concern. The concern with excess capacity, the usual justification for CON, was lacking in the case of these substitute services. To encourage the development of lower-cost substitutes for hospital care, these substitutes should not be subject to entry regulations nor any other requirements unrelated to quality, which should be similarly applicable to existing health providers.

One can readily imagine how regulating lower-cost substitutes for hospitals would hinder their growth. Unregulated, freestanding surgicenters decrease the demand for short hospital stays associated with less complex surgery, thereby providing a substitute for a service that is priced monopolistically by hospitals. To combat such cream skimming by a lower-cost method of production, hospital associations would be expected to require all surgicenters be affiliated with hospitals. This is in fact what occurred. Through affiliation, hospitals are able to control the development of potential competitors and avoid revenue loss. Permitting only existing hospitals to establish lower-cost substitutes removes any incentives that substitute organizations have to grow at hospitals' expense. The hospitals are able to limit their use and, by controlling their rates, limit the savings to be achieved by patients and third-party payors. The effect of this approach on hospital revenues, compared to the effect of keeping such substitutes independent and freestanding, is obvious.

Health maintenance organizations (HMOs) achieve their savings by reducing hospitalization. Hospital use rates of HMO subscribers are approximately one-half those of fee-for-service patients. Thus rapid growth of HMOs represent a severe threat to hospitals' revenues. Opponents of HMOs have used several approaches to retard their growth. The initial federal HMO legislation, which preempted state laws restricting HMO development, mandated that any organization wishing to qualify as a federal HMO had to offer more extensive benefits than were offered by the majority of third-party payors. A larger benefit package raises the premium of the HMO relative to other health insurance premiums, thereby decreasing its demand. This aspect of the law was subsequently changed. There was also an unsuccessful attempt to require input standards for an HMO, such as minimum ratios of beds and personnel to population served. Specifying sufficiently high inputs limits the possibility for cost reduction and substitution without necessarily assuring quality care.

Placing HMOs under CON authority would limit their growth, and HMOs such as Kaiser have opposed such moves. Kaiser and other HMOs have feared that planning agencies will view an HMO's desire to enter an area as a threat to the existing hospitals. Group Health Cooperative of Puget Sound and Kaiser, "two of the most substantial and respectable HMOs, have encountered problems in obtaining permission to construct inpatient facilities needed to serve their population in these states. Although they ultimately obtained the requisite approvals after substantial delays, it is fair to ask whether smaller or newer HMOs or HMOs organized under less impeccable auspices could survive a similar encounter" (22).

It is thus understandable why the AHA's model bill on CON placed such lower-cost substitutes as surgicenters and HMOs under CON authority. Placing constraints, other than quality assurance, on any innovation expected to lower the costs of medical care is bound to limit its growth. It is unfortunate that the existing providers of hospital care perceive these issues so much more clearly than do the proponents of medical care regulation.

Technical Competence and Performance Measures Used by the Regulatory Agency

The degree to which an agency competently fulfills its stated roles can be used to assess the accuracy of models of regulatory agency behavior. It is thus appropriate to review the evidence on the technical competence of health planning agency personnel, the criteria used by the agency for decisionmaking, and the planning agency's effectiveness.

Although health planning agencies were supposed to plan for the health needs of the community, it was understood by all that health planning is a misnomer. The agencies were concerned with facilities planning, primarily with hospitals. Ideally, when developing a plan for the community's hospital care, agency personnel should understand the factors affecting demands for care, be able to forecast those demands, estimate the costs of providing care in different-sized facilities, and incorporate in their plans the population's preferences as to travel time and cost in receiving care. Because demands, costs, and the community's preferences are always changing, the agency should be able to update its master plans continually. It is difficult to develop technical analyses, and the need to do so raised many questions. For example, what is the definition of excess capacity in an area? After all, each area requires a standby capacity that will vary by type of facility, location, and population served. In practice, most planning agencies performed technical analyses in reaction to the expansion plans submitted by hospitals. Two U.S. Government Accounting Office (GAO) studies (1972 and 1974) found that very few health planning agencies had any plans for their area (23). A later study (1975) concluded that such agencies relied on the hospitals themselves for data, which were at least two years old, and that the techniques used for planning were the old Hill-Burton projections based on obsolete data (24). The technical competence of health planning agencies had apparently not significantly improved upon the rather crude methodologies used by Hill-Burton agencies.

By relying heavily on providers for their data and by using a reactive approach to planning, an agency ensures that its decisions will be heavily influenced by providers. If existing providers wanted to control the planning agency to serve their own interest, they would prefer to have either vague criteria for investment decisions or a sufficiently large number of such criteria to enable the agency to reach and justify any decision the provider desired. Lewin and Associates' findings that planning agencies' criteria were not explicit and that they preferred "full service hospitals" —that is, existing hospitals—and were against proprietary providers support this expectation (25). The importance of controlling information as a means of dominating the decisionmaking process was also demonstrated in the studies cited. A number of agencies were found to rely on provider-dominated primary review committees, and in many instances the agencies' consumer representatives were in the minority at agency advisory meetings. One wonders how effective consumer representatives can be in a situation where they must rely on the providers for their information and presumably the expertise to determine the importance or health need of a certain capital expenditure. (The consumer representatives might also have had similar incentives as the hospitals, namely, to increase investment in beds and technology. They could then point with pride to the quality of hospital facilities in their area.) As might be expected, the studies cited found that

> [the planning agencies'] efforts to curb unnecessary investment are often not very strenuous. For example, approval rates for investment proposals generally exceeded 90 percent. Also, two thirds of the agencies studied approved additional hospital beds that would raise area bed supplies to more than 105 percent of their future need projections; in fact, half of these agencies approved new beds even though existing supplies already exceeded this level. Most surprising, however, was the finding that fewer than half of all agencies saw cost containment as the primary goal of the investment review programs and one-fifth of the areawide agencies did not consider it a goal at all (26).

Another aspect of regulatory agency behavior, observed in agencies outside the health field, is their desire to minimize conflict so as to avoid criticism. With regard to health facilities planning, the existing hospitals form the prime interest group affected by agency decisions; therefore, complaints about these decisions are most likely to come from the existing hospitals, their employees and staff, rather than a new applicant. Related to this issue of minimizing complaints against the agency is the regulatory agencies' attempt to have their own performance judged by the more obvious indicators of industry performance. Innovation and technical change in the delivery of health services in an area might offer huge potential benefits to consumers. These benefits, however, are not obvious, whereas the closing of a hospital caused by new firms entering the market will result in an obvious cost to the community and complaints from the affected hospital and its employees. Thus the health planning agency is likely to move very slowly on innovation, preferring to allow existing providers to introduce innovation if sufficient pressures arise for them to be adopted.

One example of planning agencies' selecting obvious measures of industry performance as measures of their own performance is the classic study conducted by Salkever and Bice (27). As pressures from third-party payors increase to hold down hospital capital investment, an agency would be likely to concentrate its efforts on the most obvious measure of hospital investment: beds. Salkever and Bice found that the presence of CON controls in a state resulted in a decrease in changes in the number of beds in that state, an increase in plant assets per bed, and no change in total hospital assets. The authors concluded that controls merely shifted the type of hospital investment. The authors also attempted to determine whether the existence of strong planning agency authority resulted in lower hospital costs. They concluded that there was no evidence to indicate that CON had any effect on hospital costs.

Since the initial study by Salkever and Bice, other researchers have examined the effect of CON legislation (28). The findings from all these studies are similar. CON did not have any effect on hospital investment or on the rate of growth in hospital expenditures. Some studies found a shift in hospital investment, from beds to equipment. Other studies found that CON caused an increase in hospital investment; hospitals moved their investment plans along faster in anticipation of CON legislation. Some of the studies measured the "maturity" of CON in a state; it was found that it did not matter how long a state had CON, it was still not effective. Still other studies examined the comprehensiveness of the legislation and the stringency of the CON process in a state. Again the findings were that CON did not decrease hospital investment or expenditures.

Summary

The evidence on health planning in this country does not support the traditional or public interest view of regulation, namely, that regulators will lower the price of the goods and services produced by the regulated industry. Instead, the evidence on performance of regulatory agencies in nonhealth fields appears to predict the outcome of regulation in the health field; when the regulated industry is the major group with a concentrated interest, regulatory agencies are strongly influenced by the industry they are meant to regulate. The methods used by hospitals to influence health planning agencies have varied from providing them with financial support, data, and technical expertise to functioning as the major participants in the review of their own expansion plans. The outcome of health planning regulation should have been predictable in that protection of existing providers should have been anticipated as an objective of the regulatory agencies. Older, established institutions have benefited by being able to continue their operations without being judged in the same manner as new applicants and providers. It was likely that planning agencies would disregard population movements in awarding of CON certificates, which favors existing hospitals. Not surprisingly, entry, particularly by proprietaries, has been blocked. It was predictable that the development of lower-cost substitutes for hospitals, such as free-standing surgicenters and HMOs, would be hindered. No incentives have been provided for efficient operations. The problem initially used to justify the CON legislation—to retard the increase in hospital costs and investment—has not been resolved.

Health planning has been a conservative approach to improving hospital performance. It left unchanged the method used to reimburse hospitals and it did not change the incentives facing physicians, hospitals, and patients. Moreover, once a hospital received CON approval for its investment plans (and the probability was very high that it would receive such approval), it had an incentive to undertake the most costly investment, since it would be reimbursed on a cost basis. Health planning agencies have failed to improve the allocation of resources in the delivery of medical care.

Finally, in the fall of 1986 the Congress refused to authorize funding for health planning agencies (29). The Reagan administration had been trying for several years to eliminate the program. The administration believed that the program had been ineffective and that it was inconsistent with its antiregulatory aims. Also opposing continuation of the program were aggressive hospital and medical groups which claimed that the emerging market system in health care offered sufficient incentives to prevent hospitals from undertaking unwise investments; these interests believed that they needed increased investment flexibility in the changed, competitive environment.

CON is still being used in many places in an anticompetitive manner. Thirty nine states maintained their CON laws (30). These laws are still being used to the advantage of hospitals and local health providers; for example, home health agencies desiring to enter a market to compete with existing home health agencies have to apply for a CON and in many cases have been excluded by the state planning agencies (31).

An Application of Facilities Regulation: The Issue of Hospital Bed Reduction

In the mid-1970s, it was estimated that there were between 60,000 and 100,000 excess hospital beds; as of 1985 that number had increased to approximately 160,000 (32). At approximately $130,000 a bed, proponents of hospital bed reduction point to the enormous potential savings that could be achieved if excess hospital beds were eliminated (33). These potential savings, however, are not as clear-cut as the proponents of hospital bed reduction would have us believe.

First, what is the definition of excess hospital capacity? Two definitions are generally used. The first, based on the National Health Planning Guidelines, is the number of beds that would be eliminated if the current bed/population ratio were reduced to 4.0 beds per 1,000 population (or lower). The second definition is based on the assumption that an 85 percent occupancy rate would be appropriate for the hospitals in the community. The number of hospital beds in the community should be reduced until an overall 85 percent occupancy rate is achieved.[2]

Under hospital bed reduction programs, excess hospital capacity can be achieved in one of several ways. Each hospital can reduce its capacity until the community standard of 4.0 beds per 1,000 population is achieved (or until each hospital achieves an 85 percent occupancy rate). Alternatively, the goals of bed reduction can be achieved by targeting certain hospitals for complete closure.

It is important in understanding the bed reduction issue to make explicit the value judgments underlying the use of the community standards noted above. If the actual bed/population ratio is greater than the 4 beds per 1,000 population standard, it is implicitly assumed that there is "inappropriate" hospital utilization. Therefore, reducing the number of beds will presumably reduce inappropriate utilization. If beds

---

[2]For purposes of this discussion, excess hospital capacity refers to beds that are either used or for which the hospital has staffed. If a hospital has unused beds, for which it does not staff, the costs of maintaining those beds are minimal. Most of these costs have been incurred in the past (i.e., capital investment and interest payments), and there would be little if any savings if these beds were eliminated.

are then rationed, it is assumed that only those most in need of a hospital will be admitted. However, it is not necessarily the case that only inappropriate utilization is reduced when beds are reduced. There are many factors that affect a community's utilization rate. The age of the population, the availability of (and payment for) out-of-hospital substitutes, and whether someone is able to care for the patient at home are just some of the determinants of the demand for hospital care. Placing upper limits on the community's hospital use may result in a form of cost shifting; the savings from fewer hospital beds may cause increased costs to patients (and their families) if they have to be treated in a different manner. Even in those situations where there is inappropriate utilization, the hospital and medical staff's admissions policy may not use appropriateness of admission and length of stay as the rationing criteria.

If all hospitals in the community are required to maintain an 85 percent occupancy level, it is implicitly assumed that the costs of not having a bed available are less than the costs of maintaining those additional beds. Increasing the occupancy rate lowers the probability that a patient will have access to a bed when needed; they may be forced to wait or to enter another hospital. When bed reduction is achieved through closure of a hospital, there are additional travel costs, not just for the patient but also for the patient's visitors. Travel costs should include the value of time spent in travel as well as the transportation costs.

Thus based on the two standards used for defining excess capacity, an appropriate bed/population ratio and/or a desired occupancy level, excess capacity refers to both misused and underused beds.

Perhaps the most controversial aspect of hospital bed reduction programs concerns the method used to calculate potential savings. If a hospital is closed, its total costs are eliminated. (There may be buyout costs that would reduce these savings.) However, that hospital's patients will continue to seek medical care (although some percentage of the patients may no longer seek hospital care). Those patients going to other hospitals will incur costs in those hospitals. Crucial to this entire discussion of hospital bed reduction is the assumption of what the additional costs will be in those hospitals receiving patients from the closed hospital. McClure assumed that 60 percent of a hospital's costs were fixed and 40 percent were variable costs (34). Thus if a hospital were to close and its patients entered another hospital, the receiving hospital would only incur an increase in its costs equal to 40 percent of its average cost per patient. McClure assumed that the hospital's fixed cost would not change; when marginal costs are estimated to be only 40 percent of average costs, average cost per patient would fall as more patients are admitted. If, however, the marginal costs of an additional patient were equal to 100 percent of the hospital's average cost per patient, there would be no savings (assuming that all the hospitals had the same average cost and all patients from the closed hospital went to other hospitals). Thus the estimate selected for marginal cost as a percentage of average cost is an important determinant of whether savings occur as a result of bed reduction programs.

A number of studies have estimated the ratio that marginal cost is to average cost. These results, reported in a article by Lipscomb et al., have varied from a low of 21 to a high of 100 percent of average cost (35). The majority of these studies reported marginal cost/average cost ratios to be quite high. Proponents of hospital closure, however, have used the lower range of estimates to indicate savings from hospital bed reduction programs. While the estimates of the marginal cost/average cost ratio have a wide variation, the results of these studies are not necessarily inconsistent. More important, for purposes of estimating any possible savings due to a bed reduction program, it is more appropriate to use the higher ratio estimates.

Hospitals staff for an expected level of output. However, the very nature of the demand for hospital care is such that while a hospital staffs for an expected output level, there are always unexpected changes in demand. If the number of patient days is either greater or less than the expected level, the hospital is not able to adjust its staffing pattern immediately. Thus over short periods, hospital salaries may be a fixed cost. Short-run marginal costs represent the hospital's response to these unexpected changes in utilization. It is therefore not surprising that short-run marginal costs have been estimated to be between 20 and 40 percent of average costs. Over longer periods of time, however, hospitals are able to make adjustments in their staffing patterns as well as in their other resources, such as capital and equipment. Thus, if a hospital's admissions increase, and this increase is expected to be permanent, the hospital will be able to make a complete adjustment to this change over time. Such a process of adaptation is consistent with economic theory. In the long run there are no fixed costs; all factors of production are variable. Higher estimates of the marginal cost/average cost ratio represent more complete adaptation to permanent changes in a hospital's workload. Thus estimates of the ratio of marginal to average costs in the short run are not inconsistent with the higher marginal cost/average cost ratio found in other studies. In a recent article on this subject, Friedman and Pauly estimate the marginal cost of an unexpected admission to be 35 percent of average costs, while the marginal cost of an expected admission is 98 percent of average cost (36).

Based on the discussion above, it is clear that the use of short-run marginal costs is inappropriate for estimating the savings of hospital closure. When a hospital is closed and its patients are admitted to other hospitals, the other hospitals will anticipate a higher expected patient load; they will adjust their resources and staffing patterns accordingly. The reduction in costs from closing a hospital will be its average cost multiplied by its number of patients. The increase in costs at other hospitals will be the number of additional patients received multiplied by 90–95 percent of the hospitals' average costs.

To calculate whether total hospital costs in the community will be reduced after a hospital closure requires knowledge of the average cost per patient at the hospital targeted for closure, the percent of the hospital's patients that will go to other hospitals, and the long-run marginal cost at those other hospitals.

An important factor in determining which hospitals are targeted for closure is whether or not they are small community institutions. At times, bed reduction policies are used to maintain the viability of the larger hospitals that are suffering from low occupancy rates.

"When the pressures to reduce the community's bed supply becomes too powerful to resist, the hospitals themselves may coalesce to exercise some control over the process. A common characteristic of such pressure appears to be a predictable squeezing out of smaller, often lower-cost basic institutions by the larger, complex hospitals with the result that there are fewer, larger, more comprehensive service centers usually operating at higher average cost" (37).

Under these circumstances, average cost per admission in the hospital targeted for closure may well be less than the marginal cost of adding patients to the larger institutions. A hypothetical example will clarify this. As shown in Table 11–1, Hospital X is

TABLE 11-2. Estimated Inpatient Savings from Hospital Closure: A Hypothetical Example

	Average Cost Per Patient Day (1)	Total Patient Days (2)	Estimate of Marginal/Average Cost (3)	Marginal Cost of Additional Patient Day (4)	Total Cost of Additional Patient Days (5)	Net Inpatient Savings of Closure (6)
Hospital X (targeted for closure)	$280.00	50,000	—	—	($14,000,000)	—
	300.00	50,000	.85	$255.00	$12,750,000	$1,250,000
			.90	270.00	13,500,000	500,000
			.95	285.00	14,250,000	(250,000)
	325.00	50,000	.85	276.25	13,812,500	187,500
			.90	292.50	14,625,000	(625,000)
			.95	308.75	15,437,500	(1,437,500)
Hospital Y	350.00	50,000	.85	297.50	14,875,000	(875,000)
			.90	315.00	15,750,000	(1,750,000)
			.95	332.50	16,625,000	(2,625,000)

Note: Numbers in parentheses indicate losses.

277

targeted for closure. Its average costs per patient day are $280; it serves 50,000 patient days per year. If the hospital is closed, $14 million will be saved each year. Hospital Y is typical of the remaining hospitals in the community. Three different estimates of average cost in Hospital Y are provided; three estimates of marginal cost are also assumed for each of the average cost estimates. It is also assumed that all the patients from Hospital X seek care in the remaining hospitals, and that there is no change in the case mix or number of patients in the receiving hospitals. (It is further assumed that the receiving hospitals care for the additional patients with the same style of medical practice as that received by their other patients.)

Although the example above is merely illustrative, the results are very sensitive to the following assumptions: the difference in average cost between the hospital targeted for closure and the remaining hospitals; the ratio of marginal to average cost in the remaining hospitals; and (although not shown in Table 11–1) the percentage of the patients from the closed hospital who continue to seek hospital care. According to the results of the hypothetical example, savings, when they do occur, are relatively small. Any such savings, however, should be considered as gross, not net, savings since there are additional costs to be considered.

If a hospital is closed, there are increased transportation costs and travel time by patients, their visitors, and others to another hospital. The attractiveness of the community to new residents and employers may be decreased. Physicians may leave the area if they are unable to have staff appointments at nearly hospitals. The remaining hospitals will have greater market power since there are fewer competing hospitals. Additional costs are those of the regulatory process itself and the inevitable lawsuits when a hospital is targeted for closure. Part of the hospital savings (i.e., the discounted present value) may be required to pay off obligations incurred by the hospital targeted for closure. Thus offsetting any possible gross savings are other costs, some direct, others indirect, which are likely to be shifted to patients, their families, and others. These costs, unfortunately, are not always as quantifiable, nor visible, as the savings in hospital costs; they therefore tend to be neglected or given a smaller weight in the decision process.

One study that attempted to estimate the potential savings from eliminating duplication at a national level concluded that they are "disappointingly small" (38). Net savings from hospital closure are particularly doubtful when the targeted hospitals are small, relatively unsophisticated community hospitals (39). By the time lawsuits are concluded and the state legislature has had its opportunity to develop political compromises over which hospitals are should be closed, considerable time may pass before bed reduction policies can have an effect.

Local health planning agencies continue to pursue bed reduction programs. For example, in New York City the local agency has called for a reduction of 5,028 beds or 14.3 percent of New York's bed capacity. The planning agency claims that, based on an estimated $150,000 annual cost per bed, annual savings would be $750 million (40). The Federal Trade Commission has opposed New York's proposal to use CON to achieve this reduction (41). Increased understanding of hospital costs and the competitive consequences of bed reduction programs should, hopefully, clarify such issues.

An alternative approach to reducing "misused and underutilized beds" is to strive for policies that decrease the demand for hospital care. Examples of such policies are the inclusion in health benefits of coverage for out-of-hospital substitutes, such as outpatient surgery, and policies that provide physicians with an incentive not to hospitalize their patients, such as exist in HMOs and managed care plans. The advantage of a demand approach to decreasing utilization is that the patient and/or his or her physician make the decision of whether or not to hospitalize, not based on a state planning agency's guidelines. The patient and physician are also likely to have different valuations of the costs and benefits of the various alternatives. A restructuring of patient and physician incentives (as described in Chapter 12) has a greater likelihood of achieving a more efficient use of the hospital.

Rate Regulation of Hospital Services

As CON proved to be ineffective in holding down the rate of increase in hospital costs and in reducing the duplication of hospital facilities, more direct forms of regulation were proposed. In 1971 the federal government instituted rate controls for the entire country, the Economic Stabilization Program (ESP), as part of a campaign against rising inflation. While the rest of the country was removed from these controls after a short period, they remained in effect for the health sector until April 1974. Further, in the early 1970s, several states started to institute rate regulation. As more states started their own rate setting programs, they varied along a number of dimensions. In some states it was voluntary, in others it was mandatory. Some states made the rate regulation applicable to all the payors of hospital care, while other states required it for only Medicaid patients. The unit of payment to be regulated was either the hospital patient day or the admission. The effectiveness of state rate regulation programs varied according to the dimensions above. Then in 1983, the federal government instituted its own form of hospital rate regulation, DRGs for hospitalized Medicare patients.

There are three issues of importance with regard to rate regulation. First, why was rate regulation instituted? (Based on the theory of economic regulation, one would have to consider whose interests were to be served by rate setting.) Second, what are the different methods that can be used to regulate hospital rates, and what are their likely consequences? Third, what is the empirical evidence on the performance of both state and federal rate regulation?

The Introduction of Rate Regulation

There were two federal rate control programs, the ESP in 1971 and DRGs in 1983. There were several different types of state programs, from those that were mandatory and applicable to all payors to those that were voluntary and affected only Medicaid patients. These different types of programs, and their effectiveness, depended upon the reasons for their introduction.

Hospitals have a concentrated interest in any legislation affecting their revenues or their investments. As shown in the earlier discussion of CON, hospitals were instrumental in having CON legislated in their states, in controlling its implementation, and in using CON to the disadvantage of both their competitors and innovative delivery systems. Hospitals would be expected to oppose any legislation that would make it difficult for them to achieve their goals.

As expenditures for Medicare exceeded their projections, the federal government became concerned about the potential bankruptcy of the Medicare Trust Fund. To ensure that there would be sufficient funds to pay for the benefits legislated under Medicare, the amount of the social security tax that is designated for the Trust Fund was increased, as was the applicable wage base. In 1966 the employee and the employer each had to pay .35 percent of the employees' wage, up to a maximum wage of $6,600 for the Medicare Trust Fund. By 1988, that amount had risen to 1.45 percent up to a wage base of $45,000. To forestall having to request even larger increases in the social security tax, the federal government developed a concentrated interest in holding down Medicare expenditures.

In the late 1960s the inflation rate started to rise. As public concern increased, the Nixon administration made a dramatic gesture by imposing wage and price controls on the entire economy. The resulting complications of economywide controls led to their removal one year later, however, they were kept in effect for hospitals and physicians for several more years. Hospital and physician groups had opposed these controls.

In 1979, President Carter's highest domestic priority was to reimpose price controls on hospitals. Both hospital and physician groups opposed the legislation, preferring instead a voluntary program, the Voluntary Effort, to reduce the rise in hospital expenditures. The Carter administration was defeated. In a study on congressional voting on the cost-containment legislation, the authors found that Congress members who received a larger portion of their total campaign contributions from health interest groups and those who came from states with greater than average annual percentage increases in hospital expenditures were more likely to vote against cost containment (42). Also affecting a Congress member's vote was the percent of a state's population on Medicaid; the greater the proportion of the population on Medicaid, the more likely the Congress member was to vote for President Carter's hospital cost containment legislation. The political support offered to legislators by health interest groups outweighed that offered by the Carter administration.

It was not until 1983, when the Reagan administration proposed DRGs, that hospitals became subject to rate regulation for their Medicare patients. It did not matter which political party was in control of the administration, each successive administration developed a concentrated interest in limiting the rise in hospital expenditures. By 1983, hospital and physician groups were no longer able to overcome imposition of price controls by a popular Republican administration.

The development of rate regulation at the state level was also related to whether concentrated interests developed to restrain the rise in hospital expenditures. A number of states had implemented generous (with regard to benefits and eligibility) Medicaid programs, for which they had to share with the federal government the program's expenditures. As hospital and physician prices and expenditures rose, states found that their Medicaid expenditures were increasing more rapidly than expected. Medicaid expenditures were funded from general state taxes and as the program's expenditures increased, fewer funds were available for other, politically popular state programs. To keep funding other state programs as well as the rapidly rising Medicaid program would have meant increasing taxes, a politically unpopular move. As the economy entered a recession in 1981, fewer state funds were available for Medicaid.

A study examining why certain states implemented stringent hospital rate regulation programs concluded that "Liberal states with budget deficits and large Medicaid hospital expenses were most likely to enact rate-setting laws" (43). California, which had a high probability of implementing rate setting but did not, used alternative methods to lower its Medicaid expenditures; Medicaid patients were signed up in HMOs, a federal waiver was granted to permit the state to impose copayments on

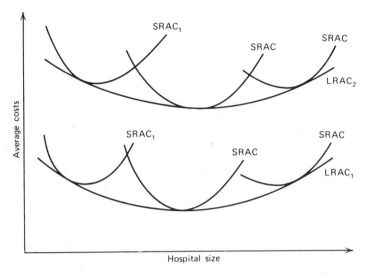

Figure 11-1. Variations in hospital costs as a result of product and size differences.

Medicaid patients, and it was the first state to implement selective contracting with hospitals for its Medicaid population.

Thus the implementation of rate regulation, at both the federal and the state levels, the stringency of the program, and its likely effectiveness are consistent with the economic theory of regulation. As groups having a concentrated interest in restraining their medical expenditures develop, it becomes more difficult for hospital and medical groups to achieve their own objectives. Political competition between opposing interest groups is likely to result in compromises; as one group becomes politically more powerful, it will be able to achieve more of what it desires by imposing its costs on those who have less political influence. The groups bearing the costs of a lower rate of increase in Medicare and Medicaid expenditures are likely to be both the hospitals and patients.

Objectives of Hospital Rate Regulation

Before examining the performance of different methods of rate regulation, the likely effects of different rate setting methods are examined. First, however, we review why hospital costs vary and the differing objectives underlying rate regulation.

The earlier discussion on hospital economies of scale described the factors, other than size, that affect hospital costs. Those factors will be reviewed here with reference to Figure 11-1. The long-run average-cost curve, represented by $LRAC_1$, shows the relationship between average cost and size of a hospital. Different hospital sizes are represented by different short-run average-cost curves (SRAC) along a given LRAC curve. It is assumed that each hospital on $LRAC_1$ is producing the same type of product, by which we mean the same case mix of patients with the same degree of severity of illness and receiving the same quality of care. When differences in quality or patients' severity of illness exist between two types of hospitals, they will be on different long-run average-cost curves; for example, if one hospital is a teaching hospital, with a more severely ill mix of patients, and the other is not, the teaching hospital will be on

$LRAC_2$ and the nonteaching hospital, with lower average costs, will be on $LRAC_1$. Thus differences in hospital size will be represented by different SRAC curves, while differences in the products that hospitals produce will be represented by different LRAC curves. Further, if two hospitals are identical in size and products but differ in efficiency, the more efficient hospital will be represented by a lower SRAC. Finally, since the prices the hospital must pay for its inputs, labor, equipment, supplies, and capital are continually increasing, a group of hospitals represented by $LRAC_1$ will find themselves slowly rising to $LRAC_2$ as the prices of their inputs rise. It will no longer be possible for those same hospitals to remain on $LRAC_1$.

The foregoing brief discussion indicates the issues with which any rate regulation agency must be concerned. The rate regulators must be able to reimburse hospitals while making adjustments for the many ways in which hospitals and their patients may differ, including size, products, and efficiency, and they must be able to determine the rate at which hospital input prices are rising, thereby moving hospitals to a higher LRAC. Unless the rate regulators are able to distinguish the sources of cost differences among hospitals and estimate the amount of those differences, the rates that are established may reward some hospitals unfairly while penalizing others. Further, unless rate regulators are able to estimate the increase in hospital input prices over time, they will either be rewarding hospitals too generously (if they allow too large a price increase) or they will penalize all the hospitals by granting them too small a rate increase. In the latter case, hospitals will not be able to remain on their original LRAC. Receiving less than the full amount of the price increase (adjusted for input substitution) will require hospitals to move to a lower LRAC, requiring that they produce a less expensive or different product. The task of a rate regulator is not easy; unless they are extremely accurate in accounting for differences among hospitals and in estimating increases in hospital input prices, the consequences of their actions will be different from what they intended.

What should be the objectives of rate regulators? Ideally, they should use regulation to achieve an outcome similar to that which would result from a well informed competitive market. In a perfectly competitive market, the following four outcomes would occur. First, each hospital would be both economically and technically efficient; technical efficiency means that the hospital would produce the maximum output for the inputs it used.[3] To be economically efficient as well, the hospital would have to use the least costly combination of inputs to produce a given level of output (the isoquant is tangent to the isocost line). The resulting internal efficiency (the lowest SRAC curve for a given hospital size and type of output) is desirable, but it cannot be the sole objective of a reimbursement scheme. Internal efficiency results in the hospital's production of output at minimum cost, but it does not identify the types and quantity of output that should be produced, or whether a particular hospital should be permitted to continue to provide hospital care. A hospital may be doing the best it can, given its size, age, and the facilities it has, but if it is too small or its facilities too old to produce its output at as low a cost as other hospitals, or if some of its facilities are underutilized, the community may be best served by eliminating the hospital or some of its facilities. Even if all hospitals were internally efficient, but economies of scale existed, total hospital expenditures could be reduced if fewer hospitals were to provide the same quantity and quality of output. Therefore, a second objective of rate regula-

---

[3]If the hospital were technically efficient, it would be operating on (rather than within) its isoquant for that particular level of output.

tion should be to strive for efficiency in the use of all the hospital resources in the community. Hospital services should be produced at minimum cost as calculated in terms of the entire system rather than just the individual hospital. (Assuming low travel costs, hospitals operating on the SRAC curve that is at the minimum point of the LRAC curve for a given type of product would be preferred.) If one open heart surgery unit were less costly than four such units, it would be economically inefficient to have multiple, higher-cost facilities.

A third objective is to determine the appropriate amount of hospital care, relative to other forms of care, for providing a medical treatment at minimum cost. Hospitals are only one setting in which a medical treatment can be provided; others include physicians' offices, nursing homes, or a patient's own home. Minimizing the cost of a treatment is likely to require substitution of care away from the hospital to a less costly institutional setting. Reimbursement schemes concerned solely with the rate at which hospitals are paid may cause distortions in the use of other services.

Rate-setting agencies are generally concerned with hospital expenditures, not with minimizing treatment costs. It would thus appear that internal hospital efficiency is the rate-setting agency's main objective. The second possible objective, minimizing the cost of hospital care for the community by eliminating unnecessary duplication, is generally a concern of the planning agency. The third possible objective, minimizing the cost of medical treatments, is usually discussed by interested persons; the rate-setting and planning agencies are generally not involved with this broader problem of economic efficiency in the provision of medical care.

A fourth objective is important to several interest groups concerned with the rate-setting process. Some proponents of rate regulation, especially federal and state governments, seek to contain the total amount spent on hospital care. It is important to recognize that success in holding down the rate of increase in hospital expenditures will not necessarily achieve any of the first three objectives. Hospitals may reduce their costs by admitting fewer patients or by releasing patients sooner, thus shifting costs of medical care to other providers or to the consumer. These practices might achieve the third objective if care can be provided adequately and at lower cost in other settings, but they could also lead to undesirable decreases in the amount of care some individuals receive. The objective of merely containing the increase in total hospital expenditures may prevent hospitals from remaining on their original LRAC as their input prices rise. A cost-containment policy that provides hospitals with insufficient funds to move from $LRAC_1$ to $LRAC_2$ as shown in Figure 11-1 (where the difference between the two LRAC curves is the result of input price increases only and not of increased quality or product differences) will force those hospitals to be on a lower LRAC than previously. The lower LRAC would represent a diminution of product in some manner, but not necessarily an increase in hospital efficiency or a desirable reduction in the hospitals' output.

The movement from retrospective (cost-based) hospital payment to prospective payment caused a change in the incentives facing hospital decisionmakers. The effect of cost-based reimbursement was to enable each hospital to move to any LRAC curve it desired and to achieve any size of facility (SRAC) on that LRAC curve. The risks of higher costs were shifted to the patients through their third-party payors. Under prospective payment, hospital rates or budgets are determined in advance and the risks of exceeding those rates are borne by the hospital. To achieve the objectives of internal efficiency (objective 1), system efficiency (objective 2), minimizing the cost of a treatment (objective 3), and limiting the increase in hospital expenditures (objective 4), hospital reimbursement must be on a prospective basis; however, not all payment systems will achieve all four objectives. The two general types of prospective payment systems used in rate setting are discussed below.

Budget Review on a Prospective Basis

Hospitals favor the budget review approach for determining hospital reimbursement. This approach assumes that it is impossible to separate out differences in products, size, and efficiency among hospitals. A representative of the rate-setting agency reviews each hospital's budget for the reasonableness of its cost increases:

> Hospitals have an opportunity to explain and defend their budgets, and the rate setting agency or program has an opportunity to question items that appear out of line. Budget review gives the agency more of a chance to influence specific hospital activities and plans before decisions about them are implemented. In short, a detailed, institution by institution examination of costs and cost influencing factors characterizes the budget review method of rate setting. To many, this is the attractive feature of this method; to others, its basic drawback. Meaningful budget reviews require considerable expertise—in accounting, economics, finance, and hospital management—which many rate setting agencies and programs do not have. Comprehensive and thorough reviews also require considerable and fairly detailed cost and statistical data; a knowledge of the assumptions, modes of operation, and plans that underlie the figures presented; a knowledge of the need for new programs and services proposed; . . . (typically, the management staffs of a few large hospitals taken together are larger than the entire agency staff) . . . (44).

The proponents of prospective reimbursement on an individual hospital basis stress that it allows for an explicit consideration of differences among hospitals and permits the elimination of waste while treating hospitals fairly. Some variations on this basic approach allow for incentives; if the hospital can keep its costs below the prospectively determined rates, it can keep a portion of the savings. If its costs exceed the rates, it must absorb a portion of the loss. Critics of this approach maintain that it poses no risk for the hospital and therefore is unlikely to result in cost savings. Because of its familiarity with its own budget, the hospital staff will find it easy to justify any of its expenditures. Further, this system offers little incentive for the hospital to hold down its costs, since it can receive a pass-through for legitimate costs such as wage increases.

Impact on Objectives. There is likely to be little effect on hospital efficiency from a prospective payment system that determines each hospital's budget without regard to the performance of comparable hospitals. Unless input ratios, costs, and patient characteristics from other hospitals can be used as a yardstick, it is difficult for regulators to question the appropriateness of a hospital's expenditures. Too often, each item may appear justifiable from the hospital's perspective, and they may be able to convince the regulators on each particular cost area, however, in aggregate the institution may be inefficient.

A hospital may operate a service that is subject to large economies of scale and yet have a relatively high unit cost because its volume is too small. The hospital may be operating that facility as efficiently as possible. If the rate regulators are concerned only with the hospital's internal efficiency, it is unlikely that the hospital would be required to merge or close its specialized facility. Usually, approval for new investments is determined by the local CON planning agency, not the rate setters. Once CON approval is granted, the rate regulators reimburse the hospital for those new facilities regardless of their cost-size relationship.

Setting hospital budgets or rates prospectively on an individual basis does not by itself provide incentives to substitute less costly forms of medical care for hospital care. Further, if the hospital is paid a set fee per patient day, it has some incentive to keep patients longer than necessary (again assuming this does not conflict with other objectives and is not prevented by effective monitoring procedures), since the marginal cost of the extra days during which few services are provided is likely to be less than the additional payment. Similarly, if the hospital is paid a fee per admission, it has an incentive to admit patients who could be treated at less cost in other settings.

Whether the budget review approach limits the rise in hospital expenditures depends on whether the rate regulators are able to impose tight annual limits on each hospital. If the state has a strong concentrated interest in limiting increases in hospital expenditures, tight controls may be imposed. The annual percent increase factor is subject to a great deal of negotiation between those groups with a concentrated interest in its outcome.

Establishing Reimbursement Levels Based on a Hospital's Performance Relative to Other Hospitals

The second basic approach used for establishing prospective hospital payment is to base the rate upon the particular classification in which a hospital is grouped. Ideally, one would want to be able to classify hospitals according to differences in their products by determining which LRAC curve they are on and then establishing a rate for the output category that reflects the minimum point on the long-run average-cost curve (assuming no travel costs). Hospitals producing similar products would receive one rate per unit of output regardless of their differences in size or efficiency. Presumably those hospitals that are internally efficient and least costly in terms of size of operation will be able to produce their output at a cost at or below the reimbursement rate. Those hospitals whose costs are above the prospectively set rate will have to merge, become more efficient, or not provide that particular service. Since high-cost hospitals may attempt to change their product line if their costs are greater than the rate established for their group, it is necessary under this approach, more so than under the previous approach, to monitor changes in their outputs, quality, facilities, and services. The difficulty is in properly determining each hospital's classification. Critics of this approach, primarily hospital administrators, claim that it is not possible to develop adequate classifications for each hospital. Hospitals vary so greatly in the services and quality of care they provide, and in their case mix of patients, that three or four major groupings will not adequately reflect the differences among them. The result of inadequate groupings will be an inequitable system of rewards and penalties. The hospital is at greater risk under this type of payment system than under the previous one.

There are several examples where rate setting has used this approach for determining prospective rates. Several states, including New York, classified hospitals into groups according to their size, type, ownership, and location.

The best known version of basing hospital rates relative to those of other hospitals is the Medicare diagnostic related groupings (DRGs) system. DRGs were based on the characteristics of the patient and the treatment received rather than on hospital characteristics, such as bed size. DRGs were first instituted in New Jersey. They were adapted by the federal government in October 1983 and phased in over a four-year period. DRGs are determined empirically; they were initially created according to whether the primary and secondary diagnosis, age, and existence of a surgical procedure affected the patient's length of stay. Within each DRG, there is assumed to be a certain resource use associated with a patient's treatment, and the use of those resources is assumed to vary according to such factors as the patient's age, sex, primary and secondary diagnoses, and discharge status. The use of DRGs is a recognition that hospitals are multiproduct firms; hospitals treat different types of patients. There are now 473 Medicare DRGs. Under DRGs, hospital reimbursement is tied to the type of patient treated. In its simplest form, a fixed amount is paid to a hospital for each patient within a given DRG. The hospital has a financial incentive to produce care at a cost below the fixed price, since it can keep the difference. If the hospital's cost for treating a patient exceeds that patient's DRG price, the hospital loses money.

Conceptually, the DRG approach is appealing. Similar types of patients in different hospitals should use similar quantities of resources. Differences in the costs of producing similar patients are either a result of differences in hospital efficiency and/or style of medical practice. Facing a fixed price, a hospital has an incentive to minimize its costs of caring for that patient; the hospital can reduce a patient's length of stay, perhaps treat them as outpatients, and not use an excessive amount of ancillary services (or other services) in treatment. Hospitals having different patient mixes would be reimbursed accordingly. Hospitals also have an incentive to specialize in those DRGs at which they are most efficient.

There are, however, a number of concerns with the DRG system. The first is with the appropriate DRG classification for a patient. Often, patients have multiple diagnoses. The DRG classification is heavily influenced by the primary diagnosis. The sequence of diagnoses proved to be a major source of error in a study conducted by the Institute of Medicine, which found a 35 percent error rate in the principal discharge diagnosis (45). One study examined the impact on hospital reimbursement if the primary and secondary diagnoses were classified according to which diagnosis maximized the hospital's reimbursement (46). Had such a reclassification actually been used for reimbursement purposes, the hospital's case-mix cost would have increased by 14 percent; the hospital would have received a windfall profit.

In many cases the diagnosis sequence may be appropriately switched. Computer programs are being marketed to hospitals claiming that in those situations in which either the primary or secondary diagnoses could be appropriately interchanged, the program will select the higher-priced diagnosis as the DRG classification. Uncertainty often exists as to the patient's diagnosis. Physicians may be "educated" to select certain DRG classifications rather than others under conditions of such uncertainty. "DRG creep" could be rationalized as being an appropriate reclassification of diagnoses. However, a financial incentive is created for unethical behavior. To prevent any such potential abuse, utilization review mechanisms must be effective. In New Jersey, a study found that 26.4 percent of the patients had been misclassified (47). Even if this error rate was unrelated to any financial incentives, such a high percentage of patients incorrectly assigned to DRGs will result in windfall gains and losses to hospitals and payors. Thus one possible response to DRGs by hospitals is to reclassify their patients into the higher-priced DRGs.[4]

A second serious concern with DRGs is that the current classification scheme does not consider the patient's severity of illness. Since the DRG is supposed to indicate the resource costs of caring for a particular patient, excluding certain patient characteristics, such as severity of illness, will result in inadequate reimbursement for hospitals that care for more severely ill patients. One study found that the degree of patient severity of illness varied greatly between hospitals and that some hospitals treated a greater proportion of the severely ill patients. Further, that teaching hospital status and the Medicare Case Mix Index did not always coincide with which hospitals treated the more severely ill patients (48). A second type of hospital response to the DRG system is to be more selective with regard to the patient's severity of illness.

There are a number of additional hospital responses to the DRG payment system that should be considered. DRGs are not based on the lowest production cost by the most efficient hospital for producing a given DRG; instead, DRGs are based on average costs over a large number of hospitals for producing a DRG. For any hospital, therefore, the DRG price may be higher or lower than its actual cost for producing that particular DRG. If the DRG price is above the hospital's own costs for that DRG, the hospital is likely to want to expand its output of that DRG. To maximize its profits, a firm will produce to the point where its marginal costs equals its marginal revenue, which in the case of DRGs, is the DRG price. To increase the number of its profitable DRGs, the hospital would be willing to increase its costs to compete for patients and/ or physicians. The analogy is the same as when airline fares and interest paid by savings and loan associations were regulated. The competing firms will engage in nonprice competition to increase their business. The same is hypothesized to occur with hospitals (49).

As shown in Figure 11-2, P_0 is the DRG price and MC_0 is the hospital's cost for caring for that DRG patient. To maximize profits, the hospital will attempt to increase its number of patients until its marginal costs equal its marginal revenue. The profit-maximizing output would be OQ_A. To compete for additional patients, the hospital would be willing to incur additional costs per patient, which would increase the hospital's marginal cost curve to MC_1. The hospital, under competition, will end up at the point where its new, higher, marginal cost curve equals the DRG price.

If hospitals were able to engage in price competition for their Medicare patients, they might lower the price to the patient by not requiring the Medicare hospital deductible. However, since the hospital cannot use price to compete for patients or referring physicians, hospitals will compete on a nonprice basis. The consequence of nonprice competition will be to increase hospital costs. If the DRG price were tied to hospital costs, nonprice competition would drive up DRG prices.

If the hospital does not have to compete for patients (i.e., the hospital has monopoly power), the hospital keeps the difference between the DRG price and its costs. How that "profit" is then spent is determined by who is in control of the institution.

---

[4]One of the most publicized examples of misclassification in the New Jersey experiment was the softball player who had injured his finger. He had to be hospitalized for two days so that the bone in his finger could be repaired with a metal pin. The DRG category assigned to this patient was "fracture with major surgery," usually reserved for serious cases such as total hip replacement. While the patient's actual charges would have been less than $1,000, the DRG classification resulted in a bill for $5,000.

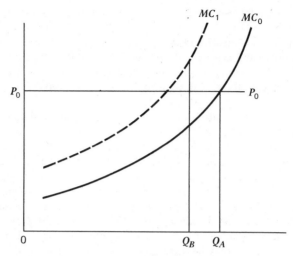

Figure 11-2. Rate regulation when patients in the same classification have different treatment costs.

When the DRG price is less than the hospital's costs for producing that DRG, the hospital is likely to respond in the following ways. Assume, again with reference to Figure 11-2, that the hospital is on marginal cost curve MC_1 and that it is caring for OQ_B patients; its marginal cost for those patients exceeds its DRG price, P_0. If the reason for the hospital's costs being greater than the DRG price is that the hospital is inefficient, the hospital could increase its efficiency (i.e., move to a lower marginal cost curve, MC_0). The reason that the hospital's costs exceed the DRG price could be because it cares for a more severely ill mix of patients and DRG prices do not reflect differences in severity. In this situation, the hospital has an incentive not to take the more severely ill patients (50). By not taking the severely ill patients, the hospital moves to MC_0 from MC_1. This practice of trying to shift the severely ill patients to other institutions has been referred to as "dumping." Since the DRG price is based on an average severity mix of patients within a DRG category, hospitals that admit only less severely ill patients receive a windfall. Senate hearings have been held as a result of anecdotal evidence of dumping (51).

In addition to dumping, there is a concern that to reduce its costs a hospital will reduce the quality of care received by a patient. In 1984, professional review organizations (PROs) were started; the PROs replaced the generally ineffective professional standards review organizations (PSROs). Whether PROs will be able to monitor quality of care provided to Medicare patients under DRGs is as yet unknown. The current publicity given by the government to overall hospital mortality rates is misleading, since no additional information is provided on which hospitals take the more complex cases, and so on. In a market where quality is not easily measured or individuals very knowledgeable, the development by the PROs of hospital quality measures, and publicizing those results, would be useful.

One response that hospitals appear to be using to maximize their reimbursement under DRGs is referred to as "unbundling" of services. Unbundling is similar to decreasing the use of inputs used in producing the treatment and charging separately for their use. (It represents another method for the hospital to lower its marginal cost curve.) For example, patients may be discharged earlier and admitted to a nursing home or to their own home; the patients would then purchase (through Medicare) additional services, such as home care or additional hospital outpatient services. Unbundling reduces costs in the regulated sector and, by shifting costs to the unregulated sector, increases expenditures in those markets. Discharging patients early also shifts part of the cost to the patient in the form of additional out-of-pocket costs and to family members who have to care for the discharged patient.

When hospitals shift part of the treatment costs out of the hospital, either to other settings or to patients and their families, the cost of the DRG system (or a state rate-setting program) will appear to be lower than when these additional costs are included (52). Broadening the payment unit, such as used in HMOs, should provide a more accurate measure of the product upon which the payment unit is based as well as provide fewer provider incentives to shift costs to other settings for which separate government payment is available. Use of a broader payment unit would also reduce the costs of monitoring which services have been unbundled, quality of care, and the appropriate patient classification.

DRG prices provide incentives for the hospital to be internally efficient and to take advantage of any economies of scale in the provision of services. Hospitals may decide to specialize in some complex DRGs, while hospitals having too little volume in those DRGs may no longer provide such treatment in their own institution. There is little incentive for hospitals to minimize the cost of providing a medical treatment under a regulated hospital pricing system. Instead, the hospital's incentive is to shift costs to markets where the price in unregulated; the resulting combination of services is unlikely to be the least costly mix. A fixed pricing system, where there is little remaining between the price and the hospital's cost of providing that service, forces the hospital to eliminate cross-subsidies. Some of the services being cross-subsidized, such as teaching or provision of complex technology, may also be valued by the community. If the community desires those services, it will be forced to make explicit subsidies to have them provided.

The DRG system is still evolving and there are a number of issues to be resolved. For example, the DRG system does not include capital costs; hospitals are still reimbursed on a cost basis for their capital expenditures. Discussions are occurring as to whether hospitals should receive a fixed percentage (e.g., 6 percent) on all DRGs for their capital. Other issues include correcting the DRG for the patient's severity of illness, determining whether there is code "creep," monitoring quality of care and dumping, including physician payment into the DRG price, and whether DRGs are an interim step in the movement toward a broader payment unit. As with any regulated pricing system, the regulatory scope is likely to be extended so as to enable it to achieve its initial intent.

Impact on Objectives. Regulatory methods that establish hospital payments based on hospital averages, such as DRGs or state rate-setting programs that group hospitals, imply that cost differences are due to differences in efficiency. Differences in hospital costs, however, are also due to differences in patient characteristics that are not easily measured. Whether the hospitals have incentives for efficiency depends upon how the payment unit was established, that is, according to the least-cost method of producing the unit or group averages, and whether hospitals are engaged in competition. If the price faced by the hospital exceeds its costs, it is likely to increase its costs as it competes for patients. Unless the payment unit is well defined, some hospitals will suffer losses and others will receive windfall gains. The administrative cost of the regulatory agency is likely to increase as it attempts to improve the definition of the payment unit and monitor hospital performance.

The cost per unit in facilities that are subject to economies of scale is likely to be lower than the regulatory price, which is presumably based on the average costs of all facilities. Hospitals should have an incentive under such a system to specialize and to merge or close facilities that are subject to economies of scale when they have insufficient volumes.

Classification of hospitals or patients for payment is unlikely to lead to producing the medical treatment at minimum cost. Unbundling hospital services and early discharge to other facilities or to the patient's home, where additional reimbursement is available, is an attempt by the hospital to maximize its reimbursement rather than minimize the cost of the treatment. Unbundling may also shift part of the treatment costs to the patient and their families.

Rate-setting programs that set prices based on group averages of either hospitals or patients are unlikely to stem increases in total hospital expenditures. A careful analysis of the Blue Cross of Western Pennsylvania experience from 1966 to 1968 by Lave, Lave, and Silverman revealed that, whereas the program apparently put some pressure on high-cost hospitals to move toward the means of their groups, it did not seem to restrict the overall average rate of cost increase in the area (53). To reduce the rise in overall expenditures, this or any other rate setting approach must be combined with an effective method of limiting the rate of increase in hospital expenditures.

Setting a Maximum Rate of Increase in Total Hospital Expenditures

To achieve the objective of lowering the rate of increase in total hospital expenditures, any rate-setting method must establish an annual rate of increase for hospital expenditures. This annual percent increase can be used as a rate-setting method by itself, as when it is applied to each hospital's budget, or it can be combined with the previous method in which the payment unit is based on hospital averages. The rate-setting agency then determines the percent increase that the payment per unit is permitted to rise. Establishing a maximum annual percent increase for total hospital expenditures provides a state rate-setting agency with an incentive to negotiate harder with the hospitals, since they cannot exceed the maximum allowable increase for all hospitals, referred to as a maxi-cap. Alternatively, the maximum allowable increase might be established so that hospitals within certain groupings would be allowed different maximum allowable increases.

The major difficulty with the annual percent increase approach is to determine the appropriate rate of increase in hospital expenditures. In a competitive market, the percentage increase from one year to the next represents the effects of shifts in demand and supply. It is, however, difficult for a regulatory agency to estimate these demand and supply shifts, even if that were the intention; more likely, the agency's goal is to limit the increase in expenditures because of its own budgetary reasons. The determination of the annual percent increase is usually a result of negotiations with the hospital associations.

Hospital associations have maintained that hospital input prices rather than an economywide measure of inflation should determine the annual rate of hospital cost inflation. Opponents of this method maintain that, in the long run, hospitals face labor markets similar to other industries, and that allowing the use of hospital input prices reduces any incentive for opposing large hospital wage increases that would affect all hospitals equally. In negotiations over the annual percent increase, hospital associations claim that if the percentage increase is too low, that is, it does not consider inflation in the appropriate input mix and allowance for new technology, the viability of the hospital system might be threatened; hospitals may be forced to shift costs out of the hospital and onto the patients and/or reduce the quality and intensity of their services.

As part of the DRG system, DRG rates were supposed to rise by a hospital "market basket" index plus 1 percent. The market basket is the rate of increase in the prices that hospitals have to pay for their inputs. The 1 percent is an "intensity" factor to allow for increases in technology. By agreeing to this formula, the government was committing itself to rates of increase in hospital prices that are greater than the CPI, but less than historical rates of increase in hospital expenses. Thus the method used by the government to limit its rise in Medicare hospital expenditures is not DRGs, but the annual percent increase in DRG prices.

Empirical Evidence on Rate Regulation

State Rate-Setting Programs

Sixteen states have established mandatory rate-setting commissions, with seven of those states having an all-payor system (54). The empirical research on the effects of rate setting has concentrated on those states having all-payor systems.[5] Generally, the more payors involved in the rate-setting process, the greater will be the constraints on hospital cost increases. Those states considered to have had a more stringent regulatory program used a formula approach for determining hospital payment. Classification of hospitals, the use of budget screens, interhospital comparisons, and development of an inflation factor are some of the methods used in the mandatory regulatory programs. Prospective reimbursement programs within a state have changed over time, and the length of time a state has had a program varies from one state to the other.

The conclusion reached in recent studies is that when hospitals do not face financial incentives to hold down their costs, mandatory rate regulation appears to have held down hospital cost increases (55). Schramm et al. compared the six states that have had mandatory rate regulation since at least 1976, and that have included a majority of non-Medicare hospital payors, to those states without such regulation over the period 1971–1984. Based on a number of measures, such as the annual rate of increase in hospital expense per admission, hospital expense per capita, admissions per 1,000, and percent change in length of stay, the authors concluded that over the period studied, rate regulation resulted in a lower rate of increase in hospital expense per admission and in expense per capita than in the nonregulated states. States with mandatory rate review programs had on average a 3 to 4 percent lower rate of increase in their hospital expense per admission, except for more recent years such as 1983–1984. With regard to hospital expense per capita, regulated states were approximately 27 percent

[5]Commercial insurance companies are proponents of all-payor rate setting since they would then pay the same price for hospital care as Blue Cross; Blue Cross would lose its discount, hence its relative price advantage.

higher than nonregulated states from 1972–1975, then the difference lessened until the difference was only 7.8 percent by 1983. By 1984, the difference increased to 11 percent. The authors claim that the disappearance of the rate-setting effects in 1984 was the result of the DRG system in nonregulated states. Several other studies, using multivariate techniques to control for the effects of other factors, have confirmed that mandatory rate setting has lowered the rate of increase in hospital expenses (56).

Table 11–2 describes the annual percentage increase in total expense per admission for mandatory-rate-review states and for all other states for the years 1971–1985. Only seven states were classified as mandatory regulatory. (The only difference between this group and those studied by Schramm et al. was Wisconsin.) Next to each of the regulated states is the date when the regulatory program in that state was initiated. In the early years of rate review, 1971–1975, the federal Economic Stabilization Program (ESP) was also in effect for all hospitals in the country. Although the ESP went through several phases between August 1971 and April 1974, its general approach was to place maximum allowable limits on increases in hospital costs and charges (57). The ESP appeared to be effective in holding down hospital cost increases. This finding is confirmed through studies that used sophisticated statistical techniques as well as a casual examination of the increases in hospital costs both before and after ESP was in effect. During the period 1971–1975 the annual percentage increase in total expense per admission was similar for both the regulated and nonregulated states. In fact, the nonregulated states had a slightly lower rate of increase in their costs per admission. Starting in 1976, however, the regulated states had a lower rate of increase in their costs. In 1977 the difference was almost 4 percent. Between 1978 and 1983, regulated states were consistently below nonregulated states by approximately 3 percentage points a year. By 1984, as DRGs took effect and businesses became concerned with their employees' health care costs, annual percent increases in hospital expenses moderated and the differences between the two groups became less.

The effectiveness of rate regulation in limiting annual rates of increase in hospital expenditures was very uneven. Some states, such as Massachusetts, varied greatly year to year. While others, such as New York, were generally more effective in that their hospital cost increases were generally below the national average. Those regulated states with consistently lower rates of increase in the post-1975 period all used stringent review methodologies. For example, New York used a formula approach combined with a maximum annual percentage increase. Hospitals in New York were grouped according to size, type, ownership, and geographic location. Hospitals faced a ceiling of 110 percent of the average routine costs for hospitals within each group. Researchers of the early New York experience found that rate regulation in New York slowed increases in cost per patient day by about 3 percent per year, and cost per case by about .5 percent per year (58).

Based on the evidence to date it appears that mandatory rate regulation can reduce the annual rate of increase in hospital expenses regardless of whether it is on the federal level, such as the ESP, or on a state level. However, unless rate regulation programs establish maximum limits on annual percentage increases on hospital expenditures or use a tight-formula approach, rate regulation will not be effective. In the early years of a rate review program, hospitals may not be adversely affected. The requirements placed on hospitals are unlikely to be very stringent, and hospitals are likely to have influence over the rate-setting process. As the fiscal constraints on the payors become more severe, as in New York and the federal government under the ESP, and currently under Medicare, tighter controls are placed on hospitals. Eventu-

TABLE 11-2. The Impact of Rate Regulation on the Annual Percentage Increase in Total Expense Per Admission for Community Hospitals, 1971–1985

Regulated State[a]	1971	1972	1973	1974	1975	1976	1977	1978	1979	1980	1981	1982	1983	1984	1985
Connecticut (1974)	13.7	10.1	8.8	7.3	17.0	14.5	11.7	10.7	8.8	12.5	16.0	16.0	10.9	7.9	13.2
Maryland (1973)	15.9	9.1	11.5	9.8	17.5	13.8	8.7	9.2	11.9	10.8	15.1	10.9	6.9	5.0	8.2
Massachusetts (1971)	14.1	10.3	9.3	12.7	17.4	15.3	14.5	8.7	9.1	15.3	15.8	15.8	22.8	7.8	12.2
New Jersey (1971)	14.4	9.8	11.5	10.2	14.8	14.1	10.6	9.1	11.2	10.5	12.2	14.6	6.7	11.8	7.9
New York (1969)	9.2	10.5	9.2	10.3	18.7	9.0	7.7	8.9	9.1	11.2	12.6	10.1	9.5	10.4	9.3
Washington (1973)	9.8	11.4	10.2	7.8	20.6	17.0	13.7	12.7	10.9	11.5	16.9	21.8	13.1	14.5	18.7
Wisconsin (1975)	13.2	10.8	9.2	9.9	16.1	19.9	13.2	13.2	11.4	13.2	18.3	13.4	12.0	8.6	10.5
Mean percent change regulated states[b]	12.9	10.3	10.0	9.7	17.4	14.8	11.5	10.3	10.3	12.6	15.3	12.5	9.3	9.8	10.5
Mean percent change all other states	10.8	10.3	8.1	11.5	17.2	16.0	15.4	13.0	12.4	14.0	18.2	14.6	14.6	8.6	11.4

SOURCE: *Hospital Statistics*, 1971–1986 editions, copyright 1971–1986 by the American Hospital Association.

[a]The numbers in parentheses are the years when rate regulation was initiated.

[b]These are weighted mean percent changes.

ally, tight controls will affect hospitals' financial position. In New York, an increased number of hospitals closed as rate regulation became more severe (59). Unfortunately, a number of these hospitals also served indigent populations.

Experience with state rate-setting programs may be summed up as follows: when the program places stringent annual percent increases on hospital expenditures and when a majority of the payors are included, such programs are likely to reduce the annual rate of increase in hospital expenditures. However, the effectiveness of these programs will still vary greatly and in some states have minimal effects. It will also take several years after the introduction of these programs before they will begin to have an effect. Finally, it is difficult to generalize these results to other states; there has to be the right environment for stringent rate regulation to be enacted and for it to be enforced. When there are important fiscal pressures on the state and other payors coalesce to form concentrated interest groups, such programs are likely to be more effective.

Effects of the DRG System

The early effects of the DRG system are likely to be more exaggerated than the long-term consequences. There are two reasons for this: first, hospitals' responses to the changed incentives may occur in the first few years, such as increases in efficiency, and in later years such increases may be minimal. Second, as a result of hospitals' performance, changes are likely to be introduced into the payment system to negate certain outcomes, such as increased hospital profitability.

One of the expectations of a fixed DRG price is that hospitals would reduce the length of stay, since the hospital receives the same price regardless of the patient's length of stay. In the pre-DRG period, length of stay (LOS) for Medicare patients was 10.5, 10.3, and 10.0 days in 1981, 1982, and 1983, respectively. In the first year of the DRG phase-in, 1984, LOS declined 9.0 percent to 9.1 days (60). In 1985 the LOS declined 3.8 percent, and in 1986, LOS increased .01 percent (61). The very slight increase in LOS in 1986 is believed to be a result of more severely ill patients, as more of the less severely ill patients are shifted to outpatient settings. The decline in LOS may have reached its low point.

The Senate Special Committee on Aging has been holding hearings on whether Medicare patients are being discharged too soon. There has been a concern that patients are being discharged "quicker and sicker." The AMA has also testified that physicians are being pressured by hospitals to discharge their Medicare patients early (62). While the evidence presented is anecdotal, it is likely that the Congress will continue to monitor this issue.

It was initially expected that under DRGs, aged admissions would increase since hospitals were paid per admission. Instead, admissions fell. Admissions per 1,000 Medicare enrollees were 386 in 1982 and had been rising approximately 2 percent per year. For the following three years, 1984–1986, the admission rate declined 3.5, 4.8, and 2.0 percent per year (63). It has been hypothesized that changes in technology and payment for outpatient services caused this shift away from inpatient care.

The decline in LOS and in the admission rate, together with similar trends for the nonaged, caused hospital occupancy rates to fall dramatically. In early 1983 (pre-DRGs), hospital occupancy rates were 74 percent. By late 1986 occupancy rates were only 63.2 percent.

The effect of these declines in hospital occupancy rates, as a result of changes in both the Medicare and non-Medicare markets, caused an increasing number of hospitals to close. In the three years preceding DRGs, approximately 25 hospitals closed each year. As occupancy rates started to decline in 1984, the number of closures increased, reaching a high of 83 in 1986. Small hospitals were most likely to be forced to close (64).

Although some small hospitals were having a difficult time, most hospitals profited from the change to DRGs. According to a government study, hospitals earned an average profit margin on their Medicare revenues of 14.18 percent in 1984, and this increased to 15.27 percent in 1985. Eighty percent of the hospitals in the government sample earned profits, while 20 percent lost money on their Medicare patients (65). The American Hospital Association acknowledged that hospital profit margins increased after DRGs. The profit margins on all inpatients doubled, from 1 to 2 percent in the first year of DRGs. The total profit margin for the hospital increased from 5.1 to 6.2 percent in 1984. The 6.2 percent was the highest since 1963, when the AHA started recording these data. These total profit margins declined in 1985 and 1986; the patient margin fell to 1.5 percent in 1985 and to .7 percent in 1986. Total profit margins similarly declined from their high in 1984 to 6 percent in 1985 and to 5.1 percent in 1986 (66). Part of the increase in hospital profits was their incentive under a fixed-price system to reduce their costs and to show the rate of increase in those costs (67).

A concern by the government, however, was whether the large increase in hospital profits was a result of DRG "creep." A study was undertaken to determine whether there had been any code "creep" since DRGs were implemented. Before DRGs were started, a Medicare Case Mix Index (CMI) was computed for each hospital based on its 1981 data. The CMI was calculated by multiplying the proportion of Medicare patients in each DRG by the DRG's payment rate, or "weight." The government, in its budget projections, estimated that the CMI would increase by 3.4 percent in 1984; the actual increase turned out to be 9.2 percent.

Analyzing the reasons for the larger-than-expected increase in the CMI, the researchers concluded that changes in medical practice, such as the shift to greater outpatient use and the trends in medical practice that had started before DRGs were introduced, were responsible for only 2.2 percentage points of the 9.2-point increase. The aging of Medicare patients did not have any effect on the CMI over this period. Changes in coding accounted for the remaining 7.0-percentage-point increase (68). It is uncertain how much of the change in coding was a result of more accurate patient classifications and how much was the result of an attempt to maximize hospital DRG payment. It is also too early to tell whether these changes in the CMI as a result of coding changes are continuing.

As reports have surfaced of the large "profits" being made by hospitals under DRGs, the administration and the Congress have been using the annual percent increase in DRG prices as a means of controlling Medicare hospital expenditures. Annual rates of increase in Medicare hospital payments are much smaller than the originally agreed-upon concept of the market basket plus 1 percent. The hospital market basket price index increased 5.4 percent in 1986 and the rates of increase being proposed by the administration and the Congress are between zero and 1.0 percent, much smaller than even the increase in the CPI. The rationalization for such small increases is to take away the excess profits earned by hospitals. While the annual percent increase is the same for all hospitals, it is not clear that all hospitals profited equally.

As inpatient utilization declined, hospitals have experienced large increases in their outpatient visits. After a growth rate of approximately 1.9 percent in the pre-DRG period (1977–1983), outpatient visits have increased by 4.8 and 8.3 percent in 1985 and 1986, respectively. In fact, Medicare outpatient revenues have increased at a faster rate than Medicare inpatient revenues. In 1970, Medicare payments for outpatient care was $93 million, this increased to $509 million in 1975, to $1.8 billion in 1980, and to $3.7 billion in 1984 (69). Hospital outpatient activities have increased in importance, particularly since they are still reimbursed on a cost basis. Medicare payments for outpatient surgery are also increasing rapidly, approximately 20 percent per year. In 1981 Medicare covered outpatient surgery as a benefit and patients did not have to pay any part of the bill; if they had the surgery performed in the hospital, they would have had to pay a large deductible. The effect was a large shift in demand to ambulatory surgery.

The shift from inpatient to other settings is also indicated by the rapid growth in home health care. Medicare payments for home health care, reimbursed to the provider on a cost basis up to a maximum amount per visit, have more than doubled in just four years, from $770 million in 1980 to $1.9 billion in 1984, and are increasing at more than 22 percent per year (70).

The DRG system is likely to have far-reaching implications for hospitals. Inpatient utilization is declining, as is hospital occupancy. The hospital is shifting more of its resources to the outpatient side. After several years of high profits, hospitals are likely to be squeezed as the government refuses to increase the rate at which DRG prices increase each year. To limit further the increase in Medicare expenditures, it is likely that the government will place constraints on nonhospital expenditures next.

CONCLUDING COMMENTS

Interest groups demand increased regulation of hospitals for various reasons. For some, increased regulation is viewed as a means of assuring access to medical care for all persons, which is the welfare argument; for others, regulation is a means of rationalizing the system of health care delivery, the efficiency argument; for others, regulation is a means of protecting consumers from incompetent providers; for still other groups, regulation is a means whereby the existing providers may be protected from possible threatening changes; and finally, for other interest groups, regulation represents a means for limiting expenditures on hospital care. The relative effectiveness of regulation when compared with alternative approaches can be judged only in terms of a common objective. It is to the advantage of regulation proponents to combine these differing health care goals and objectives and to suggest that only increased regulation can achieve all of them. Proponents claim that alternatives to regulation may be more effective in meeting certain of the desired objectives, but that only regulation can achieve all of the combined goals.

The effectiveness with which regulation is likely to achieve economically efficient medical care delivery was examined in this section. Alternative approaches for achieving the other goals are discussed in other chapters. The consequences of regulation in other industries were examined for purposes of hypothesizing the probable effects of increased regulation in the health field. It was seen that regulation in nonhealth industries led to higher, not lower prices; to cross-subsidization of services; to greater nonprice competition, which in turn led to increased costs in the regulated industry; to protection of the regulated firms, thereby lessening their incentives to strive for efficiency; and to a reluctance to introduce innovation in the delivery of services because such innovation threatens the revenues of the regulated industry. As competition arises from nonregulated industries, the regulatory agency increases its scope and authority and the number of industries over which its authority is exercised. The degree of regulation also increases as nonprice competition increases.

Either proponents of health care regulation are unaware of the experience with regulation in other industries, or else their biases against alternatives to regulation are so strong as to provide them with no alternative. Those proponents with vested interests are very aware of the consequences of regulation in other industries, and they favor it for precisely that reason.

Hospital planning was the first major attempt to regulate hospitals. Voluntary efforts were unsuccessful in achieving the goals of greater efficiency in the allocation of hospital resources, so certificate-of-need legislation was passed. Hospital planning, strengthened by CON, appears to have had some effect, which is predictable from the evidence on regulation in other industries. Proprietary institutions were more likely to be denied CON approval for starting new hospitals or for expansion of their existing facility. Innovations in the delivery of medical services that threatened the revenues of existing hospitals, such as ambulatory surgery centers and HMOs, were brought under the CON authority of the planning agencies. The growth and development of such freestanding units was retarded. Existing hospitals' expansion plans for new beds in areas that already had excess beds were approved by the CON agency, or else hospital investment was channeled into areas less obvious than beds, but hospital investment did not decline as a result of CON legislation. As hospital costs continued to increase rapidly each year, rather than admitting that CON legislation was a failure, its proponents maintained that the regulatory agencies' staff would improve, and that what was needed instead was still more hospital regulation.

A second regulatory program, which was not discussed but whose effects were similar to what would occur when there is a major group with a concentrated interest, involves utilization review programs. After Medicare and Medicaid had been passed, there was concern that the beneficiaries of these programs not receive unnecessary care and/or care of low quality. To rectify this situation, amendments to the Social Security Act were passed in 1972 establishing the professional standards review organizations (PSROs). The major emphasis of PSRO programs (over two-thirds of the program's budget) has been on appropriateness of hospital length of stay by Medicare beneficiaries. Several studies have been conducted to evaluate the effectiveness of the PSRO program. One large study compared the hospital utilizaton experience of Medicare beneficiaries from 1974 to 1976 in areas with and without an active PSRO (71). The results showed that PSROs had no overall effect on hospital utilization or admissions. Other studies reported similar findings (72).

When the Congressional Budget Office (CBO) evaluated PSROs, it reported:

The evidence that PSROs reduce Medicare utilization, however, is not firm. Considering the nation as a whole, the program's apparent effect is sufficiently small and variable that it could be an artifact of chance variation in the data./ . . . the program consumes more resources than it saves society as a whole. The 1978 data indicate that, for every dollar spent on PSRO review of Medicare patients, only $.40 in resources were recouped, for a net loss of $.60./ . . . by channeling resources into the PSRO program, society increases slightly its total expenditures for health care (73).

Also important to an analysis of the effectiveness of PSROs is whether their performance is likely to improve over time. Unfortunately, this is not likely. The CBO study found that even though the PSRO agencies matured between 1977 and 1978, their effectiveness did not increase.

The effectiveness of the PSRO program is apparently no different from other utilization review programs. While some studies indicate that there may be slight differences in use when a utilization review program is used, a review of these studies by Thomas Bice concludes that there is no conclusive evidence that they reduce per capita use of hospitals or eliminate unnecessary costs. In those cases where a study suggests that utilization review has lowered utilization, Bice states that "in nearly all instances these conclusions are questionable on methodological grounds" (74).

PROs replaced PSROs in 1984. Quality assessment techniques have improved, however, whether PROs are likely to be more effective than PSROs have yet to be determined.

Three basic approaches to hospital rate regulation have been discussed. The first was budget review on an individual hospital basis. This approach is the one most preferred by hospitals because it involves negotiation with each hospital, thereby precluding drastic revisions in a hospital's budget. It offers the smallest possibility for holding down the rise in hospital costs or for promoting greater efficiency within and among hospitals. The negotiators representing the regulatory agency are likely to be more sympathetic in such face-to-face negotiations and less familiar with the hospital's budget than the hospital negotiators.

The second rate-setting approach is to classify hospitals or their patients, as under DRGs, and apply similar rates to those in each classification. There is a greater possibility for hospital efficiency under this approach, since reimbursement rates are set with less regard for personal factors and are based on more standardized groupings. There are, however, problems with this approach; rates may be set according to group averages rather than the most efficient firm, and nonprice competition between hospitals may increase hospital costs. Further, it is difficult to develop appropriate classifications for the payment unit. As a result, some hospitals may be unjustly harmed, while others will receive a windfall.

The last approach, which is generally used in conjunction with the others, is to establish a maximum allowable percentage increase in hospital costs for the coming year. If there are groups with a concentrated interest in restraining the rise in hospital expenditures, the annual percent increase will be smaller than what would occur in a competitive market and certainly less than what hospitals would prefer. One effect of a tight expenditure lid, however, will be increased expenditures in nonregulated medical markets. The regulators will eventually have to expand their regulatory scope to restrain expenditure increases in these other areas. The multiple goals of limiting expenditure increases, increased hospital efficiency, minimizing the cost of a medical treatment, and equity across hospitals are unlikely to be achieved.

Initially, hospitals receive favorable treatment under a regulatory framework. However, as additional groups with concentrated interests in holding down health care costs develop, such as state governments, business, labor, and insurance companies, compromise decisions are reached by the legislature; and hospitals do not do as well. Their reimbursement becomes tighter and their financial position begins to decline. As other interests begin to dominate the regulatory process, hospitals will find that regulation is being used to freeze the hospital's budget. As regulation limits hospital revenue, the growth in health care expenditures will occur outside the regulated sector. Other organizations, not subject to regulatory constraints, will be able to innovate and offer profitable services. Regulated hospitals will find themselves in a shrinking market.

Rate regulation is a highly conservative approach; drastic changes in the delivery system are not encouraged. The alternative to rate setting for achieving a more efficient allocation of resources, namely, increased market competition, is discussed next.

REFERENCES

1. George J. Stigler, "The Theory of Economic Regulation," *Bell Journal of Economics and Management Sciences*, Spring 1971; Richard A. Posner, "Theories of Economic Regulation," *Bell Journal of Economics and Management Sciences*, Autumn 1974; Sam L. Peltzman, "Toward a More General Theory of Regulation," *Journal of Law and Economics*, August 1976.

2. Anthony Downs, *An Economic Theory of Democracy* (New York: Harper & Row, 1957), p. 297.

3. For a more complete discussion of policy typologies, see Michael T. Hayes, "The Semi-Sovereign Pressure Groups: A Critique of Current Theory and an Alternative Typology," *Journal of Politics*, February 1978.

4. William Jordan, "Producer Protection, Prior Market Structure and the Effects of Government Regulation," *Journal of Law and Economics*, April 1972.

5. Richard Farmer, "The Case for Unregulated Truck Transportation," *Journal of Farm Economics*, 46, 1964.

6. Roger Noll, "The Consequences of Public Utility Regulation of Hospitals," in *Controls on Health Care*, Conference Proceedings (Washington, D.C.: National Academy of Sciences, January 1974, p. 32.

7. George Stigler and Clair Friedland, "What Can Regulators Regulate? The Case of Electricity," *Journal of Law and Economics*, October 1962.

8. "The Regulators: Federal Commissions Draw Increasing Fire, Called Inept and Costly," *Wall Street Journal*, October 9, 1974: p. 1.

9. Noll, *op. cit.*, p. 33.

10. C. Vincent Olson and John M. Trapani, "Who Has Benefited from Regulation of the Airline Industry?" *Journal of Law and Economics*, April 1981.

11. Richard Posner, "Taxation by Regulation," *Bell Journal of Economics and Management Science*, 2, 1971.

12. George Eads, *The Local Service Airline Experiment* (Washington, D.C.: Brookings Institution, 1972).

13. Ann F. Friedlander, *The Dilemma of Freight Transport Regulation* (Washington, D.C.: Brookings Institution, 1969).

14. For a brief discussion of the history of health planning, see Symond Gottlieb, "A Brief History of Health Planning in the United States," in Clark Havighurst, ed.,

Regulating Health Facilities Construction (Washington, D.C.: American Enterprise Institute for Public Policy Research, 1974).

15. Joel May, *Health Planning—Its Past and Potential* (Chicago: Center for Health Administration Studies, University of Chicago, 1967). These findings are also presented in Joel May, "The Planning and Licensing Agencies," in Havighurst, ed., *op. cit.*

16. See P. O'Donoghue, A. Bryant, and P. Shaughnessy, *A Descriptive Analysis of CHP "B" Agencies* (Denver: Spectrum Research, 1974).

17. W. Wendling and J. Werner, "Nonprofit Firms and the Economic Theory of Regulation," *Quarterly Review of Economics and Business*, Fall 1980.

18. For a critical history of certificate of need (CON) legislation, see Sallyanne Payton and Rhoda M. Powsner, "Regulation Through the Looking Glass: Hospitals, Blue Cross, and Certificate-of-Need," *Michigan Law Review*, December 1980.

19. J. P. Newhouse and J. P. Acton, "Compulsory Health Planning Laws and National Health Insurance," in Havighurst, ed. *op. cit.*, 228–229.

20. William Curran, Richard Steele, and Ellen Ober, "Government Intervention on Increase," *Hospitals*, May 16, 1974: p. 60.

21. Clark Havighurst, "Regulating Health Facilities and Services by Certificate of Need," *Virginia Law Review*, October 1973: p. 117. See also Merton D. Finkler, "Changes in Certificate-of-Need Laws: Read the Fine Print," in Jack A. Myer, ed., *Incentives vs. Controls in Health Policy*, (Washington, D.C.: American Enterprise Institute, 1985).

22. Havighurst, *op. cit.*, p. 186. See also Clark C. Havighurst, *"Deregulating the Health Care Industry* (Cambridge, Mass.: Ballinger, 1982), particularly Chapter 8, "HMOs and the Health Planners." This chapter provides a legislative history of health maintenance organization (HMO) development and evidence on the regulatory discrimination against HMOs. This book also contains an excellent comprehensive discussion of a broad range of issues dealing with regulation and competition. See also William P. Brandon and Emma K. Lee, "Evaluating Health Planning: Empirical Evidence on HSA Regulation of Prepaid Group Practices", *Journal of Health Politics, Policy and Law*, 9(1), Spring 1984.

23. Comptroller General of the United States, *Study of Health Facilities Construction Cost* (Washington, D.C.: U.S. General Accounting Office, 1972); and Comptroller General of the United States, *Comprehensive Health Planning as Carved Out by State and Areawide Agencies in Three States* (Washington, D.C.: U.S. General Accounting Office, 1974.

24. Lewin and Associates, Inc., *Evaluation of the Effectiveness and Efficiency of the Section 1122 Review Process* (Washington, D.C.: Lewin and Associates, Inc., September 1975).

25. *Ibid.*, Chapt. 1, p. 7.

26. David Salkever, "Health Planning and Cost Containment: A Selective Review of the Recent U.S. Experience," paper presented at the International Conference on Programs for the Containment of Health Care Costs and Expenditures, The Fogarty International Center, National Institutes of Health, Bethesda, Md., June 2–4, 1976, 6–7.

27. David Salkever and Thomas Bice, "Certificate-of-Need and Hospital Costs," in Michael Zubkoff, Ira Raskin, and Ruth Hanft, eds., *Hospital Cost Containment: Selected Notes for Future Policy* (New York: PRODIST, 1978).

28. *Evaluation of the Effects of Certificate of Need Programs*, Final Report for the Bureau of Health Planning and Resources Development (Brookline, Mass.: Policy Analysis Inc. and Urban Systems Research, 1980); Frank Sloan and Bruce Steinwald, *Insurance, Regulation and Hospital Costs* (Lexington, Mass.: Lexington Books, 1980); F. J. Hellinger, "The Effects of Certificate of Need Legislation on Hospital Investment," *Inquiry*, June 1976; David S. Salkever and Thomas W. Bice, *Hospital Certificate-of-Need Controls: Impact on Investment, Costs and Use* (Washington, D.C.: American Enterprise Institute, 1979); Paul L. Joskow, "Alternative Regulatory Mechanisms for Controlling Hospital Costs," and Bruce Steinwald and Frank A. Sloan, "Regulatory Approaches to Hospital Cost Containment: A Synthesis of the Empirical Evidence," in Mancur Olson, ed., *A New Approach to the Economics of Health Care* (Washington, D.C.: American Enterprise Institute, 1981).

29. "Congress Ends Federal Health Planning," *Medicine and Health Perspectives*, October 6, 1986.

30. Michelle Polchow, *State Efforts at Health Care Cost Containment*, mimeographed (Denver, Colo.: National Conference of State Legislators, September 1986).

31. Keith B. Anderson and David I. Kass, *Certificate of Need Regulation of Entry into Home Health Care*, Bureau of Economics Staff Report to the Federal Trade Commission, (Washington, D.C.: Federal Trade Commission, January 1986).

32. Institute of Medicine, *Controlling the Supply of Hospital Beds* (Washington, D.C.: National Academy of Sciences. 1976), pp. 7–9.

33. Total expenditures per bed in nonfederal short-term general hospitals in 1985 were $130,309. American Hospital Association, *Hospital Statistics*, 1986 ed. (Chicago: American Hospital Association, 1986), p. 5, Table 1.

34. Walter McClure, *Reducing Excess Hospital Capacity* (Excelsior, Minn.: Interstudy, 1976), p. 20.

35. Joseph Lipscomb, Ira Raskin, and Joseph Eichenholz, "The Use of Short-Run Marginal Cost Estimates in Hospital Cost Containment Policy," in Zubkoff, Raskin and Hanft, eds., *op. cit.*

36. Bernard Friedman and Mark Pauly, "Cost Functions for a Service Firm with Variable Quality and Stochastic Demand: The Case of Hospitals," *Review of Economics and Statistics*, November 1981: p. 624.

37. Lewin and Associates, *Final Report: Societal Factors and Excess hospital Beds—An Exploratory Study*, DHEW Publication (HRA) 80–644 (Washington, D.C.: U.S. Department of Health, Education, and Welfare, 1979), p. 11.

38. William B. Schwartz and Paul J. Joskow, "Duplicated Hospital Facilities: How Much Can We Save by Consolidating Them?" *New England Journal of Medicine*, 303, 1980: 1449–1457.

39. In his study on hospital closure in Massachusetts, Shepard found that the most likely result would be a "a small *increase* in the area's annual hospital costs, because many patients are referred to more costly teaching hospitals." Donald S.

Shepard, "Estimating the Effect of Hospital Closure on Areawide Inpatient Hospital Costs: A Preliminary Model and Application," *Health Services Research*, Special Issue on Hospital Closures, Part II, 18(4), Winter 1983: 513–549. In the Fall 1983 issue of this journal, which was devoted to hospital closings and financial distress, are related articles, such as the one by Alan Sager on the impact on access to care when a community loses its hospital. Hospitals that serve minority and Medicaid populations were more likely to be closed. When the displaced patient populations are moved to more costly teaching hospitals, the result is like to be higher Medicare and Medicaid costs.

40. "14% Cut in N.Y. Hospital Beds Urged," *Modern Healthcare*, January 2, 1987: p.11.

41. "Opportunity for Mischief Exists in CON Laws-FTC," *Modern Healthcare*, February 13, 1987.

42. Paul J. Feldstein and Glenn A. Melnick, "Congressional Voting Behavior on Hospital Legislation: An Exploratory Study," *Journal of Health Politics, Policy and Law*, 8(4), Winter 1984.

43. Kenneth R. Cone and David Dranove, "Why Did States Enact Hospital Rate-Setting Laws?" *Journal of Law and Economics*, 29, October 1986: p. 298. Finkler claims that hospitals also supported rate regulation in return for barriers to entry. As evidence, states with stringent rate-setting programs had from zero to six free-standing ambulatory surgery centers. States without rate setting had from 13 to 47. For additional examples, see Finkler, *op. cit.*

44. William L. Dowling, "Prospective Rate Setting: Concept and Practice," in William L. Dowling, ed., *Prospective Rate Setting* (Germantown, Md.: Aspen Systems Corporation, Winter 1976), p. 32.

45. Institute of Medicine, *Reliability of Hospital Discharge Abstracts* (Washington, D.C.: National Academy of Sciences, 1977).

46. Donald W. Simborg, "DRG Creep: A New Hospital-Acquired Disease," *New England Journal of Medicine*, June 25, 1981.

47. Paul L. Grimaldi, "Equity and Efficiency Implications of Case-Mix Reimbursement in New Jersey," in Gerald Glandon and Roberta Shapiro, eds., *Profile of Medical Practice 1980*, (Chicago: American Medical Association, 1980), p. 94.

48. Susan Horn et al., "Interhospital Differences in Severity of Illness," *New England Journal of Medicine*, 313(1), July 4, 1985: 20–24.

49. Philip J. Held and Mark V. Pauly, "Competition and Efficiency in the End Stage Renal Disease Program," *Journal of Health Economics*, 2, 1983: 95–118.

50. Joseph P. Newhouse, "Two Prospective Difficulties with Prospective Payment of Hospitals, or, It's Better to Be a Resident than a Patient with a Complex Problem," *Journal of Health Economics*, 2(3), December 1983: 269–274. Ellis and McGuire discuss the role of the physician under both cost-based and prospective payment. The physician, as the key decisionmaker, considers the effect on the patient as well as on the hospital in making treatment choices. Under a cost-based payment system, both patient and hospital benefit when the physician prescribes additional treatments; the patient receives additional benefits for which they do not have to pay and the hospital receives additional revenues. Under DRGs, the interests of patients and hospitals may no longer be synonymous. When the DRG price is less than the costs of caring for a patient, the physician must make a trade-

off between benefits to the patient and the profits to the hospital. If the market power of hospitals is greater relative to that of physicians, because of the increased supply of physicians, and patients are not very knowledgeable, physicians may give greater weight to hospital profits than patient benefits in their decisionmaking. In such a situation, the physician becomes an imperfect agent for the patient. Randall P. Ellis and Thomas G. McGuire, "Provider Behavior Under Prospective Reimbursement," *Journal of Health Economics*, 5(2), June 1986: 129–151.

51. *Impact of Medicare's Prospective Payment System on the Quality of Care Received by Medicare Beneficiaries*, Special Committee on Aging Staff Report, September 26, 1985. For a study attempting to measure the extent of dumping on a public hospital, see Robert L. Schiff et al., "Transfers to a Public Hospital," *New England Journal of Medicine*, 314, February 27, 1986.

52. Michael A. Morrisey, Douglas A. Conrad, Stephen M. Shortell, and Karen S. Cook, "Hospital Rate Review: A Theory and Empirical Review," *Journal of Health Economics*, 3(1), 1984: 25–48.

53. Judith Lave, Lester Lave, and Lester Silverman, "A Proposal for Incentive Reimbursement of Hospitals," *Medical Care*, 11, March-April 1973: p. 88.

54. Polchow, *op. cit.*

55. Carl J. Schramm, Steven C. Renn, and Brian Biles, "Controlling Hospital Cost Inflation: New Perspectives on State Rate Setting," *Health Affairs*, Fall 1986; Craig Coelen and Daniel Sullivan, "An Analysis of the Effects of Prospective Reimbursement Programs on Hospital Expenditures," *Health Care Financing Review*, Winter 1981; Frank Sloan, "Regulation and the Rising Cost of Health Care," *Review of Economics and Statistics*, November 1981; Glenn Melnick, John Wheeler, and Paul Feldstein, "The Effects of Hospital Rate Regulation on Hospital Costs and Utilization, 1975–1979," *Inquiry*, Fall 1981.

56. David Dranove and Kenneth Cone, "Do State Rate Setting Regulations Really Lower Hospital Expenses?" *Journal of Health Economics*, 4, 1985: 159–165; Charles L. Eby and Donald R. Cohodes, "What Do We Know About Rate-Setting?" *Journal of Health Politics, Policy and Law*, 10(2), 1985: 299–313; *Constraining National Health Care Expenditures*, (Washington, D.C.: Government Accounting Office, September 1985.

57. Information on the application of ESP to hospitals can be found in Stuart Altman and Joseph Eichenholz, "Inflation in the Health Industry: Causes and Cures," in Michael Zubkoff, ed., *Health: A Victim or Cause of Inflation* (New York: PRODIST, 1976), 7–30; and Richard Berman, "The Economic Stabilization Program of the United States: August 1971–April 1974," *World Hospitals*, 12, 1976.

58. Ralph Berry, "Prospective Reimbursement and Cost Containment: Formula Reimbursement in New York," *Inquiry*, September 1976; and William L. Dowling et al., *Prospective Reimbursement in Downstate New York and Its Impact on Hospitals, A Summary* (Seattle: Department of Health Services, University of Washington, 1976).

59. Hirsch S. Ruchlin and Harry M. Rosen, "The Process of Hospital Rate Regulation: The New York Experience," *Inquiry*, 18, Spring 1981. See also Judith D. Bentkover, Richard Schroeder, and A. James Lee, "Financial Viability of New York Hospitals: A Retrospective Assessment," *Hospital and Health Services Administration*, 30, May-June 1985.

60. Stuart Guterman and Alan Dobson, "Impact of the Medicare Prospective Payment System for Hospitals," *Health Care Financing Review*, 7(3), Spring 1986: p. 103.

61. *Economic Trends*, 2(4), Winter 1987 (data are through September 1986).

62. John K. Iglehart, "Early Experience with Prospective Payment of Hospitals," *New England Journal of Medicine*, 314(22), May 29, 1986: p. 1461.

63. Guterman and Dobson, *op. cit.* and *Economic Trends, op. cit.*

64. "45% More Community Hospitals Closed in '86," *Hospitals*, May 5, 1987: p. 32.

65. *Hospitals Continue to Earn Large Profits in the Second Year of the Prospective Payment System"* (Washington, D.C.: Office of Inspector General, U.S. Department of Health and Human Services, February 25, 1987), p. 2.

66. "Margins Fall Despite Slower Inpatient Declines," *Hospitals*, May 5, 1987: 40–42.

67. Judith Feder, Jack Hadley, and Stephen Zuckerman, "How Did Medicare's Prospective Payment System Affect Hospitals?" *New England Journal of Medicine*, 317(14), October 1, 1987: 867–873.

68. Paul B. Ginsburg and Grace M. Carter, "Medicare Case Mix Index Increase," *Health Care Financing Review*, 7(4), Summer 1986.

69. Guterman and Dobson, *op. cit.*, p. 110.

70. *Ibid.*, p. 110.

71. A. Dobson et al., "PSROs: Their Current Status and Their Impact to Date," *Inquiry*, June 1978.

72. A brief review of these studies appears in Thomas W. Bice, "Health Planning and Regulation Effects on Hospital Costs," in Lester Breslow, ed., *Annual Review of Public Health*, 1 (Palo Alto, Calif.: Annual Reviews, 1980).

73. Congressional Budget Office, *The Impact of PSROs on Health Care Costs: Update of CBO's 1979 Evaluation* (Washington, D.C.: Congressional Budget Office, January 1981), pp. xi–xiv.

74. Bice, *op. cit.*, p. 154.

CHAPTER 12

Market Competition in Medical Care

THE EMERGENCE OF COMPETITION

In the last five years the delivery of medical services in the United States has changed dramatically. The trend in the late 1970s was toward increased regulation. An increasing number of states were moving toward rate regulation of hospitals, CON was used to regulate hospital investment, and there were discussions in the literature of granting hospitals public utility status. Yet rather than moving in the direction of increased regulation, market competition has become the dominant force affecting hospitals and health professionals. This change was not anticipated.

To place the movement to market competition within an economic framework, the reasons for deregulation of nonhealth industries is reviewed briefly. The economic motivation of regulated firms and their unions is to maintain their regulated benefits; market competition threatens their economic well-being. To have greater usefulness, the economic theory of regulation should be able to explain not only why firms seek and are successful at achieving regulation but also why some industries are deregulated whereas others are not.

Deregulation of Nonhealth Industries

In the late 1970s, the following industries were either completely or partially deregulated: railroads, trucking, airlines, banking, stock brokerage, and telecommunications. While these industries were being deregulated, others, such as network TV, maintained their regulatory protection. In other industries, government regulation actually increased. Deregulation, as an idea whose time had come, has been proposed as the reason for deregulation (1). However, as a theory of deregulation, this hypothesis is unable to explain why some industries are deregulated while others are not, or why the industries were initially regulated.

Consistent with the economic theory of regulation, there are two reasons why industries may lose their regulatory protection. The first is changes in relative political support for regulation; the second is the applicability of the antitrust laws (2). Each is discussed in turn.

An industry is able to receive regulatory benefits when the political support it is able to offer to legislators exceeds that offered by its opponents. A decline in political support offered by the regulated industry and/or an increase in political support offered by those adversely affected by continued regulation can change the regulatory framework affecting an industry. An increase in regulatory costs, if imposed in a diffuse manner on the public, is unlikely to be sufficient to overturn an industry's regulatory benefits. While the costs of import quotas and farm price supports are large, they are sufficiently diffuse among consumers so that it is not worthwhile for them to organize and lobby the Congress to have them removed. For regulatory change to occur, the costs of regulation must be imposed on groups with a concentrated interest in having them reduced. It then becomes worthwhile for these groups to organize and provide political support to lessen their regulatory burden.

Fixed commission rates for the sale and purchase of stocks collapsed when large institutional traders bypassed the New York Stock Exchange (NYSE) and started trading on regional exchanges. Large institutional traders had a concentrated interest in reducing their commissions and thus sought alternative ways of lowering their costs. To prevent their loss of all business from large institutional traders, NYSE firms agreed to compete by doing away with fixed commissions. The deregulation of the securities business was a recognition of changes that had occurred in the marketplace.

Savings and loan associations (S&Ls) favored regulated maximum interest rates paid to depositors since they could loan the funds out at higher rates of interest. Commercial banks and money market funds would not have been able to attract funds if they could not raise the interest they were willing to pay for those funds. These competitors to the S&Ls had a concentrated interest in lobbying for elimination of maximum interest rates to be paid to depositors.

To protect railroads from low-cost competitors (trucks) in the short-haul market, the Interstate Commerce Commission included truckers under their regulatory jurisdiction. As the regulatory influence of truckers increased, railroads began losing money; the high regulated rates on long-haul business, at which railroads were more efficient than truckers, enabled the truckers to enter the long-haul market and reduce the railroads' market share. Railroads were no longer benefiting from regulation; they wanted to be able to change their prices (increase short haul and decrease long haul prices) to compete with truckers. The bankruptcy of the Penn Central was indicative of the worsening financial position of railroads. The federal government also developed a concentrated interest in deregulating the railroads; the government was having to subsidize the railroads. Railroads were no longer willing to provide political support for a regulatory system that was causing them to lose money.

Another example where the regulated firms were no longer making monopoly profits and therefore were unwilling to provide the necessary political support to continue regulation was the airlines. Monopoly profits on certain routes were being competed away in the form of nonprice competition. As a result of experimentation with more flexible fares, airline traffic and profitability increased. Airlines believed that they could become more profitable under deregulation; as a consequence, they offered little opposition to deregulation.

As the economic value of regulation declined, so did the political support offered by the regulated firms to maintain it. In fact some firms actively promoted deregulation in their belief that they could become more profitable. Similarly, as the cost of regulation to groups with a concentrated interest increased, it became worthwhile for these groups to provide political support to lessen their burden or to increase their profits.

Unions within the regulated industry have always opposed deregulation. Unions have been able to capture part of the regulatory profits in the form of higher wages. With deregulation, the firms that were formerly regulated could not compete on price with new firms using lower-cost labor. The power of the union declined and the unionized employees have had to accept lower wages. Unions in regulated industries are therefore in the forefront of those opposing deregulation and, once deregulated, support reregulating the industry.

The antitrust laws were the second reason why some industries were deregulated. The federal judicial system is less in need of political support, hence less subject to political pressures, than are Congress or the regulatory agencies. The federal courts are therefore more likely to act regardless of an industry's economic interest when applying the antitrust laws. Although it is possible for a concentrated interest group to receive congressional exemption from the antitrust laws, it has been very difficult to do so. (There are a few exceptions, labor unions are one.) For an industry to receive such an exemption requires a much higher degree of political support than to achieve regulatory benefits where the regulatory costs are diffuse and less visible.

AT&T faced the prospect of losing an antitrust case and having to pay large damages that convinced it to settle with the government and accept deregulation. The intervention of the federal courts in several trucking cases led to greater entry in the trucking industry. When the courts become involved because of antitrust, the regulated firms are unable to prevent competitors and low-cost substitutes from eroding their profits.

When regulated firms continue to make monopoly profits and the costs of regulation are diffuse, opposing interest groups are unlikely to arise and deregulation is unlikely to occur. It is for these reasons that many industries have continued to retain their regulatory benefits.

The consequences of deregulation in the foregoing industries are that prices reflect the costs of service, wages have declined, quality has either stayed the same or increased, innovation has increased, and the method of providing the previously regulated services has become more integrated.

Under regulation, prices did not reflect the cost of providing the service. As such, some users were subsidized while others bore the burden of those subsidies. Entry and price cutting has occurred on those services where the price-cost ratios were highest. Long-haul rates for railroads, long-distance flights for airlines, large brokerage trades, and long-distance telephone charges declined with deregulation.

Wages were lower and labor productivity was higher in those firms that entered the previously regulated industry. To remain cost competitive, the regulated firms had to reduce their labor costs. AT&T released tens of thousand of employees, restrictive work rules were reduced in the railroads and the airlines, and union contracts were renegotiated in the airline, trucking, and railroad industries.

The quality of services provided to railroad shippers increased after deregulation while accidents on poorly maintained tracks decreased. In trucking, complaints by shippers to the ICC declined. With regard to airline safety, as measured by accidents and fatalities per passenger mile, there was no decrease in quality; however, passenger comfort declined as airline traffic increased sharply as a result of lower air fares.

Innovation and service delivery systems changed after deregulation. Railroads developed integrated delivery systems by combining the flexibility of trucks for local pickup and delivery with the long-haul efficiency of railroads, which were previously prohibited by the regulatory agency. New telephone systems and instruments are now available and AT&T has diversified into related lines of business, such as computers. Brokerage firms and banks now provide a more complete range of financial options for the investor, such as mutual funds, real estate, and money market funds. Airlines have moved to a hub-and-spoke system of delivery, where their own or regional airlines serve smaller cities that feed passengers into their major hubs for longer flights. There are also a greater variety of firms competing in the once-regulated industries; discount brokers compete with full-service firms and no frills airlines have emerged.

The brief discussion above of the reasons for deregulation and its subsequent effects provide a framework for analyzing the emergence of market competition in the medical industry.

The Emergence of Competition in Medical Care

Government expenditures for Medicare and Medicaid greatly exceeded their original projections. Inflation during the 1960s served to stimulate the demand for private insurance. As incomes increased due to inflation, employees moved into higher tax brackets and unions bargained for increased health benefits, which were not taxable. As insurance coverage in the private and public sectors increased, consumer concern with health costs diminished. Health providers were able to increase their prices with little fear of decreased demand. In an increasing economy with rising inflation, business firms were able to pass on their higher labor costs by increasing the prices of their goods and services.

One consequence of these rising expenditures was that federal expenditures increased from $3.6 billion in 1965, to $31.4 billion by 1975, to 62.5 billion in 1980, and to more than $112 billion by 1985. State expenditures under Medicaid also increased sharply, from $4.3 billion in 1965 to $35 billion in 1985. Expenditures in the private sector went from $31 billion a year in 1965 to $250 billion in 1985. These massive increases in health expenditures from both the public and private sectors greatly exceeded the economy's rate of inflation. These expenditures were equivalent to a huge redistribution program, from the taxpayers to those working in the health sector.

Early attempts at reducing the rise in health expenditures came from the federal government. Original expectations were that Medicare would cost only $2 billion a year. However, as an entitlement program, Medicare's benefits and beneficiaries were defined by law; no limit was placed on its overall expenditures. Successive administrations developed a concentrated interest in halting Medicare's rapidly escalating expenditures. Any administration asking Congress to change the law would lose a great deal of political support from the aged and their supporters. Equally troublesome (politically) for an administration would be to request continual tax increases for the program. Thus the federal government had only two alternatives for limiting the increase in Medicare expenditures, which were rising by approximately 15 percent a year. These alternatives were either to limit payments to providers or to place controls on utilization of services.

The federal government started chipping away at the cost-based reimbursement of hospitals in 1969, when it removed the plus 2 percent from the cost plus formula. In 1971, because of rising inflation, President Nixon placed the entire U.S. economy under a wage and price freeze (the Economic Stabilization Program). The rest of the economy was removed from this freeze after one year. However, the health sector remained under price controls until April 1974. In the first year following their removal, physician and hospital expenditures increased very rapidly, 17.5 percent and 19.4 percent, respectively (see Tables 9–2 and 10–4).

Additional regulatory methods were used to limit these rapid expenditure increases. Each one failed. Physician fee increases under Medicare were limited by the Medicare Fee Index; the result was that increasing numbers of physicians declined to participate in the Medicare program, while physicians that did participate charged for additional services, thereby negating the effect of the fee freeze. Congress passed the National Health Planning and Resources Development Act in 1974 (CON) which placed limits on hospitals' capital expenditures. Utilization review programs (professional standard review organizations) were passed by the Congress in 1972. Again empirical studies failed to find significant savings in hospital use or expenditures as a result of these programs.

In 1979, President Carter made hospital cost containment his highest legislative priority—and was unable to have his legislation enacted. His proposed legislation would have placed limits on the annual percent increase in each hospital's expenditures.

There were a number of events that provided the preconditions for market competition, but only one that made it possible to occur.

Federal Initiatives

The Increased Supply of Physicians. For approximately 15 years, through the 1950s and early 1960s, the supply of physicians in relation to the population remained constant, at 141 physicians per 100,000. During this period physicians' incomes were rising (relative to those of other occupations), as were the number of applicants to acceptances to medical schools (see Tables 13–1 to 13–4). As the demand for physicians' services continued to grow, stimulated by the passage of Medicare and Medicaid and the growth of private health insurance, an increased number of foreign medical graduates (FMGs) came to the United States.

During this period there was constant talk of a shortage of physicians. Many qualified U.S. students who could not gain admission to the limited number of medical school spaces went overseas to receive a medical education. Many middle-class families were concerned that their sons and daughters could not become physicians, while, at the same time, there was increased immigration by FMGs. The Congress responded to these constituent pressures and passed the Health Professions Educational Assistance Act (HPEA). Senator Yarborough stated the reasons for the passage of the HPEA in 1963. "It was when we were trying to give more American boys and girls a chance for a medical education, so that we would not have to drain the help of other foreign countries." And again, "To me it is just shocking that we do not give American boys and girls a chance to obtain a medical education so that they can serve their own people" (3). It took a number of years before the full magnitude of this Act took effect. New medical schools were built and existing medical schools increased their spaces. (The same occurred for other health professions.) By 1980 the supply of physicians had reached 200 per 100,000, almost a 50 percent increase from the early 1960s.

In response to their constituent interests and over the objections of the American Medical Association, Congress enacted legislation which eventually created excess capacity among physicians. It was not Congress's intention to create competition among physicians. However, their actions in passing the HPEA set the stage for it.

The HMO Act. In the early 1970s, President Nixon wanted a health initiative that would not be very costly to the federal government. His proposal was to stimulate the growth of prepaid health plans, renamed health maintenance organizations (HMOs).

When Congress passed the HMO Act in 1973, it included two provisions helpful to the development of HMOs and one that was a hindrance. First, employers with 25 or more employees had to offer their employees an HMO option if there was a federally qualified HMO available in their area. Second, federally qualified HMOs were exempt from restrictive state practices. HMOs initially had a small competitive effect. However, as more people joined HMOs, the decreased hospital use of HMO subscribers contributed to hospitals' excess capacity.

The 1979 Amendments to the CON Legislation. The initial CON legislation established planning agencies whose purpose was to limit the increase in hospital capital expenditures. HMOs needed access to a hospital to provide a full range of medical services. Some HMOs had hospitals which they wanted to expand, while other HMOs wanted to construct hospitals. HMOs began to complain to the Congress that the CON legislation was being used to block their growth. HMOs were a threat to existing hospitals and physicians in a community. "HMOs were subjected to more extensive controls than fee-for-service providers. Although financing plans and provider organizations of other kinds could be established without government approval, establishment of an HMO was subject to planning agency review" (4).

In 1979, Congress amended the CON legislation so that the Act should not be used to inhibit competition. However, these amendments did not grant all HMOs a complete exemption from the CON Act; it merely loosened the restrictions (5).

Except for the change in the CON legislation and the enactment of the HMO Act and its amendments, it was difficult for Congress to develop a consensus with the various health interest groups as to what legislative approach, if any, should be proposed to resolve the problem of rising federal health expenditures.

Some of the opponents of President Carter's cost-containment legislation, such as Representatives Gephardt and Stockman, began to propose an alternative approach, the use of market competition. Various academicians, such as Enthoven, wrote on the virtues of market competition (6). If competition had to be enacted into law, it would not have occurred. Too many powerful interest groups were opposed to organizing the delivery of health services along competitive lines (7). Organized medicine correctly foresaw that its members would be made worse off under competition. In competitive areas, such as in the Twin Cities, physicians had to accept changes in their style of practice and restrictions on their behavior. The growth of competition and prepaid health plans resulted in a decreased demand for hospital care—up to 50 percent less. Many hospitals would have preferred the security of a regulatory system. Thus hospitals, another important interest group, were unlikely to support a competition proposal. Commercial health insurers have opposed the concept. They were unsure of their future role in a system of competing prepaid health plans. The insurance companies instead preferred some form of all-payor hospital rate regulation so that the Blue Cross discount would no longer place them at a competitive disadvantage. Blue Cross was also reluctant to favor a change to market competition. Blue Cross plans with high market shares and good provider relations would have had little to gain from such a change. (Although both commercial insurors and Blue Cross were opposed to competition, they have since started many alternative delivery systems and are continually seeking ways of reducing their hospital costs.)

Business groups, which might be expected to favor competition in general, were, at most, lukewarm supporters of health care competition. Many companies believed that they had preferred-risk groups and did not want to incur increased administrative costs from offering multiple health plans to their employees.

Unions were among the most vocal of the groups opposing a competitive delivery system. Although unions have been strong supporters of prepaid group practice, those same unions have a basic distrust of competitive markets. They preferred not-for-profit health plans and wanted the government, rather than markets, to be the regulator of provider and insurer performance. Unions also opposed legislative proposals to increase competition that would have taxed employer-purchased health insurance premiums. Large unions generally have comprehensive health insurance benefits and a tax limit on health benefits would make their members worse off.

The beneficiaries of a competitive market are consumers. Their interest in pro-competitive legislation, however, is diffuse; the potential benefits of competition would not have been viewed as being sufficiently large to warrant involvement in the political process.

Elimination of "Free Choice" of Provider Under Medicaid. It was not until several years later, under President Reagan, that additional cost-containment legislation was enacted. In 1981 Congress amended the Medicaid Act (8) to provide states with greater flexibility in how they pay for their medically indigent. States were no longer required to offer their medically indigent "free choice" of medical provider. This meant that states could take bids and negotiate contracts with selected providers for the care of their medically indigent. Although a potentially powerful force for using market forces in the Medicaid program, many states moved slowly.

New Hospital Payment System Under Medicare. Then, starting in September 1983, the Reagan administration, introduced a revolutionary method to pay hospitals under Medicare, the use of diagnostic related groupings (DRGs). The hospital and medical associations were powerless against a Republican administration intent on reducing federal expenditures for hospitals. As the incentives facing hospitals changed, lengths of stay for the aged declined.

However, by the time hospitals began to experience the effect of DRGs on their occupancy rates, the move toward market competition had already started. DRGs reinforced the competitive pressures on hospitals stimulated several years earlier by declining occupancy rates.

Private Sector Initiatives

Approximately two-thirds of the population has private health insurance coverage, and most private health insurance is purchased through the workplace. The stimulus for competition started in the private sector.

In 1981 the nation was faced with a severe recession. In addition, the automobile and steel industries faced increased import competition from foreign producers. These were also the same industries that had the most comprehensive health insurance programs for their employees. The recession led to unemployment, loss of income, a decrease in health insurance benefits, resulting in a decline in elective hospital admissions. The recession also lowered tax revenues for states. Consequently, many states cut back on their Medicaid benefits, decreased the numbers of eligibles, and instituted cost containment measures, such as prior authorization for admission. These factors, which led to a decline in the hospital admission rate for those under 65 years of age, started in late 1981.

Once the recession ended, industry was still concerned with its labor costs. Those industries engaged in competition with foreign producers found that the strength of the U.S. dollar relative to other currencies forced them to reduce their costs to remain competitive.

Industry began to examine ways in which they could contain the rise in their employees' health insurance costs. Greater pressure was placed on health insurers to hold their premiums down and to institute new cost-saving programs. Also, an increasing number of business firms started their own self-insurance plans. The firms believed that they, rather than insurance companies, would be better able to control their employees' health care use. Businesses also added deductibles and coinsurance to their employees' health plans, thereby increasing their employees' price sensitivity. A survey of 1,185 companies found that the percentage of firms requiring deductible payments for their employee's inpatient care rose from 30 percent in 1982 to 63 percent in 1984; similarly, the percent of firms requiring preauthorization for hospital admission increased from 2 percent to 26 percent over that same period (9).

One of the most important changes firms (or insurance companies on their behalf) introduced was a change in the benefit package. Insurance coverage for lower-cost substitutes to hospitals was introduced. Previously, even though it was less costly to perform surgery in an outpatient setting, if this service was not covered by insurance, it became less costly *to the employee* to have the surgery performed in a hospital. Thus by adding outpatient surgery to the benefit package the insurance premium paid by the business could be reduced.

Private-sector initiatives had two effects. First, as purchasers of health care benefits, they demonstrated that they were concerned with health care costs. This concern was transmitted to the health insurers and resulted in insurers becoming more concerned with utilization review of providers. Preauthorization for admission, concurrent review, and second opinions for surgery were instituted as a means of reducing the insurance premium. Insurers, particularly the Blues, began to change their relationship with providers and became more adversarial. They began to place greater pressure on hospitals to limit their cost increases.

The second consequence of the concern by business with its employees' health costs was that hospitals developed excess capacity. The efforts to reduce hospital utilization, such as utilization controls, the growth of HMOs, and coverage of care in nonhospital settings were succeeding. Occupancy rates in short-term general hospitals declined from 78 percent in 1980 to 64.8 percent by 1985. As excess capacity increased, hospitals were willing to participate with and become part of alternative delivery systems.

The Enforcement of Antitrust Laws

Concern by business with their employees' health care costs and the creation of excess capacity among both hospitals and physicians were important preconditions for competition. However, had it not been for the application of the antitrust laws, it is unlikely that market competition would have occurred.

Medical societies and state practice acts inhibited market competition by limiting advertising, fee splitting, corporate practice, and delegation of tasks. Blue Cross and Blue Shield maintained the principle of "free choice" of provider; that is, their subscribers had no incentive to choose between providers on the basis of price. Blue Cross enrollees had a service benefit policy. Regardless of whether the participating hospital had high or low costs, Blue Cross paid 100 percent of those costs. Under Blue Shield, price comparisons by enrollees were also discouraged; Blue Shield reimbursed participating physicians according to their usual fees (up to a percentile limit).

In the past, during the 1930s, the same preconditions for market competition had existed. Physicians and hospitals had excess capacity; patients and their insurance companies were concerned with the cost of health care. Yet market competition did not occur. For example, insurance companies in Oregon attempted to lower their insurance premiums so as to compete better for subscribers. The method used to reduce the cost of the insurance premium was to place restraints on physician utilization. Preauthorization of services and monitoring of claims were used.

The response by the medical societies in Oregon to a competitive market in medical care was twofold. First, the medical societies threatened to expel from the society any physician that participated in these competitive insurance plans. Second, the medical societies started their own insurance plans. These plans did not use aggressive utilization methods. With the growth of their own insurance plans, physicians were encouraged to boycott other insurance plans. The effect of these policies by the medical societies was to cause these other insurance plans to decline. To have physicians participate in their plans, the insurance companies had to drop their aggressive cost containment efforts. The medical societies were thereby able to determine that the type of insurance programs that would be offered to the public were also those that were in the physicians' economic interests (10).

Therefore, unless the antitrust laws were applicable to the health sector, physician and hospital boycotts and other anticompetitive behavior could have prevented market competition from once again occurring.

Up until 1975 it was believed that the antitrust laws did not apply to "learned professions," which included the health professions. In 1975, the U.S. Supreme Court decided the case of Goldberg v. Virginia State Bar. The local Bar association, believing that lawyers were not engaged in "trade or commerce", established a minimum fee schedule for lawyers. The Supreme Court ruled against the bar association, thereby denying any sweeping exclusion for the learned professions from the antitrust laws. In another important precedent, the Supreme Court in 1978 denied the use of anticompetitive behavior by the National Society of Professional Engineers even if it was to prevent a threat to either the profession's ethics or to public safety. Encouraged by the Supreme Court decisions, the Federal Trade Commission (FTC) began to enforce vigorously the antitrust laws in the health field. The FTC, in 1975, charged the American Medical Association and its constituent medical societies with anticompetitive behavior. In a 1978 decision, the FTC prevailed. The AMA appealed the verdict to the Supreme Court, but was again unsuccessful.

The Supreme Court's decision, rendered in 1982, was a clear signal to health providers that they would now be subject to the antitrust laws. The FTC subsequently brought suit to prevent physician and dentist boycotts against insurors (Michigan State Medical Society and the Indiana Federation of Dentists), prevent physicians from denying hospital privileges to physicians participating in prepaid health plans (Forbes Health System Medical Staff), enabled advertising to be used (FTC v. AMA), opposed the per se rule against exclusive contracts (Hyde case), and enabled preferred provider organizations and HMOs to compete, (11).

The reasons for the emergence of market competition in health care were similar to other deregulated industries. Business and the federal government each developed a concentrated interest in holding down the rise in their medical expenditures. As a result of the 1981 recession and severe import competition, business moved toward self-insurance; their increased concern with health care costs stimulated insurance companies to introduce cost saving innovations in their benefit packages. The federal government introduced DRGs as a means of controlling rapidly rising Medicare and Medicaid expenditures. Low cost substitutes to traditional providers developed, namely HMOs and outpatient surgery clinics. These new delivery systems decreased hospital and physician revenues. The excess capacity among physicians and hospitals and the change in business incentives and in government were important preconditions for market competition. However, it is unlikely that market competition would have occurred had it not been for the applicability and enforcement of the antitrust laws. The judicial system ensured that market competition would occur when the Supreme Court upheld the applicability of antitrust to the health care industry.

HOW COMPETITION IS EVOLVING IN MEDICAL CARE

An Overview

Market competition has changed the incentives facing the purchaser as well as the supplier of medical services by transferring financial risk. Purchasers, whether they are patients, employers, or insurance companies, have an economic incentive to search for those providers that can provide a given quality product at the lowest price. Purchasers also have an incentive to consider the trade-off between price and quality; increases in quality that are worth less than their increased cost are less likely to be purchased. Regardless of whether the supplier is for-profit or nonprofit, they have an incentive to minimize the cost of the product they are producing when they face a fixed price, either market or government determined.

The economic incentives on the purchaser side of the medical market occurs when the patient is required to pay part of the provider's price, as under cost sharing, or when the purchaser of health insurance must choose among the types of plans offered. The consumer will choose among alternative plans according to the plan's premium, benefits, reputation, and accessibility. At times the purchaser is the employer, as when they self-insure, or when they contribute a given dollar amount per employee, regardless of the health plan chosen by the employee; the employer may then decide which plans are to be offered to their employees and at what premiums. Insurance companies, having to compete on premiums as well as other qualities, are also purchasers of medical services in that they have an economic incentive to be concerned with the provider's price, utilization, and quality. Another large purchaser is the federal government, which has established fixed prices for the payment of hospitals under Medicare.

Different institutional arrangements have emerged on the supply side of the market in response to the heightened concern over expenditures on the demand side. Initially, there was a large growth in health maintenance organizations (HMOs).

HMOs have become synonymous with the idea of market competition. However, market competition exhibits much broader forms of competitive behavior than just HMOs. The aspect of HMOs, or prepaid health plans, that generated opposition from organized medicine was the lack of "free choice" of physician by the HMO's subscribers. Only those physicians participating in the HMO were available to the subscribers, the physicians were part of a "closed panel." As HMOs' market share grows, those physicians not participating are "locked" out of a significant part of the market.

A delivery system must be able to exclude certain providers if it is to have control over its costs and reputation. The ability to exclude providers, such as physicians, also creates price competition among physicians. If a physician believes that joining a closed panel organization will increase the number of their patients, they would be willing to accept a lower fee for their services from the organization. The closed panel organization is then able to lower its input costs and market its services at a lower premium than the traditional fee-for-service plan.

Physician participants in a closed panel arrangement may be reimbursed in a variety of ways. An HMO can have salaried physicians, can pay their physicians according to fee for service, provide a bonus on performance, or any combination of the above. Prepaid health plans that permit participating physicians to continue to serve their other patients in their own office setting are referred to as independent practice associations (IPAs).

The Advantages of Prepaid Health Plans

Using prepayment on a capitation basis in return for delivery of comprehensive medical care is not new. It was proposed by the Commission on the Cost of Medical Care in the 1930s. Early examples of such organizations are the Kaiser Foundation Health Plan and the Group Health Association. This concept was used as the basis for the health maintenance organization (HMO) strategy,[1] which permits an organization based on the corporate practice of medicine to compete with the fee-for-service delivery system. The economic incentive of such organizations is to retain the difference between the capitation payment and the costs of providing medical services. Thus the organization and its physicians have a financial incentive to minimize the cost of medical care provided to its enrollees.

Prepaid health plans may be organized in a variety of ways. An organization can own its own hospitals and employ physicians on salary. An organization can contract separately with hospitals and physicians for their services and reimburse participating providers on a fee-for-service basis. Insurance companies may, and do, form their own prepaid plans; they market such services and bear the risk themselves and then may contract with other providers for the services. As market competition continues to evolve, so do the form of health care organizations. The most common feature of these organizations is that the participating physicians are provided with a financial incentive to minimize the use of medical services.

An important advantage of prepaid health plans is that the consumer chooses an organization for the delivery of medical services and does not have to select providers at the time of illness. The responsibility for quality rests with the organization and requires less investment by the consumer to determine the credentials of individual

---

[1]The originator of the term health maintenance organization is Paul M. Ellwood, Jr. See his "Health Maintenance Strategy," *Medical Care*, May–June 1971.

providers. Quality assurance programs are more easily developed and monitored for larger organizations than for a large number of smaller, independent providers.

The hypothesized effects of competition among prepaid health plans to provide medical services for a fixed capitation payment should be the following.

Incentives for Hospital Efficiency

Under cost-based hospital reimbursement, the physician had little or no incentive to be concerned with the cost of hospital care. Under a capitated system of reimbursement for all of a person's medical services, an HMO either operates its own hospitals or purchases hospital care from existing hospitals in the community. The HMO therefore has an incentive to be more concerned with the costs of their patients' hospital care and should select hospitals according to the hospitals' costs, the hospital's reputation, and the services required for their patients.

Less Duplication of Facilities

Hospital facilities and services that were primarily for the convenience of the physician or because they provided prestige to the institution now have a cost associated with their use. If the organization had fewer such facilities, the HMO's premium could be reduced, its benefits increased, or the savings used to reward the HMO's staff. It is not in the best interests of an HMO to own every type of facility or service. Because some facilities are subject to large economies of scale, it may be financially advantageous for an HMO to purchase such services from other institutions when the HMO's patients require them. Since there is now a cost to the HMO and its physicians for having duplicate facilities, fewer duplicated facilities are expected.

Minimizing the Cost of a Medical Treatment

Previously, financial incentives to use the least costly setting for patient treatment, when medically feasible, did not exist. Providers were separately reimbursed and Blue Cross did not cover less costly substitutes. Under a capitation system, the criteria for use of alternatives to hospitalization changes. The HMO (and the patient's physician) has an incentive to provide care in the least costly manner. When medically feasible, we expect to observe greater use of outpatient surgical care in lieu of hospitalization and shorter hospital stays, with the remainder of the patient's convalescence provided for in another setting or in the patient's home. No other reimbursement system provides incentives for minimizing the cost of the patient's entire medical treatment.

Increased Physician Productivity

Under a capitated system, there is a financial incentive for the HMO to use more auxiliary medical personnel in physician offices and in the hospital, thereby increasing physicians' productivity. As long as the revenue produced by the additional auxiliaries exceeds their cost, it is in the interests of physicians and the HMO to add auxiliary personnel. We would thus expect to observe an increase in demand for such personnel from HMOs. HMOs might even develop their own training programs or permit specially trained registered nurses to perform tasks currently undertaken by physicians. Currently, state practice acts place limits on the tasks that health professions are permitted to perform. Large, economically powerful, HMOs, in their desire to minimize their costs, have an incentive to seek changes in state practice acts to permit greater substitution of personnel in the performance of tasks. Delegation of tasks might eventually also be based on the training and experience of individuals rather than, as under current practice, whether a profession has a monopoly on the performance of those tasks.

Incentives for Preventive Care and Health Education

To the extent that preventive care delivered to an HMO's enrollees result in decreased future demand for more costly medical services, we would expect the HMO to provide a greater amount of those services than is provided under the current fee-for-service system. Similarly, to the extent that the enrollees' health habits can be improved, thus reducing future demand for medical care, the HMO can be expected to undertake health education programs. To provide them with an even greater incentive to be concerned with their enrollees' health status, HMOs should be encouraged to sell life insurance to their enrolled population (12).

Use of Generic Drugs

Assuming that drugs are a covered benefit, HMOs are expected to be more concerned with drug prices; it is thus in the economic interests of HMOs and their physicians to prescribe less costly drugs. The HMO, rather the drug companies' detailmen, have an incentive to become the source of drug information for HMO physicians. It is likely that HMOs will provide their physicians with the option of selecting generic drugs when writing a prescription.

Innovations in the Delivery of Medical Care

Innovations in the delivery of medical services are potentially threatening to physicians and to other providers. Substitutes for existing personnel, lower-cost facilities, and new treatment methods decrease the demand for existing providers. Previously, restrictions have been used to inhibit such innovations. However, under a system of competing HMOs, HMOs have an incentive to be innovative in the diagnostic area, in management techniques, and in delivering services. Greater experimentation with location and accessibility of services to the HMO's enrolled population is likely to occur. HMOs have an incentive to seek out and quickly adopt (when economically feasible) new techniques with both medical and management applications. Such techniques might enable the HMO to lower its costs or increase its services, thereby enhancing its ability to compete. The rate of innovation in the delivery of medical services is expected to increase in a market-competitive system.

Preferred Provider Organizations

Other forms of closed panel delivery systems have arisen since the development of HMOs. Preferred provider organizations (PPOs) offer their subscribers services either at a discount or include physicians that are low utilizers of hospital services. PPOs may consist of groups of hospitals, of physicians, or of combinations of the two. Often a subscriber does not have to go to a participating PPO provider, but their copayment is reduced if they do. PPOs also generally differ from HMOs in that the PPO does not market its services based on an annual capitation fee. The participating providers are paid on a fee-for-service basis and do not bear the financial risk of exceeding an annual capitation payment as does an HMO. PPOs may sell their services directly to employers or to insurance companies, which then market their services for an annual premium. The sponsorship of a PPO may be a group of providers or insurance companies, such as Blue Cross, which may form and market its own PPO. Although other delivery systems are likely to emerge in the coming years, they are likely to include the exclusion feature that is common to HMOs and PPOs (i.e., a closed panel of providers).

From the perspective of the patient, market competition is likely to result in the consumer making annual choices on health care providers, as when they choose which health plan to join. Consumers now have increased choices of types of health plans, such as HMOs, PPOs, and the fee-for-service (FFS) system, which vary according to their premiums, benefits, and access to providers. An annual choice enables the consumer to make an unhurried decision. It is also easier for the consumer to choose among different health plans than to select different combinations of providers.

There are several reasons why alternative delivery systems arise. HMOs, for example, represented a lower-cost alternative (or increased benefits at the same premium) than FFS. Some consumers were willing to accept restrictions on their choice of providers in return for lower premiums and/or increased benefits. Other delivery systems, such as PPOs, are able to accommodate those consumers willing to accept restrictions on choice of provider while still permitting other consumers to go outside the PPO (either occasionally or all the time) and pay a higher price.

Another reason for the growth of PPOs has been employer dissatisfaction with HMOs. Employers contribute, on behalf of their employees, a given amount to the traditional (FFS) plan. These contributions have been sufficiently high to require only small employee co-premiums. Employers have then been required by law to contribute an equal dollar amount on behalf of the employee to HMOs. The pricing strategy of HMOs has been to tie their premium implicitly to the traditional plan offered by the employer. If the HMO is able to produce its services at lower cost because it uses less hospital care, these savings are not passed onto the employer as long as the employer contributes an equal amount to both types of plans. To increase its market share over the traditional plan, the HMO passes the savings from its lower costs to the employees in the form of increased benefits. Thus HMOs have not resulted in the savings employers initially expected. (Ultimately, the traditional plan has to reduce the rate of increase in its premium; otherwise, it will continue losing market share.)

By contracting with a PPO (either directly or through an insurance company) an employer receives the savings of lower prices and/or decreased utilization. To ensure that it receives the PPO savings for all its employees (not just those enrolling in the PPO), an employer may become self-insured and offer only one plan to its employees.

The major savings of an HMO, which come from reduced hospital use, are able to be achieved by employers and insurance companies through their own cost-containment programs. Companies with high admission rates are able to save approximately 25 percent on their medical costs by instituting their own utilization review programs, such as preadmission review (13). The ability to control hospital costs has become so well known that a wide variety of organizations are now able to achieve these savings. The competitive advantage of HMOs in this regard has been lessened.

PPOs have been a method used to increase price competition among providers (14). Hospitals have always been in competition with one another, but not on the basis of price. Given previous payment systems and patient incentives, hospitals have competed for physicians and patients on the basis of facilities and services, amenities, and quality. With the emergence of PPOs, hospitals are now engaged in price competition. By using price, as well as other criteria, to select participating hospitals, PPOs cause the individual hospital's demand curve to become more elastic; by offering a discount to a PPO, a hospital can increase its volume and total revenues. As the hospital's demand curve becomes more elastic, with the same marginal cost curve, its profit-maximizing price falls. (While the hospital's demand curve becomes more elastic in the PPO market, the elasticity of the hospital's demand curve for other payors may be unchanged.)

PPOs have not spread uniformly around the country; California has more than twice as many (82) as the next closest state (15). The growth of PPOs, however, has been rapid; it has been estimated that as much as 40 percent of the population will be enrolled in PPOs (16). The discounts received from hospitals by PPOs, which have been between 10 and 20 percent have been passed on in the form of lower premiums. Some PPO premiums ("prudent buyer" plans) are as much as 24 percent below traditional Blue Cross premiums.

In a study of the effect of competition among California hospitals, Melnick and Zwansiger found that hospital behavior changed since 1983 (17). Using a Herfindahl index, hospitals were classified according to the degree of competition within their markets. During the period 1983–1985, total hospital expenses actually declined by 8.2 percentage points in competitive markets as compared to an increase of 3.7 percent in less competitive markets. Competitive policies were effective in reducing total hospital expenses. To maintain their revenues, however, hospitals shifted their focus to outpatient services. Outpatient services are generally not covered by PPO contracts, thus there is little price competition or utilization review in outpatient settings. Further, Medicare DRGs are not applicable to outpatient services. The consequence is that hospitals in more competitive markets had more rapid increases in their outpatient revenues, 18 versus 14 percent in 1985. Since hospitals in less competitive markets had more rapid increases in their inpatient revenues, the net effect was an increase in total real net revenues of 7.8 percent for hospitals in noncompetitive markets during the period 1983–1985 as compared to only 1.4 percent for hospitals in more competitive markets.

The growth of market competition has been more rapid in California than in other parts of the country. As expected, market competition has reduced hospital revenues. To survive, hospitals in competitive markets are reducing their inpatient expenses and shifting to other sources of revenues. As these same competitive forces increase throughout the country, similar results are expected.

The results of other studies indicating extensive duplication of complex services in highly competitive markets and the conclusion that competition encourages such duplication may be premature (18). During the period examined by these studies, hospitals were engaged in intense nonprice competition. As hospitals around the country become more price competitive, hospitals will find it more difficult to cross subsidize money losing duplicative services. Price competition will force hospitals to eliminate complex services, in which they perform few procedures, to minimize their losses. The result is likely to be an increase in quality in more price-competitive hospital markets; facilities in which higher volumes of complex procedures are performed have lower mortality rates.

THE EFFECT OF ADVERTISING ON THE MARKET FOR MEDICAL SERVICES

An important prerequisite to competition in medical services is information, which comes from advertising. However, many people, in addition to medical care providers, are opposed to advertising of medical services. Such opposition is usually based on the fear that consumers will be misled, that they will be induced to purchase unnecessary services, and that the prices of such services will be increased because the cost of advertising will be passed on to the consumer. The argument that consumers will be misled is weak. The Federal Trade Commission (FTC), which seeks to improve market competition, polices advertising claims. Existing health providers are also likely to monitor carefully their competitor's claims and report any misinformation to the FTC. Further, it seems unlikely that consumers will be more misled by providers who publish misinformation than they were under a system which suppressed information.

The claim that consumers will be induced to purchase unnecessary services is based on the assumption that providing more information from competing sources will result in greater demand creation than that which occurs when the patient is totally reliant on a single physician for advice. The recent trend toward securing second opinions for recommended surgery contradicts this claim. Surgery is an area where the patient has very little information as to prospective value; two opinions provide additional information and enable the patient to make a more informed choice, thereby resulting in a decrease in the rate of surgery.

Advertising results in lower rather than higher prices. This is often difficult to explain since advertising is an additional cost to the firm. The following discussion will therefore attempt three things: to explain why advertising of medical services results in lower prices for medical services; to provide supporting empirical evidence; and finally, to examine which population groups are likely to benefit from the removal of advertising restrictions (19).

Advertising provides price information. In an industry where each firm produces the same product but does not permit advertising of prices, wide variations in prices will exist, since it will be up to the consumer to search out the firms with the lowest prices. Since search is costly, consumers will not keep searching until they find the firm that sells its products at the lowest price. Only when the search costs approach zero will people search until the price differential approaches zero. If information were disseminated through advertising, and no additional expense, such as travel cost to purchase the product, was involved, prices would reflect the costs of producing different products. Differences in quality and variety would exist, but the different prices charged for such products would reflect their additional costs. In a world of perfect information, prices charged for what is perceived to be the same product should be the same.

In the market for medical services, however, information has been almost nonexistent. Thus each medical provider has had a less elastic demand curve. A patient is usually unawares of different competitors' quality, accessibility, and price of medical services, thereby making these other providers poor substitutes for the patient's current provider. To determine the attributes of different services and which ones are sold at lower prices, the consumer has had to spend time and money searching.

The effect of advertising on prices can be shown with reference to Figure 12–1. With little information available to consumers to judge other physicians, the physi-

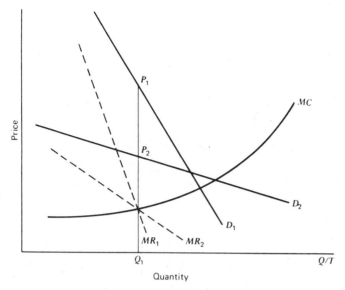

Figure 12-1. The effect of advertising on the elasticity of demand and on the firm's pricing strategy.

cian's demand curve is less elastic, shown as D_1. Assuming that the physician-firm wishes to maximize its profits, it will set its price at that point on the demand curve where the marginal revenue (MR_1) and marginal cost curves intersect. The resulting price will be P_1. With advertising, consumers have more information by which to evaluate substitute physicians and health care providers, such as the benefits provided by a prepaid plan compared to a traditional plan, physician qualifications, accessibility in terms of location and hours, and so on. Other physicians (and health plans) now become better substitutes to one another. As this happens, the physician's demand curve becomes more elastic (the closer the substitute, the more elastic the demand curve). The new, more elastic, demand curve is D_2. For the sake of simplicity, the marginal revenue curves in Figure 12-1 were drawn so that they intersected the marginal cost curve at the same point. With the same marginal cost curve, a more elastic demand curve results in a lower price, P_2 instead of P_1.[2]

The cost of advertising is not shown in Figure 12-1, since it increases the firm's average cost curve. Advertising costs may be considered a fixed cost, since they are unrelated to the cost of producing additional quantities of the particular service. Thus the cost of advertising itself does not affect the price charged by a firm attempting to maximize its profits. The price would be determined by the elasticity of demand and the marginal cost of producing that service. By causing the firm's demand curve to

---

[2]In the nonhealth field, many products are already viewed by consumers as being relatively homogeneous. One firm's soap or aspirin is considered to be a good substitute for the same product produced by another firm. In these cases, advertising is used by a firm to differentiate its product from that of its competitors. As shown in Figure 12-1, if a firm is selling a relatively homogeneous product (demand curve D_2), it advertises to make consumers believe that other products are less substitutable for its own, thereby hoping to change its demand curve to D_1.

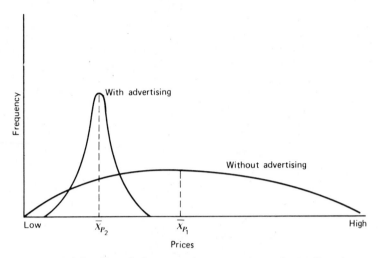

Figure 12-2. The effect of advertising on average prices and price dispersion.

become more elastic, advertising is expected to lower prices. Advertising should also increase the elasticity of demand of those providers that do not advertise.

Advertising of medical services performs three functions. First, it provides the consumer with information on the similarity and differences of services sold by different providers, enabling the consumer to evaluate the degree of substitutability of competing providers. The demand curves of the different providers are made more elastic. As shown in Figure 12-1, with a more elastic demand curve, the price would be reduced from P_1 to P_2. The second advantage of medical services advertising is that it reduces the consumer's search costs, since reading a newspaper or other publication takes less time and money than traveling to different providers to determine the quality, accessibility, and price of the services provided. These search costs are particularly high in medical care. "Price-dispersion is a manifestation of—and indeed it is a measure of—ignorance in the market" (20). Without provider information, the consumer may first have to purchase the service to determine its attributes as well as its price.[3] Although advertising is less effective when services are directly experienced, provider information on prices and qualifications still contributes to the information the consumer needs to make a choice. The consumer might then have to resort to additional sources, such as consumer groups, for information on probable satisfaction with the provider.

These two hypothesized effects of advertising are shown in Figure 12-2. Without advertising, price dispersion would be much greater; as search costs are reduced, price dispersion will decrease. As the demand for lower-priced providers increase, and as medical services are viewed as being more homogeneous, the average price will also decline.

The inability of a firm to advertise has also been used as a barrier to entry in a market. For example, large organizations, such as prepaid health plans, are subject to

---

[3]Nelson classified goods into two categories: search goods and experience goods. Search goods are those for which adequate information concerning their desirability exists prior to purchase (e.g., an airplane trip). Experience goods need to be purchased to be assessed (e.g., a dinner in a restaurant). Philip Nelson, "Advertising as Information," *Journal of Political Economy*, July–August 1974.

economies of scale, that is, they must achieve a minimum enrollment size before their premium can be competitive to those of traditional insurance plans. Their previous inability to advertise required such plans to incur large losses; they had to price their premiums competitively, but since they had such small enrollments, their costs per subscriber exceeded their premiums. Advertising enables such plans to increase their enrollments quickly so that they can take advantage of economies of scale.

Because of previous restrictions on advertising, it has been difficult to find empirical evidence in medical care to test the hypothesis that advertising leads to lower prices and less price dispersion. Until recently, advertising was prohibited by the state codes that regulate ethics in the health professions. The penalties for violating such codes were severe, including suspension of the practitioner's license. As a result of the FTC's successful suit against the AMA, health providers are beginning to advertise. Evidence on the gains from advertising that can be generalized to the entire medical sector is therefore limited. However, since restrictions on information control by optometrists have varied across states, evidence on the effects of advertising has been based on studies of optometrists.

Based on health interview survey data collected in 1970, Lee Benham and Alexandra Benham related demand factors and a set of variables measuring the degree of information control that the optometric profession maintained in each state to the prices that consumers paid for eyeglasses (21). The authors then estimated the effect of the prices paid on the likelihood that consumers would purchase eyeglasses. Several measures were used to indicate the degree of control that the optometric profession maintained over the availability of information in a state. One of these was the percentage of optometrists belonging to the state optometric association. A major prerequisite for membership was the optometrist's willingness to withhold information on prices and services rendered. It was therefore believed that the higher the percentage of optometrists belonging to the association, the smaller the amount of information available to consumers on optometric prices and services.

Commercial firms selling optometric services can advertise in certain states. Thus another measure of the degree of professional control over information was the degree to which commercial firms were restricted or prohibited by a particular state. The third measure was the percentage of eyeglass sales purchased through commercial firms. The larger the market share of commercial firms in a state, the greater was the amount of information presumably available to consumers on optometric services, and the weaker was the optometric association's control over information. These three measures—the percentage of optometrists in a state belonging to the optometric association, the presence or absence of state control over commercial firms' selling of optometric services, and the percentage of total sales by commercial firms—were indicative of the degree of professional control by a state over information on optometric services.

In addition to the professional control variables, the demand equation included the usual factors affecting demand, such as price, family income, race, age, and location (residence in an inner city or rural area). The statistical results of the demand analysis were predictable: the larger the proportion of optometrists belonging to the state association, the higher the price of the product; the price of eyeglasses was increased by $12.18, as membership proportion went from .43 to .91; the elasticity was almost .5; as the membership proportion increased, prices rose by half that percentage increase. The fewer the restrictions on commercial firms, the lower the average price in that state: specifically, $8.46 lower in the less, compared to the more, restrictive states. As the proportion of sales by commercial firms decreased from 79 percent to 0 percent, the average price increased by $11.71 (22). Thus the evidence clearly indicates that the greater the degree of professional control over information, the greater the price paid for optometric services.

These results are similar to a 1963 study conducted by Benham, in which he found that states that did not have restrictions on advertising had prices that were on average 20 percent lower ($6.70) than states with such restrictions. In that same study, Benham found that the dispersion of prices, measured by the coefficient of variation (standard deviation divided by the mean), was lower in those states that permitted advertising (23). In the later study, the Benhams also found that higher prices had a strong impact on the decision to purchase glasses. "A 30 percent increase in price associated with increased professional control implies a fall in the proportion of people obtaining eyeglasses of between 28.5 and 34.2 percent" (24).

The Benham and Benham study further determined that the effect of professional control was much greater on the less educated: that they are more likely to pay higher prices than are more educated persons in similar situations. The concern that many persons have over the supposedly negative effects of advertising should be reexamined. Although it is difficult to generalize about the quality of services the less-educated receive under a system of strong professional information control, it is clear that they are taken greater advantage of than those with higher education, perhaps because the latter are more efficient in the search process.

Benham cites a study that attempted to get at the quality issue. After price advertising began in Florida, a survey of retired persons was undertaken. One of the test questions was: "All things considered, the next time you buy eyeglasses or contact lenses, would you return to the same place where you bought your last pair?" The responses were then matched to another question which asked if the place of last purchase advertised prices. The issue, "Are consumers more dissatisfied with opticians who advertise?" was thus answered. "The results show that while 58 percent of the customers of nonadvertising opticians indicated a willingness to give the seller repeat business, 86 percent of the advertisers' customers indicated they would return . . . only 8 percent of the customers of advertising opticians said that they 'probably' or 'definitely' would not go back. A full 25 percent of the customers of nonadvertising opticians gave the same answer. . . . In brief, if there is a quality problem it is not with advertising opticians. Rather it would appear that it lies with those who refuse to advertise their prices" (25). The strong desire health (and other) professions have to maintain codes of ethics that prohibit advertising can be explained by the fact that professional control over information leads to higher prices.

The results of the Benham and Benham studies have been confirmed by a more recent study. The FTC attempted to determine what happens to prices and quality of services among providers who advertise compared to those who do not (26). Data were collected from three types of optometrists: optometrists in cities where advertising of eye examinations and eyeglasses was prohibited, optometrists who did not advertise even though advertising was permitted in their areas, and optometrists who did advertise. The FTC used seven individuals with similar visual conditions who "were trained at two schools of optometry with regard to the components of an optometric examination. They obtained examinations, recorded price, time spent, and details on the various tests and procedures performed" (27). The findings were that "the presence of advertising causes substantial and significant declines in the prices of eye examinations offered by all types of optometrists" (28). Prices were reduced, but not by as much, even for optometrists located in markets where advertising occurred but did not themselves advertise. Further, nonadvertising optometrists in advertising markets spent more time with their patients (a proxy for quality) than did advertising optometrists and even more time than did nonadvertising optometrists in nonadvertising markets.

The author concludes that advertising does not reduce quality by all practitioners in a market. In fact, enough nonadvertisers remain so that the overall market quality is higher. The removal of advertising restrictions was estimated to result in a 20 percent decrease in price without any decline in overall quality. Nonadvertisers in advertising markets compete on price and quality and apparently consumers are able to choose and differentiate between providers on the basis of prices and quality of service (29).

It is important to keep in mind that since information is costly to gather, rational consumers are unlikely to become completely knowledgeable; they will gather information to the point where the marginal benefit of additional information equals the marginal cost of collecting it. For some types of medical services, the marginal benefit of additional information will be very high; for others, there will be little advantage to investing a great deal in the search process.

Similarly, for price, product, and quality competition to occur, it is not necessary that all consumers be informed. There are few, if any, markets where all purchasers are well informed. Lack of information by the majority of purchasers or even by the average purchaser does not preclude price competition from occurring. As long as the marginal purchaser is informed and price sensitive, demand curves have negative slopes, and providing competition for these purchasers is what makes competitive markets work.

In markets where it is costly to gather information, providers attempt to develop brand name recognition for their products. Brand name products contain two elements that the consumer purchases—the product itself and information on the company's reputation as to the quality of the product. Consumers with little information are willing to pay a higher price for a product that contains both of these components than a lower price for just the product itself. In the health field it is likely that insurance companies and multihospital systems will use brand name advertising for their products. One interesting development in this regard is the purchase of university teaching hospitals by investor-owned chains; such investments are intended to provide a name recognition for quality to the firm's health care activities.

THE EFFECT OF COMPETITION ON QUALITY OF MEDICAL CARE

There is a great deal of concern that market competition will reduce quality; this concern is addressed next. The quality issue may be divided into two parts: the effect of the for-profit incentive on quality and the effect on quality of organizations, such as prepaid health plans, that have incentives to provide fewer services.

Many people believe that for-profit organizations will sacrifice quality for profit. When nonprofit providers do not perform well, it is said that they at least meant well. However, nonprofit status does not ensure high quality. When voluntary hospitals are examined, it is found that their tissue committees do not perform as they should; county nursing homes are not necessarily noted for their high quality of care; state mental institutions and Veterans Administration (VA) hospitals are not centers of excellence. Outside the health field, nonprofit status does not necessarily lead to higher quality, nor does it lead to a sensitivity to the public interest greater than that of for-profit competitors. All public schools are not necessarily of higher quality than private schools; municipal governments are often greater polluters than for-profit firms; and when nonprofit unions manage their own pension funds, they do not often receive as high a rate of return as received by for-profit funds.

Nonprofit status alone should not relieve us of a concern for quality. Quality should be monitored directly, and if this is done, it should not matter that for-profit providers exist. If only nonprofit providers are permitted, the effort to monitor quality will lessen. The advantage of permitting for-profit providers to compete in the medical market is that, precisely because they are not trusted, a greater incentive exists to develop and apply strong quality review mechanisms. These quality review mechanisms should then apply equally to all providers. [For a debate on whether health providers should be expected to be different from "purveyors of other goods and services," the reader is referred an exchange of letters on this subject between Relman and Reinhardt (30).]

It might be claimed that under a system of capitation payment for medical care, for-profit HMOs in particular might be tempted to provide minimal medical services so as to retain as much of the capitation fee as possible. Although such a situation is unlikely to occur for a number of reasons, several safeguards exist and others can be built into the system to ensure that it does not occur.

Consumer Choice

One such safeguard is consumer choice in a competitive market. Under the antitrust laws, no organization, whether it be an HMO or a large medical group, can have a monopoly over the delivery of medical services in an area. Urban areas have multiple HMOs as well as a fee-for-service system. Consumers can choose from among these alternative delivery systems and among HMOs and can renew their choice annually. The various HMOs and alternative delivery systems have to compete for new subscribers as well as to retain their existing enrollees. Some consumers make their enrollment decisions based on limited information. Other subscribers, however, are more knowledgeable; for example, unions and employers can afford to develop the necessary expertise and information to evaluate alternative medical care delivery options available to their employees. Employers are also requiring alternative delivery systems to reassure them of the quality of their care as part of an evaluation of the performance of their organization (31). The greater selectivity of better-informed groups benefits the less-informed subscribers. [All automobile purchasers are not equally knowledgeable, yet automobile companies compete on the basis of quality (e.g., increased warranty periods) as well as on price and styling, because part of their market is knowledgeable and willing to shift their purchases. The same occurs in the markets for other durable goods.] If a well-informed group were to switch from one HMO to another HMO, or to a traditional fee-for-service plan, the health plan losing subscribers would have to change its benefits, accessibility, quality, or premiums if it is to survive. The competition among health plans for the better-informed purchasers, those who are more likely to switch plans if quality deteriorates, will help those who are less well informed.

The Permanent Nature of the Organization

Large organizations or corporations are usually in business for an indefinite period. The expected long life of such organizations leads them to behave differently than small firms or those in business for a short time. Whereas an individual entrepreneur may go into business, mislead consumers, produce a poor product, and then quickly move on to another area, large corporations cannot afford such behavior. A large corporation cannot undertake those business practices that will maximize its present income at the expense of future business. It cannot afford purposely to produce a poor product. Because for-profit health plans and HMOs have their reputations at stake, pocketing the capitation fee and providing little or no service would adversely affect the reputation of the organization and decrease its future business. Poor business practices are therefore more likely to be expected of smaller organizations, for which the costs of entering and leaving a market are lower. This is as true in the medical field as it is for corporations in general. Prepaid plans such as Kaiser Foundation Health Plan, Health Insurance Plan of Greater New York, and Group Health Association, to name a few, have not been criticized for producing lower-quality health care than their fee-for-service competitors.

Spillover Effects Among Physicians in For-Profit Entities

Just as the permanence of an organization leads to attempts to maintain or increase quality, so does the size of an organization. In a for-profit organization or in an HMO comprised of a large number of physicians, the quality of care practiced by any one physician in the group affects the reputation, hence the incomes, of the other physicians. This spillover effect helps to ensure that poor medical care is not practiced by the participating physicians. More meaningful utilization review among the participating physicians is expected in such organizations. Under the traditional fee-for-service delivery system, economic incentives do not exist among physicians to monitor other physicians or to impose sanctions against physicians whose performance, when examined by utilization review and tissue committees, is revealed to be unacceptable. Quality of care is thus expected to be higher when physicians practice as part of a group than when they remain economically unaffected by the actions of an incompetent or unethical colleague.

External Quality Review Mechanisms

The states should, as part of their role to protect the health of their citizens, monitor the health and medical outcomes of all delivery systems, including HMOs. Although outcome measures have been difficult to develop, emphasizing even primitive outcome measures in the monitoring process would speed the development of improved measures and allow greater flexibility in the use of medical inputs to achieve those outcomes (32). Measuring quality in terms of inputs used or through the credentials of licensed personnel increases the costs of providing care (hence lessens the competitive advantage of new delivery systems) and would inhibit innovation in the provision of medical care.

The federal government currently uses professional review organizations (PROs) to monitor the hospital care received by Medicare patients. It is too early to judge the effectiveness of these review organizations; in the past such programs have not been effective.

In addition to continual monitoring of the quality of care provided by a state or a federal agency, health officials should publish the results of their quality reviews. For example, the Joint Commission on Accreditation of Hospitals should make available the results of its surveys. Financial penalties and other sanctions should be applied when instances of poor quality are found.[4] Publicizing the results of quality reviews would also serve as an additional stimulus to competing organizations to maintain and increase their quality. Although not all consumers will use that information in choosing their delivery system, some large, informed consumer groups will use it. Other consumers will then benefit by the actions of the better-informed consumer groups. The development of a broader range of quality measures should improve consumers' ability to choose among delivery systems on the basis of quality, access, and cost.

Additional Quality Assurance Mechanisms

Two additional mechanisms are available to assure that the quality of care provided by HMOs and other delivery systems is at least maintained. The first of these is the malpractice system. Poor quality of care is too costly to an organization if it results in an increase in lawsuits and in large awards to the aggrieved parties. The threat of malpractice suits should inhibit the provision of poor quality care.

Another approach that can be used to ensure that low-quality care is not deliberately provided to enrollees is to have a federal quality review board accredit such organizations. In determining minimum criteria for establishing an HMO or other insurance-type system, the federal agency might consider such factors as minimum financial reserve requirements; capacity to serve a minimum size of population, such as 20,000 persons,[5] and limits on the percentage or number of particular categories of the population served—for example, not more than 50 percent of the Medicaid or Medicare population.[6]

Empirical Evidence on Quality of Care

A number of studies have examined the quality of care provided in for-profit enterprises and in prepaid health plans. One indicator of hospital quality is accreditation.

---

[4]Greater use should be made of financial penalties when instances of poor quality are determined to exist. In the past, strong sanctions for poor quality, such as removal of a license to practice or of the accreditation of a hospital, have been considered so severe that they were rarely used. If less drastic measures such as financial penalties were available, it is likely that they would be applied more frequently to minor infractions of quality which would otherwise have gone unpublished.

[5]One reason for establishing a minimum size for the organization is that there is great variability in a person's medical expenses. A small organization might not be able to absorb the possible losses if certain of their patients required treatment for illnesses considered to be catastrophic. One possible remedy to the problem of size of organization is to require minimum-sized organizations to carry reinsurance.

[6]If minimum criteria had been developed for the establishment of HMOs (or prepaid health plans), and if these regulations had been enforced, many of the abuses associated with some of the early HMOs that were established in California to serve the Medicaid population, such as questionable marketing techniques and restrictions on access to enrollees, would not have occurred. See, for example, Milton I. Roemer, "Better Weather Ahead for California's Prepaid Health Plans?" *American Medical News*, October 25, 1976: 7–8. See also Paul M. Ellwood, Jr., "Alternatives to Regulation: Improving the Market," in *Controls on Health Care*, Papers of the Conference on Regulation in the Health Industry (Washington, D.C.: National Academy of Sciences, January 7–9, 1974), 61–63.

There is virtually no difference in accreditation status between investor owned and nonprofit hospital chains (33). As investor owned chains have grown by acquiring independent for-profit hospitals, whose accreditation rates are lowest, accreditation of hospitals has increased. With regard to approval of physicians for staff privileges, there is no statistical difference between hospitals in investor-owned, religious, and nonprofit systems. There was also no significant difference in board certification of staff physicians, or in the numbers of nursing personnel per patient. Independent for-profit hospitals and those owned by state and local governments fare worse on the quality indicators noted above. When outcome measures such as postoperative mortality was examined, no pattern of large persistent differences according to ownership could be detected.

Empirical evidence of capitation systems on quality, based on well-established HMOs, indicates that their quality of care is comparable to or higher than that provided under the traditional fee-for-service system (34). The most recent study in this area, by RAND, compared the health outcomes of subscribers to an HMO to those in a fee-for-service setting (35). The study was able to assign individuals randomly to an HMO or a fee-for-service (FFS) plan in Seattle, Washington. The authors concluded that despite large reductions in the use of services for individuals assigned to the HMO, their health levels were no lower than those in the FFS system; those in the HMO also received more preventive services. Further, those with higher incomes who were initially sick improved more than did a similar group in the FFS system. However, the opposite was true for low-income initially sick persons. The authors caution that this does not mean that those with low income would be better off in a Medicaid FFS plan. In the experiment many of the FFS physicians do not accept Medicaid patients, and their fees were higher than those paid by Medicaid. Thus it is unknown whether initially sick Medicaid patients in a typical FFS system would experience improved health outcomes.

As the emphasis on quality assurance is shifted from educational requirements and individual licensure of participating personnel to measurement of the outcome of medical treatment, much broader latitude should be permitted alternative delivery systems' use of various personnel to perform specified tasks. The licensing of institutions rather than individuals would enable organizations to be more flexible in their use of personnel. Various health manpower personnel would be assigned tasks that match their training and competence rather than those specified by an individual licensing process under state law, as is the current practice. Institutional licensure should, consequently, result in lower costs for providing medical services, without any diminution of the quality of care (36).

EVIDENCE ON THE PERFORMANCE OF HMOS

The performance of HMOs should be examined with respect to two markets. One market is the insurance market; HMOs compete against traditional insurance plans on the basis of their premiums, benefits, accessibility, and quality. The competitive success of HMOs in the insurance market is determined by whether HMOs have been able to increase their market share at the expense of traditional plans. HMOs are also a delivery system and attempt to produce their product at minimum cost, HMOs thus compete against hospitals and physicians that are paid on a FFS basis. If HMOs are a more efficient delivery system, their lower costs will provide them with a cost advantage in the insurance market. The effects of HMOs in each of these markets are examined.

The Efficiency of HMOs As A Delivery System

The early claims that HMOs perform better than the fee-for-service system were based on data from a few of the larger prepaid group practices, such as Kaiser, Health Insurance Plan of Greater New York, and Group Health Association. Comparative data on fee-for-service were based on either utilization surveys of the general population or, in several instances, surveys of groups of employees whose insurance companies, such as Aetna or Blue Cross, provided them with a choice between prepaid and fee-for-service plans. A major problem with many of the early studies was subscriber selectivity; if subscribers with low utilization patterns selected prepaid health plans, differences in utilization rates between HMOs and FFS could not be considered the result of the HMO, nor would it be possible to extrapolate the potential savings if a much larger segment of the population were enrolled in prepaid plans.

A number of studies have looked at the issue of whether HMOs receive a favorable or an adverse risk group (37). Using different methodologies and data, these studies have found that the HMOs examined have had favorable and unfavorable risk selection; and some studies have either found no evidence of biased selection or their results are inconclusive. These studies have investigated biased selection in HMOs among both working-age populations and Medicare enrollees. Niepp and Zeckhauser find that there is very little switching among health plans, approximately 5 percent, and that there is a great deal of persistence by the other 95 percent in their choice of health plan. Thus as plan subscribers remain with their HMO and age over time, preferred or adverse selection should not be a problem (38).

A RAND study undertook a controlled experiment to determine whether the results of HMO studies were due to biased selection or to the style of practice in the HMO (39). Also examined was the amount of out-of-plan use by enrollees in the HMO, since favorable HMO performance could be a result of high out-of-plan use. Individuals were assigned to one of three groups: two fee-for-service (FFS) groups, in one of which all services were free whereas in the other copayments were required, or a third group assigned to the HMO (referred to as the HMO experimental group). The study also examined a group that already belonged to the HMO, referred to as the HMO control group. Expenditures were imputed for use of services in the HMO so that comparisons could be made to those in fee for service.

Imputed expenditures between those in the HMO experimental and control groups were very similar, although the experimental group had a slightly higher out-of-plan expenditure, $63 versus $15. Both HMO groups, however, had much lower expenditures (including out of plan) than those of the free FFS group (23–28 percent less). The size of the expenditures in the HMO groups were comparable to those in the FFS plan, who had to pay a 95 percent copayment up to a family maximum of $1,000 a year. Although expenditures for these groups were comparable, those assigned to the FFS 95 percent copayment group had fewer face-to-face visits than did the two HMO groups. Data on the different groups are presented in Table 12–1.

The large differences between the HMO enrollees and the free FFS group occur in their hospital use rates, which were approximately 40 percent lower for the HMO group. The admission rate in the HMO was 8.4 per 100 persons compared to 13.8;

TABLE 12-1. Comparison of HMO and Fee-for-Service Plans According to Imputed
Expenditures and Use of Services

Plan	Imputed Expenditure per person[a]	Admission Rate per 100 Persons	Hospitals Days per 100 Persons	Face to Face Visits	Preventive Visits
HMO experimental	$439	8.4	49	4.3	.55
HMO control	469	8.3	38	4.7	.60
Fee-for-service					
Free	609	13.8	83	4.2	.41
25%	620	10.0	87	3.5	.32
95%	459	10.5	46	2.9	.29

SOURCE: Willard G. Manning et al., "A Controlled Trial of the Effect of a Prepaid Group Practice on Use of Services," *New England Journal of Medicine*, 310(23), June 7, 1984, Tables 1 and 2.
[a]In 1983 dollars and includes out-of-plan use for HMO enrollees.

patient days per 100 persons in the two groups were 49 versus 83. The authors attribute this lower use rate to the "style of practice" at the HMO, which is less hospital intensive. The hospital use rate for those in the 95 percent FFS plan is less than the rate for the free FFS plan, as expected. Visit rates in the HMO and free FFS plan were similar; however, the HMO enrollees had a greater number of preventive visits, approximately two-thirds of which were for well-child care and gynecologic examinations.

The findings above suggest that as HMO market share increases, it should be followed by decreases in hospital use rates. According to the earlier discussion on quality of care in HMOs, these reductions in hospital use rates are not accompanied by reductions in quality of care. Increasing copayments in the FFS sector will also reduce hospital use rates, but the style of care will be different than in the HMO studied; there will also be fewer ambulatory care visits.

The findings from the study above are supported by evidence from other studies on HMO performance (40). It appears that the total cost of medical care (premium plus out of pocket expenses) for HMO enrollees is 10–40 percent lower than for persons with comparable insurance coverage using the FFS delivery system. Further, HMOs have lower hospital use rates than those of FFS plans. Lower hospitalization is achieved primarily through lower admission rates, although there is some indication of shorter lengths of stay. In general, there are approximately 30 percent fewer hospital days among HMO enrollees as compared to those with fee-for-service coverage. Luft concludes that HMOs do not achieve their lower admission rates as a result of eliminating unnecessary or discretionary procedures; surgical cases are not reduced by a greater proportion than medical cases.

Based on the studies cited above, HMOs appear to be competitive with the FFS system. Given a fair market test, HMOs should grow and increase their market share.

The Competitive Effect of HMOs in the Insurance Market

If HMO subscribers use less hospital care than do those in traditional insurance plans, then, other things being equal, HMOs should be able to market their services at a lower premium and increase their market share. However, since HMOs restrict their enrollee's choice of provider, the HMO must provide additional benefits to offset their

TABLE 12-2. Growth in HMO Enrollment, 1981–1986

Year	Enrollment (Millions)	Annual Percent Increase
1981	10.5	
1982	11.6	10.5
1983	13.7	18.1
1984	16.7	21.9
1985	21.0	25.7
1986	25.8	22.9

SOURCE: "The Interstudy Edge," *Interstudy*, Spring 1987: 3.

greater restrictiveness. HMOs would be expected to increase their market share only if they are able to have lower relative premiums and/or increased benefits, beyond what is necessary to offset their increased restrictiveness. Based on data on HMO growth, HMOs have been sufficiently efficient to enable them to increase their market shares.

HMO enrollment growth really began in the early 1980s, as shown in Table 12-2. In the last several years the annual increases in enrollment have been greater than 20 percent per year. HMO enrollment now represents approximately 15 percent of the population under 65 years of age with health insurance. Of the approximately 26 million HMO enrollees, the majority (71 percent) are enrolled in HMOs that have been in existence for more than 6 years. The greatest percent increase in enrollment, however, is occurring in the newest plans, as shown in Table 12–3. The type of HMO is also changing. The largest increases in enrollment are occurring in for-profit plans, which currently have 42 percent of the enrollees. Along with these changes in ownership, the organization of the HMO is changing as well. IPA-type plans, which contract directly with physicians in private practice, have 37 percent of the enrollees. Network-type HMOs, with 23 percent of the enrollees, contract with independent physician groups. These types of HMOs comprise the majority of all HMOs and are also the fastest-growing models.

Increased HMO market share is expected to bring forth a competitive response from traditional insurance plans, who are losing market share. Traditional plans are likely to undertake several responses. One response is for traditional plans to start their own HMOs. In this way the insurance company is able to offer different products to consumers who have different elasticities of demand. Presumably, those subscribers with the least elastic demands will continue to purchase FFS insurance, which has the highest premium. A second response is for the insurance company to institute utilization review controls so as to reduce their enrollees' hospital use. As the insurance company is able to reduce its hospital costs, it is able to offer additional benefits to its enrollees. If HMOs and insurance companies engaged in premium competition, then instead of increased benefits, premiums would be reduced. Thus, in addition to benefiting their own enrollees, HMOs, through their competitive effects in the insurance market, should benefit all consumers in the area.

When HMO growth begins to decrease the market share of traditional insurors by a significant amount, traditional insurors will respond, with the consequence that hospital occupancy rates will fall. With excess capacity, hospitals are more likely to engage in price competition to increase their business with HMOs.

TABLE 12-3. Year-End Enrollment and Number of HMOs by Age of Plan, Profit Status, and Model Type, 1986

	Total Enrollment 12/31/86	Percent of Total Enrollment	Percent Change 6/86–12/86
All plans	25,777,130	100.0	8.9
Age of plan			
<1 year	719,145	2.8	14.9
1–2 years	3,313,588	12.9	26.8
3–5 years	3,594,288	13.9	11.2
6–9 years	4,976,512	19.3	6.9
10 or more	13,173,597	51.1	5.1
Profit status			
For profit	10,735,498	41.6	18.8
Not-for-profit	15,041,632	58.4	3.4
For profit	10,735,498	41.6	18.8
Not-for-profit	15,041,632	58.4	3.4
Model type[a]			
Staff	2,987,103	11.6	−4.7
Group	6,822,759	26.5	−4.2
Network	6,010,398	23.3	21.3
IPA	9,956,870	38.6	17.8

SOURCE: "The Interstudy Edge," *Interstudy*, Spring 1987: 6.

[a]Staff, an HMO that delivers health services through a physician group that is controlled by the HMO unit; group, an HMO that contracts with one independent group practice to provide health services; network, an HMO that contracts with two or more independent group practices; IPA, an HMO that contracts directly with physicians in independent practices.

The empirical evidence on the foregoing competitive scenario is mixed (41). Studies examining the competitive effect of HMOs are generally based on data that only go up to 1982. These studies find that hospital expense per capita either increases with HMO growth, which is contrary to expectations, or that HMOs do not reduce hospital expenses per capita (42); other studies, using more recent data from another state, find that in highly competitive areas hospital expenses per capita decline (43). As hypothesized, in market-competitive areas, traditional plans respond to HMO growth by starting their own HMOs and instituting utilization controls. Studies confirm that HMO growth is associated with lower hospital admission rates. Empirical studies of market competition have generally not had access to more recent data; thus conclusions as to the effect of market competition have been based on periods where there has been only limited competition. In the next several years a greater number of empirical studies on the effects of market competition on health care costs and use should become available.

The twin cities of Minneapolis-St. Paul have been the subject of a number of case studies as a result of rapid HMO growth. Almost 50 percent of consumers in this market belong to HMOs, which is the highest percentage of any metropolitan area. Approximately 95 percent of the physicians have an affiliation with an HMO. The effects of HMOs have been dramatic. Hospital use in the twin cities has dropped from almost 1,200 patient days per 1,000 population in 1976 to approximately 700 days per 1,000 in 1986. Enrollees in HMOs have use rates of only 385 days per 1,000 compared to 1,087 days per 1,000 for non-HMO subscribers (44). The result of excess hospital capacity has been hospital discounts to HMOs to attract their patients. To participate in these delivery systems, physicians have been willing to accept restrictions on their behavior and to change their style of practice. Traditional providers and insurors have responded to decreased market shares by starting their own HMOs and developing PPOs. HMOs have found themselves in severe competition with other HMOs and insurors. A number of the HMOs are now only marginally profitable or are losing money (45). To reduce their costs, these HMOs have begun to reduce their physicians' fees sharply. Based on anecdotal information and case studies, the experience of the Twin Cities area appears to conform with our expectations of market competition (46). One aspect of market competition that has not been consistent with expectations so far is the lack of premium competition among the various insurance plans for employee groups.

HISTORICAL BARRIERS TO THE DEVELOPMENT OF PREPAID HEALTH PLANS

The theoretical and empirical advantages of prepaid health plans lead one to expect that such plans would have developed in the past and constitute a major share of the medical services market. However, until recently, HMO market share has been very small. If the medical services market were competitive, a demand for such organizations would exist, particularly if prepaid health plans could provide medical care of a quality comparable to that of the fee-for-service system and at a lower cost. A favorable cost structure would undoubtedly lead to an increase in the supply of such plans. But since HMO growth did not occur for many years, we must examine our assumptions about the demand for such plans and possible explanations for the inadequate supply response.

Demands for Prepaid Health Plans

One way to estimate the potential demand for prepaid health plans is to examine what percentage of the population decides to enroll when a prepaid plan is offered in competition with the traditional fee-for-service system. Several prepaid plans, such as Kaiser, require that potential enrollees have a choice between their plan and an alternative, such as Blue Cross-Blue Shield. Based on studies where consumers have had this dual choice option, 20–60 percent of the subscribers chose the prepaid health plan. Choice of health plan is affected by a number of factors. The advantages of HMOs, as seen by subscribers, are their broad coverage, lower expected costs of utilization, and assured access to care. The major disadvantages of HMOs are the limitation on the choice of physician; the consumer often desires to retain the current relationship with his or her physician.

> The evidence so far appears to indicate that closed-panel HMOs are most likely to attract enrollees who do not have established patient-physician relationships, and who tend to be members of younger families with a larger number of

smaller children. These characteristics are often found in areas with high population mobility. Individuals and families new to a community have not had the opportunity to establish a private patient-physician relationship and they also tend to be younger. The closed-panel HMO offers them assured access without their having to search for sources of routine care in a new and unfamiliar community. Having the option available through the workplace, and having the ability to gain at least some information about the delivery characteristics of the HMO, reduces the burden of searching for sources of care. The open-panel HMO, on the other hand, appears to be most appealing to those who already know the physicians within it and who can enroll and simultaneously maintain an already existing patient-physician relationship. (47)

The second disadvantage of HMOs is that there may be an insufficient supply of HMO facilities and physicians in the consumers' area. Third, the prospective subscriber may have insufficient knowledge of how the prepaid plan works. The importance of information on prepaid plans in the selection process is strongly indicated by the relatively high degree of satisfaction among consumers who have joined such plans and by the fact that those consumers have generally remained with those plans. Although it is possible that the type of consumer who joins prepaid plans is different from the type who does not, which could explain the high degree of satisfaction and the low degree of turnover, a more likely explanation is that a minority of consumers select such plans because they are inadequately informed about the function and performance of prepaid plans.

Based on the percentage of consumers who choose to enroll in prepaid health plans when offered a dual choice, we would expect that the percentage of the population at large demanding prepaid plans would greatly exceed those presently enrolled in such plans. To determine why the growth in such plans has not kept up with the potential demand for them, it is necessary to examine the supply side of this market.

Supply Factors Affecting the Growth of Prepaid Health Plans

One supply factor that would affect the growth of HMOs is their efficiency relative to alternative delivery systems. A comparison of HMO costs and their premiums relative to annual expenditures for medical care in the traditional fee-for-service system indicates that HMOs could compete effectively on the basis of their premiums.

The reasons for the very slow growth of HMOs must therefore be found in nonmarket barriers that have inhibited their development. The first such barrier were the attempts by state medical associations to deny hospital privileges to participating physicians, thereby denying prepaid health plans access to hospitals (48). If a prepaid health plan could not provide its potential subscribers with hospital care when needed, the plan could not effectively compete with fee-for-service physicians in the community. According to Reuben Kessel, prepaid health plans represented a lower-priced substitute to fee-for-service physicians because the premium was the same for all persons regardless of their income. Since fee-for-service physicians attempted to price discriminate according to a patient's income, a plan that charges all patients the same premium is a form of price cutting. In the past, state and county medical associations successfully prevented the growth of many prepaid health plans by revoking the membership of, or refusing to grant membership to, physicians who desired to join them; such memberships had been prerequisites for hospital privileges. Therefore, to survive, a prepaid health plan such as Kaiser had to have its own hospitals. Although various medical societies subsequently lost antitrust suits, their actions sufficiently raised the cost to potential prepaid health plans to prevent their large-scale development.

As part of their successful efforts to prevent the growth of prepaid health plans, state medical societies were able to have legislation enacted at a state level that placed additional barriers on prepaid health plan development and on their ability to compete with fee-for-service practice. Restrictive legislation subjected HMOs to strict regulation by the state department of insurance, required physicians to be a majority of the controlling board of an HMO, required HMOs to permit the participation of any physician in the community, required HMOs to be organized on a nonprofit basis, and prohibited HMOs from advertising their benefits and premiums.

Prohibiting an HMO from advertising erects a major barrier to its growth. As discussed above, consumer ignorance of HMOs is an important reason why potential subscribers do not join. Further, HMOs are subject to greater economies of scale than are solo practitioners. An HMO must have certain minimum facilities, an organization to enroll members, and possibly its own hospital. Unless an HMO is able to enroll a sufficient number of subscribers, it will be forced to operate at relatively higher premiums (i.e., the declining portion of it long-run average-cost curve). If an HMO were prevented from advertising, it would take longer to reach the number of enrollees required to make its premium competitive with the fee-for-service sector. The time and losses required were too great an obstacle for many HMOs. Restricting the HMO to nonprofit status further removed any incentives that might have existed for nonphysicians to risk their talents and capital to start on HMO.

Federal and State Initiatives Affecting the Growth of HMOs

Federal efforts to stimulate the growth of HMOs started in 1973 when President Nixon proposed the HMO concept as an approach for restructuring the delivery of medical services. Federal policy during this period provided modest support for the development of HMOs and legitimized their existence (49). Ideally, the HMO legislation that was enacted should have removed any barriers that prevented HMOs from competing with their fee-for-service competitors, without providing either with any competitive advantages. However, although the early federal legislation did remove some barriers, it imposed greater requirements on HMOs, thereby decreasing their ability to compete. Some legislators may have preferred to allow HMOs to compete with fee-for-service medicine; others, and the interests they represented, wanted to prevent a fair market test of their ability to compete; while still other legislators viewed HMOs as a vehicle for achieving social change. No matter what the legislative motivation, requirements were placed on HMOs that increased their costs relative to fee-for-service medicine.

The favorable aspects of the HMO legislation were to exempt federally qualified HMOs from restrictive state laws, to allow the HMOs to advertise their benefits and rates, and provision for a dual-choice option. When a federally qualified HMO was available, employers were required to offer an HMO option to their employees along with the traditional health insurance coverage. To take advantage of these favorable factors, however, federally qualified HMOs had to adopt requirements that would have placed them at a competitive disadvantage. These included (a) a relatively large financial requirement; (b) placing HMOs under certificate-of-need (CON) laws;[7] (c) reimbursing HMOs either on a cost basis (thereby removing the financial incentives for HMOs to compete with fee-for-service medicine on the basis of price) or on a fixed-price basis with perverse incentives (e.g., in Oregon an HMO had to absorb all losses, while retaining none of its savings); (d) mandating a very costly benefit package (thereby increasing their premiums relative to the more usual health insurance premiums offered); (e) placing HMOs under permanent regulation by the Secretary of Health, Education, and Welfare; (f) requiring open enrollment [persons joining HMOs during the open enrollment periods incur 80 percent greater costs (50)]; and (g) requiring community rating as the basis for establishing premiums.

Based on their premiums relative to those of traditional insurers, HMOs could compete effectively with the fee-for-service system. However, the requirements necessary to become a federally qualified HMO imposed greater burdens on them than on their competitors. In more recent years, some of the more stringent requirements imposed on HMOs were loosened. For example, in 1976 Congress relaxed the HMO benefits and eligibility requirements mandated by the 1973 HMO Act. This followed complaints from HMOs that these requirements increased their premiums so that they could not be competitive with regular health insurance plans. Also, as part of the 1979 Health Planning Act, large HMOs (enrollment greater than 50,000 persons) were exempted from the CON process. Rather than this being procompetitive legislation for all HMOs, however, the main beneficiaries were the larger, established HMOs.

A recent federal effort to increase HMO enrollment has been the HMO voucher. In the last several years, Medicare and Medicaid eligibles have been given an opportunity to enroll in HMOs. A Medicare voucher works as follows: the federal government contributes 95 percent of the value of the voucher, thereby saving 5 percent, by basing the value of the voucher on the average per capita cost for a Medicare beneficiary within a geographic area (AAPC). The voucher is to be applied to the purchase of an approved health plan. Participation by Medicare eligibles in the voucher system is voluntary. It is compulsory when applied to the Medicaid population.

Medicare vouchers serve several purposes. First, they save the government money—5 percent of the AAPC. Second, the voucher limits the federal government's contributions under Medicare to a fixed-dollar amount per beneficiary per year, thereby making the government's outlays predictable and controllable. The risk of higher than expected Medicare expenditures is transferred from the government to private organizations. Second, a voucher system stimulates HMO enrollment.

The Medicare voucher system has only recently started, and there are mixed reports on its performance. Are HMOs competing by increasing benefits, or are some underserving the aged? Another concern is that some persons believe that HMOs will receive a favorable risk group and the voucher system will just cost the government more money. It has been estimated that 9 percent of the aged incur 70 percent of Medicare's expenditures, a large portion of which are spent on services to people who die within a year. Persons who are ill or who have chronic conditions are generally reluctant to leave their physician and switch to an HMO. Under such circumstances the HMO will enroll those aged who are healthier and have lower expenditures. If the

---

[7]According to an Interstudy survey conducted in 1973, 48 percent of the responding HMOs said that such CON laws represented moderate or severe barriers to their growth. Richard McNeil and Robert Schlenker, "HMOs, Competition, and Government," *Interstudy*, December 1974: p. 20.

HMO receives the AAPC for a Medicare beneficiary, a voluntary voucher system could end up costing the federal government more money. The government would continue paying for the high-cost aged, while HMOs would enroll those with lower average costs. Approaches to resolving this problem, such as adjusting the voucher amount according to health status, are being considered. If the voucher system were mandatory for all aged persons, this problem of risk selection would not occur. A number of HMOs, however, are reporting that they are losing money on the voucher program. Thus it is not clear that they are receiving favorable risk groups. It is too early to judge the utilization and cost experience of the participating HMOs.

CONCLUDING COMMENTS

Maintaining a Competitive Market in Medical Care

The concept of market competition as the basic approach for organizing economic activity in our economy has been accepted for quite some time. Until recently, however, self-regulation by the health professions has not only been the norm but also the preferred approach of the professions.

Certain rules of the game must be established and all the participants should abide by these rules if competition is to achieve its desired outcomes. The participants' behavior in the market must be monitored to ensure that they do not violate the rules. Monitoring behavior and intervening when necessary is the role of antitrust activity. Competitors may violate the rules of the marketplace so as to enhance their market position. If health care providers or third-party payors can use illegal means to achieve a monopoly position, they can increase their revenues. The public is harmed by such activities because they pay higher prices and have fewer choices.

Not all types of self-regulation by the professions are anticompetitive. Activities by professional associations that provide increased information on the quality and characteristics of health care providers, such as specialty certification, do not limit either entry or choice of provider. Such actions may improve market performance by providing the consumer with more information. In the past, however, professional regulation resulted in limits on entry and choice of provider, as well as other forms of anticompetitive behavior.

Anticompetitive behavior is illegal on either per se grounds or by virtue of the rule of reason. Per se violations are price fixing, economic boycotts, tying arrangements, and division of horizontal markets; these activities are believed to be obviously anticompetitive and their effects are clearly harmful to consumers. Price fixing occurs when two or more competitors agree on a price at which their service will be sold. An example is when a Medicaid agency requests bids and two providers agree to submit similar prices. It does not matter whether the fixed prices are minimums or maximums; they are both illegal. A boycott occurs when, for example, a medical society threatens to "departicipate" from Blue Shield or other third party payor if their payment demands are not met. "Tying" occurs when a purchaser who wants to purchase one product is also required to buy a second product (e.g., operating room and anesthesiology services as well). When competitors agree to divide up geographic markets, consumers, or services, and not compete with each other, it is illegal.

Other forms of anticompetitive behavior are analyzed according to the rule of reason, which attempts to determine whether the anticompetitive harm caused by the restraint exceeds the procompetitive benefits of not permitting the particular activity. Examples of cases brought under the rule of reason are hospital mergers (whether there would be decreased competition from among the remaining hospitals), staff privilege issues (as when a physician claims that they were denied privileges, thereby depriving them of the right to compete against current staff physicians), and the formation of PPOs (Is the PPO so large that it becomes a form of price fixing, or is the PPO a procompetitive organization?).

The application of antitrust laws to the health field is disturbing to many, for reasons of both economic self-interest and ideology. Some people have a basic distrust of market forces and of the ability of individuals to cope in such situations. Others fear that their incomes and preferred positions will be competed away.

Because of its desirable outcomes, society has decided to rely on competitive markets, the maintenance of which is a proper role of government. As new delivery and payment systems emerge in the health field, antitrust questions will be raised as to whether these new arrangements are procompetitive (e.g., take advantage of economies of scale) or whether they are a means of lessening competition among competitors. An appreciation of the economics of competitive markets is essential for understanding the probable antitrust implications of these new arrangements.

Cost Shifting

The concern by some payors with cost shifting has intensified as the government has moved to a fixed-price (DRG) system and as some payors, such as HMOs, are using their market power to receive discounts from hospitals. It is believed by some that hospitals will increase their charges to private-pay patients and to those with commercial insurance. The latter group of payors will then be used to subsidize other payor groups who may not be paying their "fair" share. The practice of raising prices to one group of patients because another group of patients do not pay their full charges has been referred to as "cost shifting" (51).

Cost shifting may be analyzed using a price discrimination model. Assume that there are two payors, the federal government and commercial insurance. The federal government as a large purchaser of hospital care for Medicare patients uses its market power and establishes a single hospital price for all Medicare patients. As shown in Figure 9–4, the hospital faces a horizontal demand curve for its Medicare patients. Assuming that the other payor group does not have as much market power as the government, the hospital faces a downward-sloping demand curve by non-Medicare patients. If the hospital sets its prices so as to maximize its profits, it will establish a price for non-Medicare patients that will be higher than the fixed Medicare price; the non-Medicare price will be at that point on the demand curve where the marginal revenues from both types of patients are equal. According to this analysis, however, if the Medicare price were decreased, the profit-maximizing strategy for the hospital would be to decrease, not increase, the price to non-Medicare patients (assuming no change in the marginal costs of treating non-Medicare patients).

The analysis above is contrary to what many persons believe happens as the government or other payors reduce their payments to hospitals. The hospital may want to increase its price to non-Medicare patients if it receives less from government. However, if the hospital is pricing to maximize its profits, then increasing its price beyond that point will reduce its profits. The only reason why the hospital may raise its prices is if its costs of serving non-Medicare patients increase (e.g., inflation or a sicker mix of non-Medicare patients). As these costs increase and the price of non-Medicare patients increase, it may be thought to be the result of low Medicare payment; however, the increased prices would have occurred anyway. The hospital may say that it will raise prices to non-Medicare patients if the government pays hospitals less; however, this may be more of an attempt by hospitals to scare non-Medicare payors into lobbying with them against government reductions in Medicare prices.

There is a situation under which cost shifting can occur (i.e., a reduction in government payment results in an increase in non-Medicare prices). The hospital could have been pricing in a non-profit-maximizing manner. The hospital could have been forgoing profits by setting prices to non-Medicare patients at less than the profit-maximizing level. With a decrease in government payment, the hospital could then decide to raise its non-Medicare prices.

How likely is it that hospitals were not setting profit-maximizing prices according to their different payor types? As discussed previously, hospitals have certain objectives. If physicians are the dominant group in control of the hospital, they would prefer that any additional hospital revenues be used to increase their productivity and income. Increased numbers of hospital personnel, interns and residents, new equipment, or even lower charges for hospital services that are complementary to their own are examples of the opportunity costs of charging "too low" a price to non-Medicare patients. Even using a different behavioral model of the hospital, there is an opportunity cost of forgoing additional profit. Given the different ways in which the forgone profit could be used—namely, to charge non-Medicare patients less or to forgo ways of achieving the hospital decisionmakers' objectives—it is more likely that the profit would be used by the hospital decisionmakers than for a group (e.g., private-pay patients or insurance companies) that is not as politically important to the hospital.

Cost shifting is the recognition that some payor groups pay higher prices relative to costs than others. This practice has existed for many years; it is not a recent phenomenon. Payors that have less elastic demands for hospital care will pay higher prices relative to costs than will payors with more elastic demands. However, hospital prices to a payor group will not be increased further when another payor group pays less, since the hospital was presumably already charging all payor groups a profit-maximizing price.

Market Competition and the Rise in Medical Expenditures

There is concern that the increase in market competition that has occurred in the last several years has not had the dampening effect on the rise in medical expenditures that was expected. Market competition is viewed, by some, as being ineffective in constraining total medical expenditures.

It is too early to judge how successful market competition will be in reducing the rise in expenditures. Some parts of the country (e.g., California and Minneapolis) are more engaged in competition than others. Businesses, insurors, and providers have not all become totally market oriented. It takes time to learn which strategies are more effective, and the pressures to adapt differ across regions of the country. The competitive strategy has emphasized decreased use of the hospital and this has been effective.

There has, however, been an increase in use of nonhospital services. It is likely that greater scrutiny will be given to the rise in ambulatory expenditures.

It is also inappropriate to judge the competitive strategy solely on whether the rise in medical expenditures can be held down to what is achieved by a regulatory system in another country. One of the forces influencing medical expenditures is the development of new life-enhancing technology (52). If the public is willing to pay for such technologies, in both the public and private sectors, expenditures will be greater than otherwise. Market incentives require providers to be efficient if they are to survive; they must also respond to consumer demands. If consumers believe that these technologies are worthwhile and are willing to pay for them, then, in a market system, they will be provided and this would be an appropriate outcome.

As discussed earlier on the determinants of the demand for medical care, it was found that medical care is income elastic; that is, an increase in income will result in at least a proportionate increase in expenditures on medical care. Quality is also presumably income elastic. Thus as incomes increase, other things held constant, expenditures on medical care should also increase. Increases in medical expenditures are thus perfectly consistent with a competitive market system. The following is an example of how this has led to increased medical expenditures.

Many employers have adopted cost-containment programs; however, after several years of small increases, their premiums have begun to increase more rapidly. One reason for this is an increase in new benefits to their employees (the income elasticity argument). As employers instituted deductibles and utilization programs in the early 1980s, hospital utilization of the nonaged declined. These declines in use rates were a one-time savings. Employers then started increasing employee health benefits, such as raising maximum annual payments for diagnostic services, adding a home care benefit, increasing substance abuse coverage, and improving catastrophic coverage by limiting the maximum out-of-pocket expenditure of the employee (53).

It is not yet clear, however, why medical expenditures are increasing at their current rate. Are there still inefficiencies in the system that have not been eliminated, are new technologies expanding, or are there changes in benefits that are being demanded? There are two other possible reasons why expenditures are increasing. The first is increased state regulation mandating new benefits. To shift the burden of health costs from the state to employers and to satisfy certain interest groups, many states are mandating health benefits on employers. There are currently over 640 mandated state benefit requirements, many of which have occurred in recent years. For a more complete discussion of this issue, see Chapter 20. Their effect is to increase employer-paid health insurance premiums.

Most employers do not separately fund their retirees' health care costs. As the number of retirees and their health expenditures increase, they are paid from current expenditures and are generally not separated from active employee premiums. The federal government has begun to shift responsibility for the retirees' health costs to the employer. For example, in 1984 the employer was made responsible for the health costs of their active Medicare eligible employees; this caused an increase in their employees' health insurance premiums. Over the next several years a clearer picture should emerge as to the likely effects of market competition and the reasons for continued increases in medical care expenditures.

A Summing Up

Increased regulation of the health sector is one approach for improving the performance of hospitals and other providers of medical care. The other approach for achieving greater efficiency in the production of medical services is to rely on market competition. The traditional belief among medical planners has been that competition is wasteful and should be eliminated. Under a system of insurance that provided first-dollar coverage, cost-based reimbursement for hospital care, and an absence of the physician's fiscal responsibility for the resources used in treatment, competition among providers led to duplication of beds and facilities, overutilization of hospitals, and rapidly increasing costs. The outcomes of competition depend upon the incentives faced by consumers and providers. Previous payment methods and patient and provider incentives encouraged higher costs.

The introduction of market competition to health care carries with it both positive and negative consequences. On the positive side, the public now has a greater choice of delivery systems. Those willing to limit their choice of provider, such as HMOs, can have lower out-of-pocket costs for medical care. There is also a great deal more innovation in methods for delivering medical services. Same-day outpatient surgery, hospices, and home care are examples of alternative methods of providing care that were previously provided in the hospital. Providers have become more responsive to the public's preferences.

Increased concern by business over employee health costs and premium competition among insurors is resulting in greater efficiency in the provision of medical services. Hospitals must be efficient if they are to compete with HMOs or if they want to form a PPO. DRGs also provide hospitals with incentives to keep costs down. The cost of duplicated facilities can no longer be passed on to third-party payors. There is also increased attention to managerial cost controls. An example of this is the development by hospitals of computer profiles on their physicians to determine whether they are prescribing too many tests or not discharging their patients soon enough.

There has always been a concern that quality of care would suffer under a price-competitive system. There is the fear that some physicians would engage in unethical behavior to increase their incomes or that HMOs and other providers would now have an incentive to provide fewer services based on consumer ignorance. It is too early to document the effect of market competition on quality. However, to the extent that HMOs and PPOs are enrolling employees directly at the workplace, unions and companies provide an oversight function. There is also likely to be greater emphasis on quality of care for those providers that are part of larger groups or that participate in alternative delivery systems. The negative effects of price competition are likely to be found among individuals that are not part of an employee group. It is more difficult for the individual to detect poor quality, and as a consequence the costs to the provider of providing less-than-optimal service are less.

It should be emphasized again that neither a market approach nor regulation alone will solve all of the concerns that people have with regard to medical care. Redistributing medical services requires government intervention; however, government involvement need not be direct. Government subsidies can be provided through a market mechanism, such as the use of vouchers. Given a redistribution subsidy, a market approach to the delivery of services can be compared to a regulatory system to determine which approach can more efficiently achieve the redistribution objective.

REFERENCES

1. Martha Derthick and Paul Quirk, *The Politics of Deregulation* (Washington, D.C.: Brookings Institution, 1985).

2. For a more complete discussion, see Paul J. Feldstein, *The Politics of Health Legislation: An Economic Perspective*, (Ann Arbor, Mich.: Health Administration Press, 1988), Chapter 5.

3. "Health Professions Educational Assistance Amendments of 1965," *Hearing Before the Subcommittee on Health of the Committee on Labor and Public Welfare*, U.S. Senate, 89th Congress, 1st Session, September 8, 1965, pp. 39–40.

4. For a complete discussion of CON and its legislative changes, see Clark C. Havighurst, *Deregulating the Health Care Industry: Planning for Competition* (Cambridge, Mass.: Ballinger, 1982) p. 222.

5. *Ibid.*

6. Alain C. Enthoven, *Health Plan* (Reading, Mass.: Addison-Wesley, 1980).

7. For a more complete discussion of these issues, see: "Tax Incentives: Competition, Round Two," *Medicine and Health Perspectives*, October 12, 1981; Donald W. Moran, "HMOs, Competition and the Politics of Minimum Benefits," *Milbank Memorial Fund Quarterly*, Spring 1981; Alain C. Enthoven, "How Interested Groups Have Responded to a Proposal for Economic Competition in Health Services," *American Economic Review*, May 1980; and John K. Iglehart, "Drawing the Lines for the Debate on Competition," *New England Journal of Medicine*, July 30, 1981.

8. *Medicaid Freedom of Choice Waiver Activities*, Hearing Before the Subcommittee on Health of the Committee on Finance, U.S. Senate, 98th Congress, 2nd Session, March 30, 1984.

9. *Company Practices in Health Care Cost Management* (Lincolnshire, Ill.: Hewitt Associates, 1984).

10. Lawrence G. Goldberg and Warren Greenberg, "The Emergence of Physician-Sponsored Health Insurance: A Historical Perspective," in Warren Greenberg, ed., *Competition in the Health Care Sector* (Germantown, Md.: Aspen Systems Corporation, 1978).

11. For a review of antitrust actions in the health field, see L. Barry Costillo, "Antitrust Enforcement in Health Care: Ten Years After the AMA Suit," *New England Journal of Medicine*, 313(14), October 3, 1985; Robert F. Leibenluft and Michael R. Pollard, "Antitrust Scrutiny of the Health Professions: Developing a Framework for Assessing Private Restraints," *Vanderbilt Law Review*, 34(4), May 1981; and Clark C. Havighurst, "Antitrust Enforcement in the Medical Services Industry," *Milbank Memorial Fund Quarterly*, 58(1), Winter 1980; and Arthur N. Lerner, "Federal Trade Commission Anti-Trust Activities in the Health Care Services Field," *Antitrust Bulletin*, 29(2), Summer 1984: 205–224.

12. For a more complete discussion of this idea, see Kenneth Warner, "Health Maintenance Insurance: Toward an Optimal HMO," *Policy Sciences 10*, December 1978.

13. Paul J. Feldstein, Thomas Wickizer, and John R. C. Wheeler, "Private Cost Containment: The Effects of Utilization Review Programs on Health Care Use and Expenditures," *New England Journal of Medicine*, May 19, 1988.

14. David Dranove, Mark Satterthwaite, and Jody Sindelar, "The Effect of Injecting Price Competition into the Hospital Market: The Case of Preferred Provider Organizations," *Inquiry*, 23, Winter 1986: 419–431.

15. "Data Bank," *Modern Healthcare*, May 22, 1987: p. 102. The next closest state was Florida with 36 PPOs.

16. Jon Gabel et al., "The Emergence and Future of PPOs," *Journal of Health Politics, Policy and Law*, 11(2), Summer 1986: 305–322.

17. Glenn A. Melnick and Jack Zwanziger, "Hospital Behavior Under Competition and Cost Containment Policies: The California Experience, 1980–1985," RAND Working Paper, June 17, 1987.

18. James C. Robinson, Deborah W. Garnick, and Stephen J. McPhee, "Market and Regulatory Influences on the Availability of Coronary Angioplasty and Bypass Surgery in U.S. Hospitals," *New England Journal of Medicine*, 317(2), July 9, 1987: 85–90.

19. For a comprehensive review of the advertising literature, see William S. Comanor and Thomas A. Wilson, "Advertising and Competition: A Survey," *Journal of Economic Literature*, 17, June 1979. For a more recent survey, see Sherman T. Folland, "The Effects of Health Care Advertising," *Journal of Health Politics, Policy and Law*, 10(2), Summer 1985.

20. George Stigler, "The Economics of Information," *Journal of Political Economy*, 69(3), June 1961.

21. Lee Benham and Alexandra Benham, "Regulating Through the Professions: A Perspective on Information Control," *Journal of Law and Economics*, October 1975.

22. *Ibid.*, pp. 433, 435.

23. Lee Benham, "The Effects of Advertising on the Price of Eyeglasses," *Journal of Law and Economics*, 15, October 1972.

24. Benham and Benham, *op. cit.*, p.438.

25. Statement of the National Retired Teachers' Association and the American Association of Retired Persons on the Economics of the Eyeglasses Industry Before the Monopoly Subcommittee of the Senate Small Business Committee, U.S. Senate, May 24, 1977. Cited in Lee Benham, "Guilds and the Form of Competition in the Health Care Sector," in Greenberg, ed., *op. cit.*

26. John E. Kwoka, Jr., "Advertising and the Price and Quality of Optometric Services," *American Economic Review*, 74(1), March 1984: 211–216.

27. *Ibid.*, p. 213.

28. *Ibid.*

29. Using data from a previous FTC study in which the FTC trained 19 professional interviewers to identify the equipment and procedures used in eye examinations, Haas-Wilson found that commercial practice restrictions used in various states in 1977 increased the price of an eye examination and a pair of eyeglasses by 5–13 percent, holding constant the thoroughness of the eye exam and the accuracy of the eyeglass prescription. Deborah Haas-Wilson, "The Effect of Commercial Practice Restrictions: The Case of Optometry," *Journal of Law and Economics*, April 29, 1986: 165–186. In another study on the effect of advertising restrictions on the price of optometric examinations, the authors found that the "price is 16 percent higher in states that ban both optometric and optician price advertising,

when examination length, procedures, and office equipment are held consistent." Roger Feldman and James Begun, "The Effects of Advertising: Lessons from Optometry," *Journal of Human Resources*, Supplement, 1978: p. 247. For a discussion of advertising prescription drugs directly to consumers, see Alison Masson and Paul H. Rubin, "Matching Prescription Drugs and Consumers: The Benefits of Direct Advertising," *New England Journal of Medicine*, 313 (8), August 22, 1985: 513–515.

30. Arnold S. Relman and Uwe E. Reinhardt, "Debating For-Profit Health Care," *Health Affairs*, 5(2) Summer 1986. This exchange was initiated as a result of the authors' participation in the following report. Institute of Medicine, *For-Profit Enterprise in Health Care* (Washington, D.C.: National Academy Press, 1986).

31. Paul M. Ellwood, Jr. and Barbara A. Paul, "But What About Quality?" *Health Affairs*, 5(1), Spring 1986: p. 137.

32. For an excellent conceptualization of the issues as well as a review of the literature on quality, see Avedis Donabedian, *The Definition of Quality and Approaches to Its Assessment*, Vol. I (Ann Arbor, Mich.: Health Administration Press, 1980).

33. A summary of studies on hospital quality is contained in Chapter 6 of the Institute of Medicine report, *op. cit.*

34. M. Roemer and W. Schonick, "HMO Performance: The Recent Evidence," *Milbank Memorial Fund Quarterly*, 51, 1973. See also F. C. Cunningham and J. W. Williamson, "How Does the Quality of Health Care in HMOs Compare to That in Other Settings?" *Group Health Journal*, Winter 1980.

35. John E. Ware, Jr., et al., "Comparison of Health Outcomes at a Health Maintenance Organization with Those of Fee-for-Service Care," *Lancet*, 1(8488) May 3, 1986: 1017–1022. See also a follow up analysis of the same data, Elizabeth M. Sloss et al., "Effect of a Health Maintenance Organization on Physiologic Health," *Annals of Internal Medicine*, 106(1), January 1987: 130–138.

36. For a more complete discussion of the idea of institutional licensure, see N. Hershey, "The Inhibiting Effect upon Innovation of the Prevailing Licensure System," *Annals of the New York Academy of Sciences*, 166, 1969: 951–959.

37. A recent survey article on biased selection in HMOs is Gail R. Wilensky and Louis F. Rossiter, "Patient Self-Selection in HMOs," *Health Affairs*, 5(1), Spring 1986: 66–80. The proceedings of a conference on "Biased Selection in Health Care Markets" (also reviewed by Wilensky and Rossiter) has been published in Richard Scheffler and Louis Rossiter, eds., *Advances in Health Economics and Health Services* (Greenwich, Conn.: JAI Press, 1985).

38. J. Niepp and R. Zeckhauser, "Persistence in the Choice of Health Plans," in Scheffler and Rossiter, eds., *op. cit.*

39. Willard G. Manning et al., "A Controlled Trial of the Effect of a Prepaid Group Practice on Use of Services," *New England Journal of Medicine*, 310(23), June 7, 1984.

40. Harold S. Luft, *Health Maintenance Organizations: Dimensions of Performance*, (New York: Wiley, 1981). See also Harold S. Luft, "How Do Health Maintenance Organizations Achieve Their 'Savings'?" *New England Journal of Medicine*, June 15, 1978: 1336–1343.

41. Richard G. Frank and W. P. Welch, "The Competitive Effects of HMOs: A Review of the Evidence," *Inquiry*, 22, Summer 1985: 148–161. A survey of the liter-

ature on competition in the health field up until 1981 may be found in Kathryn M. Langwell and Sylvia F. Moore, *A Synthesis of Research on Competition in the Financing and Delivery of Health Services* (Hyattsville, Md.: National Center For Health Services Research, 1982).

42. For an example of the latter effect, see Catherine G. Mclaughlin, "HMO Growth and Hospital Expenses and Use: A Simultaneous-Equation Approach," *Health Services Research*, 22(2), June 1987: 183–205.

43. Melnick and Zwanziger, *op. cit.*

44. Claire H. Kohrman, "Medical Practice Where HMOs Dominate: The Perspective of Physicians in Minneapolis-St.Paul," *Journal of Medical Practice Management*, 2(2), Fall 1986: p. 87. See also John K. Iglehart, "The Twin Cities' Medical Marketplace," *New England Journal of Medicine*, 311(5), August 2, 1984.

45. "Doctors Dilemma: Unionizing," *New York Times*, July 13, 1987: p. 24.

46. For a cautious commentary on the effects of market competition, see Harold S. Luft, Susan Maerki, and Joan Trauner, "The Competitive Effects of Health Maintenance Organizations: Another Look at the Evidence From Hawaii, Rochester, and Minneapolis/St. Paul," *Journal of Health Politics, Policy and Law*, 10, Winter 1986.

47. S. E. Berki and Marie L. F. Ashcraft, "HMO Enrollment: Who Joins What and Why: A Review of the Literature," *Milbank Memorial Fund Quarterly*, Fall 1980.

48. See Reuben Kessel, "Price Discrimination in Medicine," *Journal of Law and Economics*, October 1958. This article is discussed more completely in Chapter 14.

49. This discussion in this section is based on the paper by Richard McNeil and Robert Schlenker, "HMOs, Competition, and Government," *Interstudy*, December 1974. For background on the legislative aspects of the HMO Act and its various amendments, see the *Congressional Quarterly Almanac*, various years. For a detailed discussion on the early HMO legislation, see Joseph Falkson, *HMOs and the Politics of Health System Reform* (Chicago: American Hospital Association, 1980).

50. Walter McClure, "A Critique of the Health Maintenance Act of 1972," *Interstudy*, February 1974.

51. For a more extensive discussion of cost shifting, see Charles E. Phelps, "Cross-Subsidies and Charge Shifting in American Hospitals," in Frank Sloan, James Blumstein, and James Perrin, eds., *Uncompensated Hospital Care* (Baltimore: Johns Hopkins University Press, 1986); Richard W. Foster, "Cost-Shifting Under Cost Reimbursement and Prospective Payment," *Journal of Health Economics*, 4, 1985: 261–271; and Frank Sloan and Edmund Becker, "Cross-Subsidies and Payment for Hospital Care," *Journal of Health Politics, Policy and Law*, 8(4), 1984: 660–685.

52. William B. Schwartz, "The Inevitable Failure of Cost Containment Strategies," *Journal of the American Medical Association*, 1987.

53. Robert N. Frumkin, "Health Insurance Trends in Cost Control and Coverage," *Monthly Labor Review*, 109(9), September 1986. See also *Employee Benefits in Medium and Large Firms, 1985*, Bulletin 2262, U.S. Department of Labor, July 1986.

CHAPTER 13

Health Manpower Shortages and Surpluses: Definitions, Measurement, and Policies

Within the context of the overall market for medical care, the various categories of health manpower comprise separate submarkets. The health manpower professions are thus an *input* to the provision of medical services. In Chapter 3 it was shown that the overall market for medical care consists of a set of institutional markets, a set of health manpower markets, and a set of markets in which the demand and supply of health manpower education occurs. With a change in the demand for medical care, perhaps resulting from an increase in the population with insurance coverage, there will be increases in the demand for the institutional settings in which medical care is provided, and, subsequently, an increase in demand by the different institutional settings for inputs used in the production of their services. The demand for the different health manpower professions is, therefore, a *derived* demand, derived from the demand for medical and institutional services. These demands by the various institutions for different types of health manpower, together with the existing stock of trained health manpower, will determine the wages, the number of persons employed, and their participation rate (what percent of the available stock of each health manpower profession is employed). The health education institutions determine the long-run supply or stock of health manpower in each profession.

How well the different health manpower and education markets perform has an effect not only on the wages and number of health professionals, but also on the price and quantity of medical and institutional services. Since the various submarkets are interrelated and feed into the market for medical services, the efficiency with which the health manpower market performs will affect prices and outputs in each of the other markets; the more efficient a market is, the greater will be its output. Thus an important reason for examining the separate health manpower markets for different categories of health professionals is to determine how well each market performs. If the markets are determined not to perform well, we will want to examine alternative approaches for improving their performance, giving due consideration to the reasons for inadequate performance.

The market for health professional *education* will also be examined to determine whether it is performing efficiently—that is, whether the quantity of health professional education has been "optimal" over different time periods and whether health education is being produced efficiently. The market for health professional education is important not only because it determines the long-run supply of health manpower, but also because it has been the recipient of a great deal of federal and state funding. Where federal and state health manpower legislation exists in any of the separate health manpower and health education markets, it will be analyzed to determine both its purpose and how effective it has been in achieving its stated goals.

Besides analyzing the efficiency of the separate health manpower markets, the performance of the markets for health professional education, and public policies in these areas, primarily governmental funding policies, we shall examine alternative approaches for forecasting health manpower "requirements." Because forecasts of health manpower have served as the basis for much of the federal and state legislation dealing with health manpower, the usefulness of different forecasting approaches will be examined.

DEFINITIONS OF A HEALTH MANPOWER SHORTAGE

To determine how efficiently a manpower market is performing, we begin by discussing the concept of health manpower shortages, which are often used as an indication of inadequate performance and form the basis for subsequent government intervention.

Health manpower shortages may have different meanings to different people. Often, policy prescriptions are proposed to alleviate all shortage situations. Policy prescriptions, however, should vary according to the type of shortage. This section therefore will discuss different definitions of shortage, together with the appropriate policy prescription for each. Subsequent sections discuss the measurement of the various types of shortages and apply the definitions and their measurement to different health manpower markets.

Normative Judgment of a Shortage

There are several *noneconomic* definitions of health manpower shortages. An example is the statement that the demand for physicians "ought" to be greater. It has also been said that the "need" for physicians is greater than the demand or that the price of physician services is "too high", thereby preventing people from consuming all the physician services they need. A normative judgment of a shortage is that there is a shortage of effective demand relative to what it should be. The noneconomic defini-

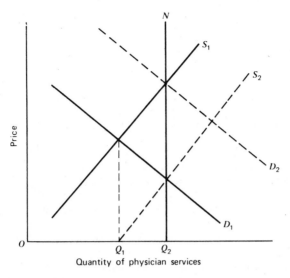

Figure 13-1. Alternative policy prescriptions based upon a normative shortage of health manpower.

tions of a shortage are based either upon a value judgment of how much care people should receive, or upon 'a professional determination of how much physician care is appropriate in the population.

Such normative judgments of shortage are based upon a determination of "need" in the population, or upon some professional estimate of health manpower requirements. For example, physician/population ratios in high-income states are contrasted with physician/population ratios in low-income states. The differences in the ratio are believed to indicate the "need" for physicians in low-income states, which is the number of physicians "required" to achieve a physician/population ratio equal to that of the high-income states. (The ratio technique is discussed in more detail below.)

The classic example of the use of professional determination to determine the number of physicians "needed" was the study by Lee and Jones (1). Lee and Jones based their estimate of the number of physicians required on estimates of the incidence of morbidity and on the number of physician hours required to provide both preventive and therapeutic services to the population. The policy proposals that result from normative definitions of a shortage of health manpower are generally the same: increase the number of trained professionals through increased federal funding.

In Figure 13-1 it is assumed that the initial situation is represented by the supply and demand diagrams S_1 and D_1, resulting in the quantity of physician services Q_1. The number of physician services for the population, based on either need or professional determination, is determined to be Q_2. The usual policy prescription to achieve an increase in physician services is to shift the supply of physicians to S_2, thereby increasing physician services to Q_2. Q_2 of physician services can also be achieved by shifting the demand schedule to D_2. This would not require a shift in supply or in the number of physicians. (A shift in demand can be achieved through a demand subsidy, such as insurance coverage for physician services.) Thus the normative judgment of a shortage of physician services, $Q_1 - Q_2$, can be alleviated either by increasing the number of physicians (shifting S_1 to S_2) or by subsidizing the demand for physician services (shifting D_1 to D_2) along a given supply curve. A movement along a given supply curve represents increased production by existing physicians; physicians either work longer hours and/or they use more auxiliary personnel.

Which policy alternative—the demand or the supply shift—is preferable depends upon the cost of each proposal, the population groups receiving the benefits, and the length of time required to achieve the increase in services consumed. Normative judgments of a manpower shortage can be alleviated in various ways; however, these judgments of a shortage say nothing about how well the market for such health professionals is functioning. The market for physicians may be functioning efficiently, although some persons may believe there "should" be more physicians; conversely, the number of physicians may be less than would be produced in an efficiently functioning market. The basic policy prescription using a normative definition of a shortage, however, is always for federal funding to achieve an increase in the number of physicians. If the market is not performing efficiently, there might be alternative ways of achieving an increase in the number of physicians or physician services *without* resorting to federal funding. Perhaps some legal barriers might be changed to permit an increase in the physician supply. To determine how well the market for health professionals is functioning, we must establish the economic definitions of a shortage and examine how such shortages may occur. Possible policy prescriptions for correcting these shortages will be an outgrowth of their analysis.

Economic Definitions of Shortages in Health Manpower

In a competitive market, market equilibrium occurs when the value placed on a good or service by its demanders equals the cost of the resources used in its production. When the value placed on that good or service exceeds its cost of production, too little of that good is produced, creating a shortage.[1] As the quantity supplied of the good is increased, the costs of its production (which include the higher prices that are necessary to attract the required resources from their other uses) will rise until the cost of production equals the value placed on it by those who demand it. In freely operating markets, shortages cannot exist in the long run.

There are two ways of looking at how an economic shortage can occur with respect to health manpower. First, the quantity demanded of a particular health profession (i.e., hospitals' demands for registered nurses) can exceed the quantity supplied at a given market price (wage). For this to occur, the wage would have to be below the equilibrium wage. The second way in which a shortage can occur is when the income of a health profession exceeds the costs of entering that profession. In the latter instance, the income of a health profession reflects the value of the services that the profession produces. The costs of entering the profession include the out-of-pocket costs of training for that profession, as well as the value of the entrant's time, that is, their opportunity costs. (Since the time streams at which the income is earned and the costs incurred differ, an appropriate discount rate must be used in equating the two.)

The latter situation may be illustrated by use of Figure 13–2. D_1 is the demand by firms for a particular health manpower occupation. S_L represents the long-run supply

---

[1]This situation also occurs when a monopolist establishes a price for its service greater than the marginal cost of producing that service.

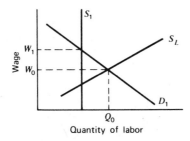

Figure 13-2. A shortage created by a restriction of supply.

curve and is the number of persons willing to enter that occupation at different wage rates. S_1 is the current number of persons in that health profession. (S_1 is unlikely to be vertical, since the supply of work effort from the current stock of trained professionals will depend upon the responsiveness of their hours worked and their participation rate to different wage rates.) With a supply equal to S_1 the wage will be W_1. If the market were operating freely, the wage would fall to W_0 as the supply of labor to that occupation increases. If the health manpower profession in question were able to establish entry barriers, S_1 would not shift to the right along S_L and the resulting wage would be W_1. Wage W_1 represents the value placed on that labor input by its demanders and it exceeds the cost of inducing additions to the supply of that health profession.

Each of the two types of static shortage—the first example, where the wage is held below the equilibrium level, and the case just considered, where the wage exceeds the wage at which persons are willing to enter that occupation—is caused by market power on either the demand or supply side of the health manpower market. When the wage is prevented from rising to its equilibrium level, the demanders of labor are exercising monopoly power; in the latter case it is the suppliers of labor services that are the monopolists. In both of these types of shortage situations, the shortage would disappear with an increase in supply. Supply would increase in the first case if the price of the service were allowed to rise, and in the second case if more persons were allowed to enter the profession.

These discussions of economic shortage indicate what information should be examined to determine whether or not an economic shortage exists or has occurred. Since each of these approaches will be used with regard to different health professions (i.e., physicians and registered nurses), these approaches are discussed in more detail.

When quantity demanded exceeds quantity supplied at a given market price, as in Figure 13-3, the price will rise (to P_2), and there will be no excess demand. All who are willing to pay price P_2 will be able to purchase as much as they want of the commodity they are seeking. (There may be persons who cannot afford to buy as much of the commodity as others believe they should purchase at the new, higher price; however, such a normative judgment can still be handled using a market mechanism by providing subsidies directly to such persons.) An economic shortage would occur in the situation above if, with an increase in demand from D_1 to D_2, the price of the service were prevented from rising to its new equilibrium point P_2. With an increase in demand and a price of P_1 the demand would be for Q_3 units of service. However, at a price of P_1 the supply of that service would be Q_1. The shortage would be the excess of demand over supply at the prevailing price, of $Q_3 - Q_1$.

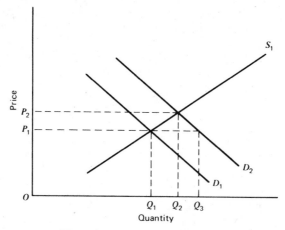

Figure 13-3. An economic shortage.

There can be two types of economic shortage: a temporary (dynamic) shortage or a static (long-run) shortage. Both types of economic shortage are believed to have existed at one time or another in the health professions.

A Dynamic Shortage

A dynamic or temporary shortage occurs when, as in Figure 13–3, there is an increase in demand but the new price has not yet reached its new equilibrium point of P_2. Demand will exceed supply at the old price of P_1. Not everyone who is willing to pay P_1 will receive as much as he or she wants. In the long run, however, this form of temporary or dynamic shortage will work itself out; the price will rise to the equilibrium level and there will no longer be a shortage. If demand continues to increase, it will take longer to achieve the equilibrium situation. There will be continued claims of a shortage while the price is rising, although supply will also be increasing. *Increases in quantity supplied, as well as rising prices, distinguish a dynamic shortage from a static shortage.*

How long will a dynamic shortage persist? In their article on dynamic shortages, Kenneth Arrow and William Capron claim that "the amount of shortage will tend to disappear faster the greater the reaction speed and also the greater the elasticity of supply (or demand)" (2). The reaction speed is the time it takes for price to reach its equilibrium level given the excess of demand over supply. It will take time for firms to realize that there is a shortage at the old price and that they must raise wages to attract more personnel. Firms must also decide how many more persons they want in the event that they have to pay higher wage rates. It also takes time for employees to react to these higher salaries. If demand and supply are relatively elastic, it will take smaller price increases to bring about a new equilibrium situation. Thus, in a dynamic situation where demands are increasing, temporary shortages can exist. The magnitude of the dynamic shortage will depend upon how fast demand is increasing, the reaction speed of increased prices to the excess demand, and the elasticities of supply and demand.

The policy prescriptions for a dynamic shortage differ from those prescribed for a shortage based on a "normative" judgment or for a static shortage. Increasing infor-

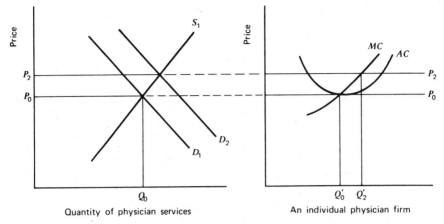

Figure 13-4. The market for physician services and for an individual physician firm.

mation to both demanders and suppliers in a market where dynamic shortages exist will make the equilibrium situation occur more quickly. Career information given to prospective applicants in professions where demand is increasing, and similar information given to prospective employers regarding the higher wages they will have to pay for such personnel, will bring about a quicker adjustment process. Massive supply subsidies to finance additional applicants entering those professions for which demands are increasing cannot be justified on grounds of economic efficiency. Such subsidies would have to be justified on the basis of other reasons, such as a normative shortage.

Static Economic Shortages

A static or long-run shortage occurs because supply does not increase; market equilibrium is therefore not achieved. In the typical case of a static shortage, prices are controlled and prevented from rising to their equilibrium level. If prices are not able to rise, the suppliers cannot pay higher prices to attract personnel away from other occupations. Similarly, a given health professional will not increase the amount of time that he or she is willing to work if the wage rate per hour does not increase; at some point the person will prefer leisure to more work. Thus suppliers will not increase the services they offer unless the prices paid for their services rise. The available supply in such situations is rationed by other methods: there may be long waiting lines to see a physician and only those willing to wait (those with low time costs) will see the physician; there may be a decrease in quality (i.e., physicians may spend less time with each patient); physicians may also refuse to see new patients.

It is possible that either a static shortage or a market equilibrium situation could exist in the physician *services* market, while in the market for physician *manpower* there could also be either an equilibrium or a static shortage situation. It is important to keep the analysis of these two markets—the services and manpower markets—separate. For example, in Figure 13-4, the left-hand diagram represents the market for physician services, while the right-hand diagram represents a typical firm (i.e., a physician in solo or group practice) within the overall market for physician services. Starting from an equilibrium situation in both markets, with price equal to P_0 and quantity of physician services equal to Q_0, the physician as a firm faces a price of P_0 and produces a quantity of services given by Q'_0, which is the intersection of the physician firm's marginal cost curve (MC) and the market price P_0. (For simplicity, we are assuming a competitive market in both the production and demand for physician services.) The physician firm is in equilibrium (physicians will neither leave the industry nor enter it) since they are earning a normal rate of return, with no excess profits, as shown by the position of the physician firm's average cost curve (AC) and the market price P_0.

Given the foregoing initial equilibrium position in both the services and manpower markets, let us assume that there is an increase in demand for physician services, possibly as a result of increased income in the population. The demand for physician services will increase from D_1 to D_2. Given the same number of physicians, physicians will either work longer hours or increase their productivity by hiring auxiliary personnel. This increased output is shown by a movement up the industry's supply curve (S_1), which is the sum of the physician firms' marginal cost curves. The market price will rise to P_2, and each physician will be making excess profits (the distance from P_2 to the firm's average cost curve at output level Q'_2). The increase in price and output in the market for physician services is the short-run reaction to the increase in demand for physician services.

In this situation there is no shortage in the physicians' services market. If there is an increase in the number of physicians (i.e., firms) in the long run in the manpower market because of excess profits, the industry supply curve will shift to the right, and each physician firm will be producing at the point where the new price equals average cost and marginal cost. The increase in the number of physicians in the long run will also bring about an equilibrium situation in the manpower market, and no shortage will exist in either market.

If, however, with an increase in the demand for physician services the price is *prevented* from rising, a static shortage will occur in the services market. Equilibrium could still exist in the physician manpower market, since there will not be an excess of profits (or losses). Alternatively, if the price is allowed to reach its equilibrium level in the services market but new physicians are not permitted to enter the manpower market, a shortage situation will exist in the physician manpower market. Physicians will be earning excess profits and we would observe little, if any, addition to the number of physicians. *A static shortage in the number of physicians will be represented by high rates of returns (excess profits) to physicians and little or no entry into the physician market.*

The policy implications for a static shortage situation are to allow the price to rise if the shortage is in the services market. If the shortage is in the physician manpower market, then easing the entry barriers will result in an increase in the number of physicians. With an increase in the number of physicians, excess profits per physician will fall until profits are "normal" and there will no longer be an economic shortage of physicians. If a static shortage exists because of barriers to entry, providing subsidies to the new entrants will not resolve the static shortage. The entry barriers are not eliminated by such subsidies. Subsidizing the limited number of new entrants will merely increase their return in a profession whose profits are currently considered to be excessive.

The Definitions of a Surplus of Health Manpower

The discussion above defined a shortage in the physician manpower market as occurring when the physician earned an above-normal rate of return, or excess profits. A surplus of physicians would exist when the opposite occurs, that is, when physicians are earning a below-normal rate of return. (The price would be below the average-cost curve; thus the physician would not be covering all their costs, including a normal return.)

A surplus situation can occur if one or both of the following situations occur. The price of physician services may increase at a slower rate than the increase in physicians' costs. Physician fees may be held down by the government or other third-party payors while the cost of a physician's practice may increase more rapidly (e.g., increases in malpractice insurance premiums). The rate of return to physicians would thus fall. Fewer prospective physicians would enter the profession. Another way in which a surplus could occur is if the supply of physicians increased faster than did increases in the demand for physician services.

Surpluses are resolved more easily than are static shortages. As prospective applicants perceive a lowering in their rate of return to a medical education, fewer will apply to medical school. Over time, the smaller increase in the physician supply will bring about a new equilibrium situation. In situations of both surpluses and static shortages, dissatisfaction occurs; currently, practicing physicians receive lower incomes when there is a surplus of physicians, while prospective qualified applicants are denied a medical education when there is a static shortage.

THE MEASUREMENT OF HEALTH MANPOWER SHORTAGES AND SURPLUSES

In defining and distinguishing between normative, dynamic, and static shortages, we see that the latter two are different types of economic shortages, and that the normative shortage is based upon either a professional determination or a value judgment of how many professionals of a particular type of manpower are needed. We have also indicated the alternative policy prescriptions for the different types of shortages. In this section the methods by which each of these types of shortages has been measured is discussed. The measurement of a shortage is important, since it enables us to distinguish between the different types of shortages.

Professional Determination

Noneconomic shortages have traditionally been measured in one of two ways: The first is professional determination. The earliest approach, used by Lee and Jones, calculated the number of physicians required in the population based upon an estimate of the number of physician hours needed, as determined by professional judgment, to provide medical care to the population. The authors developed a table of annual expectancy rates for diseases and injuries; they then asked leading physicians to determine the number of services required to diagnose and treat a given illness; the number of physician hours required to provide care for each illness category was then estimated; finally, assuming a 40-hour workweek per physician, the authors translated these hours into a requirement of 165,000 physicians, or a proposed physician/population ratio of 135 per 100,000 population. The difference between the current number of physicians and the number of physicians arrived at by the foregoing method was the "shortage" of physicians.

One of the problems with using such an approach for estimating shortages and for proposing government intervention to subsidize increases in the number of needed physicians is that the additional physicians do not necessarily go where they are most needed. Further, those persons most in need of physician services may not be able to pay for them even if they are made available. There are additional problems with this approach. What if the current number of physicians exceeds the professionally determined estimate? If such a "surplus" of physicians were to be eliminated, an *economic* shortage might occur.

It was a concern among physicians with a possible surplus that led to the 1980 Graduate Medical Education National Advisory Committee (GEMENAC) report to the secretary of Health and Human Services on the future supply and requirements for physicians (3). The approach used by the GEMENAC committee was similar to the methodology used by Lee and Jones in the 1930s.

Estimates of future supplies of physicians were generated based on estimates of current numbers of medical school graduates, foreign medical graduates, residents, and deaths and retirements. No attempt was made to relate entry into medicine, into different specialties, or entry by foreign medical graduates to economic factors or to any other causal factors. Instead, it was implicitly assumed that such factors would not change over the period studied. Nor did this approach consider changes in physician productivity that might be occurring. It was a mechanical approach to generating future estimates of physicians and their specialty distribution.

The estimates of physician requirements was developed by combining data on current utilization and the "need" for physicians. Within each physician specialty, physicians were asked how many physicians were needed in that specialty. Again such an approach does not explicitly consider patient preferences for care or economic factors such as changes in insurance coverage, factors which in the past have been important determinants of physician utilization.

The "desired balance" between physician supply and requirements in 1990 did not consider any equilibrating mechanisms such as changes in physician prices or hours worked. The GEMENAC report states that there will be a physician "surplus" of 70,000 physicians by 1990.

The Ratio Technique

The second and most popular approach to determining health manpower shortages has been the ratio technique. This method generally uses the existing physician/population ratio (or other health manpower/population ratio) and compares it with the physician/population ratio that is likely to occur in some future period. To calculate the future ratio, the proponents of this approach estimate the future population and then calculate the likely number of additions of graduates to the stock of physicians, less the expected number of deaths and retirements. The difference between the existing physician/population ratio and the future physician/population ratio is the difference that must be made up. (Until recently, the future ratio has always been found to be less that the current ratio.) The policy prescription that always results from a finding that increases in the number of physicians are required is for federal subsidies to health professional educational institutions to produce more graduates.

There are variations on the use of the ratio technique for determining the number of physicians needed. For example, the highest regional or statewide physician/population ratio observed might be used as the ratio to be achieved for the entire country in some future period.

The ratio technique has served as the basis for much of the health manpower legislation in this country. It has been used for physicians, dentists, and registered nurses. Other health professional organizations also make use of this approach in their requests for federal subsidies. Since this approach has had such an important legislative role and has resulted in many billions of dollars of subsidies both by the federal and state governments, it deserves a critical evaluation.

One way of thinking of the physician/population ratio is that it is the outcome of an equilibrium situation. At any point in time there is a demand for physicians and a supply of physicians; the intersection of the demand and supply curves result in the physician's income and in a physician/population ratio. Attempts to change the physician/population ratio generally ignore the fact that this ratio is the result of demand and other supply factors. Any significant change simply in the number of physicians should cause changes in the demands for other inputs (substitutes for and complements to physicians) as well as in the demands for physicians themselves, which would mean a movement down the physician demand curve.

Three basic problems are associated with the use of the ratio technique for estimating shortages (or for forecasting manpower requirements). The first problem is that the method does not consider any changes that may occur in the demand for physician (or other health manpower) services. If demand were to increase, then even maintaining an existing ratio (or striving for a higher ratio as found in other states) might result in an *increase* in the price of physician services (i.e., the shift in demand is greater than the increase in the physician/population ratio). Since this approach basically ignores the demand side, differences between the future ratio of physicians to population and the ratio that would be demanded will be resolved through changes in the *price* of physician services. Some persons will be even less likely to buy physician services if the price of those services has increased. Thus, maintaining a given ratio says nothing about whether the future price of physician services will be the same; it may be higher or lower, but it is highly unlikely that it will be the same. Since the future price is likely to be different, and generally will be higher than the current price because of increasing demand, what is the real purpose of maintaining a given ratio? If the objective were to provide more services to certain population groups or to the entire population, it would be important to lower the price of the service so as to increase consumption. The ratio technique and its basic policy prescription of changing the number of physicians does not even consider price or alternative ways to affect consumption of services.

The second problem with the use of the ratio technique is that it does not consider productivity changes that are likely to occur or that are possible to achieve. The ratio of farmers to the population has fallen drastically in the last 100 years (from a ratio of 60 farmers to every 100 persons in 1860 to fewer than 4 in 100 persons today), yet few people would maintain that there is a shortage of farmers or that it would be desirable to retain the previous farmer/population ratio. Because of enormous increases in farm productivity, it takes fewer farmers today to produce more food than their predecessors did. Although productivity gains in medical care appear to be more limited than what has occurred in agriculture, it is still possible to achieve an increase in physician services without increasing the number of physicians. Lesser-trained personnel can be used to relieve physicians of many of the tasks they perform; delegation of tasks would permit an increase in the number of physician visits. If increased productivity is considered, a smaller physician/population ratio would be needed in the future. Increasing productivity is an alternative approach for achieving an increase in the quantity of physician services; policies to increase productivity require smaller subsidies than do policies to increase the number of physicians.

The third problem with the use of the ratio technique is that no indication of the importance of the shortage of physicians is provided. For example, the Bane Report estimated that if the 1959 physician/population ratio were maintained (140 per 100,000), an additional 11,000 physicians would be needed by 1975. These projections assumed that without federal support for medical education there would be 319,000 physicians with a resulting shortage of 11,000 physicians (4). How much is it worth (in terms of governmental subsidies) to reduce this shortage to 7,000 physicians or to no shortage whatsoever? It is difficult, if not impossible, to use the ratio technique to compare the additional cost of decreasing the estimated shortage of physicians with their marginal contribution to medical care or to increased health.

There are a number of technical difficulties inherent in using the ratio technique that can cause variations in its estimates; it is necessary to exclude research physicians from the physician/population ratio, to correct for the age distribution of physicians (since it may affect productivity), and to develop an accurate forecast of the population in a future period. However, the three conceptual problems inherent in this approach—no consideration given to demand or productivity changes and no understanding of the importance of the shortage estimate—are more significant shortcomings.

The Rate-of-Return Approach

Three types of market situations can exist in the health manpower market: an equilibrium situation, a dynamic shortage, or a static shortage. An equilibrium situation is one in which physicians are earning normal profits. If there were an increase in demand in the physician services market, physicians would, in the short run, experience higher prices, leading to excess profits, and in the long run we would expect an increase in the number of physicians, thereby returning their profits to a normal level.

This analogy of the physician as a firm is useful because it helps to delineate what we expect to observe. Normal profits or excess profits mean that the rate of return to a medical education is either normal or high compared with equivalent investments. Although not all, nor even perhaps most, physicians seek a medical education because of its value as a remunerative investment, enough persons do so that if one profession becomes more lucrative than another, some persons will change their preference as to the occupation they wish to enter. This just means that as some professions and occupations become relatively more rewarding financially, some potential applicants who are relatively indifferent between one occupation or another will switch their preferences to the more rewarding profession. This switching between occupations and professions will, on the average, equalize returns among different occupations. (Because there are always large variations in skills, returns *within* an occupation or profession will vary. In the long run, however, the average return should be similar among different occupations.)

When viewing medical education as an investment, one calculates the rate of return by estimating the costs of that investment and the expected higher financial returns. Thus one can compare its profitability with alternative investments, educational and otherwise. The costs of purchasing a medical education are the direct outlays, such as tuition, laboratory, and book fees, and the income a student forgoes had he or she gone to work immediately upon graduating from college. These opportunity costs of the student's time are the more significant costs of securing a professional education. The high return of an investment in a medical education is the higher income that a physician will earn compared with the income from an alternative occupation. Since these higher incomes occur in the future, they are worth less than if they occurred immediately; the difference in financial returns between being a physician and entering an alternative occupation must be discounted to the present. The comparison between these higher returns and the costs required to receive them is the rate of return to a medical education. [More precisely, the internal rate of return is that discount rate which, when applied to the future earnings stream, will make its present value equal to the cost of entry into that profession (i.e., the present value of the expected outlay or cost stream).]

A normal rate of return might be similar to the rate of return on a college education or on the return the individual could have received had he or she invested a sum of money comparable to what was spent on a medical education. It is necessary to compare the rate of return on a medical education with an alternative rate of return to be able to determine whether or not physicians are receiving a normal return. Returning to our analogy of the physician as a firm, if physicians were receiving "excess" profits, this would be translated into a high relative rate of return to a medical education. If rates of return to medicine are higher than those received in other occupations, we expect to observe a greater number of applicants to medical schools. As the number of physicians increase over time, the rate of return to a medical career will become comparable to other occupations or investments.

To distinguish between a dynamic and a static shortage, we want to examine both the rate of return to a medical education, relative to some standard or to another profession, and whether there is an increase in the number of physicians. A dynamic shortage would be characterized by a high relative rate of return in the short run, increases in the number of physicians, and eventually normal rates of return. A static shortage would also be characterized by a high relative rate of return, but it would persist since there would be little or no entry into the profession to drive these rates of return down. If rates of return remained relatively high and there was a large increase in the supply of physicians, there might be a persistent dynamic shortage. The key difference between the dynamic and static shortage is whether additions to the stock of physicians occur over time. A dynamic shortage will eventually resolve itself; a static shortage requires intervention, since entry into the profession is prevented.

The main indicators of the performance of the physician market, as well as other health manpower markets, are data on relative rates of return and additions to the stock of physicians (or other health manpower). Other indications of a shortage situation, such as greater use of substitute manpower, may be observed; however, such substitution could occur because of changes in the relative wages of different occupations and be unrelated to a shortage situation. For example, if wages and costs of entering a profession increased, the rates of return between occupations could be similar but their relative wages would differ; hence substitution would occur. Thus the main method whereby different types of shortages are distinguished is in the use of relative rates of return and entry into the profession.[2]

The concept of rate of return is also important for public policy. If it is desired to increase the number of persons entering a profession, subsidies can be provided to offset the applicant's training costs. Assuming a normal rate of return, lowering the training cost to enter a profession will result in a higher rate of return and, consequently, an increased demand for that profession. For purposes of both policy and forecasting demand for professional education, it is important to determine empirically the elasticity of lowering training costs with respect to expected increases in the number of applicants to that profession.

Empirical Estimates

Several studies have attempted to estimate the rate of return to a medical education. The earliest economic study of the physician shortage was by Milton Friedman and Simon Kuznets (5). They studied several professions during the early 1930s and found that for two of the professions, dentistry and medicine, physicians earned, on the average, 32 percent per year more than dentists did. This higher income for physicians was, in part, offset by the 17 percent higher cost of becoming a physician. Friedman and Kuznets attributed part of the increased income of physicians to greater entry barriers into the profession. The greater return to physicians represented a relative shortage of physicians; that is, their marginal value as represented by their incomes exceeded the costs of producing additional physicians.

A subsequent study by W. Lee Hansen found that by 1939 there was a slight *surplus* of physicians and dentists. However, by 1949, physicians and dentists had a 16 percent greater rate of return than did college graduates, indicating a shortage. By 1956 the shortage had decreased slightly: physicians' rates of return were only 10 percent greater than for college graduates; the comparable figure for dentists was 4 percent. This is shown in Table 13–1, which is reproduced from Hansen's work.[3]

Several additional studies have estimated the internal rate of return to a medical education; the results are presented in Table 13–2 (6). These estimates are for all physicians and separately for general practitioners. The "all physicians" estimate includes general practitioners as well as the various physician specialties. Two of the studies (7, 8) determine that general practitioners earn higher rates of return than specialists. Dresch (9), on the other hand, finds that the decision to specialize was profitable,

---

[2]Another approach suggested for measuring whether or not a shortage exists is to examine changes in relative incomes. If one profession's income rises more rapidly than another profession's, a relative shortage is said to exist. (See, for example, Elton Rayack, "The Supply of Physicians' Services," *Industrial and Labor Relations Review*, January 1964.) The problem with this approach is that it does not consider differences in the relative costs of entering different professions. If training times have increased, or if there is a decrease in the number of working years, we would expect higher relative incomes for this profession in order for the relative rates of return to be similar. Another problem in using the relative income approach is that the base year for making comparisons among professions is quite important. Depending upon which base year is used, the relative income approach can show a shortage or a surplus of the manpower in a particular profession. Finally, the relative income approach cannot distinguish between relative shortages in all professions and a shortage situation in only one profession.

[3]There is a difference in the method used by Hansen and the other studies. Hansen's income and cost streams begin at the first year of undergraduate college, and his forgone earnings are based on those of a high school graduate. The other studies are based on the forgone earnings of a college graduate and begin the income and cost streams at the first year of medical school.

TABLE 13-1. Internal Rates of Return to Male College Graduates, Physicians, and Dentists, and Ratios of Internal Rates of Return of Physicians and Dentists to Male College Graduates, United States, 1939, 1949, and 1956

	1939		1949		1956	
	Rates	Ratios	Rates	Ratios	Rates	Ratios
Male college graduates	13.7	1.00	11.5	1.00	11.6	1.00
Physicians	13.5	.98	13.4	1.16	12.8	1.10
Dentists	12.3	.90	13.4	1.16	12.0	1.04

Source: W. Lee Hansen, " 'Shortages' and Investment in Health Manpower," in *The Economics of Health and Medical Care* (Ann Arbor, Mich.: University of Michigan, 1964), p. 86.

although it varies greatly by specialty, from 40.5 percent for internal medicine to − 5 percent for pediatrics.

The rates of return to both general practitioners and to all physicians over the period 1955–1980 were sufficiently high to make medicine a financially attractive profession. These internal rates of return were approximately twice as great as those received by lawyers (10).

The 1976 estimate by Dresch (11) of 17.5 percent is relative to that of a teacher (i.e., a college graduate). He found that the rates of return varied greatly depending

TABLE 13-2. Internal Rate of Return, All Physicians and General Practitioners, 1955–1980

Year	All Physicians		General Practitioners
1980	—	14.0[a]	16.7[a]
1976	17.5[b]	13.3[a]	16.4[a]
1970	22.0[c]	14.7[a]	16.8[a]
1965	17.5[d]		24.1[e]
1962	16.6[d]		—
1959	14.7[d]		23.7[e]
1955	13.5[d]		29.1[e]

SOURCES:

[a]Philip Burstein and Jerry Cromwell, "Relative Incomes and Rates of Return for U.S. Physicians," *Journal of Health Economics*, 4, 1985: 63–78, p. 74.

[b]Stephen Dresch, "Marginal Wage Rates, Hours of Work, and Returns to Physician's Training and Specialization," in Nancy Greenspan, ed., *Health Care Financing, Conference Proceedings: Issues in Physician Reimbursement*, (Washington, D.C.: Department of Health and Human Services, 1981), pp. 199–200.

[c]Roger Feldman and Richard M. Scheffler, "The Supply of Medical School Applicants and the Rate of Return to Training," *Quarterly Review of Economics and Business*, Spring 1978: 92, Table 1.

[d]Frank Sloan, *Economic Models of Physician Supply*, unpublished doctoral dissertation, Harvard University, 1968, p. 164.

[e]Frank Sloan, "Lifetime Earnings and the Physician's Choice of Specialty," *Industrial and Labor Relations Review*, October 1970: 6.

upon which occupation was compared to medicine. For example, the rate of return to a medical education was over 100 percent greater than for that of a college professor.

What can we conclude based on these rate of return data? In the pre-World War II period there appeared to be a slight surplus of physicians and dentists. The rate of return to a medical and dental education was lower than for comparable investments. After World War II, however, the rate of return to a medical and dental education increased. The rates of return during this period were sufficiently high to indicate a shortage situation. With increasing rates of return, we would expect to observe increased demands for a medical education. If large increases in the stock of physicians were occurring, we would conclude that a dynamic shortage existed. If, however, the rates of return remained high, and in fact increased, and there were few or no additions to the stock of physicians, then we would have to conclude that a static shortage situation existed and that barriers prevented an adjustment process from occurring. To determine whether a dynamic or a static shortage of physicians existed through the late 1940s, the 1950s, and the 1960s, we turn to an examination of data on changes in the stock of physicians during these periods, as presented in Table 13-3.

In 1950 there were 209,000 active physicians in the United States. By 1965 the number of active physicians reached 277,000, which is a rate of increase of less than 2 percent per year. When the increase in the number of physicians is adjusted for increases in the population, the physician/population ratio remained virtually unchanged between 1950 and 1963 (141 physicians per 100,000 population and 140 per 100,000, respectively). After 1963 the total number of active physicians began to increase at a slightly more rapid rate, averaging between 1.5 and 3.7 percent per year until 1975, when the annual increase was 4.5 percent. The physician/population ratio also began to show a gradual annual increase during this same period, reaching 170 physicians per 100,000 in 1974. Part of the increase in physicians over this period was a result of increases in foreign medical graduates (FMGs). In 1960, 5.8 percent of the total number of active physicians were FMGs; by 1973, FMGs comprised almost 20 percent of the number of active physicians. In 1973 the number of FMGs entering the United States exceeded the number of U.S. medical graduates (USMGs) in that year (12,285 FMGs, 10,391 USMGs). When the physician/population ratio is adjusted for the number of FMGs, then between 1960 and 1974 the ratio was virtually unchanged.

The Immigration Act of 1965 facilitated the immigration of foreign-trained physicians (FMGs) into the United States. As a result, there was a rapid rise in FMGs between 1966 and 1976. During this period, approximately one-third of the permanent increase in physician supply was attributed to the inflow of FMGs.[4]

---

[4]There are two main classifications of FMGs: those that have permanent immigrant status and those that have exchange visitor status. Exchange visitor FMGs are supposed to return to their own countries after they have received graduate medical training. However, until 1976 many exchange visitor FMGs extended their stays indefinitely, thus clouding the difference between themselves and FMGs permanently immigrating. The annual increase in exchange visitor FMGs exceeded the number of FMGs permanently immigrating up until the mid-1970s. Exchange visitor FMGs were an important component of total FMGs and they were becoming a significant portion of all physicians.

In 1976, as part of the renewal of the Health Professions Educational Assistance Act (HPEA), Congress changed the immigration laws affecting FMGs. Newly entering FMGs were now required to pass more rigorous medical exams, as well as exams in written and oral English. The legislation also restricted the number of FMGs who can remain indefinitely by requiring exchange visitor FMGs to return to their own countries after two years of U.S. graduate medical education (a one-year extension is possible). This legislation had its greatest

Not all active physicians are involved in patient care. When the growth in the number of physicians is adjusted to determine those in patient care activities and the number of FMGs is excluded, the physician/population ratio for U.S. physicians engaged in patient care actually *declined* between 1960 and 1975, from 115 to 110 per 100,000 population.

Demand for physicians had been increasing during the period from 1950 to 1965, as indicated by the relatively high rates of return to a medical education. We would therefore expect to observe large increases in the number of physicians. However, rather than increasing, U.S. physicians engaged in patient care as a ratio to the population actually decreased during this 15 year period; the absolute increase in the number of U.S. trained physicians was extremely small.

The small increase in the number of physicians was not the result of a lack of applicants to medical schools. As shown in Table 13–4, the applicants/acceptances ratio during this period was continually greater than 1.

In 1965, Congress passed the Health Professions Educational Assistance Act in response to claims of a "shortage" of physicians and other health manpower. As a result of this legislation, which provided generous subsidies to health professional educational institutions, medical schools were required to increase their enrollments to qualify for federal funds. The effect of this legislation began to be felt by the late 1960s, when the number of U.S.-trained physicians began to increase at a more rapid rate.

By 1980, the total number of physicians per 100,000 population reached 199 and continued increasing to 215 in 1985. Even when adjusted for the increase in FMGs, the physician/population ratio is greater than it has been for many years. The expansion in medical school spaces resulting from the previous manpower legislation is still having its effect. The physician/population ratio should continue increasing into the 1990s. However, even with the increase in the number of physicians, the ratio of applicants to acceptances is still greater than 1; after reaching a level of 2.8 in the mid-1970s, the applicants/acceptances ratio is declining—it is now approximately 2.0.

What can we conclude from the data on rates of return, physician to population ratios, and the ratio of applicants to acceptances to medical schools? During the entire post-World War II period, rates of return to medicine were high and rising. Based on these higher returns, we would have expected greater entry into the profession and, consequently, an increase in the number of U.S.-trained physicians providing patient care; however, it appears that there was very little entry into the profession by U.S.-trained physicians. Although there was a sufficient number of students demanding a medical education, as indicated by the applicant/acceptance ratio, very few additional physicians were produced. Even after the introduction of federal legislation that led to increases in the production of physicians, there was still an excess demand for a medical education. The only possible conclusion, based on the minimal increase

---

impact on newly entering FMGs with exchange visitor status; their numbers decreased from 2,563 in 1976, to 1,578 in 1977, to 951 in 1978, and finally to 544 in 1982. The number of newly entering permanent immigrants also declined from 4,410 in 1976 to 2,336 in 1978. As a percentage of total new licensees, FMGs decreased from 36.0 percent in 1976 to 17.9 percent in 1985. The data seem to indicate that the annual increase in FMGs has been significantly reduced. U.S. Department of Health and Human Services, Division of Health Professions Analysis, *Report to the President and Congress on the Status of Health Professions Personnel in the United States* (1981 and 1986) (Washington, D.C.: U.S. Government Printing Office, 1981), pp. III-20, III-143; (1986), pp. III-36, III-38.

TABLE 13-3. Number of Physicians and Physician/Population Ratios, United States, 1950–1985

Year	Active Physicians[a]	Annual Percent Change[b]	Physicians per 100,000 Population[c]	Annual Percent Change[b]	Foreign-Trained Physicians[d]	Foreign-Trained Physicians as a Percentage of All Active Physicians[c]	Physician/Population Ratios Excluding Foreign-Trained Physicians (Physicians per 100,000 Population)[c]
1950	208,997		141				
1955	228,553	1.9	141	NC			
1960	247,257	1.6	140	-.1	15,154[e]	5.8	132
1963	261,728	1.9	140	NC	30,925	11.3	124
1965	277,575	3.0	145	-1.8			
1967	294,072	3.0	150	1.7	45,816	15.0	127
1969	302,966	1.5	151	.3	53,552	17.0	126
1970	311,203	2.7	158	4.6	54,404	16.8	131
1971	322,228	3.6	161	1.9	59,499	17.8	132
1972	333,259	3.4	165	2.5	64,701	18.7	134
1973	338,111	1.5	166	.6	67,141	19.1	134
1974	350,609	3.7	170	2.4	70,940	19.5	137
1975	366,425	4.5	176	3.5	76,205	20.0	141
1976	378,572	3.3	180	2.3	78,295[f]	20.0	144
1977	381,969	.9	180	NC	81,386[f]	20.5	143
1978	401,364	5.1	188	4.4	83,976	20.1	150
1979	417,266	4.0	191	1.6	89,210	20.5	153
1980	435,545	4.4	199	4.2	90,803	20.1	159
1983	479,440	3.4	207	2.3	106,111	22.1	167
1985	511,090	3.3	215[g]	2.1	112,668	22.8	168

sources: U.S. Department of Health and Human Services, Office of Research, Statistics and Technology, *Health, United States, 1980*, DHHS Publication (PHS) 81-1232 (Hyattsville, Md.: U.S. Government Printing Office, 1980), p. 188; Department of Health and Human Services, *Supply and Characteristics of Selected Health Personnel*, Publication (HRA) 81-20, 1981, p. 36; *Physician Distribution and Medical Licensure in the United States*, Department of Statistical Analysis, Center for Health Policy Research (Chicago: American Medical Association, 1977). *Physician Characteristics and Distribution in the United States*, 1981 and 1986 eds., Division of Survey and Data Resources, (Chicago: American Medical Association, 1982); U.S. Department of Health and Human Services, Bureau of Health Professions. *A Report to the President and Congress on the Status of Health Professions Personnel in the United States*, Draft, April 27, 1981; pp. 111–141, Table 7, pp. 111–143, Table 9; *Foreign Medical Graduates*, 1986 ed., (Chicago: American Medical Association, 1986); Bureau of the Census, *Statistical Abstract of the United States*, 1986, 106th ed., (Washington, D.C.: U.S. Department of Commerce, various years).

[a]M.D.s only. Excludes inactive and temporary foreign physicians, and those with unknown addresses.

[b]Calculated as an average for each year in a multiyear period (e.g., 9.4 percent increase for 1950–1955 averages to 1.9 percent per year), NC, no change.

[c]Physicians in these columns refers to the sum of M.D.s and Doctors of Osteopathy (D.O.s). The number of D.O.s has fluctuated between 11,000 in 1950 and 17,000 in 1982. Population refers to civilian population.

[d]Includes active physicians and 90 percent of those unclassified. It excludes inactive, temporary foreign physicians, and those with unknown address.

[e]Figure for 1959.

[f]Estimated through interpolation.

[g]Based on population estimate.

365

TABLE 13-4. Ratio of Applicants to Acceptances, 1947–1948 to 1985–1986

Year	Applicants/Acceptance Ratio
1947–1948	2.9
1950–1951	3.1
1955–1956	1.9
1960–1961	1.7
1965–1966	2.1
1970–1971	2.2
1975–1976	2.8
1980–1981	2.1
1985–1986	1.9

SOURCES: American Medical Association, "Medical Education in the United States, 1971–1972," *Journal of the American Medical Association*, 222, November 20, 1972: 979, Table 12; "Undergraduate Medical Education," *Journal of the American Medical Association*, 256(12), September 26, 1986: 1561, Table 5. Copyright 1971, 1986, American Medical Association.

in the number of U.S.-trained physicians until the mid-1970s, and the continued high rates of return, is that a static shortage situation existed.

The rapid rise in the physician/population ratio is currently causing concern among a number of persons, particularly the medical profession, that there will be a "surplus" of physicians in coming years. If an economic surplus were to occur, we would expect to observe declining applicants to acceptances to medical schools, to a ratio of less than 1, and a decline in the relative rate of return to becoming a physician, similar to the situation that existed in the 1930s, as shown in Table 13–1. The mechanisms used by the medical profession to create and maintain a static shortage of physicians for so many years is discussed next in Chapter 14.

REFERENCES

1. R. I. Lee and L. W. Jones, *The Fundamentals of Good Medical Care* (Chicago: University of Chicago Press, 1933).
2. Kenneth J. Arrow and William.M. Capron, "Dynamic Shortages and Price Rises: The Scientist-Engineer Case," *Quarterly Journal of Economics*, 73, 1959: 299.
3. *Summary Report of the Graduate Medical Education National Advisory Committee to the Secretary, Department of Health and Human Services*, Vol. I, DHHS Publication (HRA) 81–651, 1980, 48–56. Volume II contains a more complete description of the Modeling, Research, and Data Technical Panel.
4. *Physicians for a Growing America*, Report of the Surgeon General's Consultant Group on Medical Education, Public Health Service, U.S. Department of Health, Education, and Welfare (Washington, D.C.: U.S. Government Printing Office, 1959).

5. Milton Friedman and Simon Kuznets, *Income from Independent Practice* (New York: National Bureau of Economic Research, 1954).

6. The rates of return shown in Table 13-2 are unadjusted for the number of hours worked by physicians. There has been substantial debate about whether the internal rates of return, unadjusted for hours worked, adequately reflect the true internal rates of return to a medical education. Lindsay claims that a physician, because of his or her training, will receive a relatively high market wage. This high wage will induce the physician to substitute work for leisure; consequently, he or she will work more hours than someone with a lower market wage. Lindsay believed that there should be an adjustment for the number of hours worked before the income and cost streams are calculated. When Lindsay adjusts Sloan's data for hours worked (he assumes a 60-hour week for physicians and a 40- to 45-hour week for the alternative occupation), the internal rate of return is reduced.
   Sloan's response is twofold: first, he claims that Lindsay overestimated the number of hours that physicians work; second, Sloan claims that being a physician provides intangible benefits, such as increased status in society, which compensate the physician for any additional hours worked. For this reason, Sloan argues, it is not necessary to take into consideration these extra hours when calculating the income and cost streams.
   For a more detailed discussion of the Sloan and Lindsay debate see: Cotton M. Lindsay, "Real Returns to Medical Education," *Journal of Human Resources*, 8, Summer 1973: 331–348; "More Real Returns to Medical Education," *Journal of Human Resources*, 11, Winter 1976: 127–130; and Frank A. Sloan, "Real Returns to Medical Education, A Comment," *Journal of Human Resources*, 11, Winter 1976: 118–126.

7. Frank Sloan, "Lifetime Earnings and the Physician's Choice of Specialty," *Industrial and Labor Relations Review*, 6, October 1970.

8. Philip Burstein and Jerry Cromwell, "Relative Incomes and Rates of Return for U.S. Physicians," *Journal of Health Economics*, 4, 1985: 63–78, p. 74.

9. Stephen Dresch, "Marginal Wage Rates, Hours of Work, and Returns to Physician's Training and Specialization," in Nancy Greenspan, ed., *Health Care Financing, Conference Proceedings: Issues in Physician Reimbursement* (Washington, D.C.: U.S. Department of Health and Human Services, 1981), 199–200.

10. Burstein and Cromwell, *op. cit.*, p. 74.

11. Dresch, *op. cit.*

CHAPTER 14

The Market for
Physician Manpower

In Chapter 13 a dynamic shortage was differentiated from a static shortage according to whether or not there was entry into the market. Persistently high rates of return, it was suggested, could continue only if there were barriers to entry. Based on the small growth in the number of physicians until the mid-1970s, and the continual excess of applicants to acceptances to medical schools (as well as the rapid growth in foreign medical graduates entering this country and the increasing number of U.S. students studying medicine overseas), it was concluded that entry barriers must have existed to prevent an equilibrium situation from occurring in the market for physician manpower.

Three entry barriers to the physician's market have been suggested: licensure, graduation from an approved medical school, and continual increases in training, such as the movement to a three-year residency program. There is, however, an alternative hypothesis to explain why barriers in medicine exist: rather than serving to increase the economic returns to physicians, the barriers increase the quality and competence of practicing physicians. It is rationalized that these entry barriers enhance the public interest in a variety of ways. Consumers have very little information on the quality and competence of physicians. Gathering this information is costly and the consumer may be irreparably injured if the physician is incompetent; licensure provides the consumer with protection by reducing the uncertainty as to the provider's training. Occupational licensure has also been rationalized on grounds of "neighborhood effects"; an incompetent physician may harm persons other than the patient being treated if, for example, the physician were to cause an epidemic. Licensure is thus a means of protecting others from bearing the costs of incompetent practitioners; that is, the social costs exceed the private costs (1).

Given these alternative hypotheses to explain the reasons for entry barriers to becoming a physician—namely, to increase physician incomes or to provide consumer protection from incompetent practitioners—which is the more accurate justification? If the barriers are reduced because they are believed to provide physicians with monopoly incomes, will the public lose its protection from incompetent providers? Similarly, if it is public policy to maintain such entry restrictions in the belief that they reduce consumer uncertainty and protect society from incompetent providers, but if in fact such barriers are meant to provide physicians with monopoly incomes, is the public really protected from incompetent practitioners? Could the public be better protected using other approaches, and at a lower cost?

To determine which hypothesis best describes the reasons for entry restrictions in medicine, one must determine how consistent each of these hypotheses is with regard to the assurance of quality or the achievement of monopoly power. If the restrictions are for consumer protection, the medical profession should also be expected to favor other measures that have the effect of improving quality and/or offering consumers protection from incompetent practitioners. If, on the other hand, the entry restrictions are meant to provide physicians with a monopoly, and to increase their incomes, the profession would only favor those quality measures that are in the economic interests of physicians; the profession would be expected to oppose quality measures that would adversely affect physicians' incomes.

BARRIERS TO ENTRY IN MEDICINE

The first step in controlling entry into a profession is to establish a licensure requirement. Each state has the authority to license occupations under the power granted to it to protect the public's health. A license to practice medicine, therefore, can be granted only by a state. Beginning in the mid-1800s, when the American Medical Association (AMA) was formed, and extending until 1900, the medical profession sought and received licensure in each state (2). The states, in turn, delegated this licensure authority to medical licensing boards, which have the authority to determine the requirements for licensure. These state licensing boards also have the authority to set the conditions for suspending or revoking a license once it has been granted. The conditions for licensure and for maintaining a license can be placed on the quality of care that the physician provides and/or they can be used to impose restrictions on who can practice, thereby limiting the number of persons entering the profession. The membership of the medical licensing boards in each state consisted of physicians who were either nominated by or were representatives of the state and county medical associations. It was in this manner that county and state medical associations influenced the conditions for licensure in each state.

The earliest requirement for licensure was an examination. Examination by itself, however, is a weak barrier to entry. A person may try to pass the examination many times and the number of people taking the examination is not limited (3). A more effective barrier is one that raises the cost to those wishing to take the examination. Not everyone would be willing to bear this cost, particularly if there was uncertainty as to whether they would pass the licensure exam. The second barrier to entry into the medical profession, therefore, became the imposition of an educational requirement and a limit on the number of institutions that could provide such an education.

The second stage began in 1904 with the AMA's founding of its Council on Medical Education. This group had the task of upgrading the quality of medical education offered by existing medical schools. Of the 160 medical schools in 1906, the Council on Medical Education found only 82 offering a fully acceptable medical education (4). To achieve greater recognition of its findings, the Council on Medical Education induced the Carnegie Commission to survey the existing medical schools and publish a report. The resulting report, popularly known as the Flexner Report, recommended the closing of many medical schools and an upgrading of the educational standards in the other schools. "Flexner forcefully argued that the country was suffering from an overproduction of doctors and that it was in the public interest to have fewer doctors who were better trained" (5).

The result of the Flexner Report was that state medical licensing boards instituted an additional requirement for state licensure: before taking an examination for licensure, an applicant had to be a graduate of an approved medical school. The approval of medical schools was conducted by the AMA's own Council on Medical Education. In the years that followed, as expected, the number of medical schools decreased, from 162 in 1906, to 85 in 1920, to 76 in 1930, to 69 in 1944. The number of physicians per 100,000 similarly declined. The graduates of those medical schools that were closed continued to practice. No attempts were made to rectify any supposed inadequacies in their educational backgrounds. Whenever standards are raised, grandfather clauses protect the right of existing practitioners, regardless of their abilities. The AMA now had control over entry into the profession in two ways: first, through its Council on Medical Education, the AMA was able to limit the number of approved medical schools and hence the number of applicants for licensure exams; second, entrants into the profession then had to pass state licensure exams and any other prerequisites promulgated by the individual state medical licensing boards. Thus the AMA, through its Council on Medical Education, was able to determine the "appropriate" number of physicians in the United States.

The third method used by the medical profession to restrict entry, which is also meant to increase the competence of the new physician, is to lengthen the training time required for the student to become a practicing physician. Before entering medical school, a student has to have four years of undergraduate education. Medical school is four years and the time spent in internship and residency programs continually increase; medical school graduates usually take a minimum three-year residency. For students desiring to enter certain specialties, more than three years is required. The effect of continually increasing the training required before entering a profession is to raise the costs to the entering student. Not only are tuition costs higher the longer the requirements for undergraduate and medical school education, but more important, the income forgone because of the additional years of training is very large. These increased costs reduce the rate of return to prospective physicians. The emphasis in terms of quality is always on the *entering* physician and not on those currently in the profession. It is in the economic interests of current practitioners that the costs of entering the profession continually increase; since their training occurred in the past at a lower cost, they will receive higher prices and higher incomes in the form of economic rent (6).

Until recently, the market for physicians was not competitive, that is, advertising was not permitted and there was no price competition. More highly trained physicians could not advertise their increased training and more recent knowledge; thus they could not receive a higher price for their services than physicians without this additional training. To prevent new physicians from receiving higher returns than existing physicians, who had less training, it was necessary for the medical profession to maintain the fiction that *all* physicians are of uniform quality. To enforce this impression among patients, the medical profession discouraged any intraprofessional criticism and, until recently, prohibited the advertisement of differences in training or any other quality differentials among physicians. Whether or not a person was permitted to perform certain medical tasks depended upon whether or not they were a physician. A physician was provided with an unlimited scope of practice; it did not matter whether the physician had specialized training. Anesthesiologists, for example, can be physicians who are board certified in anesthesiology, they can be physicians with additional training but who are not board certified, or they can be physicians without any additional training in anesthesia. Merely being licensed is sufficient to allow physicians to undertake tasks performed by other physicians who have had additional training.

This third barrier to entry, which has taken the form of continual increases in the training costs for entering physicians, suggests that measures to increase the quality of physician services were independent of demands by consumers for increased quality and instead were related to the income considerations of the medical profession.

In addition to entry barriers, it was necessary for physicians to control productivity increases among themselves if they were to receive monopoly profits. Otherwise, it would be possible for some physicians to greatly increase their output, with a corresponding loss of business to other physicians, and consequently, a decrease in their rate of return. Productivity increases were (and, in some cases, still are) limited in two ways. First, only licensed physicians are allowed to perform certain tasks, thereby severely limiting the ability of physicians to increase their output by delegating tasks to other personnel. Second, when new types of health personnel, such as physician's assistants, were trained to undertake certain tasks, previously the sole prerogative of the physician, state boards of medical examiners retained the authority to certify their use on an individual physician-by-physician basis. In this manner, a particular physician would not be able to hire a large number of such personnel and greatly increase his or her output. The medical licensing boards' control over physician's assistants can be used to approve their use in situations where demand for physician services has increased, or in areas where physicians are not available, such as in rural areas; their employment can be limited where physician's practices, from the standpoint of the physicians, are underutilized.

The foregoing methods, which have been used successfully by the medical profession to restrict both entry into the profession and productivity, have been adapted by other health professions as well. The American Dental Association (ADA), after successfully achieving state licensure of dentists, had a study conducted on dental education, which resulted in the Gies Report in the early 1920s. As a result of this report, applicants for state dental examinations had to be graduated from approved dental schools, with the accreditation being conducted by the ADA's own Council on Dental Education. The number of dental schools declined as standards, mandated by the ADA and carried out by its Council, were increased. The length of the training time to become a dentist has also increased; and recently the ADA has called for a hospital residency requirement for new dentists.

Increased educational requirements increase the investment cost of becoming a physician, thereby decreasing the rate of return to entering physicians. The extent to which the price of physician services and physicians' incomes will rise in response to higher entry costs and fewer physicians will depend upon the elasticities of the demand and supply of physician services. Barriers to entry in the physician market are consistent with a monopoly model that would confer higher incomes on physicians.

We now turn to an examination of these barriers as a means of protecting the consumer from incompetent providers. For this hypothesis to be an accurate description of the justification for such restrictions, the medical profession, through its representatives in county, state, and national organizations, should favor *all* policies, not just entry barriers, to protect the consumer from incompetent practitioners. If the AMA is not consistent in its support of quality measures and only favors those that favorably affect its members' incomes, while opposing those that adversely affect its members' incomes, we must conclude that the real motivation for such measures is to enhance the monopoly power of its members.

If the AMA were in favor of protecting consumers from incompetent physicians, one measure the AMA would be expected to favor would be reexamination and relicensure of physicians. One justification given for increased training requirements for new physicians is that there has been an explosion of medical knowledge. Some physicians received their medical education 30–40 years ago; reexamination and relicensure would ensure that existing physicians have kept up with this increase in knowledge. Reexamination for relicensure is required in other areas, such as for renewal of driver licenses and for commercial airline pilots. There can be little justification for favoring increased training for new physicians but not for existing physicians if quality and consumer protection is of concern to the medical profession. Yet the AMA is opposed to reexamination and/or relicensure. If reexamination and relicensure were required, then unless the passing level were set so low that everyone always passed, either a large number of physicians would fail the reexamination and be unable to practice, or different levels of licensure would be established to recognize what exists in practice.

Not all physicians should be permitted to undertake all tasks even though they are licensed. With the realization that licensure should exist by tasks or levels would come the recognition that it is possible to prepare for different levels by using different educational requirements. It should be possible to have lower training requirements for some tasks; as the complexity of the task to be performed increased, so would the training requirements. One would expect, therefore, that the number of entrants would be greater the lower the training requirements. If different levels of licensure were to exist, barriers to entry would be lowered and the incomes of practicing physicians would be decreased. Since such an approach to increasing quality among physicians would decrease the monopoly power of physicians, we would therefore expect the AMA to oppose reexamination and licensure by task.

The emphasis on quality control in medicine is on the "process" of becoming a physician and not on the care that is provided ("outcome") once a person has become a physician. Controlling quality and competency of physicians through process measures, which require an undergraduate education, four years of education in an approved medical school, a minimum of three years in residency, and throughout this period, a series of examinations, is consistent with constructing barriers to entry and raising training costs, thereby lowering the entering physician's rate of return. Once the physician has met all these requirements, there is no monitoring of the care that he or she provides. Physicians may be well trained when they begin practicing, but this does not mean that they will be ethical. A number of studies document the amount of "unnecessary" surgery; other studies show that more than one-half of all surgery is undertaken by unethical or unqualified practitioners. Virtually no quality control programs have been instituted by the medical profession that are directed toward practicing physicians. It was for precisely this reason that Congress passed the professional standards review organizations (PSROs) legislation in an attempt to develop peer review mechanisms to monitor the quality of care provided by physicians. The AMA opposed this legislation. If the medical profession were concerned primarily with quality rather than with monopoly power, there would be at least some emphasis by the profession on the quality of care provided by practicing physicians.

Requiring citizenship for physician licensure, as a number of states did (it is now unconstitutional), is another example of the use of entry barriers to achieve monopoly power instead of promoting quality. If a prospective physician has met all the educational and licensure requirements, a citizenship requirement can *only* be viewed as a means of preventing entry into the profession by foreign-trained physicians. Although the quality of foreign-trained physicians varies, examinations and other procedures, such as monitoring of care, would be a more direct and accurate measure of quality than whether or not the person is a U.S. citizen.

Similar to citizenship is the requirement by some professional associations (e.g., state dental associations) of residency in a state before a person is permitted to practice. A year's residency is imposed on dentists who wish to locate in Hawaii. Such a requirement, which forces the practitioner to be without income for a year, decreases the attractiveness to dentists in other states of moving to that particular location. Such a barrier to entry is unrelated to quality, since it does not differentiate among the educational or performance backgrounds of the persons wishing to locate there. It is solely a device to enhance the monopoly power of the practicing professionals in that location.

It would appear, therefore, that the concern of the medical profession (as well as of other health professions) with quality is selective. Quality measures that might adversely affect the incomes of their members, such as reexamination and relicensure, are opposed, as are any measures that attempt to monitor the quality of care delivered. The hypothesis that quality measures are instituted to raise the rate of return to practicing physicians appears to be consistent with the positions on quality taken by the medical profession.

It has been claimed that the selective approach to quality favored by the medical profession may actually have served to *lower* the quality of care available to the U.S. population (7). Once entry into a profession is restricted, the prices of those services are higher than they would be otherwise, and there is an increase in the growth and use of substitutes for that profession. Patients begin searching for lower-priced substitutes, such as chiropractors and faith healers. Patients also substitute self-diagnosis and treatment for the physician's services. Some of these alternatives may be of lower quality than if the restrictions on medicine were lower. Fewer, more highly trained physicians mean that a smaller percentage of the population will have access to medical care. If only physicians are permitted to perform certain tasks, even though other trained personnel might be equally capable of performing them, this will again mean that a smaller percentage of the population will have access to such services. A relevant measure of the quality of care in society should not be confined to the care received only by those persons receiving physician services; it should incorporate the size of the population that does not receive any (or many fewer) physician services or that uses poorer substitutes.[1]

---

[1]Milton Friedman also states that quality has been adversely affected because there is less experimentation in treatment, which tends to reduce the rate of growth in medical knowledge, since a person desiring to experiment in treatment must be a member of the medical profession. The profession also encourages conformity in medical practice. The medical profession has also discouraged malpractice suits against physicians by discouraging physicians from testifying against one another. This action has also limited the consumer's protection against unethical and incompetent practitioners. The possibility of high malpractice awards against them would discourage incompetent practitioners from practicing, thereby providing protection to future patients.

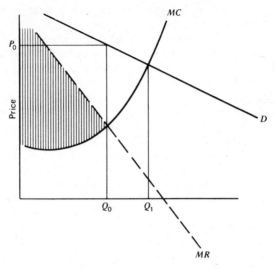

Figure 14-1. Determination of price and output by a profit-maximizing monopolist.

The current system of medical licensure, with its attendant requirements and emphasis on entry into the profession, imposes certain "costs" on society. The presumed successes of such a system of licensure in protecting consumers against unethical and incompetent practitioners are uncertain. What is desirable is the least costly system for alleviating consumer uncertainty and for meeting society's demand for protection. Several proposals in this regard will be discussed at the conclusion of this chapter.

THE PHYSICIAN AS A PRICE DISCRIMINATING MONOPOLIST

The establishment of barriers to entry in medicine provides physicians with a greater rate of return than if such barriers did not exist. However large the economic returns are from monopolizing an industry, the monopolist can earn still greater returns if it is possible to become a price-discriminating monopolist. Profit-maximizing monopolists charge one price to all of their consumers; that price and the resulting output would be determined by the intersection of their marginal revenue and marginal cost curves. This situation is shown in Figure 14-1. The profit-maximizing price and output would be P_0 and Q_0, respectively. The amount of "profit" in this situation is the striped area between marginal revenue (MR) and marginal cost (MC). If, however, the monopolist above is now able to become a price-discriminating monopolist (e.g., first degree) and can charge each patient a separate price, the monopolist's demand curve is also the marginal revenue curve. A lower price does not have to be charged to *all* patients to sell more services. If the demand curve is now also the marginal revenue curve, then with the same marginal cost curve, the monopolist's profit will have increased: instead of being just the striped area, the profit now includes the entire area between the demand and marginal cost curve. The price-discriminating monopolist's output is also

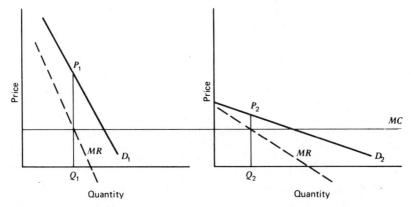

Figure 14–2. Determination of prices and outputs by a price-discriminating monopolist.

larger (Q_1), since he or she will produce to the point where the marginal cost curve intersects the demand curve, which is equivalent to the marginal revenue curve.

No single price is charged to everyone; the price-discriminating monopolist may charge each patient a different price. Because the profit can be greater if the monopolist can charge different prices to different purchasers for essentially the same service, we would expect monopolists to try to become price-discriminating monopolists. Two conditions, however, must be met if price discrimination is to be applied successfully in any market. The first is that the different purchasers of the service must have different elasticities of demand for the same service. Unless the elasticities of demand are different, the profit-maximizing price will be the same for each purchaser. The second condition is that it is necessary to separate the different markets in which the service is sold, so that the purchaser paying a lower price for the service cannot resell it in the higher-priced market. If such markets are not kept separate, prices will eventually become the same for all purchasers. Figure 14–2 is an illustration of price discrimination. Each diagram represents a different purchaser or market. Assuming a constant and similar marginal cost curve for serving each market, the profit-maximizing prices would be P_1 and P_2.

We hypothesize that since price discrimination results in greater profits than would result from setting the same price for each purchaser, physicians will attempt to maximize their "profits" by becoming price-discriminating monopolists. The necessary conditions for price discrimination are rather easily met in the physician sector. Patients paying lower prices for a physician's services cannot resell those services, thereby keeping the markets separate. The elasticities of demand for physician services differ, since persons with higher incomes are willing to pay more than are persons with lower incomes for the same services. The price-discriminating model would predict that as insurance coverage for physician services increases, physicians will still try to maintain their ability to price discriminate.

An alternative model to explain physician pricing behavior is as follows. Differences in prices charged for the same services to different patients means that the physician is acting as a charitable agency. By charging higher prices to those who can afford them, the physician can provide services to persons with lower incomes who cannot afford to pay as much. The physician thus acts as a charitable agency in determining who receives care and how much each is charged. This charity hypothesis has often been used by the medical profession to rationalize the different prices charged for the same services performed. However, the charity hypothesis should predict that as insurance coverage (both private and public) becomes more widespread among those with low incomes, there should no longer be a need for the physician to maintain their ability to practice price discrimination. There would be less of a need for the physician to subsidize the care of the poor.

When public and private insurance coverage for physician services is examined, however, we observe that physicians are still able to practice price discrimination. When treating a patient, physicians have had the option of accepting assignment under Medicare or becoming a participating physician under Blue Shield. Physicians can do so on a case-by-case basis. When the physician either accepts assignment or is a participating physician, he or she agrees to abide by the particular fee schedules. For patients that have a greater ability to pay, the physician can decide not to be a participating physician. In this situation the patient pays the physician's fee and applies to either Medicare or Blue Shield for partial reimbursement. The physician receives a greater amount and the patient pays a greater amount out of pocket than if the physician accepted assignment or was a participating physician. An illustration of this form of price discrimination was shown in Figure 9-4.

To distinguish further between the two hypotheses and to test whether physicians have acted as price-discriminating monopolists, the past behavior of county and state medical societies is examined. In this way we can determine whether the societies' actions and political positions have consistently been directed toward maintaining a situation that enables individual physicians to price discriminate. Unless a cartel like organization such as a medical society were able to enforce sanctions against price cutters, price discrimination could not survive in what would otherwise be a competitive market. One might assume that even though entry barriers existed, there is still such a large number of physicians that their market would be price competitive. If one physician charged a higher price for a given surgical procedure, for example, other physicians would be able to increase their market share by offering to sell the procedure at a lower price; price discrimination in a competitive situation could not exist. Patients with higher incomes, when charged higher prices, would seek out lower-priced, equally qualified physicians. Prices for medical services would become similar to patients with different incomes. Differences in prices for medical services would be related only to differences in the costs of providing those services, not to differences in the patient's price elasticity of demand. To shed light on the price discrimination hypothesis of physician pricing, it is necessary to ascertain why, even though there are restrictions on the number of firms (physicians) entering the industry, physician services were not priced as would be expected in a competitive industry. To determine how price discrimination could exist in what could have been an essentially competitive industry, we must look for *sanctions* that could be applied to physicians if they were to price their services competitively.

In his classic article entitled "Price Discrimination in Medicine," Reuben Kessel claimed that control over physician pricing behavior was related to the physician's need for hospital privileges and the prerequisite requirement of membership in the county medical society (8).

Internship and residency programs were offered only in hospitals approved by the AMA. Physicians wanted the hospitals they were associated with to be approved for such programs, since interns and residents increase the physician's productivity and income; the availability of interns and residents in a hospital enables a physician to see more patients and/or to have more leisure time. Interns and residents are thus demanded by physicians. The hospital pays the salaries of interns and residents, while the physician receives the benefits of the services of a resident; the resident cares for the physicians' patients in the hospital. The Mundt resolution, which was declared unconstitutional in the mid-1960s, required that the entire attending medical staff in the hospital be members of the county medical society if the hospital were to be approved for intern and residency training. Membership in the county medical society thus became important to physicians if they wished to have hospital privileges, which are a necessity for almost all specialties of medicine. Membership in the county society was also a prerequisite if a physician wanted to take an examination to qualify for a specialty board. If a physician engaged in any form of competitive behavior that was branded "unethical," the county medical society, which determined its own rules for membership, could deny such a physician membership in the society, thereby denying that physician hospital privileges and access to specialty certification.

Those physicians who potentially offer the greatest threat to the existence of price discrimination are new physicians in the community. To establish a market, new firms must advertise their availability, competence, and specialty, and they must also offer lower prices to attract consumers away from established firms. To prevent such competitive behavior from occurring, county medical societies gave new physicians probationary membership. If the new physician engaged in any of the above "unethical" activities to become established in the community, the county medical society would revoke membership and thereby deny hospital privileges to that physician. Probationary status was granted, not just to recent graduates, but also to physicians who had been in practice for a long time in another area (and were members of another county medical society) and had recently moved into the community.

After the invalidation of the Mundt resolution, the sanctions available to medical societies for use against physicians who wished to compete on price were state laws that delegated authority to medical licensing boards to determine the conditions for medical licensure. Included in such state laws were severe penalties for advertising and fee splitting. Although the mechanism for inhibiting price competition among physicians shifted from control over hospital privileges by county medical societies to state laws that prohibited such behavior, the effect was the same. Strong sanctions and penalties were available to organized medicine (which may be viewed as a cartel) to inhibit price competition, which would have eroded the physician's ability to price discriminate.

The above discussion indicates that medical societies had the ability to control price discrimination; however, is there any evidence to suggest that the available sanctions were used to support price discrimination by physicians? Does the evidence indicate whether the sanctions were imposed for reasons of "quality" or whether they were consistently imposed on physicians who attempted to engage in price competition? The AMA's position with regard to health insurance is the first evidence that Kessel examines in his test of the price discrimination hypothesis. Insurance coverage to pay for physician services would generally be favored by physicians, since it increases both the demand for physician services and the patient's ability to pay for those services. Health insurance varies with regard to the manner in which the physician is reimbursed. Indemnity plans reimburse the patient a certain dollar amount and allow the physician to charge the patient whatever he or she believes the patient can pay. Such plans are the most conducive to price discrimination by physicians. Health insurance plans that guarantee medical services rather than dollars if the consumer becomes ill would be opposed by the medical profession because they are sold at the same price to consumers regardless of their incomes. Such plans are a form of price competition, since high income persons can purchase the same medical service at the same price as can a person with low income. If the charity hypothesis were the more accurate explanation of physician pricing behavior, medical societies would not be expected to oppose such plans. The only conceivable reason for the medical profession's opposition to such medical service plans is that they undercut the ability of physicians to price discriminate. Examples of such medical service plans are prepaid health plans (PHPs), where the consumer pays a yearly capitation fee, regardless of family income, and is then entitled to hospital and medical services when ill. It is interesting, therefore, to examine the sanctions that local medical societies have applied to prevent the development of PHPs.

The opposition mounted by organized medicine against PHPs was unaffected by the location of these plans or their sponsorship. The first type of sanction, aimed at putting such plans out of business, was to deny hospital privileges to physicians associated with such plans. If the physician was already a member of the county medical society, the medical society would disband and reestablish itself without including the particular physician. New physicians entering the area with the intention of joining a PHP in the community would not be permitted to join the county medical society. Whether or not a PHP had its own hospital determined whether it was able to survive. It is for this reason that Kaiser Foundation, a well-known PHP on the west coast, operated its own hospitals; otherwise, it could not have offered hospital care to its subscribers and would not have been able to compete. The county medical societies tried other tactics against the Kaiser Foundation. The State Board of Medical Examiners in California tried Dr. Garfield, the medical director of Kaiser, for unprofessional conduct and suspended his license to practice. In subsequent legal rulings the suspension was overruled; the board's action was considered arbitrary in that Dr. Garfield did not have a fair trial.

Another approach used by medical societies to inhibit the development of PHPs was to have a higher proportion of physicians who belonged to PHPs drafted during World War II. (The medical society played a strong role with regard to the drafting of physicians at that time.) A number of physicians serving during World War II were unable to qualify as officers in the Navy and had to serve as enlisted men because they could not obtain a letter from their county medical society stating that they were members in good standing. These physicians believed they were discriminated against because they were associated with PHPs. In other instances where local medical societies ousted physicians belonging to PHPs, successful lawsuits were brought against the medical societies under the Sherman Anti-Trust Act (9).

In addition to attempting to terminate PHPs through the use of sanctions against physicians associated with them, medical societies attempted to legislate them out of business. State medical societies sponsored legislation in many states, and were successful in more than 20 states, in having restrictions placed on PHPs, thereby inhibiting their growth. These restrictive statutes permitted only the medical profession to operate or to control prepaid medical plans. (Federal legislation on health maintenance organizations specifically preempted such restrictive statutes if the HMO qualified under the federal HMO law.)

Another example of the medical profession's interest in maintaining the physician's ability to price discriminate among patients is the type of medical insurance plan favored by organized medicine. Blue Shield plans were developed and controlled by state medical societies and offered physician coverage to consumers under the following terms. If a subscriber's income was less than a certain amount, generally $7,500 a year, the participating physician would accept the Blue Shield fee as full payment for services provided to the patient; however, if the patient's income was in excess of the stated amount, the physician could bill the patient an amount in excess of the Blue Shield fee for that service. The medical profession favored Blue Shield because physicians would be assured of payment from low-income subscribers and would still be able to price discriminate among higher-income subscribers. If the physicians were charitable agencies, they would not need to charge higher-income patients an additional amount once the lower-income patient was able to pay the full fee for their services. During the 1970s, some medical societies dropped their sponsorship of Blue Shield plans because the plans raised the income limits below which the Blue Shield fee would represent full payment for the patient's use of physician services.

Additional evidence that the charity hypothesis is inapplicable to explain physician pricing behavior is provided in the following statement by Kessel:

> Most of the "free" care that was traditionally provided by the medical profession fell into three categories: (a) work done by neophytes, particularly in the surgical specialties, who wanted to develop their skills and therefore require practice; (b) services of experienced physicians in free clinics who wish to develop new skills or maintain existing skills so they can better serve their private, paying patients; and (c) services to maintain staff and medical appointments which are of great value financially. The advent of Medicare has reduced the availability of "charity" patients used as teaching material, and has led to readjustments in training procedures, particularly for residents. (10)

The sanctions available to the medical profession to prevent price competition have changed over time. Advertising can no longer be prohibited by state practice acts. That the medical profession had been successful in inhibiting price competition is evidenced by the successful suit brought by the Federal Trade Commission (FTC) against the AMA and several medical specialty societies (decided by the Supreme Court in 1982). The FTC claimed that the AMA's "Principles of Medical Ethics," which banned advertising, price competition, and other forms of competitive practices, resulted in a situation in which "prices of physician services have been stabilized, fixed, or otherwise interfered with; competition between medical doctors in the provision of such services has been hindered, restrained, foreclosed and frustrated; and consumers have been deprived of information pertinent to the selection of a physician and of the benefits of competition" (11).

Over time the medical profession has been successful in acting in the economic interest of its members. The continually high rates of return to an investment in a medical education and the excess of applicants to acceptances in medical schools are evidence that there had been a static shortage of physicians. To achieve these monopoly profits, the medical profession constructed entry barriers into the profession. Under the guise of controlling quality of care and eliminating unqualified practitioners, the medical profession emphasized "process" measures of quality control. Quality assurance was present only at the point of entry into the profession by means of requiring attendance at an approved medical school, licensure examinations, and longer minimum times spent in postgraduate training programs; virtually no quality control measures were directed at practicing physicians.

With the authority delegated to the medical licensing boards by the state, the medical profession was able to go beyond the establishment of a simple monopoly. The medical profession, acting as a cartel to protect the economic interests of its members, was able to establish and enforce the necessary conditions to enable physicians to practice price discrimination. The sanctions used by the medical profession against members who participated in prepaid medical plans were sufficiently severe as to retard the development of such plans for many years. The consequences to society of these actions by organized medicine were that prices of medical services were higher than they would be otherwise, the availability of such services was less, and importantly, consumers were (and still are) not as well protected from unqualified and unethical practitioners as they have been led to believe.

PROPOSED CHANGES IN THE PHYSICIAN MANPOWER MARKET

The objective of proposing changes in the market for physicians is twofold: first, the demand for consumer protection should be achieved in the least costly manner possible, and second, the market for physicians should perform efficiently. The key to improving market performance is to deal first with the concern to consumer protection.

Entry into The Medical Profession

If a prospective physician can pass the licensing examination, it is not clear why he or she also has to have attended an approved medical school to be licensed. The only logical reason for also requiring attendance at an approved medical school is that the licensing examination is not a sufficient assurance of the physician's knowledge. If this is the case, the examination process should be improved and less emphasis placed on the number of years of education required and on attendance at approved schools.

A second approach to lowering the cost of licensure, while also achieving a certain performance level of entering physicians, is to have "task" licensure. Currently, physicians are either licensed or they are not. Once licensed, they are permitted to undertake many tasks and practice the full scope of medicine; a number of tasks for which they might not be well trained, such as in the case of the practitioner who is legally permitted to perform surgery, provide anesthesia services, and provide medical care to the patient. Instead of such a "zero–one" level of licensure, physicians should be licensed to perform specific tasks. Such task or specific-purpose licenses would recognize what exists in the real world: namely, even though physicians are licensed, the public would be better protected if they performed only those tasks they are qualified to perform. Task licensure would mean that all physicians would not need to take the same educational training; it might be possible to provide alternative levels of training (or train certain types of physicians) in a much shorter period. Different educational requirements would lower the costs of a medical education, since both educational and opportunity costs would be reduced. If physicians wanted additional specific-purpose licenses, they could return to school and receive additional training before taking the qualifying examination for that license. (In this way a career ladder could be developed for medicine.) Under such a proposal, the training requirements to enter the medical profession would not be determined by the medical profession itself but would be related to the *demand* for different types of physicians and the least-cost manner of producing them.

Continuing Assurance of the Quality of Physician Services

As discussed earlier, once a physician is licensed, the medical profession undertakes virtually no quality assurance mechanisms. Several proposals to deal with the issue of unethical and unqualified physicians should be considered. First, periodic reexamination and relicensure would require physicians to maintain their qualifications. Rather than mandating a certain number of hours of continuing education, reexamination would determine the appropriate amount of continuing education on an individual basis.[2] It would also be a more direct measure of whether or not the physician has achieved the objectives of continuing education. Periodic reexamination and relicensure would be consistent with the earlier proposal of task or specific purpose licensure.

If physicians were reexamined and relicensed every few years for specific-purpose licenses, we would have greater assurance that physicians were practicing in the fields of medicine in which they were qualified. There would still be concern, however, regarding the physician who may be qualified but is unethical in performing unnecessary services and in charging for services not performed. Continual monitoring of the care provided by physicians, with a state agency taking responsibility (with the cooperation of the medical profession) would help to ensure that a minimum of unethical and unqualified actions were undertaken. Penalties assessed by state quality review agencies should be financial and should vary according to the severity of the misbehavior. Penalties that remove or suspend the physician's license are usually considered to be so severe that they are rarely undertaken. Financial penalties would be more likely to be imposed for actions that are not sufficiently flagrant to call for removal of the physician's license but are in need of redress.

Another approach for safeguarding consumers is recourse to the courts. However, because malpractice premiums have been rising so rapidly recently, medical societies have been lobbying for legislation that would have the effect of reducing their malpractice premiums. Although there may be problems associated with the current system of malpractice, such as the uncertainty of future awards, it would be preferable to improve the current malpractice system rather than to eliminate its deterrent effect. A well-functioning malpractice system should serve as an incentive to physicians to confine themselves to tasks they are qualified to perform (12).

The Future Supply of Physicians

An important policy debate currently is whether there is a surplus of physicians and, if so, the appropriate mechanism to deal with it. As a result of congressional action in the late 1960s to expand the number of medical schools and spaces, medical school enrollments and graduates have increased. U.S. citizens studying overseas (USFMGs) and non-U.S. citizens graduating from foreign medical schools (alien FMGs) contributed to the rapidly increasing supply of physicians. The consequences of this increased supply were that the physician/population ratio started rising, the ratio of applicants to

---

[2]After speaking to a hospital's medical staff on the "Economic Outlook for Physicians," I received a letter awarding me continuing medical education credits, which my audience had also received.

acceptances in medical schools started declining, and physicians' income, adjusted for inflation, declined in the latter half of the 1970s. Medical schools, medical societies, and the federal government became concerned with the consequences of this increased supply. Medical societies were concerned about the economic interests of their members. Medical schools were concerned about their survival; several dental schools had to close as their applicant pool diminished. In 1985–1986 a decline occurred in the number of medical school applicants and the applicant/acceptances ratio fell below 2. Once again, the "appropriate" number of physicians became the subject of a policy debate (13).

In 1980 the Graduate Medical Education National Advisory Commission (GMENAC) forecast a surplus of 70,000 physicians by 1990 (approximately 15 percent more than "needed") and 145,000 (or a 30 percent surplus) by the year 2000. The GMENAC approach, as discussed earlier, was to rely on expert panels to determine the number of physicians "required" in each specialty. Each physician specialty panel determined the needs for care in its specialty, the percent of those needing care that would be seen by their specialty, the amount of technological change occurring that would affect care within their specialty, and productivity changes. Together with estimates of the likely number of specialists in 1990 and 2000, GEMENAC reached its conclusion regarding the number of surplus physicians.

Given the approach used by GMENAC to determining the appropriate number of physicians, it would appear logical for the medical education community to suggest that the solution is to decrease the number of residency positions in each specialty; an agency such as GMENAC has been proposed to determine both the number and size of residency programs for each specialty. A second approach has been the proposal to phase out residency opportunities for alien FMGs. Reducing residency positions for USFMGs is more controversial but has also been proposed. The third approach to reduce the future supply is the suggestion by the Association of American Medical Schools that medical school enrollments be reduced. Further, to offset the decline in medical school tuition as a result of having fewer students, the federal government should provide "decapitation" grants to medical schools.

Attempts by the federal government to reduce its Medicare expenditures would also have the effect of reducing the number of residency positions in teaching hospitals. Medicare reimburses teaching hospitals for their residents. Reducing these payments would decrease the value of residents to these institutions. Other third-party payors, such as Blue Cross, are also reducing their payments for residents when they form PPOs and use nonteaching hospitals in those organizations because they are less costly. The motivation of these purchasers is to reduce their expenditures, not necessarily to decrease the demand for residents, but the effect of their policies is the same.

The GMENAC approach for determining a surplus and the use of a quasi-governmental organization for establishing the number of physicians in each specialty is not favored by those who would prefer a market-oriented approach. Special commissions to establish "requirements" and forecast future supplies have been used before and their forecasting performance has not been very accurate (14). The GMENAC study has already been proven inaccurate in a number of dimensions; the percent of physicians employed in HMOs is quite different than forecasted, with the consequence (according to GMENAC) that the number of physicians in the non-HMO sector are greater than anticipated. Females as a percent of total physicians were underestimated, thereby overestimating (according to GMENAC) overall physician productivity; female physicians were estimated to have a 78 percent lifetime productivity of male physicians. GMENAC has also been inaccurate with regard to its specialty requirements (e.g., the number of cesarean deliveries have been much greater than anticipated).

It is difficult for any group to consider all the changes that may occur; who foresaw the spread of AIDS and the consequent requirements for medical care, or the growth in transplants? It is also difficult for an agency to make the appropriate adjustments in medical school spaces and in residency positions once changes occur in their underlying forecasts.

More important, the GMENAC approach is not an economic approach for determining a surplus. An increase in the supply of physicians is causing a decline in physicians' incomes, however, this does not necessarily mean that there is a surplus. Whether or not there is a surplus depends on the rate of return to a medical and specialty education.

It is unlikely that a market approach or a regulatory approach for determining the appropriate number of physicians will always be accurate. Permitting prospective applicants to decide whether or not they wish to enter medicine and, similarly, allowing the specialty decision to be made by residents places the burden as well as the benefits of that decision on the individuals rather than on an agency. Improved information would enable these individuals to make more informed choices. Individual decision-making, based on professional and economic incentives, results in a rapid self adjusting mechanism to changes in the marketplace. We observe that individuals are adjusting to the new environment and changing their demands for a medical (and dental) education. These adjustments are quicker and more accurate than an agency whose constituency (medical schools and the medical profession) has its own economic objectives.

Having too many or too few physicians has costs and benefits to different groups. Using regulation to determine future supplies is likely to result in too few physicians because current physicians want to have high rates of return and medical schools want excess demand for their spaces. The representatives of these constituencies will dominate the regulatory body as they have with GMENAC and as they have in the past in determining the number of medical school spaces. Too few physicians imposes a cost on society; fewer physicians means that the price of their services are higher, access to care by those with low incomes is reduced, fewer physicians would locate in underserved areas, and fewer physicians would be available to work in innovative organizational settings such as HMOs.

Consumers bear the cost of too few physicians, whereas physicians bear the cost of too many. Thus whether greater caution should be placed on eliminating a surplus or a shortage depends upon one's economic perspective.

REFERENCES

1. A discussion of the reasons offered for licensure may be found in Thomas G. Moore, "The Purpose of Licensing," *Journal of Law and Economics*, 4, October 1961: 93–117; and Simon Rottenberg, "Economics of Occupational Licensing," *Aspects of Labor Economics*, National Bureau of Economic Research (Princeton, N.J.: Princeton University Press, 1962), 3–20. K. Leffler, "Physician Licensure: Competition and Monopoly in American Medicine," *Journal of Law and Eco-*

nomics, April 1978: 165–186 hypothesizes that the restrictions cited are in response to consumer demand.

2. Reuben Kessel, "Price Discrimination in Medicine," *Journal of Law and Economics*, October 1958: 25–26.
3. Milton Friedman, *Capitalism and Freedom* (Chicago: University of Chicago Press, 1962), p. 151.
4. Kessel, *op. cit..*,, p. 27.
5. *Ibid..*
6. This aspect of licensing board behavior is discussed in Rottenberg, *op. cit..*
7. Friedman, *op. cit..*, 155–158.
8. Kessel, *op. cit..*, p. 29.
9. This example of Group Health Association in Washington, D.C., and other examples cited are from Kessel, *op. cit..*, 30–41.
10. Reuben Kessel, "The AMA and the Supply of Physicians," *Law and Contemporary Problems* (Chapel Hill, N. C.: Duke University Press, 1970), p. 273.
11. United States of America Before Federal Trade Commission in the Matter of the American Medical Association, a corporation, The Connecticut State Medical Society, a corporation, The New Haven County Medical Association, Inc., Docket 9064, p. 3, December 1975.
12. For some readings on malpractice, see Patricia M. Danzon, *Medical Malpractice: Theory, Evidence, and Public Policy* (Cambridge, Mass.: Harvard University Press, 1985); and Simon Rottenberg, ed., *The Economics of Medical Malpractice* (Washington, D.C.: American Enterprise Institute for Public Policy Research, 1978).
13. The following discussion is based on the following articles in the *New England Journal of Medicine* by John K. Iglehart, "Federal Support of Graduate Medical Education," 312(15), April 11, 1985: 1000–1004, "Reducing Residency Opportunities for Graduates of Foreign Medical Schools," 313(13), September 26, 1985: 831–836, "Federal Support of Health Manpower Education," 314(5), January 30, 1986: 324–328; and "The Future Supply of Physicians," 314(13), March 27, 1986: 860–864.
14. See James H. Sammons, "Health Manpower in the Medical Marketplace," *Health Affairs*, 1(4), Fall 1982: p. 21, Table 1.

CHAPTER 15

The Market for Medical Education: Equity and Efficiency

In Chapter 14 it was shown that barriers to entry into medicine contribute significantly to the high rate of return from becoming a physician. Perhaps the most important barrier to entry into the health professions is the requirement of having graduated from an approved educational institution. Since such educational institutions determine the number of new graduates, it is important to examine the performance of the medical education sector. Medical schools, dental schools, and other health professional education institutions are the main determinants of the number of health professionals in the United States. They have also been the recipients of large sums of federal and state monies. Because of their combined role as the only approved health professional training institutions, as the determinants of the number of health professionals, and as the recipients of public funds, their performance should be examined in terms of (a) the economic efficiency with which this sector performs, and (b) whether there are any redistributive effects (the equity issue) in the manner in which this sector is financed.

THE ECONOMIC EFFICIENCY OF THE MEDICAL EDUCATION SECTOR

Every market performs certain functions; we are interested in two aspects of efficiency with respect to medical (and other health) education. First, is the industry producing an "optimal" number of health professionals? The appropriate or optimal rate of output in medical (or other health professional) education is concerned with both the number of graduates and their type (i.e., the level of training). Second, is the output (a physician or other health professional) being produced at minimum cost? Efficiency in production is judged on the basis of the extent of economies of scale in medical education (the number of schools) and whether each school is minimizing its costs.

To establish an appropriate yardstick by which to evaluate the performance of the medical education sector, we turn to a model of a purely competitive market. In examining the medical education sector as if it were similar to a competitive market, we look for any divergences between a competitive market and the current system of medical education to determine the reasons (and justification) for such differences. Using the yardstick of a competitive model and any possible economic rationales for differences between the two, we will evaluate the performance of the market for medical education and, if need be, offer proposals for improving its performance.

Medical Education in a Competitive Market

Both economic and noneconomic determinants affect the demand for a medical education. The major economic determinant of an investment in a medical education is the expected rate of return. One component of the rate of return is the price, or tuition, of a medical education. If other factors, such as physician incomes and the opportunity cost of attending medical school, are held constant, a change in the tuition level would cause movement along the demand curve for a medical education. If physician incomes were to increase, or if the opportunity cost of attending medical school were to decrease, these changes would cause a shift (to the right) in the demand for a medical education. Tuition, in a competitive market, would be the equilibrating mechanism. In the short run, with a given stock of medical education capacity, changes in demand for a medical education would cause a shift along a given supply curve of medical education; the tuition level would rise, and at the higher levels of tuition all those demanding a medical education would receive it. The level of tuition would serve as a rationing device and there would be no excess demand (applicants over acceptances). The demand and the supply of medical education would jointly determine the number of enrollments and the tuition level.

The supply response in a competitive market would be as follows. In the short run, each medical school facing an increased demand for its spaces would raise its prices (tuition). The higher tuition levels would enable the schools to attract more resources, namely to hire additional faculty by raising salaries. As a response to higher tuition levels, more medical schools might also be started. The long-run effect of the increased tuition would be increased medical school capacity.

Each school would not necessarily increase its capacity as demand increases; some schools might prefer to remain small and offer a "higher"-quality product than other schools, such as more inputs per student or longer training times. Tuition levels in such schools would be higher than in those schools that had much larger class sizes and lower training requirements. Whether or not such differences in types of schools could exist would depend upon whether there was a demand on the part of students for such differences in the quality of education. Presumably, just as there are differences in tuition levels and in the perceived quality of undergraduate and graduate schools, there would be a demand for different types of medical education at different levels of tuition. In a competitive system, as in pre-Flexnerian days, the graduates of the diverse educational institutions would have to pass a licensing examination. Some schools would have a much higher passing rate for their graduates than would other schools. Presumably, the schools would advertise such differences as they would their tuition levels and other educational requirements.[1]

Not all schools under such a competitive situation would be for-profit. Some schools might be nonprofit and have objectives similar to those of medical schools today, such as prestige maximization. As long as entry was permitted into the medical education market, differences in a school's "product"—educational requirements, pass rate on licensing examinations, and perceived quality of that institution—would have to justify the higher input costs, which would, in turn, be passed on to prospective students in the form of higher tuition levels. Unless students (or their parents) were willing to pay for such differences in quality, these educational institutions would either exit from the industry or, more likely, change their product to conform to what was being demanded.

The supply side of the medical education sector, then, would consist of many firms; economies of scale in medical education such as in library and clinical facilities are not large enough to result in only one school's being sufficiently lower in cost to preclude competition from other firms. Further, it would be expected that the schools would take advantage of any economies of scale that might exist in medical education, since that would improve their competitive position. Each school, in addition to moving to that size of operation that was of lowest per unit cost (for the type of product it was producing), would also attempt to minimize its own costs of operation. Again, the incentives for cost minimization would come either from the school's desire to increase its revenues or from competition from other schools offering prospective students lower tuition levels. Needless to say, schools would be forced to compete among themselves for prospective students.

Thus a competitive system in medical education, with the only entry barrier into the profession being a licensing examination, would result in a system of medical schools offering a variety of medical education (different training times, different input ratios of faculty to students, and so on) at tuition levels reflecting the minimum costs of producing different levels of "quality" of education. In a system of education where differences in inputs and outputs were permitted, there would presumably be a higher rate of innovation in teaching methods and in curriculum than in a system where inputs and outputs of the educational process were highly structured and little deviation from the norm exists. Such a system should result in efficiency in production, both for the individual school and for the system as a whole.

A competitive system in medical education, as just described, would also result in production of the "optimal" number of medical school graduates. The optimal number of medical school graduates, according to economic criteria, would occur when the benefits of a medical education to the student equaled the costs of that education. The demand for a medical education, at a given level of tuition, would represent the perceived private benefits of that education to the student; tuition would also reflect the costs of producing that education. As the equilibrating mechanism under such a system, tuition would reflect both the costs of producing the education and the bene-

---

[1]Not all professional schools are considered to be similar. Graduates from the Harvard and Stanford business schools are in greater demand than graduates from other business schools. The job opportunities for graduates of law school are also dissimilar. A similar quality spectrum would exist among medical schools. Graduates from higher-quality medical schools would, in addition to having higher pass rates on licensing exams, also find it easier to enter certain residency programs and to gain admission to the staff of certain hospitals.

fits received from it. The resulting number of medical school graduates would therefore be optimal, inasmuch as the costs of education would equal the benefits from it.

It may be argued that the private benefits under such a system are less than the social benefits of having a greater number of physicians in society. Under such a circumstance the number of physicians would be too few. If there are external benefits to having a greater number of physicians (this will be discussed shortly), subsidies can be provided under a competitive system to increase the demand for a medical education. The subsidies can be given directly to students, which, in lowering their tuition, would increase their demand, or they can be provided to the suppliers. If given directly to the students, students would still have an incentive to seek out those medical schools that will provide them with the type of education they desire, at minimum cost.

The foregoing scenario describes how a competitive system for medical education would perform in achieving, at minimum cost, the optimal rate of output of medical school graduates and the different levels of quality in medical education. The crucial role of tuition in this scenario is in equilibrating demand and supply and providing signals to both the demanders and suppliers of medical education.

The Current Market for Medical Education

Tuition, under the current system of medical education, does not serve as an equilibrating mechanism. Medical schools, on the average, receive only 5 percent of their income from tuition payment, as shown in Table 15-1. (For public medical schools tuition is only 3.2 percent of their income while for private schools it is 8.8 percent.) Further, for many medical schools, the amount of funds they receive from the university with which they are associated is unrelated to changes in their enrollment levels. Since medical schools are not very reliant on tuition as a source of revenue, it is not necessary for them to respond to changes in demand for a medical education. They are able to survive and to produce the type of medical education they want because they receive large, relatively unrestricted government subsidies. (Revenues from state and local governments represent 31 percent of public medical schools' unrestricted support.) The large educational subsidies received by the schools (and research grants and contracts that have also been used to subsidize educational activities) permit the schools to set tuition levels below actual costs of production. According to a study by the Institute of Medicine (IOM) and calculations performed by George Wright, tuition and fees covered less than 10 percent of the cost of education in 1972 (1). When these figures were updated to 1980, tuition and fees consisted of approximately 17 percent of the cost of education (2).

The effect on the demand for a medical education of subsidized tuition levels is to cause demand to be greater than it would otherwise be. The increased demand for a medical education resulting from the subsidized tuition is, however, not satisfied. The number of applicants admitted by the medical schools is determined by the number of available spaces. The number of spaces, in turn, is unrelated to the demand for a medical education or to tuition levels; the number is determined by the goals and objectives of the schools themselves. There is thus a continual excess demand for medical education by qualified students, given the high rates of return to a career in medicine and subsidized tuition. This situation is shown schematically in Figure 15-1. With an initial demand for medical education shown by the demand curve D_1, and the supply

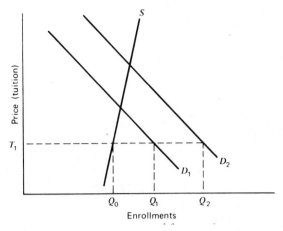

Figure 15-1. The excess demand for a medical education.

of spaces shown by S, the amount of excess demand for medical school spaces would be $Q_1 - Q_0$, when the tuition level is T_1, which is below the equilibrium level. As physician incomes increase (or other demand shift variables change), there is an increase in the demand for a medical education to D_2. Again, since tuition does not serve its rationing function, the excess demand for a medical education increases to $Q_2 - Q_0$.

On what basis does the medical school ration its spaces, since it does not rely on tuition to perform this function? It is hypothesized that the medical school will select those students who are most compatible with the goals of the school. Because all approved medical schools are nonprofit, they must have an objective other than trying to make the most money. It is hypothesized that their objective is one of prestige maximization, which is accomplished by retaining a faculty that is interested in research, a low student/faculty ratio that allows more time for research, and training medical students to be teachers and researchers rather than family practitioners. The average medical school is likely to try to emulate Johns Hopkins and Harvard medical schools, with their small class sizes, low student/faculty ratios, and emphasis on research. To achieve these goals, medical schools and their faculties want to select students based on high academic qualifications rather than on their future work preferences, such as desiring to work in rural areas. (There is little prestige among medical schools in having the highest percentage of its graduates become primary care practitioners in a rural area.) The excess of applicants resulting from setting tuition levels below the equilibrium level allows the faculty to select those students who most closely correspond to their goals.[2]

Attaining the goal of prestige maximization requires medical schools to be free from competitive pressures. If a school has to compete, then, as we have seen in the

---

[2]It has been claimed that the reduction in the number of medical schools as a result of the Flexner Report and the consequent excess demand for spaces enabled medical schools to discriminate against certain population groups in society (i.e., Jews, blacks, and women). Reuben Kessel, "The AMA and the Supply of Physicians," *Law and Contemporary Problems*, Duke University, Spring 1970: 270–272. In the 1970 Carnegie Commission Report on Medical Education, *Higher Education and the Nation's Health*, they suggest that medical schools "Refrain from discrimination on the basis of race, creed, or sex and also pursue positive policies to encourage the admission of members of minority groups" (p. 69).

TABLE 15-1. Patterns of Support for General Operations of Public and Private Medical Schools, 1968–1969, 1973–1974, 1979–1980, and 1984–1985 (Millions of Dollars)

	1968–1969		1973–1974		1979–1980		1984–1985	
	Public Schools							
Number of medical schools reporting	47		62		73		75	
Total restricted support	$330	(52.0)	$ 589	(44.6)	$1,102	(34.7)	$ 1,736	(31.5)
Total unrestricted support[a]	305	(48.0)	732	(55.4)	2,076	(65.3)	3,778	(68.5)
State and local government appropriations and subsidies	171	(26.9)	448	(34.0)	1,078	(33.9)	1,728	(31.3)
Professional fee (medical service plan) income	38	(6.0)	121	(9.1)	359	(11.3)	784	(14.2)
Recovery of indirect cost on contracts and grants	38	(6.0)	61	(4.6)	105	(3.3)	268	(4.9)
Tuition and fees	16	(2.5)	35	(2.6)	89	(2.8)	179	(3.2)
Income from college services	3	(.5)	17	(1.3)	36	(1.1)	87	(1.6)
Endowment income	1	(.2)	3	(.2)	2	(.1)	15	(.3)
Gifts	2	(.3)	6	(.5)	31	(1.0)	15	(.3)
Hospitals and clinics					191	(6.0)	323	(5.9)
Other income	36	(5.6)	41	(3.1)	185	(5.8)	379	(6.9)
Total public school support	635	(100.1)	1,321	(100.0)	3.178	(100.0)	5,514	(100.0)

Private Schools

	44		45		46		50	
Number of medical schools reporting								
Total restricted support	$450	(62.8)	$ 731	(70.7)	$1,283	(50.9)	$ 1,884	(41.2)
Total unrestricted support[a]	272	(37.2)	473	(39.3)	1,240	(49.1)	2,682	(58.7)
State and local government appropriations and subsidies	17	(2.3)	51	(4.3)	82	(3.3)	109	(2.4)
Professional fee (medical service plan) income	28	(3.8)	80	(6.6)	311	(12.3)	885	(19.4)
Recovery of indirect cost on contracts and grants	56	(7.7)	100	(8.3)	215	(8.5)	432	(9.5)
Tuition and fees	36	(4.9)	77	(6.4)	219	(8.6)	403	(8.8)
Income from college services	19	(2.6)	47	(3.9)	23	(.9)	38	(.8)
Endowment income	31	(4.2)	44	(3.6)	52	(2.1)	108	(2.4)
Gifts	21	(2.9)	23	(1.9)	49	(1.9)	52	(1.1)
Hospitals and clinics					189	(7.5)	371	(8.1)
Other income	64	(8.8)	51	(4.3)	100	(4.0)	284	(6.2)
Total private school support	731	(100.0)	1,204	(100.0)	2,523	(100.0)	4,566	(100.0)
Total medical school support private and public	$1,366		$2,525		$5,701		$10,080	

SOURCE: American Medical Association, *Journal of the American Medical Association*, Education Issues, various years.

[a]The percentages for the categories listed under "total unrestricted support" represent percentages of the total public and private school support. These percentages sum to the percentage shown on "total unrestricted support." For example, for 1968–1969 for public medical schools the percentages sum to 48 percent.

discussion of the competitive model, it will be forced to respond to the demands of students. Essential to freeing the school from competition are huge outside subsidies that relieve the school of reliance on tuition as a sole source of revenue. Also important are limits on entry into the medical school market by new medical schools that might have different objectives. The manner in which this restriction is achieved is through the accreditation process of new medical schools. It would be very difficult for a new medical school to start if its stated intention was to produce its graduates in a vastly shorter period, using a different curriculum and different input ratios to train its students. Because it might produce graduates at a much lower cost with the same probability of their passing the licensing examination, such a school would be a potential threat to other schools, and therefore it would be in the other schools' interests to see that such a school was not allowed to start.

What are the consequences of the current system for producing physicians? On the supply side of the market, the educational requirements for producing physicians are determined by the suppliers themselves without regard to demands for such an education. The product is relatively standard and many years of education are required: four years of undergraduate education before admission to a four-year medical school. The product is relatively costly to produce and there are large variations among schools in their costs of production (3). There are strong indications, based on the wide variations in cost data, that the schools are not minimizing their cost of production, nor do they have any incentive to do so as long as they are the recipients of large government subsidies. It thus appears that efficiency in production is the exception rather than the rule.

It is also highly unlikely that the current system of medical education produces the appropriate number of graduates. Since tuition is set way below the actual costs of education, the demand is much greater than it might be otherwise. [Although the price elasticity of demand for a medical education with respect to the tuition rate has been estimated to be approximately -.4, that is, price inelastic (4), if tuition were to reflect the actual costs of production, demand for such an education would be less than it is currently.] The number of medical school spaces is unrelated to the demand for such spaces, which have increased very slowly over time. As shown in Table 15–2, between 1946–1947 and 1965–1966, the number of medical school enrollments increased by less than 2.0 percent per year. Throughout this period there was a continual excess demand for medical school spaces. The number of physicians produced could not have been related to society's demands, or even to private demands, for physicians. The number of physicians was determined by the suppliers of education, either in conjunction with other organizations' requirements or solely in response to their own.[3]

The result of the constraint on the number of medical school spaces was twofold. First, there was a large demand by American students for a foreign medical education. Large numbers of qualified, but rejected medical school applicants went overseas to study medicine and then reentered the United States to practice. These American students were willing to pay a much higher tuition level in places such as Guadalajara, Mexico, to spend additional years in residence (thereby increasing their

---

[3]The goals of medical schools appear to have been synonymous with the objectives of the American Medical Association. The AMA also prefers small additions to the stock of physicians. It is therefore in the AMA's interest that medical schools be nonprofit. The schools' incentive thereby changes from cost minimization and responding to increased demands for spaces to becoming prestigious.

TABLE 15-2. U.S. Medical School Enrollment, First-Year Students and Graduates, 1946–1947 to 1985–1986

Academic Year	Students Total	Students First-Year	Graduates	Number of Schools
1946–1947	23,900	6,564	6,389	77
1950–1951	26,186	7,177	6,135	79
1955–1956	28,639	7,686	6,845	82
1960–1961	30,288	8,298	6,994	86
1965–1966	32,835	8,759	7,574	88
1970–1971	40,487	11,348	8,974	103
1975–1976	56,244	15,351	13,561	114
1980–1981	65,497	17,204	15,667	126
1985–1986	66,604	16,929	16,191[a]	127

sources: American Medical Association, *Journal of the American Medical Association*, 226, November 19, 1973: 910; and 256, September 26, 1986: 1561. Copyright 1973, 1986, American Medical Association.

[a]Estimated in April 1986.

opportunity costs), and to receive an education considered inferior to that received in U.S. medical schools. Second, as a result of increased demands for medical care during this period, the rates of return for practicing medicine were much greater in the United States than in other countries; consequently, there was a large influx of foreign medical graduates (FMGs) into this country. These FMGs came predominately from less-developed countries to work on hospital staffs, and in many cases, they provided the medical care for the urban poor in the United States.

The U.S. Congress reacted to demands by U.S. citizens for a medical education and also to stem the inflow of foreign-trained physicians by passing the Health Professions Educational Assistance Act (HPEA) in the mid-1960s. The effect of this Act was to increase the supply of medical school spaces. It was, therefore, the perception of Congress that the medical education market was not producing an appropriate number of physicians. To achieve an increase in the supply of physicians, funds were provided for new medical schools, and existing medical schools received capitation funds on the condition that they increase their enrollments. Although the AMA and medical schools opposed mandatory enrollment increases, medical schools were in need of additional funds. These congressional financial incentives to medical schools proved to be effective. As a result of the HPEA legislation, enrollments and graduates began to increase. In 1965–1966 there were 32,835 medical students in 88 medical schools. By 1985–1986, the number of students more than doubled to 66,604 and the number of schools increased to 127 (see Table 15-2). The consequence of this increase in medical school enrollment was to cause a 50 percent increase in the number of physicians between 1965 and 1980. Between 1980 and 1990 the number of physicians is expected to increase by an additional 30 percent.

By the late 1970s, these large projected increases in the supply of physicians led to a concern, particularly among organized medicine and government, that "too many" physicians were being produced. As a result, the preferential immigration treatment for FMGs was removed, making it more difficult for FMGs to enter this country, and the HPEA financial assistance to medical schools began to be phased out in the early 1980s.

As seen in Table 15-2, medical schools are slowly beginning to reduce their enrollments. The number of first-year students in 1985–1986 is 275 fewer than in 1981. This reduction in admissions is expected to continue but is unlikely to have much of an effect on the total supply of physicians for many years.

Efficiency, Externalities, and the Optimal Number of Physicians

The optimal quantity of output in an industry occurs when the cost of producing the last unit equals the additional benefits from consuming it. The price that people are willing to pay for that output is an indication of the marginal benefits they hope to receive from consuming it. When price is equal to marginal cost, as would occur in a competitive market, the marginal private benefits equal the marginal private costs of production, and the optimal quantity of that good or service is produced (assuming no external effects). Those persons receiving the benefits of the good or service are paying the full costs of producing it. When this concept is applied to the number of physicians, the optimal number of physicians are produced when the cost of producing physicians is equal to the price (tuition) of a medical education. The price that a student is willing to pay for a medical education reflects the private benefits the student hopes to receive as a result of that education. If the price that prospective students are willing to pay for a medical education is greater than the price charged for a medical education, too few physicians are being produced. More resources should flow into that industry until the cost of producing additional physicians equals the price that students are willing to pay for that education.

Under the current system of medical education, however, the costs of producing physicians are greater than they would be in a system where there were fewer artificial educational requirements, such as minimum years required both before entering and during medical school, and where incentives for efficiency were not lacking. Even if the price charged for a medical education were equal to the higher costs of a medical education, too few physicians would be produced under the conditions of the present system. The price that students would be willing to pay for a medical education (reflecting their expected marginal private benefits) would be equal to the minimum costs of producing a physician. If the price is greater than minimum cost, additional physicians could be produced if the producers were more efficient.

It has been alleged, however, that in addition to the private benefits gained by the student receiving a medical education, there are benefits to the public at large from having a greater number of physicians (5). According to this argument, basing the demand for a medical education on just the private benefits to be received by students would result in too low an estimate of the demand for a medical education. The existence of additional benefits, to be received by persons other than students, would result in a greater demand for a medical education when added to the private demand by students. For example, as shown in Figure 15-2, *MPB* represents the marginal private benefits received by students from a medical education. *MPC* represents the marginal private costs of producing additional physicians. The intersection of these marginal private benefit and cost curves would result in Q_0 number of physicians. Q_0 physicians is believed by some persons to be a nonoptimal number, i.e., too few, because the external benefits to others from having physicians (*MEB*) are excluded from

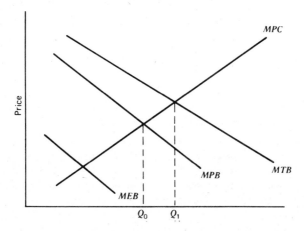

Figure 15-2. An illustration of external benefits in medical education.

this calculation. If these external benefits are included, the sum of both the private and external benefits, shown by the line *MTB*, would intersect the *MPC* curve at the point to the right of Q_0 physicians, thereby indicating that Q_1 quantity of physicians would be the optimal quantity. The manner in which these external benefits would be included in the foregoing calculation would be to provide a government subsidy, the size of which would reflect the magnitude of the external benefits. This government subsidy could be distributed to prospective medical students, which would lower their tuition costs and increase their demand for a medical education, or else the subsidy could be provided to the medical schools, thereby lowering their cost of producing physicians.

It is important to determine whether or not there are external benefits from having additional physicians. If there are external benefits, this would justify government subsidization of medical education so as to achieve an optimal number of physicians. (It would still be necessary to calculate the size of the external benefits in order to calculate the number of additional physicians that would have to be produced and the consequent size of the government subsidy.)

Before attempting to answer the question of whether external benefits exist with regard to the number of physicians, it would be best to define an externality. When someone undertakes an action, such as purchasing or producing a good or service in the private market, and this action has side effects on other persons or firms not directly involved in the market, an externality is said to have occurred. Since the allocation decisions of others are affected by the initial private decisions that created the externality, failure to consider these secondary allocation decisions would result in either too few or too many resources in the market. There are different types of external effects, both positive and negative, as well as externalities in consumption and in production. For public policy purposes it is important to distinguish between technological and pecuniary externalities. The former occur outside the market transaction; as a result of producing a product, a firm pollutes the water, thereby imposing a cost on those using the stream. Pecuniary externalities occur within the market: as a result of an increase in demand by some participants in the market, the price is increased to all other participants in the market. Government intervention is required only in the first case (technological externality) to correct what would otherwise be a misallocation of resources (6). When externalities occur, the government, by calculating the extent of external costs and/or benefits and using a system of taxes and subsidies, should attempt to achieve the optimal allocation of resources. Such a process of nonmarket decision-making would involve the use of methodologies such as cost-benefit analysis.

It is not easy to determine the extent of externalities, if any, in medicine. With regard to medical research, traditional public health programs, and water fluorida-tion, the case for externalities seems clear. Individuals undertaking medical research do not collect from all who benefit from such knowledge. And since all those who benefit do not contribute to the production of that research, too little research would be undertaken if it were based solely on support from those who contribute. The gov-ernment should, therefore, calculate the size of external benefits, levy the appropriate set of taxes, and subsidize the production of medical research. Only in this manner would the optimal quantity of research be undertaken.

What are the external benefits as a result of having a greater quantity of medical education or a larger number of physicians?[4] Is it possible to specify the benefits that accrue to others, or to society as a whole, in addition to those who purchase physician services? Without government subsidies to medical education, there would exist a cer-tain stock of physicians. The number of physicians would be determined by the pri-vate demand and private costs of producing them. Are there external benefits to hav-ing more physicians than would be provided under the private market? (The total contribution of physicians may be large, but their marginal contribution has been esti-mated to be small.) The case for public subsidies as a result of externalities in educa-tion has generally been made with regard to grade-school education: everyone in a democratic society benefits from having a better-educated electorate. The case for public subsidies to higher education is weaker, and for a professional or technical edu-cation it is not at all clear that a case can be made for such subsidies (7).

It is not enough to assert that there are external benefits to having a greater number of physicians and then to call for massive government support for medical schools. Since there is neither clear evidence nor strong argument that external benefits exist in medical, dental, or veterinary education, the case for public subsidies to the health professions' educational institutions on grounds of externalities should be reexamined.

There might be other grounds for providing public subsidies to the health profes-sions, such as attracting a certain mix of students, or locating medical graduates in a particular area. Such subsidies are based upon societal value judgments rather than on externalities. The case for subsidies to medical education on other grounds will be dis-cussed subsequently. These grounds include the improvement of equity in the dis-tribution of medical care to the recipients, or the redress of possible market imperfec-tions if medical education were to be financed through a full-cost tuition program. The equity of the current system of financing education (i.e., who receives the subsi-dies and who bears the cost) will also be discussed.

---

[4]The situation where an individual includes in his or her utility function the access to medical care by others is an example of external benefits in personal medical care. Government intervention in such a situation should seek to increase the consumption or availability of medical care by low-income persons. This can be more di-rectly achieved through some form of demand-increasing program to such persons rather than by indirectly subsidizing medical schools, which may have little or no effect on increasing the availability of care to such persons.

Some Proposals for Improving the Efficiency of the Current Market for Medical Education

An important defect in the current market for medical education is that there is no link between tuition and the role such a price variable should play on both the demand and the supply side. If tuition acted as a price on the demand side, as would occur in a competitive market, then all who were willing to pay that price would have access to a medical education and there would be no need for 6,000 Americans to be paying higher costs to study medicine overseas. If medical schools were not provided with large educational subsidies, tuition would have to reflect all the costs of a medical education. Allowing tuition to serve as a true price of medical education would encourage the suppliers to be efficient in production. If they were not, and had to charge more than $30,000 a year, which is the educational cost per student per year in some medical schools, they would have difficulty in filling their spaces. Eliminating or sharply reducing supply subsidies and allowing entry by new suppliers of medical education would enable tuition to become an accurate signal of the number of physicians that would be appropriate (assuming no external benefits). We would then have efficiency in consumption as well as in production.

If tuition reflected all the costs of education and prospective students had to pay all these costs, low-income students might be precluded from becoming physicians. Only students from high-income families would be able to afford what would be very high tuition costs (e.g., possibly in excess of $100,000 for four years of medical school). However, in a competitive system where quality was based on a number of examinations prior to entering the profession rather than on specific educational requirements prior to a licensure exam, full-cost tuition would probably be much lower than it is at present.

The cost per graduating student in a competitive system is likely to be lower for two reasons. There would be greater incentives to reduce educational costs, and greater innovation in curriculum and in teaching methods would occur. As a result, the opportunity costs of entering the profession are likely to be greatly reduced. Other countries, such as Great Britain, do not require a four-year undergraduate degree before entering a four-year medical school (8). The training times for entering the profession could be reduced (9); the opportunity costs associated with these long educational requirements are more costly than increased tuition levels. In addition to receiving such an income one to two years earlier, the student would save undergraduate tuition and fees if he or she were to enter medical school after two to three years of undergraduate education. Further, the 1970 Carnegie Commission Report on Medical Education has recommended reducing the number of years in medical school from four to three. Thus medical school tuition would be paid for only three years instead of four. If a starting physician were to earn approximately $60,000 a year, each year that the educational process could be reduced saves tuition and adds to the physician's income. Tuition could be increased by approximately $15,000 a year to offset the benefit to the student of entering practice one year earlier. If the student entered medical school after two years of undergraduate education and medical school were reduced by one year, tuition could be greatly increased without adversely affecting the rate of return to a medical education.

An important concern to many persons, however, is that under a system of full-cost tuition the medical profession would still be the province only of children from high-income families. To determine whether such a concern is justifiable and, if so, how to address it, it is necessary to examine the "equity" of the current system of financing medical education.

EQUITY IN THE CURRENT SYSTEM OF FINANCING MEDICAL EDUCATION

In the preceding section we were concerned with the economic efficiency of the medical education market. It was determined that under the current structure of medical education, it was highly unlikely that (a) the optimal number of physicians would be produced, and (b) the production of medical education would be efficient. This section is concerned with the equity (i.e., who received the benefits and who bears the costs) of the large governmental subsidies that support the current system of medical education.

According to two studies, it was estimated that the annual average cost of medical education in 1972 was between $12,650 and $20,370 per enrolled student. During that period, medical students paid, on average, approximately $1,200 a year in tuition and fees. Thus the average medical student received a subsidy of approximately $45,000 from all sources, government and nongovernment, during four years of training (10). The average annual cost of medical education was estimated to be approximately $25,000 per student in 1980. Average tuition and fees were approximately $4,280 (11). Thus the average subsidy for four years of medical school in 1980 was approximately $82,000—about double what it was in 1972. These subsidies are in addition to those received during the student's four years of undergraduate training, since higher education is also subsidized by government funds. The subsidies received by medical students are generally larger than those received by students in higher education or in other professional schools. The reason is that the costs of medical education are greater than the costs in other departments within the university. With such large subsidies going to each medical student, it is legitimate to question the equitableness of these subsidies. Do such subsidies have desirable redistributive effects, or are they neutral with respect to their effect on incomes in society?

Income redistribution is based upon a societal value judgment that persons with lower incomes should be made better off by being subsidized at the expense of persons with higher incomes. The provision of such subsidies (and the taxes to finance them) may be direct, in the form of cash grants, or indirect, in the form of grants in kind, such as lower prices for specific goods and services. Education is an in-kind subsidy to all those using it. For an in-kind subsidy to have desirable redistributive effects, low-income persons should receive a proportionately greater share of the subsidy, while the costs of financing it should come from the predominantly higher-income persons in society. Some redistributive schemes may have perverse effects, as when a greater proportion of the cost is borne by lower-income persons and a greater proportionate share of the benefits is received by higher-income persons. Such was the case at times with respect to community rating and the manner in which certain services in the hospital were priced. In the typical market situation where a person purchases a good or service, that person receives the benefits from the purchase and pays the cost of producing it. The benefits are fully received and the costs are fully borne by the purchaser, assuming no externalities. With regard to medical education, therefore, are the sizable subsidies that go to each medical student neutral in their redistributive effects, or, if not, which income groups end up subsidizing which other income groups?

TABLE 15-3. Average Family Incomes, Average Higher Education Subsidies Received, and Average State Taxes Paid by Families, by Type of California Higher Education Institution, 1964–1965

	Families Without Children Enrolled in California Higher Education	Families with Children Enrolled in California Public Higher Education	
		University of California	California State College
Average family income	$7,900	$12,000	$10,000
Average higher education subsidy per year	0	1,700	1,400
Average state taxes paid	182	350	260
Net subsidy	– 180	+ 1,350	+ 1,140

Source: Based on data in Table IV-12, p. 76, in W. Lee Hansen and Burton A. Weisbrod, *Benefits, Costs, and Finance of Public Higher Education* (Chicago: Markham Publishing Co., 1969).

There is a growing accumulation of evidence that subsidies to higher education, particularly to medical education, result in a large redistribution of income; however, the costs are borne by low-income persons and are used to subsidize the highest-income groups in society. Such redistribution, if correct, would be inequitable. First, with regard to higher education, Hansen and Weisbrod, in an examination of the financing of higher education in California and in Wisconsin, have shown that the size of the subsidy received by families that send their children to these state-supported schools is greater than the state taxes they pay for all state-supported services (12). These families have higher incomes, on average, than families that do not send their children to such schools. As shown in Table 15–3, which is based on the Hansen and Weisbrod study, the average family income of families with children enrolled in the University of California system was $12,000 in 1964–1965. The average family income for families with children enrolled in the California State College system was $10,000. The average for families without children in either system was $7,900. The average amount of state taxes paid by each of these families was $350, $260, and $182, respectively; the *net* subsidy to each of these family groups was + $1,350, + $1,140, and – $180. Because more children from higher-income families attended California's public higher education institutions, these families were subsidized by the remainder of the families, whose income, on average, was lower. Hansen and Weisbrod make two additional comments that are relevant to our discussion on financing medical education. First, the additional state taxes paid by the subsidized students, once they begin working and earning higher incomes as a result of their subsidized education, are less than the value of the subsidy they received (on a present-value basis). Second, a number of subsidized students never repay any of their subsidy, since they leave the state. If the evidence in other states is similar to what was demonstrated in California and Wisconsin, it is clear that prospective medical students (and others) receive substantial subsidies before they even enter medical school.

How are the subsidies in medical education distributed with regard to family income? Table 15–4 presents a comparison of family incomes for medical students with family incomes in the rest of the population for the period 1974–1975. Based on data from this table, it is obvious that the family incomes of medical students were higher

TABLE 15-4. Family Income of Medical Students, All U.S. Families, by Control of Medical School, 1974–1975

Family Income[a]	Private Schools	Public Schools	All Medical Schools	All U.S. Families[b]
Total	100%	100%	100%	100%
Less than $5,000	5	6	6	13
$5,000–9,999	10	11	11	23
$10,000–14,999	16	19	18	24
$15,000–19,999	14	16	15	18
$20,000–24,999	13	14	13	10
$25,000 or more	42	34	37	12
Estimated median	$21,972	$19,315	$20,249	$12,836

Source: Reproduced from *Descriptive Study of Enrolled Medical Students 1974–75*, DHEW Publication No. (HRA) 76-97, prepared by the Association of American Medical Colleges, p. 26.

[a]Based on students who supplied data.

[b]U.S. Department of Commerce, Bureau of the Census, *Money Income and Poverty Status of Families and Persons in the United States 1974*, Series P-60, No. 99, July 1975.

than those of all U.S. families. There were three times as many families of medical students with incomes of $25,000 or more than there were in the population at large. Similarly, there were twice as many families in the population with incomes less than $15,000 than among the families of medical students. The estimated median income of families of medical students was almost twice as great as the median family income in the general population. The large subsidies going to medical students, therefore, appear to be going to students whose family incomes are much higher than those in the rest of the population. It is also highly unlikely that the taxes paid to the state by the families of medical students are, on the average, greater than the subsidies received. The redistributive effects of the current method of financing medical education appear to be similar to the earlier examples of higher education in California and Wisconsin.

The redistributive effects of the medical school subsidies shown in Table 15–4 are actually an improvement over what they were in the past. In 1967, 20 percent of the medical students came from families with incomes greater than $25,000 a year, incomes that compared with only 2 percent of the families in the general population, a ratio of 10:1. Similarly, 42 percent of the families of medical students had incomes greater then $15,000, whereas only 12 percent of the families in the population had comparable incomes (13).

Data on family incomes of medical students published since 1974–1975 are surprisingly misleading. According to a 1978 publication, the highest income level used was "$20,000 or more," which characterized 46 percent of all medical student families (14). Since inflation has been causing incomes to rise generally, a larger portion of the population also ends up in that highest-income category. Thus there is only a 50 percent difference in the proportion of families in that highest-income category. If higher income categories were used, the disparities in incomes would become much more obvious. A more recent study attempted to determine whether the family incomes of prospective medical students relative to the population has been changing. After attempting to control for the problem of income categories with the highest income category being $50,000 and greater, the author concluded: "it appears that the incomes of families of students taking the MCAT (Medical College Admissions Test) have neither increased nor decreased to any substantial degree relative to the rest of the population over the period 1977-1983" (15). Although it is undoubtedly true that some medical students came from families with low incomes, the major portion of the subsidy going to medical students goes to those with high family incomes.

Another factor bearing on the inequity of the current system of financing medical education is that once medical students graduate, they enter the top 10 percent of the income distribution in society. It would seem unnecessary to subsidize medical students through their undergraduate and medical education to enable them to enter the highest income distribution, but on top of that, the students who are being selected to receive the subsidy come from the highest-income families in the first place.

In light of the foregoing discussion, the proposals of the Carnegie Commission Report on Medical Education (1970), suggesting federal subsidies to medical students and medical schools to result in a uniform level of tuition for all schools of $1,000, would worsen rather than improve the performance of the current system of medical education. At such low tuition levels, the excess demand for medical education would become greater than before. Since schools would all charge the same tuition levels, there would be no competition among schools on costs to the students and this would favor the most costly, prestigious schools: if the price is the same, why not go to the "best" school? Such a system would also provide no incentives for schools to be concerned with their costs because they would receive sufficient subsidies to enable each school to charge only $1,000 tuition per year. A more desirable proposal could not have been developed by the deans of the most prestigious, high-cost, medical schools themselves.

Are there any justifiable reasons for continuing a method of financing medical education that has the effect of worsening rather than improving the income distribution? Three rationalizations are offered for continuing the present subsidy system. The first states that if it is a societal value judgment to have physicians locate in rural and underserved areas, it is necessary to subsidize medical education (16). Similar to this argument is the one that if a change in the mix of physicians is desired, subsidies to medical schools are necessary. Compatible with this general line of reasoning is the belief that since medical students leave the state that provided them with a subsidy, to prevent the state that is acquiring them from benefiting, that state should also subsidize its medical students. The common fallacy in each of these arguments is the failure to recognize that subsidies can be provided on a selective basis: for example, only those physicians locating in a rural area would be subsidized by not having to pay all or part of their educational costs. Why should all physicians be subsidized, especially since most of them locate in high-income, urban areas? Similarly, since a small fraction of medical students are classified as minority students (i.e., approximately 10 percent), why should the remaining 90 percent of medical students receive subsidies as well? If the reason a state subsidizes its medical students is that it wants its physicians to locate within its borders, then if medical students were charged full-cost tuition, with those remaining in the state having all or part of their costs forgiven, those medical students leaving the state would have paid their debt by having paid their full educational costs. This last argument can be applied to all persons, including lawyers, accountants, and teachers, who have received subsidized training and then leave the state to practice elsewhere.

If a state explicitly states the reasons for which it wants to provide a subsidy, it may generate discussion as to whether that is a value judgment with which others agree.

Once a policy has been decided upon, it would be possible to achieve its goal in a much less expensive manner by providing the subsidies directly to persons fulfilling society's needs rather than by providing a generous subsidy to all medical students. Similarly, for a total subsidy expenditure that provides for an equal amount to all medical students, more money would be available to meet society's objectives if the subsidies went only to those participating in a particular agreed-upon program.

A more sophisticated argument favoring subsidies to all students is that the sums of money required to pay for a medical education are so large that very few persons would be able to afford it. Banks would be unwilling to provide loans for tuition and living expenses with no collateral. Further, persons from low-income families have a higher rate of time preference (i.e., income today has a much higher value to the poor than income in the future). As a result, the poor will be less likely to invest in their own human capital (i.e., higher education) than would those with higher incomes. Also, undertaking an investment involves some risk that it will not pay off. Medical education is expensive, and future physician incomes may not be as attractive. If physicians have large debts to pay off, so some persons would say, they may select only the most lucrative forms of practice instead of serving certain population groups or perhaps undertaking research.

If all medical students were to be charged full-cost tuition, then such a policy would have to be accompanied by loan programs. A type of loan program that has been advocated by a number of persons is an "income contingent loan repayment plan" (ICLRP). The way in which an ICLRP would work is as follows. Students would take out a loan during the period they are in medical school to cover both tuition and living expenses. Once they have graduated and have started to earn an income, they would annually repay a fixed percent of their adjusted gross income. The fixed percent that would be assessed would depend upon how much the student borrowed (17).

By relating the ICLRP to the income of the physician, the program would not distort the preferences of physicians as to the population they serve or the type of practice they enter. A loan repayment plan similar to the one described would also minimize the risk to the student as to the size of the loan that would have to be repaid.[5] Physicians' incomes have, in any case, been consistently high during the last 30 years. As investments go, an investment in a medical education would carry minimal risk and would be fairly predictable, as attested to by the continual excess demands for spaces and the willingness of large number of students to pay higher costs to receive such an education overseas.

If, as has been proposed, medical students are charged the full cost of their education (and medical schools are no longer provided with education subsidies), what will happen to the demand for a medical education? Will the increase in tuition result in a

---

[5]A problem with previous student loan programs was that former students nullified their debts by declaring bankruptcy. In 1977, however, "a new federal law went into effect that binds graduates to their student loan obligations even if they declare bankruptcy," *New York Times*, November 26, 1977: p. 25. A revolving medical student loan fund has been set up by Congress with the amount of funds available to medical students based upon the repayment of previous loans. A General Accounting Office study found, however, that medical schools were ineffective in collecting loans from their graduates. "Doctors Lagging on School Loans: Senate Panel Staff Finds Many Higher-Income Physicians Fail to Make Payments," *New York Times*, December 7, 1981: p. 13. For a current status report on federal loan programs to medical students, see John K. Iglehart, "Federal Support of Health Manpower Education," *New England Journal of Medicine*, 314(5), January 30, 1986: 324–328.

large decrease in the number of medical school applicants? The rate of return to a medical education was estimated to be between 15 and 22 percent in 1970 and between 14 and 17 percent in 1980; for many medical specialties, it was higher than that (See Table 13-2). If full-cost tuition were charged, it was estimated that the rate of return in 1976 would have declined to 13.5 percent (18). Even at this lower rate of return, an investment in a medical education would still be very worthwhile in that there would still be an excess rate of return to medicine. In any case, if full-cost tuition were combined with a reduction in the length of the undergraduate program and one year of the medical school, as discussed earlier, large increases in tuition should be possible to offset the benefit the student would receive from entering practice one to two years earlier. Thus there should still be an excess demand for medical school spaces at the current level of supply.

If full-cost tuition were implemented, medical schools would have to compete with one another for students. Once students have to pay a substantial cost of their education, they will become increasingly concerned with the school they select. Even if subsidies for medical education were provided to some students, the schools would have to compete for them. Medical schools would have to compete on the basis of their tuition, since it would affect the size of a student's ICLRP, and on their quality. It is likely that under such circumstances the schools will reexamine the number of years of undergraduate and medical education required (19). Medical and other educational institutions would much prefer to be subsidized themselves, since the student would have to go to that institution in order to receive subsidized training. It is for this same reason that schools prefer to distribute loans and scholarships rather than have the government or some other central agency distribute them. If the school distributes the funds, students can receive them only if they attend the institution distributing them. If students receive these funds and can then choose the school they wish to attend, the different schools are forced to compete for students.

This section has examined the equity of the present system of financing medical education. It was shown that medical students are subsidized through undergraduate education and medical school, and then enter the top 10 percent of the income distribution in society. These same medical students often come from the highest-income groups to start with. Proposals to improve the equity of the current system were suggested, such as having those students who benefit from an investment in a medical education bear the full cost of such an education. Specific value judgments of society, such as having physicians locate in certain areas, should be subsidized directly instead of rewarding all medical students regardless of whether they participate in the particular programs. A method to implement the concept of full-cost tuition, namely, income-contingent loan repayment plans, was suggested.

REFERENCES

1. George Wright, "How Should We Finance Medical Education?" Health Manpower Policy Discussion Paper Series, School of Public Health, University of Michigan, May 1974, p. 1.
2. The earlier IOM estimates were updated by multiplying the 1972 figures by the increase in the Medical Care Price Index between 1972 and 1980. As a rough check on this approach, these results were compared to those arrived at by calculating the ratio of the IOM estimate of educational expenditures per student to

total revenue per student (in 1972) based on AMA data and then applying that ratio to 1980 AMA data on revenue per student. Both estimates differed by less than 7 percent with the first method being the lower of the two. Data on tuition and fees are from Senate Committee on Labor and Human Resources, U.S. Congress, *State Support for Health Professions Education*, (Washington, D.C.: U.S. Government Printing Office, 1981), p. 20.

3. Institute of Medicine, National Academy of Sciences, *Costs of Education in the Health Professions*, Report of a Study, Parts I and II (Washington, D.C.: National Academy of Sciences, 1974). The costs of education vary by approximately 100 percent among schools.

4. Thomas Hall and Cotton Lindsay, "Medical Schools: Producers of What Sellers to Whom," *Journal of Law and Economics*, April 1980. K. Leffler and C. Lindsay, in their article "Student Discount Rates, Consumption Loans, and Subsidies to Professional Training," *Journal of Human Resources*, 16, Summer 1981: 468–475, argue that subsidies are necessary to compensate for imperfections in the market for human capital. However, they conclude that current subsidies exceed those necessary to alleviate imperfections in this market.

5. Rashi Fein and Gerald Weber, *Financing Medical Education*, A General Report Prepared for the Carnegie Commission on Higher Education and the Commonwealth Fund (New York: McGraw-Hill, 1971), 131–132.

6. For more discussion on this subject, see E. K. Browning and J. M. Browning, *Microeconomic Theory and Applications*, 2nd ed. (Boston: Little, Brown, 1986), 603–612.

7. See Theodore W. Schultz, "Optimal Investment in College Instruction: Equity and Efficiency," *Journal of Political Economy* Special Issue: "Investment in Education: The Equity-Efficiency Quandry," 80(3), Part II (May–June 1972.

8. For some suggestions on how educational and opportunity costs might be reduced under a different system for providing medical education, see Reuben Kessel, "The AMA and the Supply of Physicians," *Law and Contemporary Problems*, Health Care Part I, School of Law, Duke University, Spring 1970: 276–278.

9. Robert H. Ebert, "Can the Education of the Physician Be Made More Rational?" *New England Journal of Medicine*, 305, November 26, 1981: 1343–1346.

10. George Wright, "Why Should We Subsidize Medical Education," Health Manpower Policy Discussion Paper Series, A-6, (Ann Arbor, Mich.: School of Public Health, University of Michigan, February 1974), p. 32, fn. 6.

11. See ref. 2.

12. W. Lee Hansen and Burton A. Weisbrod, *Benefits, Costs and Finance of Public Higher Education* (Chicago: Markham Publishing, 1969), p. 76.

13. U.S. Department of Health, Education, and Welfare, *How Medical Students Finance Their Education*, (Washington, D.C.: U.S. Government Printing Office, 1970), pp. 8–9.

14. W. F. Dube, *Descriptive Study of Enrolled Medical Students, 1976–1977*, final report from the Division of Student Studies, Association of American Medical Colleges for the Bureau of Health Manpower, Department of Health, Education, and Welfare, (Washington, D.C.: U.S. Government Printing Office, February 1978), p. 55.

15. Paul Jolly, "Family Income of Students Taking the Medical College Admissions Test," unpublished paper. (Washington, D.C.: Association of American Medical Colleges, February 17, 1987). The ratio of median family incomes of U.S. families to MCAT examinee families was 1.374 in 1983.

16. An important reason why early loan forgiveness programs for physicians locating in rural and underserved areas were ineffective was that it was relatively inexpensive given the heavily subsidized cost of education, for students to buy their way out of their contracted obligations. For a more complete discussion of this topic, see Jack Hadley, "State and Local Financing Options," in Jack Hadley, ed., *Medical Education Financing: Policy Analysis and Options for the 1980s* (New York: PRODIST, 1980). See also *State Support for Health Professions Education, op. cit.*, 42–54.

17. The idea of an ICLRP is not new. It was proposed over 20 years ago as a means of financing higher education. Yale and Duke universities have experimented with such plans. A good theoretical discussion of the ICLRP is presented in Marc Nerlove, "Some Problems in the Use of Income-Contingent Loans for the Finance of Higher Education," *Journal of Political Economy* , 83, February 1975: 157–183. The author also discusses the Yale Plan. A proposal to use such a plan for medical students has been proposed by Bernard Nelson, Richard Bird, and Gilbert Rogers, "An Analysis of the Educational Opportunity Bank for Medical Student Financing," *Journal of Medical Education*, August 1972. A computer simulation of such repayment plans to indicate their feasibility is performed in William C. Weiler, "Loans for Medical Students: The Issues of Manageability," *Journal of Medical Education*, June 1976. In 1986 Congress approved an ICLRP as a pilot project for 10 universities.

18. Stephen P. Dresch, "Marginal Wage Rates, Hours of Work, and Returns to Physician Training and Specialization," in Nancy Greenspan, ed. *Health Care Financing Conference Proceedings: Issues in Physicians Reimbursement* (Washington, D.C.: Department of Health and Human Services, 1981), p. 199.

19. Robert Ebert, formerly Dean of the Harvard Medical School, has said, "Apart from the Interface Program, (funded by The Commonwealth Fund in the mid-1970s to encourage experimentation in teaching at the interface between college and the preclinical years of medical school) remarkably little that is new has been introduced into the medical school curriculum during the past decade. Medical schools seem more concerned with survival than with innovation, yet it may be that survival is really dependent on a radical reexamination of what medical education is all about. The Interface Program was a start, and asked the question, Does the sharp separation between the last two years of college and the first two years of medical school make any sense since it neither enhances general education nor education in the basic sciences? Perhaps the first year or year-and-a-half of medical school should be part of a college education.

Closely related is the question of the relationship between the clinical years of medical school and the first three years of residency training. I have suggested a way that these might be integrated, but there appears to be no interest whatsoever in the suggestion, not, as nearly as I can judge, for educational reasons, but rather for reasons of turf and control." Robert H. Ebert, "The Medical School Revisited," *Health Affairs*, 4, Summer 1985: 56–57.

CHAPTER 16

The Market for Registered Nurses

In past years there have been numerous claims of a shortage of registered nurses in the United States. The evidence used to support such claims has been data that establish the ratio of registered nurses to the population and vacancy statistics of unfilled nursing positions in hospitals. For example, in 1956, it was estimated that there was a shortage of 70,000 nurses in the United States. By 1966 that estimate had increased to 125,000 and it was estimated (in 1963) that by 1970 the magnitude of the shortage would reach 200,000 nurses (1). Vacancy rates (as a percent of total positions) were increasing from between 13 and 16 percent in the mid-1950s to 23 percent by 1962 (see Table 16–1). As a result of these claims of nurse shortages, the U.S. Congress in 1964 passed the Nurse Training Act (NTA), which provided $300 million over a five-year period to alleviate the alleged shortage. The NTA was subsequently renewed and amended in 1966, 1968, 1971, 1975, 1979, and 1983. In all, more than $2 billion has been authorized by the U.S. government to alleviate the nurse shortage.

Since there has been such a large federal commitment to nursing education, it is important to understand the bases for public policy in this area. The first step toward understanding the various claims of shortages and the subsequent massive support for nursing education is to investigate the performance of the market for registered nurses. If this market had been functioning well, then there would be no reason for any government intervention, let alone the large federal support that has been devoted to increasing the supply of nurses. If such federal support occurred when the market for nurses was performing efficiently, then we must look for other reasons to explain the demand for subsidies to nursing education. One example of such an alternative explanation would be a value judgment that medical care should be more readily available to the population and that one way to achieve this increase in availability is to subsidize one input (nurses) to the supply of medical care. If such a value judgment is the basis for federal support to this area, it should be evaluated by comparing this supply subsidy to alternative supply subsidies to determine which subsidy program achieves the largest increase in supply of medical care per dollar spent. Alternatively, such supply subsidies should be compared to demand subsidy programs that would also

TABLE 16-1. Vacancy Rates in Hospitals for
General-Duty Nurses

Year	Vacancy Rate	Year	Vacancy Rate
1953	14.6	1969	11.2
1954	13.0	1971	9.3
1956	16.8	1980	10.6
1958	13.0	1983	6.4
1961	23.2	1984	5.1
1962	23.0	1985	6.3
1967	18.1	1986	13.6
1968	15.0		

SOURCES: Reprinted by permission of the publisher, from Donald E.
Yett, *An Economic Analysis of the Nurse Shortage* (Lexington, Mass.:
Lexington Books, D.C. Health Co., 1975); copyright 1975, D.C.
Health Co.), p. 138, Table 3-13. Data on 1980–1986 vacancy rates pro-
vided by the American Hospital Association from its Survey of Hospital
Nursing Personnel.

achieve an increase in quantity of medical care consumed for a particular beneficiary
group.

If, on the other hand, it is found that the market for registered nurses has not been
functioning well, certain policy prescriptions might be called for. Depending upon the
particular reasons for its poor performance, federal subsidies might be one policy alternative; other forms of government intervention, not requiring the use of federal
subsidies, might also be appropriate. Only after examining the performance of the
market for nurses can it be determined whether there was or is any justification for
federal subsidies to nursing education and, if not, what possible explanations might be
offered for the use of such subsidies. Also, by examining the effect of the federal subsidies we might gain some insight into their intended as opposed to their stated purpose.

MEASURING THE PERFORMANCE OF THE MARKET
FOR REGISTERED NURSES

If the market for nurses were performing relatively efficiently, we would expect it to
operate as shown in Figure 16–1. Starting from an initial equilibrium point, with the
demand for registered nurses (RNs) represented by D_1 and supply by S_1, the equilibrium wage would be W_1 and the number of RNs employed, Q_1. The assumption that
the demand for RNs has been increasing over time would be represented by the shift in
the demand curve to D_2. With a higher demand for RNs, we would expect wages to
increase to W_2 and the quantity of RNs employed to increase to Q_2. The increase in
RNs employed would come from the existing stock of RNs (i.e., the total number of
trained nurses). A measure of the increase in number of those RNs in the existing stock
of RNs who are working is the "participation rate" (i.e., the percent of the stock of

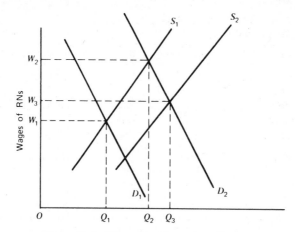

Figure 16–1. The market for registered nurses.

RNs that are employed).[1] Thus the short-run effects of an increase in demand on the market for nurses is an increase in their wages, from W_1 to W_2; an increase in their employment, from Q_1 to Q_2; and an increase in their participation rate (not shown in Figure 16–1). The long-run effect of the increase in demand, from D_1 to D_2, is an increase in the supply of nurses, which is shown in Figure 16–1 by a shift in the supply curve to the right, to S_2. The reason for the shift in the supply curve is that as the wage of RNs is increased, from W_1 to W_2, nursing becomes a relatively more attractive profession when compared with, for example, teaching. Assuming that all the factors that affect the demand for a nurse's and a teacher's education do not change, with the exception of the increase in nurses' wages relative to the wage of teachers, some prospective applicants for a teacher's education may decide to enter nursing. This change in career patterns does not mean that all candidates will switch their educational choices, nor does it mean that the persons who do change are motivated solely by financial return. What it means is that *some* people are indifferent between two professions; a change in the relative incomes of the professions will mean that more of these people select the profession with the highest income. How many people switch depends upon the difference in relative incomes and how many people are relatively close to the margin in their choices.

Thus, the long-run effect of the increase in demand is that we would expect to find an increase in the wages of RNs, relative to other occupations with similar training costs, and an increase in the number of persons entering nursing. The performance measures of an efficiently operating market that we would look for with an increase in demand are:

---

[1]For the majority of trained nurses who are women, a number of factors influence whether or not she will seek employment. Her wage is only one such factor. Whether or not she has young children and what her husband's income is are additional factors. However, if nurses' wages increase, while all other factors remain unchanged, some inactive nurses will decide to become active. The elasticity of the participation rate with respect to nurses' wages will indicate the percent increase in employment for a given percent increase in nurses' wages. This will be discussed in more detail later.

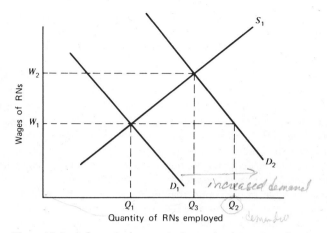

Figure 16-2. A dynamic shortage in the market for registered nurses.

- an increase in the wages of RNs;
- an increase in the rate of return to one who becomes an RN, both in absolute terms and relative to other occupations;
- an increase in the number of registered nurses employed and in their participation rate; and
- an increase in the use of substitutes. As RNs' wages increase, RNs become relatively more expensive to use. We would expect to observe their employers substituting *away* from the use of RNs to the use of other nursing personnel whose wages have not increased as rapidly.

If we wanted to test whether the market for RNs is adjusting to changes in the demand for RNs, we would collect data on each of these measures. Before turning to an examination of the data, however, we should discuss the indications that a market is not performing efficiently. In this way we will be able to determine the efficiency with which this market is operating and the possible reasons for inadequate performance, if that should be the case.

As we observed in Figure 16-1, with an increase in demand from D_1 to D_2, we would expect the wage to rise, and this would bring about an increase in the number of nurses employed—in the short run through an increase in their participation rate, and in the long run through an increase in the number of persons becoming nurses (a shift to the right in the supply curve). One possible market imperfection, therefore, would be that nurses' wages do not increase, or do not increase sufficiently to reach a new equilibrium level. Such a situation could be the result of a dynamic shortage. With an increase in the demand for nurses, the major employers of nurses may not know how much they have to increase nurses' wages to bring about an increase in their employment; similarly, it takes time for working nurses to learn which hospitals are paying higher wages and for inactive nurses both to learn of the increase in wages and to decide to become active again.

A dynamic shortage for RNs is illustrated in Figure 16-2. With the increase in demand from D_1 to D_2, the demand for RNs will initially be Q_2, which is at the old wage W_1 on the new demand curve D_2. Thus, in a dynamic shortage, until information becomes available to both nurse employers that they have to raise wages if they are to hire more nurses and to nurses that they could receive higher wages if they were to become active, there will be a shortage of magnitude $Q_1 - Q_2$. As the wages of RNs increase, the shortage will begin to decrease, which means that those employers who are willing to pay the higher price will be able to employ more nurses. The existence of a dynamic shortage is a temporary phenomenon and should disappear with time. Unless demand for RNs continually increases faster than the increase in the supply of RNs, equilibrium will eventually occur in the market. The only indication that a dynamic shortage existed (or continues to exist) would be that together with continued vacancies for RNs (budgeted but unfilled positions) there would also be observed in the market for nurses higher wages, increased rates of return, and increases in employment, in participation rates, and in use of substitutes.

Another possible imperfection that might occur in the market for nurses (and which is more serious than a dynamic shortage) is a static shortage. In a situation of a static shortage, nurses' wages are prevented from increasing to an equilibrium level. Because the wages are below the market clearing wage, there will be a continual shortage that unlike the situation of a dynamic shortage, will not be temporary and work itself out. A static shortage can also be illustrated with use of Figure 16-2. With an increase in demand from D_1 to D_2, the quantity of nurses demanded at the old wage would be Q_2. If the wage is prevented from rising, the shortage $Q_1 - Q_2$ will not disappear. In distinguishing between whether there has been (or is) a static or a dynamic shortage, we would expect to observe measures of shortages (e.g., vacancy rates for nurses) in both cases, but in a static shortage we would *not* expect to observe large increases in nurses' wages, in their participation rates, or in their rates of return. In both cases we would expect substitution away from the use of RNs to occur, since it is more difficult to employ as many RNs as the employers would like, in one case because nurses' wages have gone up and they have become relatively more expensive to employ, in the other because employers cannot hire all the nurses they would like to at the old wage.

Having specified the measures of performance to be used in determining which of the foregoing market descriptions best characterizes how the market for nurses has operated in the past, we now turn to an examination of the data; we now know which data to look for and how to interpret them.

The Performance of the Market for Registered Nurses

Nurses are predominantly employed in hospitals. As shown in Table 16-2, of the 1,485,725 registered nurses employed in 1984, 68.1 percent were working in hospitals. The remaining places of employment and their respective percentages were: nursing homes (7.7 percent), occupational health (1.5 percent), nursing education (2.7 percent), private duty and office (8.1 percent), and public health and schools (9.7 percent). (2.0 percent were employed in other nursing fields or did not report.) Thus what happens in the hospital sector has the largest effect on the employment of registered nurses. The demand for hospital care (hence the demand for RNs) has been changing over time, as described in Chapter 10. Admissions and patient days in short-term general and other special hospitals (which have approximately 80 percent of all hospital admissions) have been increasing (until the early 1980s) as a result of a number of factors: the age distribution of the population has become older; incomes and

TABLE 16-2. Number and Distribution of Active Registered Nurses by Place of Employment, 1984

Place of Employment	Number of Active RNs	Percentage of RNs
Hospitals	1,011,955	68.1
Nursing homes	115,077	7.7
Schools of nursing	40,311	2.7
Private duty	22,675	1.5
Community health	101,430	6.8
School nurses	43,144	2.9
Occupational health	22,890	1.5
Offices	97,374	6.6
Other and not reporting	30,871	2.0
Total	1,485,725	100.00

SOURCE: *National Sample Survey of Registered Nurses*, November 1984, Report 86-3 (Rockville, Md.: U.S. Department of Health and Human Services, 1986), p. 15.

health insurance coverage have increased, and Medicare and Medicaid, which started in 1966, lowered the cost of hospital care to the poor and aged. Advances in medical knowledge changed the nature of the hospital, from a place that provided chronic care to an institution that provides acute care. Also, modern medical technology increased demands for RNs per patient day—for example, in intensive care units. There has thus been an increase in use of medical care, and more of this care has been provided in hospitals. There has also been a greater demand for nurses as a result of a shift to providing more of the nursing care by RNs. An increase in the responsibilities delegated to RNs for tasks that were formerly performed by physicians in hospitals added additional burdens. These factors resulted in a 65 percent increase in the use of general duty nurses per patient (in nonfederal hospitals) between 1949 and 1966 (2).[2]

As a result of such forces, which increased the demand for RNs, we would expect to observe increases in nurses' salaries and in rates of return to a nursing education, substitution toward the use of nonregistered nurses, and increases in the nurse participation rate. According to Table 16–3, between 1946 and 1980 average annual salaries of "all active nurses" increased 649 percent, from $2,136 per year in 1946 to $15,992 per year in 1980. Salaries, however, also increased in other occupations in which women were predominantly employed over that same period. When we examine the increase in salaries both before and after the introduction of Medicare and Medicaid in 1966, we see that nurses' salaries increased by 154 percent between 1946 and 1966. However, teachers' salaries increased 233 percent and salaries of "female professional, technical, and kindred workers" increased 187 percent over the period 1946–1966. After 1966, nurses' salaries had the largest percentage increase: 194 percent between 1966 and 1980, compared with only 131 percent for teachers and 171 percent for "female professional, technical, and kindred workers." Thus when we examine nurses'

[2]A demand function for RNs in short-term hospitals was estimated by Donald E. Yett et al., and it was determined that the effect of a 1 percent increase in patient days would result in a .86 percent increase in RNs in hospitals of 200 or more beds. The effect of a 1 percent increase in RN wages would lead to a − 1.75 percent decrease in number of RNs employed, and the cross-elasticity of demand for RNs with respect to the wages of aides was 1.43. D. Yett, L. Drabek, L. Kimball, and M. Intriligator, *A Forecasting and Policy Simulation Model of the Health Care Sector* (Lexington, Mass.: Lexington Books, 1979), p. 95.

TABLE 16-3. Percentage Increase in Nominal Incomes of Registered Nurses, Teachers, Female Professional, Technical, and Kindred Workers, and Licensed Practical Nurses

	(1)	(2)	(3)	(4)	(5)	(6)	(7)
Year	Female Professional, Technical, and Kindred Workers (%)	Teachers (%)	LPNs (%)	RNs (%)	Hospital RNs General-Duty Position (%)	Nurse Educators (%)	School Nurses (%)
1946–1980	187	671		649	736	804	567
1946–1966		233		154	157	244	215
1966–1980	171	131		194	225	163	112
1966–1972	52	44	85	77	88	63	39
1972–1975	22	22	27	21	22	21	17
1975–1978	24	20	23	22	23	18	17
1978–1980	18	9	10	12	16	13	11
1980–1984	32	26	11	37	—	18	12

SOURCES: Columns 1, 2, 4, 5, 6, 7, rows 1, 2, 3, 4: Donald E. Yett, An Economic Analysis of the Nurse Shortage (Lexington, Mass.: Lexington Books, 1975), pp. 154–57, 184–186, 188–189; Column 1, rows 5, 6, 7: Department of Commerce, Bureau of the Census, Current Population Reports, Series P-60, Nos.: 90, p. 138; 103, p. 23; 123, p. 255; 132, p. 199; Column 2, rows 5, 6, 7: W. Vance Grant and Leo J. Eiden, eds., Digest of Education Statistics, 1981 (National Center for Educational Statistics), p. 60; Column 3, rows 2, 3, 4, 5, 6, 7; and column 5, rows 5, 6, 7: U.S. Department of Health and Human Services, Public Health Service, Health Resources Administration, The Recurrent Shortage of Registered Nurses: A New Look at the Issues, DHHS Publication (HRA) 81-23 (Washington, D.C.: U.S. Government Printing Office, 1980), p. 3; Columns 6, 7, rows 5, 6, 7: American Nurses Association, Facts About Nursing, 1972–1973 ed., pp. 10, 34, 145, 152; 1974–1975 ed., pp. 124, 137; 1976–1977 ed., pp. 40, 165, 179, 186; 1980–1981 ed., pp. 14, 197, 203, 230; Columns 5, 6, 7, row 7: U.S. Department of Health and Human Services, Public Health Services, Health Resources Administration, Bureau of Health Professions, Division of Health Professions Analysis, The Registered Nurse Population, An Overview from National Sample Survey of Registered Nurses, November, 1980 (Revised June 1982), Report 82-5, p. 21. Column 1, row 8: U.S. Department of Commerce, Bureau of Census, Current Population Reports, Series P-60, No. 95, p. 142. Note: "Female professional, technical, and kindred workers" is no longer a category reported in the census. The population-weighted average salary of the subcategories previously listed under "female professional, technical, and kindred workers" was computed from the 1984 census and used to calculate the 1984 percent increase. Column 2, row 8: Digest of Education Statistics, 1985–1986, (Washington, D.C.: Office of Educational Research and Improvement Center for Statistics, 1986), p. 56. Columns 3, 4, 5, 6, 7, row 8: Facts About Nursing, 1982–1983 and 1984–1985, pp. 201, 212, 208 (1982–1983); pp. 141, 147, 153 (1984–1985).

Note: The percentage changes in income do not include changes in benefits. According to the Department of Health and Human Services, The Recurrent Shortages of Registered Nurses: A New Look at the Issues, pp. 5–8, nurses' benefits were comparable to those in similar occupations by 1978, whereas in 1960 they were considered to be inferior. Values were determined by taking a weighted average of the salaries of nurses in various nursing fields.

TABLE 16-4. Ratio of All Registered Nurses' and Hospital General-Duty Registered Nurses' Salaries to Those of Teachers and Female Professional, Technical, and Kindred Workers

Year	Female Professional, Technical, and Kindred Workers		Teachers	
	All RNs	Hospital RNs	All RNs	Hospital RNs
1946	1.05	.97	1.03	.95
1948	1.00	.95	.92	.87
1951	.97	.92	.86	.82
1954	.89	.82	.82	.76
1957	.91	.85	.79	.74
1961	.86	.79	.77	.70
1963	.90	.87	.75	.73
1966	.93	.87	.79	.73
1969	1.02	.95	.87	.81
1972	1.10	1.08	.97	.96
1975	1.08	1.08	.96	.96
1978	1.07	1.06	.98	.97
1980	1.02	1.04	1.00	1.03
1984	.98	.99	1.01	1.02

SOURCES: Donald E. Yett, *An Economic Analysis of the Nurse Shortage* (Lexington, Mass.: D.C. Heath Co., 1975), pp. 154, 160, 188. Department of Commerce, Bureau of the Census, *Current Population Reports*, Series P-60, Nos.: 90, p. 138; 103, p. 23; 123, p. 255; 132, p. 199; W. Vance Grant and Leo J. Eiden, eds., *Digest of Education Statistics, 1981*, (National Center for Educational Statistics, p. 60. U.S. Department of Health and Human Services, Health Resource Administration, *The Recurrent Shortage of Registered Nurses: A New Look at the Issues*, Department of Health and Human Services, Publication (HRA) 81-23 (Washington, D.C.: U.S. Government Printing Office, 1980), p. 3. U.S. Department of Health and Human Services, Division of Health Professions Analysis, *The Registered Nurse Population, An Overview from National Sample Survey of Registered Nurses*, November 1980 (revised June, 1982), Report No. 82-5, p. 21. Column 1, 1980–84, comes from U.S. Department of Commerce, Bureau of Census, *Current Population Reports*, Series P-60, No. 95, p. 142. Note: "Female professional, technical, and kindred workers" is no longer a category reported in the census. The population-weighted average salary of the subcategories previously listed under "female professional, technical, and kindred workers" was computed from the 1984 census and used to calculate the 1984 percent increase. Column 2, 1980–84, comes from *Digest of Education Statistics, 1985–1986* (Washington, D.C.: Office of Educational Research and Improvement Center for Statistics, 1986), p. 56. Columns 3, 4, 5, 6, 7, 1980–84, comes from *Facts About Nursing*, 1982–1983 and 1984–1985, pp. 201, 212, 208 (1982–1983); pp. 141, 147, 153 (1984–1985).

wages relative to the wages in comparable professions, it appears that the overall percent increase has been similar for the entire 1946–1980 period; however, nurses' wages increased less rapidly before Medicare and more rapidly afterward. The ratio of nurses' salaries to those of teachers was 1.03 in 1946, declining to a low of .75 in 1963, and thereafter increasing to 1.00 in 1980 (see Table 16–4). Nurses' wages were 1.05 to those of "female professional, technical, and kindred workers" in 1946, declining to .86 in 1961, rising to 1.10 in 1972, and then declining to 1.02 in 1980 and .98 in 1984.

Based on these data on relative wages, it would appear that since the wages of other female workers increased more rapidly during the period before 1966, there was a relative *surplus* rather than a relative shortage of nurses during this period! This same observation is supported by the data on relative rates of return to a nursing education when they are compared with "females with one to three years of college training." In 1946 there appears to have been a sizable shortage of nurses; that is, the rate of return was higher for nurses than for the comparison group. By 1959, however, the relative rate of return to nursing declined, thereby indicating a *surplus* of nurses; that is, women could receive a higher rate of return by entering an occupation other than nursing. By 1966, however, the relative rate of return to nursing had increased, indicating a shortage situation again (3).

What is of interest in the period 1946–1966 is that wage increases to nurses have not been uniform according to place of nurse employment. Wages (nominal) increased much more rapidly between 1946 and 1966 for nurse education (224 percent) and school nurses (215 percent) than for hospital employed nurses (157 percent). After 1966 the opposite occurred, as hospital nurses experienced the largest percent increase in their wages.

When we examine the increase in supply of nurses over this period, we observe that there has been an increase in the number of nurses employed in nonfederal hospitals, an increase of 109 percent between 1949 and 1966. However, as we would expect, the increase in the number of nurses employed in nurse education positions and in other areas that have had larger percent increases in their wages was much greater, 254 percent, over the same period (4).

It thus appears that within nursing there have been increases in wages but that these wage increases have been more rapid for nonhospital-based nurses. Similarly, the percent increase in nurse employment has been greater in the nonhospital sector, which employs only about 23 percent of all nurses. It appears that particular submarkets within nursing adjusted more rapidly than the hospital sector; there were relatively larger increases in nurses' wages in those markets and corresponding larger increases in nurse supply. It is perplexing that nurses in the nonhospital sector should experience higher increases in their wages. If there are no barriers to movement between the two sectors and if the training costs are similar, we would expect wage increases to be similar in both the hospital and nonhospital sectors (or if training costs differ, the relative rates of return to be similar in the two different sectors).

With regard to substitution of other nurses (e.g., aides and licensed practical nurses) for registered nurses, we observe (according to Table 16–5) that although the relative salary differential of registered nurses to practical nurses changed very little in the period 1949–1978 , a great deal of substitution within nursing has been occurring. From 1949 to 1966 the ratio of licensed practical nurses (LPNs) to registered nurses increased by 181 percent, from .16 in 1949 to .45 in 1966. Substitution would be expected if salary differentials increased or if there was a change in relative productivity (if their productivity changed, this should have been reflected in a change in relative salaries). However, the increase in RNs' relative incomes over this period was slight. The upward trend in the use of LPNs relative to RNs began to reverse itself beginning in the early 1970s, with the use of LPNs relative to RNs decreasing from .51 in 1970 to .37 in 1980 and .27 in 1985. There was, however, virtually no change in their relative salaries over this same period.

What can we conclude about the market for nurses based upon the foregoing data? Starting from the late 1940s, the base period for comparison with changes over time

TABLE 16-5. Ratio of LPNs' to RNs' and the Ratio of LPNs' to RNs' Salaries in Nonfederal Short-Term General and Other Special Hospitals

Year	Employment	Income
1949	.16	
1955	.29	
1959	.37	
1960		76.6
1962	.40	
1963		74.6
1966	.45	72.1
1968	.50	
1969		70.2
1970	.51	
1972	.50	73.3
1973	.49	
1974	.48	
1975	.46	76.1
1976	.45	
1977	.43	
1978	.41	76.2
1979	.39	
1980	.37	
1981	.37	74.1
1982	.35	73.0
1983	.33	72.0
1984	.30	73.2
1985	.27	73.9

SOURCE: The employment and income ratios for the years 1949–1978 came from the U.S. Department of Health and Human Services, Public Health Service, Health Resources Administration, *The Recurrent Shortage of Registered Nurses: A New Look at the Issues,* DHHS Publication (HRS) 81-23—data on relative employment rates are on p. 6, and data on relative wage rates are on p. 5. The employment ratios for 1979 and 1980 were derived with permission from data in: American Hospital Association, *Hospital Statistics* (Chicago: AHA), © 1980, p. 21. The income ratio for 1981 was derived from preliminary reports of the Department of Labor, Bureau of Labor Statistics, *Industry Wage Survey: Hospitals* (1981). The data for 1981–1985 are reproduced from *Hospital Statistics,* 1980–86 editions, copyright 1980–86 by the American Hospital Association, pp. 21, 22, 23.

and other occupations, nursing appeared to be a relatively attractive profession from a financial standpoint. Its rate of return was relatively higher than comparable professions; one might even say that there was a slight shortage of nurses at that time. However, from that base period to the mid-1960s the attractiveness of nursing as a profession declined relative to comparable professions. This could be interpreted in the following way. Although there was an increase in demand for nurses, it was smaller than the increase in demand for comparable occupations, therefore wages rose faster in other professions. With a smaller increase in wages, and a decline in relative rates of return, few persons would be expected to enter nursing. Such a model would not explain a shortage situation but instead one characterized by a relative surplus of nurses.

This characterization of a surplus situation (i.e., demand increasing less rapidly than supply, resulting in a decline in the relative wage of nurses) does not coincide with what many people believed was occurring during this period. The common belief was that there was a shortage rather than a surplus of nurses. The indications of a shortage were the substitution of practical nurses for RNs and the increasing vacancy rates of RNs in hospitals. If the market were characterized by a dynamic shortage, then as demand increased faster than supply, we would expect an increase in vacancies as hospitals found that they could not hire as many nurses as they would like at the prevailing wage, and substitution toward less expensive personnel would begin. However, a dynamic shortage would also be characterized by rising wages of RNs and higher wages for RNs relative to practical nurses. Thus the data would be most characteristic of a dynamic shortage situation except for the fact that hospital nurses' wages (and their rates of return) were not rising more rapidly.

The only type of market situation that logically incorporates these contradictory data is one characterized by a static shortage. In a static shortage we might start from a point of equilibrium (1946–1949), represented by the intersection of the demand and supply curves, D_1 and S_1, as in Figure 16–2. As the demand for hospital and medical care rises, bringing with it an increased demand for RNs, the demand curve shifts to D_2. If nurses' wages, instead of rising to the new equilibrium point, were kept below it in some way, $Q_1 - Q_2$ would represent the shortage (i.e., vacancies in hospitals); hospitals would have to substitute toward greater use of practical nurses because they could not employ all the RNs they would want at the RNs' previous wage. Similarly, hospital RNs' wages, relative to those of RNs in other nursing employment, would increase less rapidly if they were held down in the hospital sector but not in other nurse employment sectors. As RN wages were prevented from increasing, they would begin to fall behind those in comparable occupations and the RNs' relative rate of return would similarly decline.

A static shortage situation, where RNs' wages show some increase but less than was necessary to clear the market and less than what was occurring in other areas of nursing or comparable occupations, would also explain why hospital nurse employment has gone up less than in the nonhospital sector; with a rising supply curve for RNs, a small increase in hospital wages would result in only a small increase in the number employed in hospitals.

The data appear consistent with somewhat of a static shortage in the hospital market for RNs during the late 1950s and early 1960s. Given this explanation or hypothesis of what has occurred, it is necessary to explain how such a static shortage could have persisted, that is, what mechanism would have prevented nurses' wages from reaching the equilibrium level, and second, why the static shortage disappeared in the period after 1966.

Imperfections in the Market for RN Services

The explanation for a possible static shortage of nurses in the hospital sector prior to 1966 is that hospitals have acted as a cartel in setting nurses' wages and are monopsonists or oligopsonists with respect to the employment of registered nurses. Ten percent of all hospitals are the only hospital in an area, 31 percent of hospitals are located in areas where there are only one or two hospitals, and 47 percent of hospitals are in areas where there are fewer than four hospitals; more than 60 percent of hospitals are in areas where there are fewer than six hospitals (5). As purchasers of nurses' services, therefore, hospitals have a great deal of market power; they employ 75 percent of all nurses (both hospital-based and private duty nurses), and since there are few hospitals in any one area it is relatively easy for them to collude in setting nurses' wages. In most sectors where a firm is only one of many other firms hiring people in a certain occupational category, it is difficult for the firms to collude or to ensure that each firm does not violate the collective agreement. When there are many firms, it is in the interest of any one firm to raise the wage slightly and attract people from other firms. Hospitals, however, can quickly find out whether or not another hospital in the area has changed its wage policy. Also, since they employ almost all of the active nurses, it is difficult to attract nurses from other, nonhospital firms. Facing an increase in the demand for their services, hospitals believed that the short-run supply of nurses is relatively inelastic (i.e., increasing the wage would result in only a small increase in the number of nurses seeking work, either through a change in their status from inactive to active or from immigration from other areas) and therefore decided to hold down nurses' wages. RNs' wages represent a significant portion of a hospital's budget (25 percent); increasing the wage rate to attract new nurses would require an increase in the wage to all existing RNs as well.

RNs employed in nonhospital settings represent a small portion of the total cost in these other settings. RNs would therefore be expected to receive higher wages in these other settings because the employers would be more willing to pay higher RN salaries to enable hiring as many RNs as needed. Further, in some employment situations (e.g., government) the RN's wage would be related to the wages of other occupational groups and would increase at the same rate as these other personnel categories.

To test the hypothesis of hospital collusion in the setting of nurses' wages, Donald Yett conducted a survey of the 31 largest hospital associations to determine whether or not they had wage stabilization programs. Fourteen of the 15 hospital associations that responded reported that they did have wage stabilization programs (6). [The one hospital association that did not have one asked how it could start one (7).] Additional evidence of the attempt by hospitals to fix nurses' wages in their area is the following statement that appeared in the *Los Angeles Times*: "The majority of hospitals fix wages for nurses on recommendations from the Hospital Council of Southern California. The Council's recommendations have always been accepted and are based on recommendations from the management consulting firm of Guffenhagen-Kroeger Inc." (8).

As hospitals found it difficult to hire more nurses during the period of continued shortage (pre-1966), they intensified their efforts to increase their number of nurses along two other lines. Hospitals began recruiting foreign trained nurses and they lobbied for legislation to subsidize an increase in the number of registered nurses.

Before evaluating how effective the subsequent nurse training legislation was, it is interesting to examine what happened to the market for nurses in the post-1966 period. After 1966 two events occurred that substantially changed the market for nurses. The first, and perhaps most important, was the passage of Medicare and Medicaid. The second was the increase in collective bargaining among hospital nurses.

When Medicare and Medicaid were passed, the demand for hospital care increased because the aged were provided with hospital coverage. At the same time, hospitals were reimbursed on a "cost-plus" basis. The effect was to increase the demand for RNs and, at the same time, to make the demand more inelastic with respect to their wages. If hospitals hired more nurses and increased their wages, these costs could then be passed on to the government (on a proportional basis according to the "ratio of charges to charges to cost" of aged patients). Depending upon what portion of their hospitalized population was covered under some form of cost reimbursement (e.g., government, Blue Cross, or other third-party reimbursement), hospitals were relieved from pressures to contain their costs. Wage increases to hospital employed nurses increased rapidly in the post-Medicare period, more rapidly than wage increases to nonhospital-employed nurses and to persons working in nonhealth field occupations with comparable training. Nurses' wages, which were artificially held down for a number of years, were allowed to rise. Thus by 1969 rates of return to hospital-employed nurses were comparable to other occupations.

Registered nurses employed in nonprofit hospitals were expressly exempt from the legal provisions of the National Labor Relations Act between 1947 and 1974 and therefore did not have legal protection of their rights to organize or support a union. Hospitals were under no obligation to engage in collective bargaining with their employees. (In 1974, an amendment to the Taft-Hartley Act repealed hospitals' exempt status.) Collective bargaining on behalf of hospital nurses therefore started slowly. In addition to the impediments to collective bargaining contracts which legally permitted hospitals to refuse to bargain with unions representing hospital employees, the American Nurses' Association (ANA) had not been a strong proponent of unionization. In 1970 approximately 38,000 RNs were included under collective bargaining agreements (9), which represented only about 5 percent of employed RNs. By 1977, 200,000 RNs, more than 20 percent of employed nurses, were included under collective bargaining agreements, a substantial increase over 1970; by 1985, 31 percent of all RNs were unionized (10). The effects of collective bargaining agreements, however, are felt beyond the numbers of nurses covered. To forestall such agreements, hospitals may offer higher wages to RNs.

The effect of unionization in a market dominated by monopsonists will be to increase wages and possibly employment; whether or not increased employment will occur will depend on how much the wage is increased. Such a situation is described in the appendix to this chapter.[3] This monopsonistic hospital control over nurses' wages was weakened by the growth (both actual and expected) of nurses' unions.

To sum up, then, the effects of Medicare and Medicaid and the increase in (as well as the threat of) nurse collective bargaining after 1966 resulted in an increase in wages for nurses at a rate that was more rapid than had been the case both in the past and for nurses not employed in hospitals. The effect of those wage increases was to decrease the reported vacancies in hospitals (refer to Table 16–1) so that by 1971 the vacancy

---

[3]Several studies have estimated the effect of a monopsonistic market on nurses' wages and then the effect on wages in these markets of collective bargaining. One study, using 1973 data, found that "Unionization of at least 75 percent of the nursing workforce is associated with an addition to yearly starting salaries of $803. The size of the negative monopsony effect remains statistically significant but is again reduced to $383." Charles Link and John Landon, "Monopsony and Union Power in the Market for Nurses," *Southern Economic Journal*, 41(4), April 1975: 655. See also Richard W. Hurd, "Equilibrium Vacancies in a Labor Market Dominated by Non-profit Firms: The 'Shortage' of Nurses," *Review of Economics and Statistics*, May 1973.

rate dropped to 9.3 percent from its high of 23.2 percent in 1961.[4] From 1969 on, the various market indicators no longer suggest a static shortage but rather, a situation characterized more by a market adjusting toward an equilibrium situation. It appears, therefore, that in the past there was probably a static shortage of registered nurses, created by the collusion of hospitals to keep nurses' wages from rising. Such a situation no longer exists. The appropriate public policy in the past would have been to allow nurses' wages to rise, which would have resulted in increased hospital costs— a normal occurrence in an industry experiencing a rising demand for its services and facing a rising supply curve for its factor inputs.[5] Allowing nurses' wages to rise would have brought forth an increase both in the stock of nurses and in their employment (participation rates). Federal legislation to increase the supply of nurses would not have been necessary.

By the late 1960s, there no longer appeared to be a static shortage of nurses (11). It would thus appear to be unnecessary to continue federal assistance to increase the supply of nurses. Yet new federal funding for support of nurse training was renewed in late 1975 (Congress overrode President Ford's veto of that legislation in order for it to become law) and again in 1979 and 1983. To better understand the probable intent of the federal legislation to support nurse training and how effective it was in achieving its stated goals of increasing the supply of nurses, it is worthwhile to examine the Nurse Training Act in some depth.

FEDERAL SUPPORT FOR NURSE TRAINING

The stimulus for the Nurse Training Act of 1964 was the estimate of the impending shortage of nurses that would occur without federal legislation. The Surgeon General's Consultant Group on Nursing, appointed in 1961 to study the problem, concluded in its report in 1963 that indeed there was a serious shortage. The shortage forecast was made using the ratio technique and was thus unrelated to any economic criterion of shortage. The forecast was also not based on any conclusion regarding the performance of the market for nurses.

Support for federal legislation on nurse training came from several groups: Congress recognized the potential political rewards of backing health legislation; the federal bureaucracy—specifically, the Division of Nursing in the U.S. Public Health Service—helped to justify the need for the legislation with an eye toward an expanded role in administering it; hospitals believed they would gain from such legislation because it would increase the supply of nurses, thereby slowing down the rate of increase in nurses' wages; and support came also from the American Nurses Association, which must have perceived the effects of the federal legislation to be different from the ef-

---

[4]There is some evidence to suggest that vacancy statistics are overstated. One independent survey of nurse vacancy rates made by the U.S. Employment Service (USES) in April 1966 found a 5 percent vacancy rate, as contrasted to the American Nurses Association estimate for that same period of 13.5 percent. If the ANA statistics are roughly twice as great as the USES vacancy statistics, then this would suggest that in 1971, when the American Hospital Association (AHA) reported a vacancy rate of 9.3 percent, a more realistic vacancy rate was half that amount, approximately 4.5 percent. Such a low vacancy rate suggests that there is no shortage of registered nurses. John Edgren, "The Federal Nurse Training Acts," *Health Manpower Policy Studies Group Discussion Paper Series* (Ann Arbor, Mich.: School of Public Health, University of Michigan, 1977), 6–7.

[5]Claims of a "shortage" in this type of situation are merely a matter of employers not wishing to pay higher prices for their inputs. Government intervention in such situations is not economically justified.

fects perceived by hospitals, if we are to interpret nurse training as being consistent with the goals of the ANA membership. Among other things, the ANA seeks to increase its members' incomes. If the legislation were to have the effect desired by hospitals, namely, an increase in the supply of nurses, then it would inhibit the rise in nurses' wages, which would be the opposite of the ANA's objective. It must therefore be assumed that the ANA saw the legislation as an opportunity to change the role of registered nurses. If the educational subsidies provided under this legislation could be redirected toward producing fewer, more highly trained nurses who could undertake more responsibilities, the effect of these fewer nurses, each with more training, would be a greater increase in nurses' wages.

Thus the reasons for federal subsidies for nurse education varied. Such legislation would not have improved the functioning of the market for nurses; in an economic sense there was no justification for federal legislation. The true intent of the legislation was to benefit either hospitals (by providing them with cheaper inputs) or nurses (by changing educational requirements and graduating fewer nurses capable of performing more tasks). By analyzing how the legislation was implemented and what its effects were we can determine who actually benefited from the legislation.

Two broad purposes were stated in the Nurse Training Act (NTA) of 1964: to increase the quantity of nurses and to improve their quality. These two goals matched the separate interests of the ANA and AHA. The goals and programs enacted in the NTA of 1964 were those recommended in the Surgeon General's report of 1963. To achieve both an increase in the quality and quantity of nurses, there were four broad areas of federal support in the NTA of 1964, which were continued in subsequent renewals and amendments to that act. The two most important areas, comprising 93 percent of the total funds expended on nursing training between 1964 and the present were, first, a program of grants to schools of nursing for distribution in the form of scholarships and loans to students (40 percent of total funds were for this purpose). The second area of federal support was for grants to the nursing schools for construction, planning or initiating programs of nursing education, or for general financial support (53 percent of the funds went for this purpose).

With regard to the quantity objective of the nurse training legislation (i.e., an increase in the number of nurses), the 1963 Surgeon General's report stated that with the federal support requested, 680,000 nurses would be a "feasible" goal by 1970. In updated estimates made in 1967, it was predicted that 1,000,000 RNs would be needed in 1975. To achieve these increases in the number of nurses, it was proposed that schools of nursing increase the number of their graduates to 53,000 a year by 1969, which represented a 75 percent increase over 1961 (12).

The goal of 680,000 RNs by 1970 was surpassed; it was achieved a year earlier than expected. The number of nurses in 1975 was also very close to what was desired. Although it would appear that the nurse training legislation achieved its goals, upon closer examination it is doubtful whether these achievements were a result of the federal support for nurse training. The number of graduates being produced by schools of nursing in 1969 was 42,196, not the 53,000 per year that was supposed to occur as a result of the federal program. In fact, the number of graduates was only 1,196 more than what the Surgeon General's report estimated would have been the case *without* any federal legislation (13). Although the quantitative goals underlying the NTA were achieved, the funding of nursing schools and students did not achieve the increase in graduates believed necessary to achieve these goals. How, then, were the desired goals met?

An increase in the number of RNs employed can occur in one of two ways: a) an increase in the number of nursing graduates, or b) an increase in the number of trained nurses (the stock of RNs) who are employed (i.e., the participation rate).[6] The federal program was directed exclusively at increasing the number of nursing graduates and thus probably had no effect on the nurse participation rate.[7]

The number of nurse graduates could have been increased under the federal programs as a result of a) funding for new construction to result in an increase in the number of spaces in nursing schools, b) the loan and scholarship programs to induce people to enter nursing who would otherwise not, and c) financial assistance to the nursing schools, which could have resulted in either more attractive facilities or lower tuition rates to attract potential students. Several economists have estimated the increase in the number of nursing graduates as a result of the federal support for nursing education. Donald Yett estimated that "the increase in enrollment of marginal entrants resulted in approximately 2,660 graduates over the years 1968 to 1970" (14). John Edgren estimated a total increase of 6,813 additional graduates between 1966 and 1972 as a result of the federal subsidy program.[8] It would appear that the federal subsidies led to an increase of fewer than 1,500 new graduates a year.

Why was the increase in nurse graduates so small, given the large federal subsidy program? Nursing education is typically provided in one of three types of settings: diploma schools, community colleges offering a two-year associate degree, and four-year colleges offering a baccalaureate degree. Diploma schools, generally located in or associated with hospitals, have in the past provided the majority of nurse graduates.[9] While attending classes, students in diploma schools work in hospitals and receive a stipend. Hospitals subsidize the cost of their diploma schools to assure themselves a supply of nurses upon graduation. However, as the mobility of nurses has increased, hospital diploma schools have become a diminishing source of nurses for the particular hospitals subsidizing them. Hospitals could no longer be assured that their subsidies to such schools would be repaid when the nurses left to work elsewhere. As tuition costs to the students in diploma schools rose, enrollments declined (15).

---

[6] An increase in nurse employment can also occur if there is a change in the rate at which nurses retire or die and also if there is a change in the immigration of foreign-trained nurses.

[7] It might be argued that the loan forgiveness portions of the loan and scholarship program might have increased the participation rate of new graduates; however, the majority of nurses are active anyway immediately upon graduation.

[8] The 6,813 additional graduates between 1966 and 1972 were out of a total of 247,753 graduates over that same period. Edgren, "The Federal Nurse Training Acts," p. 26.

[9] Of the approximately 1,472,634 employed RNs in 1985, 62.3 percent or 917,450 graduated from diploma nursing schools and associate degree programs; 32.7 percent or 481,551 graduated from a four-year baccalaureate degree program; and 5.0 percent or 73,631 graduated from masters and doctorate programs.
As of 1950, there were 1,314 state-approved schools of nursing. Of these, 1,118 were diploma schools, 195 were B.A. programs, and 1 was an associate program. By 1965 there were 1,193 programs; of these, 821 were diploma schools, 198 were B.A. schools, and 174 were associate degree schools. By 1978, there were a total of 1,374 programs: of these, 344 were diploma schools, 353 were B.A. schools, and 677 were associate degree schools. *Source Book of Nursing Personnel* (Bethesda, Md.: U.S. Department of Health, Education, and Welfare, Division of Nursing, DHEW Publication (HRA) 75-43, December 1974); American Nurses Association, *Facts About Nursing*, 1980–1981 ed., p. 152; U.S. Department of Health and Human Services, Bureau of Nursing, *Report of the Secretary of Health and Human Services on the Supply and Distribution of and Requirements for Nurses as Required by Section 951, Nurse Training Act of 1975*, April 27, 1981, p. 156; U.S. Department of Health and Human Services, Division of Health Professions Analysis, *The Registered Nurse Population, An Overview: From National Sample Survey of Registered Nurses, November 1980*, Report 82–5, p. 11; and unpublished data from the American Nurses Association.

After World War II diploma schools of nursing declined rapidly, from 1,118 in 1950 to 244 in 1985. Hospitals hoped that the federal subsidies under the NTA would be used to increase the number of nurses graduating from diploma schools of nursing. There was sufficient capacity in those schools to accommodate increases in enrollment. However, the American Nurses' Association stated in 1965 that they wanted nursing education to occur in institutions of higher learning. The National League for Nursing (NLN) was designated as the accrediting agency for dispensing federal support to schools of nursing; its goals were, of course, similar to those of the ANA. Until 1968, payment to diploma and associate degree schools under the NTA fell short of what Congress authorized (50 percent), while payments to baccalaureate programs were approximately equal to what was authorized (16).

Although the number of diploma school programs declined, graduates from these programs still made the largest contribution to the number of new active nurses during the period from 1950 to 1972. (From 1972 to 1985 more nurses have graduated from associate degree programs than from diploma programs.) The number of baccalaureate degree programs increased from 195 to 293 over the 1950–1972 period (and to 403 in 1985), yet the number of new active nurses they contributed was only twice as great as the number of graduates from associate degree programs, which grew in numbers from one program in 1950 to 541 in 1972 (and to 746 in 1985). The large growth in associate degree programs began before the funds for the NTA became available. Graduates of associate degree programs were less than 10 percent of total nurse graduates in 1965–1966. By 1984 they represented 55 percent of all nurse graduates. The number of graduates from each of these programs is shown in Table 16–6.

It appears that in administering the NTA, no attempt was made to maximize the number of nurse graduates. If that had been the goal, the funds would have been allocated differently according to the different types of nursing schools. Instead, there appears to have been a conscious decision to favor growth in the number of nursing graduates from baccalaureate degree programs. From the ANA's point of view, such graduates would be more likely to take on additional responsibilities. Shifting away from diploma schools to baccalaureate schools would also coincide with the ANA's goals, since a likely result would be a smaller increase in the number of nurse graduates, thereby resulting in an eventual increase in their wages. The starting salaries of nursing graduates are similar regardless of the type of school from which they are graduated. A graduate from a baccalaureate school spends more time in school compared with graduates from associate degree or diploma schools, yet the wage differential does not compensate baccalaureate graduates for the additional training time or foregone income. Several recent studies confirm that the rate of return to the nurse with a baccalaureate degree working in a hospital setting is less than for a nurse with only a two-year associate degree (17).

The growth in demand for associate degree education was related to its relatively high rate of return compared with comparable occupations (18). It is thus likely that associate degree programs would have grown without federal NTA support (19). The diploma school enrollments probably declined because the higher rates of return in these programs, relative to B.A. and A.A. degrees, were not high enough to offset "certain non-financial disadvantages (e.g., apprenticeship-type work requirements, restrictions on social life, little or no access to job opportunities other than in nursing, etc.)" (20). The rate of return to a B.A. degree program was lower than the diploma or associate degree programs. To compensate for this lower rate of return, the ANA attempted to provide such students with greater direct financial support and indirect

TABLE 16-6. Nursing Graduates by Type of Nursing School Program

Academic Year	Total		Diploma		Associate Degree		Baccalaureate	
	Number	Annual (% Change)	Number	Percent of Total Graduates	Number	Percent of Total Graduates	Number	Percent of Total Graduates
1952[a]	29,016		26,720	92.1	298	1.0	1,998	6.9
1955[a]	28,729	- .3	25,826	89.9	199	.7	2,704	9.4
1960–1961	30,019	.9	25,071	83.5	917	3.1	4,031	13.4
1965–1966	34,909	3.1	26,072	74.7	3,349	9.6	5,488	15.7
1970–1971	46,455	5.9	22,065	47.5	14,534	31.3	9,856	21.2
1975–1976	77,065	10.7	19,861	25.8	34,625	44.9	22,579	29.3
1976–1977	77,755	.9	18,014	23.2	36,289	46.7	23,452	30.1
1977–1978	77,874	.2	17,131	22.0	36,556	46.9	24,187	31.1
1978–1979	77,132	- 1.0	15,820	20.5	36,264	47.0	25,048	32.5
1979–1980	75,523	- 2.1	14,495	19.2	36,034	47.7	24,994	33.1
1980–1981	73,985	- 2.0	12,903	17.4	36,712	49.6	24,370	32.9
1981–1982	74,052	.1	11,682	15.8	38,289	51.7	24,081	32.5
1982–1983	77,408	4.5	11,704	15.1	41,849	54.1	23,855	30.8
1983–1984	80,312	3.8	12,200	15.2	44,394	55.3	23,718	29.5

SOURCES: For 1952 and 1955, U.S. Department of Health, Education, and Welfare, Division of Nursing, Source Book of Nursing, DHEW Publication (HRA) 75-43 (Washington, D.C.: Government Printing Office, 1974), p. 98. For 1960–1980, National League for Nursing, Nursing Data Book, 1981 (New York: National League for Nursing, 1982). For 1981–1984, National League for Nursing, Nursing Data Review, 1986 (New York: National League for Nursing, 1987). Used with permission.

[a]These represent calendar years.

423

support through payments to the collegiate schools for construction and operating expenses, to result eventually in lower tuition levels. The reasons, therefore, for the small increase in nurse graduates as a result of the federal legislation was the change in educational emphasis in nursing toward baccalaureate degrees and the allocation of the federal funds to promote this change in the type of nursing graduate. Whether or not this is a desirable federal objective is another issue.

If the federal subsidies for nurse education produced few additional nurses, then how were the quantitative goals for the number of nurses achieved? Based upon an econometric model of the nursing sector, which was used to simulate changes that have occurred in nurse employment over time, one author concluded:

> The predicted nurse graduations, which by 1969 are equal to 39,250, are not even close to the 53,000 set as the 1969 goals by the Surgeon General's Consultant Group on Nursing, necessary to achieve the 680,000 employment figure. In fact, the model's predictions of nursing school graduations are considerably below this level throughout the forecast period. Therefore, the achievement of the 1969 level of nursing is to be attributed to the increase in participation rates and the change in the age distribution of the stock of nurses, as well as increased graduations, and none of these events are even remotely influenced by the existence of the subsidy programs in question. (21)

Labor force participation rates for nurses increased from 48.8 percent in 1950, to 55.3 percent in 1960 (22), to 65.2 percent in 1966, to 70.5 percent in 1972, to 76 percent in 1980, and to 79 percent in 1984 (23). There was a net increase of 414,815 employed RNs from 1966 to 1977. It has been estimated that the sources of this net increase in employed RNs were: a change in the participation rate and in reinstatements (RNs who have renewed their lapsed licenses), 33.9 percent; foreign-trained RNs, 9.1 percent; and new graduates, 57.1 percent (24). Graduates from associate degree programs represented 3 percent of graduates in 1960–1961, 9.6 percent in 1965–1966, 31.4 percent by 1970–1971, and 55.3 percent by 1983–1984. The higher nurse participation rates were in large part due to the increase in nurses' wages. During the period that the federal subsidy program to nurse education was in effect, there were large increases in the wages of nurses as a result of the Medicare and Medicaid programs. It is believed that these wage increases resulted in a higher nurse participation rate, which was a major contributing factor in the increase in nurse employment. It appears, therefore, that the achievement of the employment goals underlying the NTA of 1964 was the result of other factors (e.g., increased nurse participation rates) rather than the federal subsidy program itself.

It is possible to compare the costs of increasing nurse employment through subsidizing nursing education, as under the nurse training legislation, with an approach that would subsidize nurses' wages directly. The cost (in terms of federal subsidy dollars required) for increases in the number of employed nurses is several times lower if direct wage subsidies are provided to nurses instead of providing federal subsidies to nursing schools to increase their number of nursing graduates. For example, earlier it was estimated that the number of additional nurses employed as a result of the federal support to nursing schools was approximately 1,500 nurses per year or 24,000 for the

16-year period 1965–1981.[10] The estimated federal expenditures under nurse training legislation during that time period were $1.57 billion. This comes to $65,000 per employed nurse as a result of the federal subsidy program. If an alternative federal program for increasing the supply of active nurses were implemented, namely, simply to provide a wage subsidy to all employed nurses, how much would this cost? Several studies have attempted to estimate the elasticity of the participation rate with respect to nurses' wages, holding other factors constant. These studies have derived elasticity estimates ranging from a negative elasticity to an elasticity of 2.8 (25). In our example we use an elasticity estimate of 1.0; that is, a 1 percent increase in nurses' wages leads to a 1 percent increase in the number of active nurses.

If the wage elasticity with respect to the nurse participation rate were 1.0, it would require a 1 percent increase in nurses' wages, multiplied by all the employed nurses, to achieve a 1 percent increase in the number of employed RNs. In 1963 there were approximately 550,000 active RNs receiving an annual wage of $4,714. A 1 percent subsidy to increase their wage would be $47 per nurse multiplied by 550,000 active nurses, for a total subsidy cost of $25 million. This would result in a 1 percent increase in the number of active RNs, or 5,500 additional nurses. The federal subsidy per additional nurse employed under this program comes to $4,545. Table 16–7 shows the federal subsidy per active nurse under this type of a program for different time periods. As the number of active RNs increase, so does the annual number of subsidy dollars required to produce an additional active RN under this approach—from $4,545 per active RN in 1963 to $7,936 per active RN in 1969. To produce an equivalent 24,000 nurses through a wage subsidy program would have taken approximately four years at a total subsidy cost of $120 million, for an average cost of $5,000 per additional nurse. When compared with the cost of $65,000 per active RN produced under the actual nurse training legislation, the cost per active RN under this alternative subsidy program is approximately 10 times less expensive. Even if one were to vastly change the assumptions used in these calculations (i.e., the elasticity of the nurse participation rates or the number of nursing school graduates produced under the NTA), this alternative subsidy program is still less expensive.[11] (The attractiveness of this program would be increased further if the subsidies *were discounted*.)

Other advantages of the alternative subsidy program are that the administrative costs of this subsidy program are lower and that the increase in active nurses will occur much more quickly than it would as a result of a subsidy program that relies on increased nursing graduates. Also, under the alternative subsidy program, the federal government does not make a *continuing* commitment of financial support to schools of nursing. Once federal funds have subsidized these institutions, a new constituency for federal support has been created and it is difficult to reduce support even when there is no longer a nursing shortage.

---

[10]The number of nurses produced as a result of the NTA would be lower than this estimate, since a long lead time is necessary before the federal funds have their effect. Legislation enacted in 1964 contained authorizations for 1965 and began to affect nursing schools in 1966. First graduates from associate degree programs would appear in 1967, and graduates from baccalaureate programs, which were the recipients of a large part of the funds, would not appear until 1969.

[11]If a .25 elasticity estimate were assumed, a wage subsidy program would have taken 14 years at a total subsidy cost of $888 million to produce 24,000 nurses—almost half the cost of the program adopted by the government.

TABLE 16-7. Cost of an Alternative Federal Subsidy Program to Increase the Number of Active RNs

Year	Annual Wage	1 Percent Increase in Wage	Number of Active RNs	Total Cost of 1 Percent Increase Col. 3 × Col. 4	1 Percent Increase in Employed RNs	Cost per Additional RN Col. 5 ÷ Col. 6
1963	$4,714	$47	550,000	$25,000,000	5,500	$4,545
1966	5,763	57	600,000	34,000,000	6,000	5,666
1969	7,815	78	630,000	50,000,000	6,300	7,936

An important difference between the nurse training legislation and the alternative subsidy program is that the more successful the federal government is in increasing the number of nursing graduates, the lower will be the increase in nurses' wages. The increased supply of new nurses will hold down potential increases in nurses' wages; this dampening effect will have an adverse impact upon the participation rate. Thus the subsidy to nursing schools could well be self-defeating!

AN ECONOMIC ANALYSIS OF COMPARABLE WORTH

According to the 1964 Civil Rights Act, a person must receive equal pay for performing equal work; discrimination in employment is illegal. Comparable worth goes beyond that concept; its proponents want equal pay for work of comparable value. If two people are performing different jobs, but it is judged that their work is of equal value, they should be rewarded equally. The proponents of greater pay equity base their argument on the empirical observation that certain jobs that are filled predominately by women are paid less than jobs that are filled predominately by men. The value of each job should be determined, not by the marketplace, but by fact-finding commissions. The crux of the debate regarding comparable worth is over the appropriate mechanism for setting wages. Nurse associations are in the forefront of the movement to legislate comparable worth throughout the country.

Comparable worth is analyzed by first reviewing the determination of wages in a competitive market and the effects on wages and employment of noncompetitive restrictions. Two alternative theories are then used to explain observed wage disparities between males and females. Next, the consequences of using comparable worth to achieve pay equity are discussed, and finally, alternative strategies to increase nursing salaries are presented.

The Determination of Wages

In a competitive market, wages and employees' incomes are determined by the firm's demand for employees and by the number or supply of those employees. The wage is the equilibrating mechanism; it is the price of labor. At higher or lower wages, the firm would be willing to hire fewer or more persons, respectively. Also, the higher the wages or income, the greater are the number of people willing to enter that occupation or profession.

In addition to wages, the value of an employee's output determines how many employees a firm will hire. The value of an employee's output consists of two parts: the productivity of the employee (i.e., how much output one person can produce) and the price at which that output can be sold in the marketplace. An employees' productivity is affected by his or her education, skill, and experience. Thus even within a given profession, differences in income exist. The higher the price at which the output can be sold, the greater is the value of the employee producing that output. For example, if a nurse practitioner is reimbursed for a physical at a lower fee than a family practitioner, the value of the output produced by the nurse practitioner is lower. (Changes in either employee productivity or the price of the output cause shifts in the demand for labor.)

In a competitive market, therefore, a person's income depends on three things: the type of output or service the person is able to produce, the value or price of that service in the market, and the number of people in the profession.

Market restrictions may either increase or decrease employees' incomes. For example, restrictions as to who can enter the profession will increase the incomes of those in the profession while decreasing the incomes of those who must work in other, unrestricted occupations. These restrictions are often sanctioned by the government, such as with licensing, or by nongovernment groups, such as unions, when they determine, for example, who can become plumbers. The effect of these entry restrictions is to have a smaller supply of professionals in the restricted market and a larger supply in the unrestricted market, causing a large wage differential between the two markets.

Similar to entry restrictions are restrictions on the tasks that health professionals may perform. There often are tasks that a person is capable of performing (either by experience or training), but the profession is prohibited from doing so by state practice acts. A profession prohibited from performing highly remunerative tasks thereby produces an output that has a lower economic value (the demand for their services is shifted to the left).

Another type of restriction that makes a market noncompetitive is when employers collude on the setting of wages, as apparently occurred during the 1950s and early 1960s, when hospitals colluded in the setting of nurses' wages. The effect of such monopoly power by the purchasers of services was to hold down the rate of increase in nurses' salaries.

Finally, if a firm does not face competition in the sale of its product, then the firm does not have to be as concerned with its costs of production (i.e., the wage rates they pay or whether they employ the best people for the job). This would happen, for example, in regulated companies (such as utilities) or in state and local governments. Similarly, prior to enactment of prospective payment legislation (DRGs), hospitals were not constrained to produce in cost-minimizing ways. Medical schools that are heavily subsidized and that have excess demand for their places can also be less efficient. A firm that is a monopolist in the sale of its product can pass on higher wages and the additional costs of hiring less competent personnel. It is precisely in such situations that firms can also practice discrimination in hiring.

In a competitive industry, if a firm paid higher wages or hired less competent workers than its competitors, its costs would be higher. The firm could not compete on price and would either be forced to go out of business or to change its employment practices. Discriminatory practices are therefore more likely to occur in industries or among firms that do not have to be as concerned with costs (26).

Theories to Explain Wage Disparities

Women, on average, earn less than men. Some occupations are also filled predominately by either women or men, with women earning less. Why does this occur?

According to the "crowding" theory, women are channeled by either their own expectations or by those of others into certain professions that are predominately female (27). The exclusion of women from higher-paying male dominated jobs causes a surplus of women within particular jobs, thereby leading to lower wages in the female-dominated jobs.

How valid is the crowding theory to justify eliminating the market and substitute fact-finding commissions to determine wages? Little evidence seems to exist to support the premise that women's occupations, such as nursing or clerical work, are more crowded than men's occupations. Moreover, for the crowding theory to be a valid explanation of differences in male/female wages, the market would have to be non-competitive in some manner. Otherwise, some women would enter male-dominated professions to receive a higher rate of return. The mobility between occupations would equalize wages.

The most accepted explanation by economists for wage disparities is based on the theory of human capital (28). There are nonmonetary reasons why people select certain jobs; preferences as to the type of work and location may have an influence on a person's employment preferences. Wages reflect these differences in preferences. Second, individuals have different abilities, resulting in different incomes. However, an individual's productivity is not fixed; it can be increased with additional training and education. Therefore, wages also differ according to the individual's investment in education, training, and experience. Thus if females anticipate leaving the work force, they may invest less in education; married women who have undertaken traditional home responsibilities have found this to be an obstacle in making a full commitment to their careers.

How well does the above explain male/female wage differentials? In 1983 the wage differential between males and females was approximately .72 (29). The ratio was closer for younger age groups, .89 for 20 to 24 year olds, and lower for those 35 years and older, .65. *According to empirical studies, most of the differences in male/female wage ratios can be explained by differences in the total number of years of work experience, the years of tenure on the current job, and the pattern or continuity of previous work experience* (30). These studies do not deny that discrimination may exist, however, it is not an important determinant of observed wage differences.

As differences in human capital between males and females lessen, so should differences in their wage rates. Career patterns and expectations have changed significantly during the 1970s; for example, the proportion of women in medical school has reached 30 percent. As educational levels, work roles, and work expectations of males and females become similar, so should their relative wages.

Determination of Wages Through Comparable Worth

What would happen if wages were based on comparable worth instead of being left to the marketplace? Consultants and committees would be used to conduct job evaluations on each position within an organization or firm. These evaluations would involve assessment of the relative worth of each position according to skill required, effort involved, working conditions, and level of responsibility. Points would be assessed for each of these factors and salaries would be determined by the total number of points in each position.

The implementation of a wage determination system based on comparable worth would result in a number of problems. First, the complexity of categorizing people would be tremendous, particularly if one were trying to establish a nationally applicable system affecting tens of thousands of jobs in hundreds of thousands of places. Further, these job evaluations would have to be updated as tasks and job conditions change. The cost of such a system would be enormous, not only in terms of the time involved but also the cost of hiring the consultants and establishing job evaluation committees. An additional very large cost would be that arising from the resolution of identified pay inequities. This may well be in the billions of dollars.

Second, if comparable worth were instituted, wage equity would not be achieved by lowering wages in certain job classifications, even if job evaluations indicated that certain groups were being overpaid, since individuals in those groups would protest. Instead, occupations in which employees were currently being underpaid would have their wages increased. When the employer is a state government, the state can increase taxes to pay the increased costs; however, if taxpayers or their legislators are unwilling to vote for higher taxes, the effect would be similar to imposing higher wages on private industry. Less money would be spent on other programs or the employer would be forced to reduce employment in those occupations where wages were raised. Moreover, it is in female-dominated occupations that wages would be increased and, consequently, where fewer people would be hired. Although those remaining on the job would receive higher wages, some would be let go.

Third, wages determined by a commission would not reflect supply and demand conditions. The result would be shortages and surpluses of workers in different occupations. How would this be resolved? In those occupations experiencing shortages will it be possible to increase wages? Jobs in surplus professions will have to be rationed; what criteria will be used? Rationing provides an opportunity for discrimination, as has previously been the case with medical school admissions.

In summary, while comparable worth may be conceptually appealing to those that distrust the market, its implementation would be costly and likely not to achieve the goals its proponents desire. Problems that would emerge are politicization of wage determination, a large bureaucracy for evaluating all positions in the economy, lower levels of employment for women in those occupations in which wages have been increased artificially, increased costs of services and a smaller output in those industries with a greater portion of women, a decreased incentive for women to move into other professions, and continual shortages and surpluses.

Alternative Strategies for Increasing Wages

There are alternative strategies that society should favor to achieve greater pay equity. The first is the enforcement of current laws against discrimination; females desiring to enter male-dominated professions should be able to do so. A shift in the number of females from female-dominated professions to male-dominated professions should increase the wage in the former and depress wages in male-dominated professions. Differences in wages would more closely reflect either preferences for some types of occupations or differences in investment in human capital.

Next should be the elimination of the many restrictions that prevent labor markets from operating competitively. Legal restrictions that prohibit certain persons from undertaking tasks even though they are qualified to perform those tasks result in higher prices to society and in lower wages to those who are prohibited from performing them. For example, a nurse could receive increased income if he or she became a nurse-midwife. However, when a hospital denies the nurse-midwife staff privileges, or if the insurance company refuses to pay the nurse-midwife unless the bill is submitted by a physician, these actions prevent the growth of nurse-midwifery services, raise the cost to patients desiring such services; and prevent nurses from increasing their incomes. In many instances, restrictive nurse practice acts unnecessarily limit the nurse's ability to perform certain functions.

The increasing trend toward competition in the delivery of health services should prove beneficial to the career goals of nurses. Large organizations, such as health maintenance organizations, must be able to compete on their premiums if they are to increase their market share. The managers of such organizations will be more willing to look for less expensive methods of providing services, more willing to innovate, and less bound to traditional tasks and roles than were not-for-profit hospitals reimbursed on a cost basis. In a price-competitive system, nurses are moving into new settings and performing additional tasks previously denied them.

In conclusion, the marketplace does not place the same value on people or services as many would prefer; however, years of experience with trying to control the market through wage and price controls have demonstrated that it is costly and eventually ineffective to try and do so. Therefore, an alternative is to understand the criteria used by the market to establish incomes and to use those criteria to help achieve the desired goals. Enforcing current laws on discrimination, removing economic restrictions, and providing access to educational and training opportunities would increase job opportunities and incomes for women while benefiting society through increased availability of services.

CONCLUDING COMMENTS

The measures used to evaluate the performance of the nursing market were the rise in the number of hospital-employed nurses, their rate of return compared with other nurses and other occupations with comparable training, the increase in the number of nurses entering nursing, and the participation rate of nurses. In an efficiently operating market, as the demand for nurses increases so would their wages, their relative rate of return, the number of students entering nursing, and the percentage of trained nurses who are active.

Initially, in the late 1940s, the nursing market appeared to have been in equilibrium. However, during the late 1950s and mid-1960s there was a shortage; the demand for nurses by hospitals exceeded the supply of nurses at the market wage. From an analysis of changes in relative wages of hospital employed nurses relative to other nurses, it appeared that there was a static shortage caused by hospital collusion to prevent nurses' wages from rising. This collusion, motivated by hospitals to keep their costs from increasing, led to intensified recruiting of foreign-trained nurses and to greater substitution of practical nurses and nurse aides by hospitals. Hospitals also lobbied for federal subsidies to increase the supply of nurses. The "shortage" began to disappear when Medicare and Medicaid were enacted. As the demand for hospital care (and the consequent demand for nurses) increased, hospitals were able to pass on to the government both the increased costs of higher wages and an increase in the number of nurses employed. Collective bargaining agreements between hospitals and nurses began several years later. Nurses' wages in the post-Medicare period increased rapidly, as did nurse participation rates; the high rate of return to nursing led to increased enrollments in associate degree programs. The rate of return to nursing again became comparable to other occupations. (The rate of return varied, however, depending upon the type of degree received by the nurse.)

Federal legislation to support nurse training starting in 1964 and continuing for many years thereafter coincided with the increased demand by prospective nurses for associate degree programs. The original manpower goals underlying the 1964 Nurse Training Act were achieved, although it appears that they would have been achieved without the federal subsidy program. What further justification is there for continued federal subsidies for nursing education? If the objective of continued subsidies is to raise the educational level of nurses so as to be able to undertake additional responsibilities, it is questionable whether this is a sufficient criterion for federal intervention in the nursing market and for use of public funds. If there is a greater demand for such personnel, and if state practice acts permit nurses to undertake additional responsibilities, the increased return from doing these tasks would justify increased investment by nurses for this training. It is not clear why federal subsidies are required. The goals used by the nursing profession to justify subsidies to nursing education should be made explicit so that it can be determined whether it is a goal agreed to by the rest of society and whether the proposed approach is the least expensive way to achieve it.

A proposal by the American Nurses' Association, if implemented by each state, should have an important effect on the supply of nurses. The ANA has proposed that all nursing graduates who wish to obtain a R.N. license should receive a B.A. degree. Nursing students who graduate from two year programs would only receive a technical nursing license. If the ANA is successful in having each state increase nurse educational requirements in this manner, there should be a sharp reduction in the number of new graduates each year. Currently, graduates with a B.A. degree represent only 31 percent of new nurse graduates. If implemented today, this policy would result in a loss of 54,000 graduates per year. The impact of this policy over time would be an increase in salaries of nurses, with a consequent rise in hospital costs. These higher costs would, in part, be shifted to patients, government, and other third-party payors.

After years of relative equilibrium in the nursing market, it appears that an economic shortage is again occurring. This shortage is different from the earlier one in that it appears to be a dynamic one. As shown in Table 16–1, the nurse vacancy rate in hospitals increased sharply from 6.3 percent in 1985 to 13.6 percent in December 1986 (the time of the survey). Although hospital utilization is declining, several other factors are increasing the demand for nurses. Other organizations are increasing their demand for RNs, such as home health care agencies, HMOs, and insurance companies (for utilization review). Hospitals are also increasing the proportion of RNs per patient as the acuity level of their patients are increasing. From 1984 to 1985 the percent of RNs as a proportion of all nursing personnel increased from 53.3 to 67.4 (31). As the demand for RNs has increased, enrollment at nursing schools has been declining. The decline in enrollment is related to changes in demographics (i.e., a smaller female age cohort), as well as to increased career opportunities for women. The consequence of this dynamic shortage is likely to be increased nurse wages in coming years.

APPENDIX: THE EFFECTS ON WAGES AND EMPLOYMENT OF REGISTERED NURSES OF UNIONIZATION IN A MONOPSONY MARKET

A monopsonist, with a demand curve D_1, will face a rising supply curve for nurses described by S_1 in Figure 16–3. Since the monopsonist must pay a higher wage to all

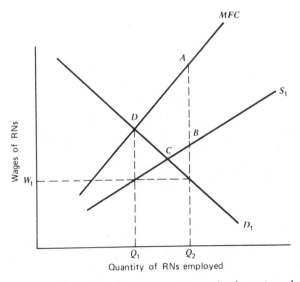

Figure 16-3. An illustration of a monopsonistic market for registered nurses.

currently employed nurses each time it pays a higher wage for an additional nurse, it faces a marginal factor cost (MFC) curve which lies above the supply curve. The MFC curve represents the cost to the monopsonist of hiring an additional nurse. At each point on the supply curve, the MFC curve indicates the additional cost in terms of higher wages that must be paid to all nurses hired previously. Thus the equilibrium quantity of nurses the firm will hire and the wage it will pay under such circumstances are given by the intersection of the demand curve and the MFC curve. Drawing a line down to the supply curve will indicate the wage the firm would pay and the quantity of RNs employed. At the equilibrium wage, W_1, the monopsonist would be willing to hire Q_2 quantity of nurses, which is the point on the firm's demand curve at a wage of W_1. However, if the firm were actually to hire Q_2 number of RNs, it would have to pay a wage much higher than W_1 to attract them. The new wage would be at that point on the supply curve above Q_2 shown by B. The cost to the firm of that wage and Q_2 number of nurses would be point A *on the MFC curve.* Since point A on the MFC curve exceeds the firm's demand, the firm would not want to hire Q_2 nurses at a wage represented by point B on the supply curve. Thus W_1 and Q_1 are equilibrium points for the monopsonist. However, at that wage, W_1, the firm will report $Q_1 - Q_2$ vacancies for nurses. These are the number of nurses it would be willing to hire at wage W_1. Vacancies are thus expected and quite normal in a monopsony situation.

In a monopsony or oligopsony situation, if a union were formed and set a minimum wage for its employees, the supply curve for nurses would change. It would become horizontal up to the point of the minimum wage on the original supply curve. This would indicate that under the collective bargaining agreement, nurses cannot be paid below a certain minimum union wage. The hospital can hire all the nurses it wants at that wage. The MFC curve would also change. It would become equal to the new minimum wage, since there is no additional cost to the hospital as it hires an additional nurse; that is, it does not have to increase the wages of those nurses currently employed. Up to the point where the negotiated wage intersects the original supply

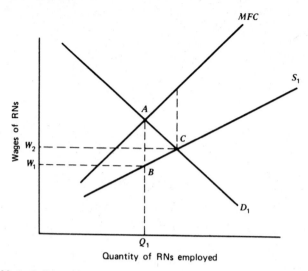

Figure 16–4. Collective bargaining and a monopsony market for registered nurses.

curve, the hospital can hire all the nurses it wants at the negotiated wage. Beyond that point the hospital will have to increase its wages and also pay higher wages to its existing nurses. Thus at that point the hospital will again face a rising supply curve and a rising *MFC* curve. In situations involving a monopsony purchaser and a union representing the employees, it is possible for the union to set a wage that is higher than the previous wage and also increase employment. This is illustrated in Figure 16–4. If the union sets a wage rate anywhere between *A* and *B*, it will raise the wage (since the current wage is W_1) and it will increase the number of nurses hired. Any wage between *A* and *B* will make the supply curve and the *MFC* curve horizontal up to that point. For example, a wage rate of W_2 is the point where employment of RNs is greatest. The new wage rate intersects the demand curve at the same point that the supply curve does. Therefore the wage rate (W_2) is the new *MFC* and supply curve up to the point where it intersects the original supply curve. To hire more nurses after that point, the firm will have to pay a higher wage and thus face a rising *MFC* and rising supply curve. Above point *A* on the demand curve, a union wage will decrease employment of RNs, unless the demand curve shifts to the right.

REFERENCES

1. Donald E. Yett, *An Economic Analysis of the Nurse Shortage* (Lexington, Mass: D.C. Health, 1975), p. 19.
2. *Ibid.*, p. 110.
3. *Ibid.*, p. 182.
4. *Ibid.*, p. 199.
5. *Ibid.*, p. 221.
6. *Hospital Statistics 1986* (Chicago: American Hospital Association, 1986), p. 196. F. Sloan and R. Elnicki constructed a model to test the monopsony hypothesis and

several other hypotheses about nurses' wages for the year 1972. Their model and conclusions may be found in Frank Sloan and Richard Elnicki, "Determinants of Professional Nurses' Wages," in Richard Scheffler, ed., *Research in Health Economics*, Vol. 1 (Greenwich, Conn.: JAI Press, 1979), 217–254.

7. Yett, *op. cit.*, p. 221.

8. *Ibid.*, p. 221.

9. Stuart Altman, *Present and Future Supply of Registered Nurses*, U.S. Department of Health, Education, and Welfare Publication (NIH) 72–134, Division of Nursing (Washington, D.C.: U.S. Government Printing Office, November 1971), p. 15.

10. Communication from the American Nurses Association, April 29, 1987.

11. Several studies in the early 1980s also concluded that an economic shortage of nurses no longer existed. See National Academy of Sciences, Institute of Medicine *Report by the Committee of the Institute of Medicine for a Study of Nursing and Nursing Education* (Washington, D.C.: National Academy of Sciences, 1983); and Jesse S. Hixson, Jack Reid, Jack Rodgers, and Stephen Boehlert, "The Shortage of Nursing Personnel—A New Look at the Issues," mimeographed, Division of Health Professions Analysis, Bureau of Health Professions, Health Resources Administration, February 26, 1981.

12. Yett, *op. cit.*, p. 246.

13. *Ibid.*, p. 247.

14. *Ibid.*, p. 248.

15. *Ibid.*, p. 29.

16. *Ibid.*, pp. 32–33.

17. Stephen T. Mennemeyer and Gary Gaumer, "Nursing Wages and the Value of Educational Credentials," *Journal of Human Resources*, 18, Winter 1983: 32–48; Lavonne A. Booton and Julia I. Lane, "Hospital Market Structure and the Return to Nursing Education," *Journal of Human Resources*, 20, Spring 1985: 184–195.

18. Yett, *op. cit.*, p. 251.

19. *Ibid.*, p. 249.

20. *Ibid.*, p. 249.

21. Robert T. Dean, "Simulating an Econometric Model of the Market for Nurses," unpublished doctoral dissertation, Department of Economics, University of California at Los Angeles, 1971, p. 218. A further discussion of the ineffectiveness of the Nurse Training Act (NTA) may be found in Robert Deane and Donald Yett, "Nurse Market Policy Simulations Using an Econometric Model," in Scheffler, ed., *op. cit.*

22. Altman, *op cit.*, p. 102.

23. *The Registered Nurse Population: An Overview*, from a national sample of registered nurses, November 1980, U.S. Department of Health and Human Services, Bureau of Health Professions, Division of Health Professions Analysis, Report 82–5 Rockville, Md.: U.S. Department of Health and Human Services, December 1981. Recent data are from *Facts About Nursing* (Kansas City, Mo.: American Nurses Association, 1986), p. 2.

24. John Edgren, "The Federal Nurse Training Acts," *Health Manpower Policy Studies Group Discussion Paper Series* (Ann Arbor, Mich.: School of Public Health, University of Michigan, 1977), p. 39.

25. The reasons for the differences in the estimates relate to the types of data used, aggregate versus micro, characteristics of the nurses, and the econometric methods employed. For a further discussion of these estimates, see Frank A. Sloan, *Equalizing Access to Nursing Services: The Geographic Discussion*, Department of Health, Education, and Welfare Publication (HRA) 78–51 (Washington, D.C.: U.S. Government Printing Office, March 1978); and Charles R. Link and Russell F. Settle, "Wage Incentives and Married Professional Nurses: A Case of Backward-Bending Supply?" *Economic Inquiry*, 19, January 1981: 144–156.

26. Gary Becker, *The Economics of Discrimination*, 2nd ed. (Chicago: University of Chicago Press, 1971).

27. Barbara Bergmann, "Occupational Segregation, Wages and Profits When Employers Discriminate by Race or Sex," *Eastern Economic Journal*, 1, 1974, 103–110.

28. Gary Becker, *Human Capital* (New York: Columbia University Press, 1964).

29. June O'Neill, "An Argument Against Comparable Worth," in *Comparable Worth: Issue for the 1980s*, Vol. 1 (Washington, D.C.: U.S. Commission on Civil Rights, 1984), 177–186. The ratio used by O'Neill is adjusted for hours worked. When unadjusted for hours worked, the ratio in 1982 was 62 percent.

30. *Ibid.*, p. 179.

31. *Survey of Hospital Nursing Personnel* (Chicago: American Hospital Association, 1984), p. 34; (1985), p. 10.

CHAPTER 17

The Pharmaceutical Industry

INTRODUCTION

Drugs provide society with enormous benefits. They reduce mortality and morbidity, relieve pain and suffering, are less expensive forms of treatment than surgery and hospitalization, are more readily accessible to a larger portion of the population than are more expensive technologies, and have enabled physicians to see more patients with improved treatment outcomes.

Many serious diseases have had their incidence and severity greatly reduced by modern drugs. For example, penicillin and the antibiotics have caused a large decline in the mortality and morbidity associated with infectious diseases such as pneumonia, meningitis, and tuberculosis. Pneumonia used to be a widespread, greatly feared, and often fatal disease. Tranquilizers and chemotherapy of mental patients have resulted in changes in the treatment of mental illness and large reductions in use of mental institutions, enabling many who would have been incapable of functioning adequately to work and live at home. Antihypertensive drugs reduced the death rate from hypertensive heart disease from 44 per 100,000 in 1960 to 8.6 per 100,000 in 1985. Synthetic hormones and birth control pills have had a worldwide impact. People have been able to plan their families conveniently. Many childhood diseases, such as measles, diphtheria, and polio, that are potentially fatal or crippling have been virtually eliminated by the use of vaccinations. Table 17-1 provides an indication of the success of drug therapy in reducing once-feared diseases.

Drugs also reduce the direct and indirect costs of illness. They reduce the need for hospitalization and the length of time needed as an inpatient when it is required, a very large savings of the direct cost of illness. By reducing both the length and severity of illness, drugs enable the patient to return to work sooner, thereby lowering the indirect costs of sickness. Drugs are an integral part of medical treatment, whose benefits in medical, social and economic terms would be incalculable should their availability be withdrawn.

For all of their enormous impact on health status and in the alleviation of pain, personal expenditures on drugs have been rising less rapidly than personal medical

TABLE 17-1. Death Rates per 100,000 Population, 1920–1985

Cause of Death	1920	1940	1960	1978	1985	Percent Decline 1920–1985
Tuberculosis, all forms	113.1	45.9	5.9	1.3	.7	99
Dysentery	4.0	1.9	.2	.0[a]	.0	100
Whooping cough	12.5	2.2	.1	.0	.0	100
Diptheria	15.3	1.1	.0[b]	—	.0	100
Measles	8.8	.5	.2	.0	.0	100
Influenza and pneumonia	207.3	70.3	36.6	26.7	27.9	87

SOURCE: Ernst B. Chain, "Academic and Industrial Contributions to Drug Research," *Nature*, November 2, 1963: 441; and U.S. Department of Health, Education, and Welfare, Public Health Service, Health Resources Administration, "Final Mortality Statistics, 1978," *Monthly Vital Statistics Report*, 29(6) and 34(13) September 17, 1980 and September 1986. Partially reprinted from Henry Grabowski, "Public Policy and Innovation: The Case of Pharmaceuticals," *Technovation*, 1, 1982: 168.

[a]Bacillary dysentery and ambeiasis.

[b]1959 (figures for 1960 and 1978 not available).

care expenditures over the past 30 years. Drug (and medical sundry) expenditures were $3.7 billion in 1960, $8.0 billion in 1970, $18.8 billion in 1980, increasing to $28.5 in 1985, for an average annual rate of increase of 9.1 percent over the last 10 years [1]. This is in contrast to the increase in total personal health care expenditures, which rose from $23.6 billion in 1960 to $371.4 billion in 1985, for an average annual rate of increase of 12.2 percent from 1975 to 1985. As a percentage of total personal health care expenditures, drugs have fallen from 15 percent in 1960 to 7.7 percent in 1985. This is shown in Table 17-2.

Drug prices have also been subject to less price inflation than have medical care prices. According to the Bureau of Labor Statistics, the drug price index has increased from 115.3 in 1960 to 256.5 in 1985. Over this same period, the Medical Care Price Index has risen from 79.1 in 1960 to 403.1 in 1985, while some components of this index, such as hospital services, have increased from 57.3 to 710.5 over this period. These data are shown in Table 17.3.

Given the impact that drugs have had, their relatively small proportion of total health expenditures, and their small annual rates of increase in prices, why has so much attention been given to the ethical drug industry, which consists of drugs promoted and distributed primarily to health professionals and which are available to consumers by prescription only? There are two reasons for such attention. First, there has been concern that selling costs and profits in this industry are too high and that this is indicative of monopoly power among pharmaceutical companies. Second is the concern that the drugs manufactured and marketed by this for-profit industry should be safe.

---

[1]Drug and medical sundry expenditures include expenditures for both prescription and nonprescription drugs. Approximately 56 percent of drug and medical sundry expenditures are for prescription drugs. See the footnote to Table 17-2.

TABLE 17-2. Personal Expenditures on Drugs and Personal Health
Care Expenditures, 1950–1985 (Billions of Dollars)

Year	Personal Health Care Expenditures	Drug and Medical Sundries[a]	Drug Expenditures as a Percentage of Personal Health Care Expenditures
1950	$ 10.9	$ 1.7	15.9
1960	23.7	3.7	15.4
1965	35.8	5.2	14.5
1970	65.1	8.0	12.6
1975	116.8	11.9	10.1
1980	217.9	19.2	8.8
1985	371.4	28.5	7.7

SOURCES: Robert Gibson and Daniel Waldo, "National Health Care Expenditures,
1980," *Health Care Financing Review*, 3, September 1981: 20–31; Daniel R. Waldo,
Katherine R. Levitt, and Helen Lazenby, "National Health Expenditures, 1985,"
Health Care Financing Review, 8, Fall 1986: 14, Table 2.

[a]Includes spending for prescription drugs, over-the-counter drugs, and medical sundries dispensed through retail channels. Expenditures for drugs purchased or dispensed by hospitals, nursing homes, other institutions, physicians, and dentists are excluded. About 57 percent of all dollars for drugs and medical sundries are spent for prescription drugs alone, and another 31 percent are spent for over-the-counter drugs. Whether prescription expenditures as a percentage of personal health care expenditures parallel the trend exhibited by drug and medical sundries as a percentage of personal health care expenditures was examined by studying the annual survey of prescription sales published by the *American Druggist*. The *American Druggist* estimates for dollar volume of retail prescription sales should approximate the total consumer expenditures for prescriptions. The *American Druggist* estimates show that the dollar volume of prescription sales is a declining percentage of personal health care expenditures, over the period 1955–1979. It declined from 8.21 percent in 1955 to 7.74 percent in 1965, to 5.22 percent in 1975, to finally 4.75 percent in 1979. It appears then that, in relation to personal health care expenditures, drug and medical sundries and prescription expenditures do behave similarly.

The issue of drug safety and efficacy have been dealt with in the Food, Drug and Cosmetic Act of 1938 and in the 1962 Kefauver-Harris amendments to that act. In the second half of this chapter, the federal regulations to improve drug safety and efficacy and their effect on the industry's rate of drug innovation are analyzed. The first part of this chapter is devoted to an analysis of the economic performance of the industry. Public policies that have been proposed to improve the industry's performance will also be evaluated. Policies to change the economic performance of the industry, such as curtailing promotional expenditures, reducing prices, and lowering the rate of profits, also affect the industry's rate of drug innovation. For purposes of analysis, however, each of these effects on drug innovation will be discussed separately.

THE ECONOMIC PERFORMANCE OF THE PHARMACEUTICAL INDUSTRY

Critics of the pharmaceutical industry have been concerned by what they perceive as monopoly power and its attendant abuses. They cite many examples of these abuses: the continuous high rates of profit, the extraordinary large and wasteful amounts that

TABLE 17-3. Selected Average Consumer Price Indices,
Calendar Years 1950–1985

Year	Medical Care	Prescription Drugs	Hospital (Semiprivate Room)	Physicians' Services
1950	53.7	92.6	30.3	55.2
1955	64.8	101.6	42.3	65.4
1960	79.1	115.3	57.3	77.0
1965	89.5	102.0	75.9	88.3
1970	120.6	101.2	145.4	121.4
1975	168.6	109.3	236.1	169.4
1980	265.9	154.8	418.9	269.3
1985	403.1	256.5	710.5	398.8

SOURCES: Two sources were used. Data for 1950–1970 came from U.S. Department of Labor, Bureau of Labor Statistics, *Handbook of Labor Statistics, 1975—Reference Edition* (Washington, D.C.: U.S. Government Printing Office, 1975), pp. 326–336; data for 1970–1985 came from U.S. Department of Labor, Bureau of Labor Statistics, *Consumer Price Index Detailed Report*, various years. Also Bureau of the Census, *Statistical Abstracts of the United States, 1986* (Washington, D.C.: U.S. Department of Commerce, 1986), p. 478.

are spent on detailing and other promotional expenses, the high prices at which drugs are sold in relation to their costs of production, and the existence of price discrimination, as evidenced by the fact that the same drugs are sold for less to large purchasers, such as hospitals, than they are to retailers, and that brand name drugs sell for so much more than generic drugs. These measures of inadequate industry performance are believed to be a result of a highly concentrated industry, caused by high entry barriers, and consequently little competition among its members.

If an industry were competitive, profits would be normal, similar to what is earned in other industries, and there would be a greater degree of price competition: price discrimination would also therefore be less likely. High promotion expenditures would not be necessary, as firms competed more on price.

Thus critics of the pharmaceutical industry and earlier economic studies have viewed the industry from a traditional perspective. They concluded that high profits, prices, and promotion expenditures could exist only in an industry characterized by monopoly power. With an emphasis on these aspects of monopoly power, they proposed policies that would change both the structure of the industry and the behavior of firms in the industry. For example, decreasing the effective life of patents would lessen one source of monopoly power. Having the federal government reimburse for drug prescriptions according to the price of generic drugs only (the maximum allowable cost regulations) would result in a lowering of drug prices. Contrasting the performance of the pharmaceutical industry to that of a theoretically competitive industry led the critics of this industry to propose wide-ranging policies to change what they perceived as an inadequate performance.

This traditional or static view of the pharmaceutical industry has come under sharp attack for two reasons. First, emphasizing the more visible monopoly abuses neglects the tremendous beneficial impact that product innovation has had, not only on society, but also on industry competition. A more dynamic analysis of the drug industry, based on the competitive effects of product innovation, suggests an entirely different picture of the industry's performance. Second, economists have recently begun to question whether the indicators of monopoly power are in fact accurate. It has been suggested that industry profits are greatly overstated using traditional accounting methods, that there is in fact a great deal of price competition, and that high promotion and selling expenses serve important economic functions, such as providing physicians with information and as an important means by which firms enter new markets, rather than being a barrier to entry.

The "dynamic competition" view of the pharmaceutical industry reaches quite opposite conclusions on the industry's performance. Further, when the policy prescriptions of the traditionalists are examined in this new light, the impacts of their proposals are seen to be quite harmful in terms of their effects on product innovation and competition.

In analyzing the drug industry, the structure of the industry is examined first. Examples of structure are the conditions of entry into the various therapeutic markets and the importance of economies of scale in determining firm size. Structural characteristics determine the number of competing firms, given the size of the market. This information is usually summed up in the measure referred to as the *concentration ratio*, which is the percentage of the industry's sales accounted for by the four (or eight) largest firms.

After industry structure, the pharmaceutical firm's behavior is examined. Examples of firm behavior are the degree of price competition, product promotion, and product competition. Last, we attempt to evaluate the industry's performance.

While viewing the drug industry within this traditional framework, the importance of dynamic competition, as manifested through product competition, is examined in terms of how it influences the industry's structure, conduct, and performance. Within this context, the accuracy of profitability, which has been the basis of much of the criticism of the pharmaceutical industry, will also be discussed.

Characteristics of the Drug Industry

When economists examine the structure of an industry, the concentration ratio is used as an indication of monopoly power. The concentration ratio is the percentage of total industry sales provided by a small number of firms. Thus a four-firm concentration ratio indicates the percentage of total sales supplied by the four largest firms. If this concentration ratio is high, it is often assumed that these firms have monopoly power; that is, the fewer the number of firms there are, the easier it is for these firms to collude in the setting of prices. A low concentration ratio suggests that the market shares of firms are generally small and that there is more competition among firms. Scherer claims that "when the leading four firms control 40 percent or more of the total market, it is fair to assume that oligopoly is beginning to rear its head" (1).

The determinants of the concentration ratio depend on how easy it is to enter that industry. The greater the barriers to entry, the higher the concentration ratio. Entry barriers may differ by industry; some may involve control over the resources used in production, such as was the case with bauxite, which is used in the production of aluminum. The more typical entry barrier is economies of scale in production. In the drug industry it has been suggested that patents are the prime barrier to entering a therapeutic market. Other barriers that have been mentioned are economies of scale in research and development and high promotion expenditures, which are used to differentiate a brand name drug in the minds of physicians.

There are approximately 1,000 drug firms in this country. The four-firm concentration ratio in the pharmaceutical industry (as of 1973) was 27.8 percent. This is certainly lower than for automobiles, which is 99 percent; cigarettes, 84 percent; and soaps and detergents, 62 percent (2). Further, no one firm accounts for more than 8 percent of total drug sales in the United States. (3). However, it is not appropriate to look at the concentration ratio with respect to total drug sales because there are many separate markets within the overall drug industry in which firms either cannot or do not compete. The question, then, is what is the relevant market over which concentration ratios should be calculated? One analyst has observed that one should not

ignore the fact that the overall drug market is fragmented into a number of separate, noncompeting therapeutic markets; antibiotics are not substitutes for antidiabetic drugs, and tranquilizers are not substitutes for vitamins. Manufacturers do not compete on an industrywide basis, and hence concentration must be evaluated within the various therapeutic groups of drugs in which competition does occur (4).

A more general definition of markets has been proposed by Stigler:

An industry should embrace the maximum geographical area and the maximum variety of productive activities in which there is a strong long-run substitution. If buyers can shift on a large scale from product or area B to A, then the two should be combined. If producers can shift on a large scale from B to A, again they should be combined.
Economists usually state this in an alternative form: All products or enterprises with large long-run cross-elasticities of either supply or demand should be combined into a single industry (5).

Thus even though therapeutic markets appear to be a more relevant definition than overall industry sales, there is still the problem of which are the relevant therapeutic markets. For example, one investigator, Vernon, classified drugs into 19 therapeutic markets after consulting with various marketing people in the drug industry (6). The criteria used for categorizing drugs was the degree of demand side substitutability between different drugs. In another study, Hornbrook classified drugs into 69 therapeutic markets. The criteria used by Hornbrook was whether the drugs produced essentially the same therapeutic effects; if so, they were then classified into the same therapeutic market (7). In still another study the investigators developed their definition of therapeutic markets by evaluating physicians' prescribing habits (8). This study resulted in only 10 economic markets.

Each of the studies cited above is based on demand-side substitutability. None fulfill the supply-side criterion suggested by Stigler, namely, if a producer in market A can shift on a large scale to producing product B, both should be combined into a single market. Thus if a firm is currently producing antibiotics and it can quickly shift and produce antiarthritics, they should then be included in a single market definition. Supply-side substitution is more difficult for researchers to determine than demand-

TABLE 17-4. Concentration of Sales in the U.S. Ethical
Drug Industry, by Therapeutic Markets, 1968

Therapeutic Market	Four-Firm Ratio
Anesthetics	69
Antiarthritics	95
Antibiotics–penicillin	55
Antispasmodics	59
Ataractics	79
Bronchial dilators	61
Cardiovascular hypotensives	79
Coronary–peripheral vasodilators	70
Diabetic therapy	93
Diuretics	64
Enzymes–digestants	46
Hematinic preparations	52
Sex hormones	67
Corticoids	55
Muscle relaxants	59
Psychostimulants	78
Sulfonamides	79
Thyroid therapy	69
Unweighted average	68

Source: John M. Vernon, "Concentration, Promotion and Market Share Stability in Pharmaceutical Industry," *Journal of Industrial Economics* 19 (July 1971): 246–266. Reprinted with permission by Basil Blackwell Publisher, Ltd.

side substitution. The supply-side definition would be likely to result in lower concentration ratios than a market definition based on demand-side substitution alone.

Using Vernon's classification of therapeutic markets, as shown in Table 17-4, the four-firm concentration ratio is quite high. The lowest four-firm concentration ratio in a therapeutic market was 46 percent. There are several in the 90 percent range, and the unweighted average was 68 percent. These concentration ratios indicate a high degree of market concentration by a few firms.

If we were to rely on the traditional method of analyzing monopoly power in an industry, namely high concentration ratios, we would conclude that drug firms possess a high degree of monopoly power in various therapeutic markets. This conclusion, however, has been disputed by a number of economists. Concentration ratios are a "static" measure of market power. While particular therapeutic markets may have high concentration ratios at a given point in time, there is a high rate of turnover in market shares. Instability in market shares is a result of intense competition among firms through new product innovation and is indicative of "dynamic" competition. Unless this dynamic aspect of competition among drug firms is analyzed, the use of static concentration ratios provides a misleading impression of monopoly power over time.

An investigation of the instability of market shares among 20 different industries (in the early 1970s) was undertaken using an index of market instability. Of the 20 different industries examined, only the petroleum industry had a higher index of market instability than the drug industry (9).

Another indication of the degree of product competition in the drug industry and its effect on market shares was a study of entry and exit in different therapeutic markets. Seventeen therapeutic markets were studied over the period 1963–1972. In 15 of the 17 markets there were more than five new entrants. The market shares of new entrants exceeded 10 percent and in some cases went as high as 33 and 43 percent. Exit from the industry also occurred in 16 of the 17 therapeutic markets (10).

Although concentration ratios in the various therapeutic markets are high, it is necessary to examine changes in market shares over time to better understand the degree of competition in the drug industry. As evidenced by the turnover of leading firms and the instability of market shares, these findings suggest that monopoly power is eroded over time. It is through new product development that firms compete in various therapeutic markets.

New Product Competition

Patents provide a firm with protection against competitive suppliers providing the identical compound. Since a large proportion of prescription drugs, more than two-thirds, have patent protection, entry into specific therapeutic markets requires some kind of chemical product differentiation (11). However, the importance of patent protection for achieving monopoly power in a therapeutic market can be overstated. The various therapeutic markets are not monopolized by single drugs. It is through the development of both major and minor chemical modifications and new dosage forms that firms enter markets and compete.

Critics of the drug industry claim that much of the product differentiation are for minor modifications that provide little social value and that large promotional expenditures are used to establish brand name loyalty among physicians. Further, most of the product innovations were derived from discoveries at universities and in nonindustrial settings. The drug industry, of course, disputes these criticisms. How important are the products produced by the drug industry?

Several studies have attempted to assess the relative importance of the drug industry to other institutions and organizations in their contribution to new drug discoveries. In one study, Schnee determined which drugs were important drug discoveries over different periods by using data on significant drug discoveries prior to 1963 from a study conducted by the Commission on Cost of Medical Care of the American Medical Association. The commission determined significant drug discoveries by asking "400 physicians and pharmacologists to select the most important advances from a preselected list of eighty-nine drugs introduced after 1934. His selection of important drug introductions in the 1963–1970 period was largely based on a survey by *The Medical Letter* of 170 physicians at medical schools" (12). Schnee found that the share of important drugs discovered by the drug industry has been increasing over time. As shown in Table 17–5, the drug industry's share has increased from more than 50 percent in the period 1935–1949, to 69 percent between 1950 and 1962, and to 82 percent between 1963 and 1970. The drug industry, according to Schnee, had always been an important source of drug discoveries and is now the prime source in the development of significant new chemical entities.

Another study, with similar results, was undertaken by the Food and Drug Administration (FDA) in 1974. The FDA determined those drugs introduced in the periods 1950–1962 and 1963–1970 that in its opinion represented important gains in medicine.

TABLE 17-5. Schnee's Distribution of Drug Discoveries,1935–1970

Source	1935–1949	1950–1962	1963–1970
Industry	52	69	82
Universities, hospitals, or research institutions	34	16	9
Other	14	15	9
Total	100	100	100

Source: Based on Jerome Schnee, "The Changing Pattern of Pharmaceutical Innovation and Discovery," mimeographed (New York: Columbia University, Graduate School of Business, 1973). This table was reprinted with permission from David Schwartzman, *Innovation in the Pharmaceutical Industry* (Baltimore, Md.: The Johns Hopkins University Press, 1976), p. 77.

As shown in Table 17-6, the distribution of those new drugs attributed to development by the drug industry was 69 percent and 82 percent, respectively, for the two periods studied (13).

A more recent study confirms the findings of the earlier studies and concludes that the pharmaceutical industry is the source of an even greater percentage of new chemical entities. Between 1970 and 1978, Grabowski and Vernon attribute 93 percent of new chemical entities to the pharmaceutical industry (14).

All product innovation and competition are not the result of significant medical discoveries. However, as a source of new drug discoveries, the drug industry has played a leading role in the past, and in recent years its role has increased to the point where it is the major source for such drug discoveries. Different studies, using different definitions of major drug discoveries, reach similar conclusions. In addition to major drug discoveries, minor modifications and different dosage forms can have important social and economic advantages. For example, "the modification of an injectable drug to permit oral self-administration is an economic advance, if not a major medical advance" (15).

Expenditures on Research and Development

An indication of the importance of product competition to the drug industry is its expenditures on research and development. The drug industry spends approximately

TABLE 17-6. Percentage Distribution of Discoveries of Important New Drugs Introduced in 1950–1962 and 1963–1970, Selected by FDA

Source	1950–1962	1963–1970
Drug Industry	69	82
Other	31	18
Total	100	100

Source: Commissioner Schmidt's statement to the Subcommittee on Health of the Senate Committee on Labor and Public Welfare, August 16, 1974, appearing in August 26, 1974, FDC Reports. Discoveries assigned by Paul de Haen, *Nonproprietary Name Index*, and the *Merck Index*. This table was reprinted with permission from David Schwartzman, *Innovation in the Pharmaceutical Industry* (Baltimore, Md.: The Johns Hopkins University Press, 1976), p. 79.

15.0 percent of its sales on research and development. This percentage has varied between 10.5 and 15.0 percent since 1965. These expenditures were approximately $4.1 billion dollars in 1985. The drug industry's research and development expenditures, at 15 percent of sales, is exceeded by only two other industries, information processing and semiconductors (16). Approximately 70 percent of drug research and development is funded by the drug companies themselves, 10 percent by universities (often in conjunction with leading drug companies), and 20 percent by the government and other sources (17).

It has been suggested that research and development expenditures serve as a barrier to entry into various therapeutic markets. If there are large economies of scale in research and development, product competition will only occur among the same large firms. However, several studies have concluded that research and development as a percent of sales was similar for different-sized firms in the period before 1962. With respect to the output of research and development expenditures, i.e., product innovation, it was also determined that small firms were not at a disadvantage. In fact, the "firms that contributed the most innovations, relative to their size, were not the largest firms but somewhat smaller ones" (18).

These findings with respect to expenditures on research and development and product innovation changed when data from the post-1962 period were examined. Schwartzman found that in the period 1965–1970 larger firms spent a larger portion of their sales on research and development than did smaller firms. Similarly, larger firms had an advantage over smaller firms in terms of the number of product innovations produced (19). These findings are reinforced by another study.

Grabowski and Vernon examined production of innovations in three different periods, 1957–1961, 1962–1966, and 1967–1971. The number of firms having a new chemical entity declined in each of these three periods from 51, 34, and 23 firms, respectively. Also the four largest firms in terms of sales have increased their output of new chemical entities, from 24 and 25 percent in the first two periods to 48.7 percent of innovational output in the 1967–1971 period. It would thus appear that innovational output is becoming more concentrated in the largest drug firms (20).

These findings, which indicate economies of scale in the post-1962 period, suggest that the 1962 FDA Amendments (which are discussed more fully later) may have provided an advantage to larger firms. The time and resources required for developing and testing new products as a result of the FDA Amendments have been increased (21).

Promotional Expenditures

The role of promotional expenditures is controversial. Its critics believe it to be wasteful, as a means of providing physicians with information, a relatively inefficient mechanism with its reliance on detail men and heavy journal advertising. Many people oppose large advertising expenditures, not only in the drug industry but also for automobiles, breakfast cereals, and other products; they believe that advertising is misleading and that it attempts to manipulate consumers into choosing products they do not need.

In perfectly competitive markets advertising is viewed as unnecessary, since buyers have perfect information and products are homogeneous. In oligopolistic markets, advertising expenditures are viewed as a means by which the competing firms avoid price competition. Advertising is used to differentiate the firm's products. Again, persons opposed to advertising consider it wasteful, if not misleading, in these uses as well. Traditionally, advertising within the drug industry has been analyzed within a similar context. Within therapeutic markets, products have been considered to be relatively homogeneous, and large promotional expenditures are seen as an attempt by the firm to create product differentiation and brand loyalties in the minds of physicians.

In recent years, drug industry promotional expenditures have undergone a reevaluation. Promotional expenditures are seen as serving two important purposes: information and as a means of achieving entry for new product innovations (22).

When prescribing, physicians should be aware of which drugs are most appropriate for treatment, the correct dosages, the appropriate dosage form, and the effects of such patient characteristics as weight, age, other drugs being taken, the patient's health condition, and the price to the patient of the drug. Learning about all the possible drugs that might be used for all the physicians' patients is a formidable task. There are many thousands of drugs available to choose from. New drugs, modifications, and changes in dosage are constantly coming on the market. There are a number of ways that physicians may stay informed: medical journals, *The Medical Letter*, and books such as the *Physician's Desk Reference*. To stay abreast of the literature is very time consuming for a physician.

Based on several studies, it appears that marketing efforts by drug firms play an important role in keeping physicians informed. One study, published in 1982, surveyed physicians in the Boston area and concluded that a majority of the practitioners received their information from advertisements and detail men (23). A previous survey of physicians also found that physicians regarded detail men as either a very good or fairly good source of information (24); further, it was found that 60 percent of the reporting physicians believed the information provided by the detail men was sufficiently valuable as to warrant seeing all the detail men who tried to make appointments with them.

Promotion by itself does not guarantee success for a new drug. Physicians are apparently able to distinguish among claims for various drugs. Schwartzman cites the case when a number of drugs were heavily promoted and yet their sales turned out to be less than their promotion costs. These were new drugs that were ranked by the FDA as having little or no therapeutic gain over existing drugs (25). Similarly, drugs that were rapidly accepted as a result of strong promotion efforts were of significant benefit compared to alternative available. In fact, it has been estimated that at times too little has been spent on promotional activities. Peltzman examined the consequences of failure by physicians to adopt drugs due to a lack of information. When certain innovations in drug therapies occur, there is a benefit to society if physicians are sufficiently knowledgeable to prescribe such drugs as soon as possible. He cites the case of tuberculosis (TB), estimating that if the use of TB drugs had spread as rapidly as the Salk vaccine, 80,600 lives would have been saved. Similarly, if major tranquilizers had been more heavily promoted, this might have resulted in a savings of 645 million patient days in the hospital (26).

Drug industry promotion may not be the ideal way of disseminating information to physicians. Physicians differ on what sources they rely on for information. Patients who go to physicians who keep up with developments in drug therapies through the medical literature bear the cost of heavy drug promotion that attempts to reach other physicians who rely on the drug companies for their information. There is, unfortunately, no way of lowering the price of drugs to the patients of physicians who do not rely on drug company promotion (27). If drug promotion expenditures are to be reduced in the future, there must be changes in the incentives and/or costs to physicians for relying on other sources of information on drugs.

In addition to providing information, promotional expenditures enable firms to enter new markets. Contrary to the previous belief that promotional expenditures served as a barrier to entry, more recent studies have concluded the opposite. Telser studied drug entry in 17 therapeutic markets over the period 1962–1972 in order to determine whether promotional expenditures deter or facilitate entry into the market for new drugs. Entry in a market was measured by the percentage of sales in a market as of 1972 for a drug which did not have any sales in that market previously. Using multivariate analysis, Telser found a positive relationship between promotional expenditures and entry. He therefore concluded that promotional expenditures facilitate entry, without which new products would be unable to compete with existing drugs (28). In another study, Hornbrook found similar results and concluded that "promotion has a procompetitive effect, other things being the same, in that it acts as a means of entry—a market penetration tool—more effectively, on balance, than as a barrier to entry" (29).

What would be the possible savings to consumers if all promotional expenditures were eliminated? Schwartzman estimates that if all promotional expenditures were eliminated, the amount of the savings that would eventually be passed on to consumers would represent approximately 5 percent of their drug bill (30). This potential savings, however, must be offset by a cost to physicians (and most likely shifted to their patients) of the costs to replace the information previously provided by the drug companies. Another cost would be a delay in introducing new products into highly concentrated markets. Product competition would undoubtedly decline as the marketing of new products becomes more difficult without promotional expenditures. Both nominal and quality-adjusted prices would remain high with less product competition. The slower dissemination of new drug innovations also results in a cost to patients: the forgone benefits they may have received had they had earlier access to a new, more beneficial drug.

Price Competition

It has been commonly believed that there is no price competition among drug companies. The reasons for this belief are, first, that patents provide a firm with monopoly power, hence protection against close substitutes. Second, physicians do not pay for the drug and are therefore less sensitive to drug prices. Physicians also prescribe by brand name, thereby limiting the patient's choice. Further, there are legal restrictions (i.e., antisubstitution laws) that limit competition in those cases when close substitutes may exist. And finally, given the high degree of concentration in therapeutic markets, it is easier for drug firms to collude on pricing policies. Their desire for wanting to maintain high drug prices is that the price elasticity of demand for drugs is low. Thus if a firm were to engage in price competition and the other firms were to follow, total sales revenue in that market would fall.

The evidence offered in support of this lack of price competition is that drugs are sold at prices much higher than their marginal costs of production. Second, based on a study over the period 1949–1959, Markham observed a great deal of price inflexibility.

Of the 308 drugs examined, more than 50 percent did not change their price over this period (31). If prices were competitively set, they would change in response to changing demand and cost conditions. Also, price discrimination appears to exist in the pricing of drugs; prices are higher in retail markets than for hospitals, and prices differ in domestic and international markets.

To understand the degree of price competition in the drug industry, it is again necessary to view it within a dynamic framework. At a given point in time, prices are "high" in relation to their marginal costs. However, over time different forms of price competition emerge. Close substitutes enter markets, not protected by patents, and prices begin to decline. In other cases, improvements occur in competing drugs that sell for similar prices as existing drugs; hence their quality-adjusted prices decline. Over time both the number and closeness of substitutes within a therapeutic market increase. As this occurs, the price elasticity of demand for each of the drugs increases, and prices begin to decline. There is thus a life cycle to therapeutic markets.

Drugs that are considered to be major innovations (i.e., to have large therapeutic gains and not having any close substitutes), can obtain a high market share despite a high relative price. However, drugs that are considered to be minor innovations are more likely to be introduced at low prices relative to other drugs in that market. Such pricing strategies are consistent with pricing according to the perceived elasticity of demand for that drug. The closer the substitutes (the case of a minor innovation), the greater the price elasticity of demand, hence the lower the price to obtain a share of the market.

Multiple-source drugs, which are generic type drugs supplied by several manufacturers under their own brand names, comprise more than 44 percent of total prescriptions (32). Once a patent has expired, entry into that market is relatively easy. FDA approval is required before a new drug can be marketed. But if the drug is a duplicate of an existing drug, FDA approval is more easily acquired. Under the Drug Price Competition and Patent Restoration Act of 1984, generic drug manufacturers are no longer required to present data showing that a generic version of a drug is safe and effective. Instead, generic versions can now be approved by the FDA on the basis of data showing that the particular generic drug is "bioequivalent" or therapeutically identical to the original brand name drug that has already been approved by the FDA. By speeding up the approval process for generic drugs, there should be a large increase in competitive drugs for those drugs facing patent expiration. (Previously, generic drugs were treated as "new" drugs. Generic drug manufacturers were required to conduct the full range of safety and efficacy tests required for approval of a completely new chemical entity.)

For a new entrant to gain a share of a market, with a similar type of product, it usually lowers price. Even though price cutting will have an adverse impact on profits, it may be the only way for a new multiple-source drug to gain a share of the market. Given the low price elasticity of demand for drugs, the total number of drugs sold in the market is unlikely to change as a result of lower prices. Changes in market sales will be at the expense of existing firms. The pattern appears to be that as more duplicate drugs are offered in a market, the later entrants reduce their prices much more than the earlier entrants; eventually, the original drug manufacturer and others must match these price reductions at least in part.

Demand elasticity also increases over time. In markets where price exceeds marginal cost, there is an incentive for firms to enter. As more and closer substitutes enter a market, the price elasticity of demand of the original firms increases and prices are eventually reduced. For example, with respect to tetracycline, there were five major manufacturers. Lederle, which had an 85 percent share of the market in 1962, declined to 72 percent in 1964, at which time Squibb started sharply reducing its prices, from $15.00 to $3.98. Squibb's market share increased over the next several years. One of the major losers was Lederle, which did not respond to price cutting; its market share declined from 72 percent to 33 percent before it finally started to compete on price (33).

Evidence of greater price elasticity over time is also provided by data on overall drug price trends. Drug prices have declined even though there has been inflation in the general economy as measured by the rise in the Consumer Price Index. Thus the "real" price of drugs has declined even faster than their nominal prices.

Still another approach that has been used to indicate price competition in different therapeutic markets is to adjust drug prices by a quality measure. When the prices of different drugs are compared, it is usually assumed that the brands are of equal quality. If the newer drug is improved compared to existing drugs, and it is sold for a similar price, the actual price (i.e., the nominal price divided by quality), has actually declined. Just looking at nominal prices therefore can be misleading.

To understand the reason behind drug manufacturers' willingness to engage in price competition, it becomes necessary to reexamine our beliefs as to the prescribing habits of physicians and the role of pharmacists. Apparently, drug manufacturers assume that at least some physicians are price conscious when they prescribe for their patients and that some pharmacists are willing to act as the patient's agent. This behavior among physicians and pharmacists will serve to increase price competition among drug firms. "Pharmacists will use a low-priced drug rather than the original brand to fill a generic prescription. This is not universally true, but the proportion of generic prescriptions filled with low-priced drugs is much higher than the proportion of prescriptions that specify a brand accounted for by the low-priced brands. Substitution occurs. The pharmacist, in effect, acts as a price agent for the consumer" (34).

A recent study finds that although there are savings as a result of generic drugs, these savings are not always passed on to the consumer. The cost per pill to pharmacies is always less for generics and, on average, its price is less than for the brand name drug. (The median price per pill to the consumer was higher for the brand name than for the generic version in 18 of the 21 pairs of drugs studied.) However, given the lack of consumer price information and the time to shop, wide variations exist in the prices of drugs (35). Thus pharmacies may also benefit from the price competition of generics.

Also, antisubstitution laws are not as great an inhibiter of price competition as is believed:

> Before it was legal to do so, pharmacists did substitute; and frequently they did so without asking permission from the prescriber. For example, there was brand substitution in 33 percent of all ampicillin prescriptions, and the pharmacists did not obtain permission to make such substitutions in 82 percent of these cases; they were doing so illegally. When they are substituted, they tended to substitute a low-priced brand for the prescribed brand. Again they were acting as a price agent. (36)

These findings suggest much more price flexibility and competition than previously believed. It is possible to reconcile the foregoing evidence on price competition with the earlier evidence on price inflexibility cited by Markham through the findings that there is a difference in the manufacturer's posted prices and the price at which transactions occur. Apparently, Markham was observing posted prices rather than "real" prices.

Patented drugs and major innovations provide greater monopoly power in pricing a drug. Uniqueness in the short run, however, gives way to imitations and a greater number of substitutes over time. As price elasticity increases, there is greater price competition. "Historically, no leading product has maintained its market share position for more than a limited number of years. Preeminence is temporary" (37).

Profitability in the Pharmaceutical Industry

One of the criticisms of the drug industry is the high rate of profits that are made as a result of other people's illnesses, many of whom are of low incomes. Most critics will acknowledge that a normal rate of return is appropriate so as to enable the industry to continue to supply drugs and to provide for an incentive for research. However, published data on profitability of the drug industry, compared to other industries, show that drug companies receive an "excessive" rate of return. The average rate of return on equity for all manufacturing companies over the period 1958–1975 was 11.1 percent. For drug companies it was 18.1 percent (38). Since these "excessive" profits have continued over a large number of years, it is used as evidence of the drug companies' monopoly power.

Recently, economists have reexamined the rate of profit received by drug companies. The conclusion of many of these studies is that published profit data are seriously in error and that they *overstate* the true rate of profit earned by drug companies. When corrections are made to the published data, the rate of return earned by drug companies are approximately comparable to rates of return earned in other industries. It has been further said that since the passage of the 1962 FDA Amendments the true rate of return to drug firms has been falling.

To the extent that these new findings on drug industry profitability are correct, there are important public policy implications: Previous estimates of the relatively high rate of return to drug firms have been the impetus for policies to lower prices, require the cross-licensing of patents, and reduce the patent life of new drugs. If implemented, each of these policies would decrease drug industry profitability. If drug firm profitability has not been excessive, policies to decrease profitability in this industry further would cause the rate of return to be below that earned in other industries; with a lower return on investment, there would be a consequent decline in research and development, hence drug innovation would fall.

The finding that drug industry profitability is relatively normal also suggests that there are no strong barriers to entry into various drug markets; although firms might have temporary monopoly power, it is eroded over time.

To understand this change in perception of drug industry profitability, it is necessary to examine how profits are calculated and to discuss some of the determinants of industry profitability.

The manner in which accountants calculate profitability (R_{acc}) is to subtract all expenses (E) from sales revenue (S) and divide this by the firm's capital or the stockholders' equity (C).

$$R_{acc} = \frac{(S - E)}{C}$$

Net income $(S - E)$ is the income remaining after all expenses and taxes have been paid. This accountant's definition of profitability is the method used to compare profitability between different industries. According to the definition above, advertising, research and development, and promotional expenses are all treated as current expenses; they are deducted from sales revenue in the year they are incurred. Economists have argued that these expenditures are more than current expenses. They are, in fact, intangible capital, since their effect continues beyond the year in which they are incurred. For example, research and development expenditures might not yield any benefit in the current year; but if a successful drug is developed, benefits will accrue in future years. It takes a number of years before a successful drug is finally marketed. The testing process to receive FDA approval alone may take a few years. These expenditures are incurred so as to receive future benefits. A similar case can be made for advertising and promotional expenditures; their effects are longer lasting than for the year in which they were made. Because the foregoing types of expenditures provide future benefits, their economic life is greater than one year. They are a form of intangible capital of the firm and should therefore be depreciated rather than expensed all at once.

In accordance with conservative accounting principles, such expenditures are expensed since there is uncertainty as to the future benefits they may provide and over how many years such future revenues may accrue. Therefore the most conservative approach is to assume that there are no benefits in future periods from these expenditures.

If the economists' definition of profitability (R_{acc}) were to be used, and these expenditures were treated as intangible assets (A), then a certain portion of these assets should be depreciated (D) each year (i.e., treated as an expense). The remainder, that is, the undepreciated portion of the asset, should then be added to the firm's capital investment. Thus the economists' definition of profitability would be stated as follows:

$$R_{econ} = \frac{(S - E - D)}{C + (A - D)}$$

The effect of this change in the treatment of advertising, research and development, and promotional expenditures is to cause net income to be greater than it would otherwise be, since only a part of the expenditure is deducted from sales revenue rather than the entire amount. However, the capital base of the firm is increased by the amount of the undepreciated asset.

Each year new expenditures are incurred for research and development, advertising, and promotion. At the same time, previous year's expenditures are being depreciated. To see why failure to capitalize these expenditures leads to an overstatement of profitability, one has merely to think of a situation when the amount being depreciated in a given year is equal to that year's expenditures on intangible capital. Under the accountants' definition of profitability (R_{acc}) the capital base is smaller than under the economists' definition of profitability (R_{econ}); the economist includes the undepreciated asset as part of capital while the accountant does not. Therefore the accountants' definition will show a higher rate of profitability than would the economists'.

In accordance with generally accepted accounting principles, the accountants' definition of profitability is used by all industries. The pharmaceutical industry, however, is more affected by this definition of profit than any other industry. As a percentage of sales, expenditures for advertising, promotion, and research and development are greater in the drug industry than for any other industry. For example, the pharmaceutical industry spent 5.3 percent of its sales for research and development during the period 1961–1971. For other industries such as food, the comparable percentage was .4 percent. (For 1985, the respective figures are 15 percent for pharmaceuticals and 3 percent for other industries.) With respect to advertising, no other industry had as high a percent of sales as did the drug firms, which were 3.7 percent over the period 1949–1971 and 15 percent in 1985. Companies that were relatively high on research and development (as a percentage of sales) were generally low on advertising expenditures (as a percentage of sales), although the pharmaceutical industry was highest in both categories (39).

How large an overstatement of accounting profitability is caused by a failure to include these expenditures as intangible capital depends upon several factors: which expenditures should be considered as current versus capital outlays, the depreciation schedule for each category of expenditure, and how rapidly the capital base of the firm is growing over time. As the economic life of intangible capital increases, the effect is a decrease in the rate of return to the industry (40).

Several studies have estimated "corrected" rates of return to the drug industry using the economists' definition of profitability. The differences between the corrected and uncorrected rates of return are striking. The accounting rate of return for the drug industry in the late 1960s was estimated at greater than 18 percent a year. The economic rates of return for those same years was less than 12 percent. Over the 10-year period, 1965–1974, the average rate of return, using the accounting definition, was 17.2 percent; the estimated economic rate of return for that same period was 11.1 percent (41).

When similar corrections for intangible capital are made to rates of return in other industries, it can be observed that while the rate of return is still higher for the drug industry, they are much closer to those of other industries. These data are shown in Table 17–7.

There are a number of other factors that have been suggested as the reasons for the remaining differences in the rates of return between the drug industry and other industries. One reason to expect higher rates of return in the drug industry is that they have faced a continual rising demand for their products. Drug sales have risen at a faster rate than many other industries. Since the 1950s, drug sales have increased more than twice as fast the gross national product. Growth in overseas sales has also been increasing at more than twice the rate of sales in this country (42). Some of the reasons for the high rate of growth in sales, in addition to the therapeutic benefits of new drugs, has been changes in payment mechanisms, such as Medicare, Medicaid, and the growth of health insurance. Changes in the demographic composition of the population, such as the increasing portion that is aged, has led to increased demands for medical care and consequently an increase in the demand for drugs.

Another reason for increased returns in the drug industry is the greater risks in returns. In competitive markets the rate of return would move toward the opportunity cost of capital adjusted for risk. Those industries with less predictable returns on their investment would require a greater risk premium to attract investors. The uncertainty of returns to research and development expenditures contains an element of risk that is perhaps greater than in other industries.

Several studies have attempted to empirically estimate the effect on drug industry profitability of higher-than-average growth in sales and a premium for greater risk.

TABLE 17-7. Average Accounting and Corrected Rates of Return on Net Worth, 1959–1973 (Percentages)

Industry	Accounting Rates of Return	Corrected Rates of Return	Difference
Pharmaceuticals	18.3	12.9	−5.4
Electrical machinery	13.3	10.1	−3.2
Foods	11.8	10.6	−1.2
Petroleum	11.2	10.8	−0.4
Chemicals	10.6	9.1	−1.5
Paper	10.5	10.1	−0.4
Office machinery	10.5	9.9	−0.6
Motor vehicles	10.5	9.2	−1.3
Rubber products	10.1	8.7	−1.4
Aerospace	9.2	7.4	−1.8
Ferrous metals	7.6	7.3	−0.3
Average	11.2	9.6	−1.6
Variance	7.5	2.5	

Source: Kenneth W. Clarkson, *Intangible Capital and Rates of Return* (Washington, D.C.: American Enterprise Institute, 1977), p. 64. Reprinted by permission from *Issues in Pharmaceutical Economics*, edited by Robert I. Chien. Lexington, Mass.: Lexington Books, D.C. Heath and Company, Copyright 1979, D.C. Heath and Company.

These studies suggest that drug industry rates of return are several percentage points higher than in other industries because of these two factors (43).

After the effects of these factors (i.e., growth in demand and higher risks), on rates of return in the drug industry are allowed for, Schwartzman concludes that the effects of patents as a means of providing monopoly profits are surprisingly small. He estimates that they provide only a normal rate of return on investment, contrary to what is commonly believed:

> The average realized rate of profit of pharmaceutical manufacturers has not exceeded the average realized rate of all manufacturing after adjustment for expensing research and development, riskiness of investment, and the growth of sales, despite the importance of patents for this industry. The patent protection has resulted in a large investment in research and development rather than a high expected rate of profit. The public policy of granting patents has had the intended effect of increasing investment in research which has reduced the profit rate to the same level as in other industries where patent protection is unimportant. (44)

An important implication of capitalizing intangible capital has occurred since the passage of the 1962 FDA Amendments. The effect of these Amendments has been to increase the time and resources required to develop and test a new drug before it can be marketed. This is to increase the probability that there are no harmful side effects and that the proposed drug is effective in treatment. The effect of the increased time and resources required to bring a new drug to market is an increase in the capital (undepreciated assets) of the drug firm (the ratio of research and development capital to other capital increases) with a consequent decrease in the economic rate of return to the firm. (The accounting rate of return may be unchanged.) One study has estimated that an increase of two additional years for development time would decrease the economic rate of return by 2 percent while leaving unchanged the accounting rate of return. Another study estimated that the 1962 FDA Amendments will cause a 50 percent decrease in the economic rate of return (45). If investment in research and development is related to the expected economic rate of return to be earned by the firm, the effect of the 1962 Amendments will be a decrease in investment in research and development. The effect of the 1962 Amendments on drug firm profitability is also discussed below with regard to its effect on the rate of drug innovation.

One other unintended consequence of the 1962 Amendments with respect to profitability is that entry barriers have been increased. It now costs more and takes longer for drug firms with competitive products to enter a given therapeutic market. Drug firms with established products will be able to earn larger profits for a longer period of time until competitive products are introduced.

Published data on drug industry profits, based on the accounting rate of return, showing continual high rates of profitability, have been one of the reasons for proposals to change the structure of the industry. It would be unfortunate, not only for the drug firms but for consumers of drugs as well, if public policies to reduce industry profitability were based on misleading profitability data rather than on the more accurate economic rate of return measures.

FEDERAL REGULATION OF DRUGS

History of Federal Drug Legislation

The passage of the Pure Food and Drugs Act of 1906 was the beginning of federal regulation over drugs. The major emphasis of this legislation was not on drugs but was instead concerned with abuses in food adulteration and with patent (secret) medicines. Under this law the government had control only over the labeling of drugs; it was not concerned with advertising, testing, or even the content of the drug. The government sought to protect the public from medical quacks and the false claims made for patent medicines (46).

It was not until the 1930s that the modern drug era began. As new drugs were introduced in this period, a tragedy occurred and was the impetus for new drug legislation. A company seeking to make a liquid form of sulfanilamide for children, the first therapeutic discovery of the modern era, dissolved it in ethylene glycol (antifreeze). The company was unaware of its toxic effects and did not test it on animals. This resulted in the death of more than 100 children (47).

The passage in 1938 of the Food, Drug and Cosmetic Act (FDC) not only increased the government's control over the advertising and labeling of foods, drugs, and cosmetics, but also, for the first time, said a drug had to be considered safe. The Food and Drug Administration was given the authority for judging safety. The 1938 law was intended to protect the public from unsafe, potentially harmful drugs. Before the FDA gave a company approval for a new drug, the New Drug Application (NDA) had to indicate that the drug was safe for the use suggested on the label. Drug companies instituted premarket testing to prove the safety of the drug. (Drug testing was also in the companies' interest since it would limit their potential liability by excluding potentially hazardous drugs from the market; thus it is likely that they would have instituted such safety procedures in the absence of any legislation.) It was left up to the drug companies to decide the amount of clinical research necessary to prove that a drug was safe. The FDA did not specify the procedures for premarket testing.

The next step in the federal regulation of drugs, and the most controversial, was the 1962 Amendments to the FDC Act. Starting in 1959, Senator Kefauver held hearings on the drug industry. Pervasive throughout these hearings was the belief that existing regulations permitted new drugs to be sold, at high prices, that were of questionable efficacy. Senator Kefauver apparently believed that it was possible to sell drugs at high prices, of dubious quality, because of patent protection, heavy promotion by the drug companies, consumer and physician ignorance, and minimal incentives for physicians to be concerned with their patients' drug costs. Heavy promotion and extravagant claims for their effectiveness, it was believed, misled physicians and patients into purchasing their drugs. Underlying this attitude of drug company behavior was the belief that much of their research was for minor innovations. Senator Kefauver believed that only if the federal government regulated drug company claims about their effectiveness would the public receive accurate information (48).

A number of people believed that the 1962 Amendments would not have passed had it not been for another drug tragedy, this time thalidomide. Thalidomide was a tranquilizer and was first distributed in Europe. An American drug company began to distribute it in this country to some physicians on an experimental basis. The 1938 legislation permitted such limited distribution to qualified experts as long as the drug was labeled as being under investigation. The American drug company withdrew the drug from use after reports from Europe that deformed babies were born to mothers who had taken the drug during their pregnancy. Thalidomide was effectively kept off the U.S. market by the 1938 legislation. However, there was great concern that there was insufficient testing of new drugs. These concerns, in addition to the earlier concerns arising from the Kefauver hearings, led to the 1962 Amendments (49). In response to these concerns, the Amendments made two major changes in the 1938 legislation. There was now greater specificity over the premarket testing of new drugs, and second, the criteria for introducing new drugs were changed.

The 1962 Amendments enabled the FDA to specify the testing procedures that a drug manufacturer must use to produce acceptable information for evaluating the drug company's NDA. Extensive data on animal tests were now required before the FDA would permit testing on human subjects.

Although the thalidomide tragedy was the event that led to the 1962 Amendments, it is quite possible that had the Amendments been in force during that time, the problem with thalidomide would not have been discovered. Subsequent animal studies failed to reveal thalidomide's effect in a number of studies. The FDA might have approved the drug under the new guidelines had they been applicable during 1962, had it not been for the results of its use in Europe. "Ironically, even though the thalidomide disaster was widely interpreted as evidence of the need for longer premarket review, it actually illustrated the basic unreliability of premarket studies. Had other nations adopted the same cautious policies as the FDA in reviewing thalidomide, the United States itself might well have suffered disaster" (50).

With respect to the new criterion for introducing new drugs, a proof of efficacy was added to the proof of safety that was required under the 1938 legislation. Previously, under the 1938 law, the FDA had to determine that it was safe to market a new drug (the proof being left to the drug company), but now under the 1962 Amendments, the FDA also had to find that the drug was effective in its intended use. Effective was interpreted as achieving the claims made for it by the drug company. To prove efficacy, drug companies were required by the FDA to conduct double-blind "experiments" (i.e., neither the patient nor physician was aware of the drug therapy being administered).

Numerous other changes were made with regard to regulation of drugs in the 1962 Amendments such as those with respect to advertising and promotion. Generic names were required on drug labels and advertised claims were restricted to those approved by the FDA. However, the increased emphasis on premarket testing (and its specificity) and the proof of efficacy were the two most important changes. It was toward these two aspects that much criticism has been directed.

A Framework for Analyzing the 1962 Amendments

How can anyone oppose increased testing requirements for new drugs and proof that the claims made by the drug companies are in fact accurate? Any additional benefits accruing to the public as a result of the 1962 legislation, however, are not without additional costs. Public policy that attempts to increase benefits without regard to their costs may in fact make the public worse off than they were before. Increasingly, researchers, including economists, pharmacologists, and others, are suggesting that this is what has occurred as a result of the 1962 Amendments. To understand how increased testing of drugs and proof of efficacy can result in greater harm to society, it is necessary to have a framework within which the 1962 Amendments can be evaluated.

As a result of increased federal regulation over drugs, there has been an increase in both the benefits and costs to the public. First the presumed benefits will be discussed and then the costs.

The positive aspects of the legislation were expected to be threefold: Ineffective drugs will no longer be marketed, thereby saving consumers money. Second, because of the more stringent testing procedures and the requirements for animal testing, it was expected that drug safety would be enhanced. And third, greater control over the accuracy of drug claims and the dissemination of information on their benefits and risks was expected to stimulate price competition among drug companies. Drug companies would be less able to differentiate their products "artificially," thereby decreasing promotional expenditures and consequently drug costs. If these lower prices are passed on, consumers should benefit through lower drug prices.

In a classic study, Peltzman has attempted to quantify the value of these benefits to consumers (51). To estimate the savings due to keeping ineffective drugs off the market, Peltzman attempted to compare the change in demand curves of new drugs both before and after the 1962 Amendments. If ineffective drugs were introduced before 1962, their demand curves should decline over time as physicians discover that they are ineffective drugs. Demand curves in the post-1962 period should not decline but should instead increase since they are "effective" drugs. Other factors also affect the demand for drugs. However, once these other factors are controlled for, we would expect the pre-1962 demand curves growing less than post-1962 demand curves. Peltzman found that there was no substantial difference between pre- and post-1962 Amendment new drugs with respect to their market shares or prices. "If pre-amendment efficacy claims were substantially exaggerated, it would be expected that pre-1962 new drugs would not hold their market share as well as post-1962 new drugs, or that they would do so only if their prices were reduced once the exaggeration was revealed by experience in use. But [the data] suggests the experience with them did not generally cause doctors and consumers to regard their initial evaluations as exaggerated" (52). Peltzman claims the reasons for such a small regulatory effect on ineffective drugs is that, "The penalties imposed by the marketplace on sellers of ineffective drugs before 1962 seems to have been sufficient to have left little room for improvement by a regulatory agency" (53).

The issue of efficacy from the perspective of patient treatment was addressed by Professor Wardell as follows:

> Failure to show a difference in efficacy between a new drug and an older one should not be taken to mean that the new drug cannot be a worthwhile advance . . . . First, each drug's efficacy may be exerted on a different segment of the population; if both drugs were available, the proportion of patients treatable might be much higher than if either drug were available alone. By the same argument, a drug that is "on average" less effective and more toxic than existing therapy may still be highly desirable for some segments of the population. Our current simplistic statistical concepts of efficacy and safety usually fail to take this into account. Second, it is common to find that the spectrum of side effects differs for each drug, or that the pharmacokinetics are different enough to confer different dosage regimens upon each drug. Third, in the actual treatment of many types of conditions, a patient should receive several drugs in turn on a trial-and-error basis until the one that is best for his needs is determined empirically. These realities of therapeutics for individual patients are generally ignored in the current requirements for evidence of drug efficacy. All these factors can be crucial for tailoring therapy to an individual patient to achieve maximal efficacy, safety, comfort, convenience, and compliance with the therapeutic regimen. To achieve these goals it is desirable to have a number of alternative therapies from which to choose. (54)

With respect to the benefits from increased testing requirements, Peltzman expected to observe fewer health risks (reduction in loss of life and morbidity) and a consequent reduction in medical expenditures as a result of safer drugs. To calculate the expected value of increased safety requirements, Peltzman estimated the losses that would have been prevented if the 1962 Amendments had been in effect earlier. He examined those cases where drugs were implicated in either fatal or harmful effects to patients. "Thalidomide-type products do not appear to have been introduced frequently in the years before 1962" (55). In estimating the consequences of a thalidomide disaster in this country Peltzman assumed it would have been on a scale that occurred in West Germany, even though thalidomide was kept off the U.S. market by the 1938 FDC Act in 1961. (He further assumed that such drug tragedies occurred once every decade.)

The yearly savings due to all of the benefits above was estimated by Peltzman to be less than $100 million (56).

Turning to the cost side, Peltzman lists a number of negative consequences as a result of the 1962 Amendments.

1. Since fewer new drugs are introduced and the time required to do so increases, older drugs can command higher prices for a longer period of time than previously.

Barriers to entry increased and fewer new drugs led to a decline in price competition.

2. As a result of the increased testing requirement, there is now a greater delay in the introduction of new drugs. Because of an increased delay, physicians have had to use older drugs that were less safe than newer ones to which they did not yet have access.

3. The cost of developing a new drug has now increased because of the more stringent testing requirements. This has led to a permanent decrease in the number of new drugs.

Peltzman estimates the cost to consumers of higher prices as a result of the decline in price competition at $50 million. A much larger cost, estimated at $300–400 million, results from the reduced flow of new drugs. The net cost of the drug amendments from these "measurable effects add up to a net loss of $250–350 million, or about 6 percent of total drug sales" (57).

Each of the "costs" cited above is discussed in more detail.

Effects on Price Competition

It was believed by its proponents that the 1962 Amendments, with its proof of efficacy and controls over drug advertising, that price competition would be increased. Drug companies would be less able to differentiate their products; drugs would be seen as having closer substitutes. In setting their prices, drug companies would be more sensitive to the prices of close competitors. However, if there are fewer new drugs entering a market and there is a longer period before drugs can enter, a barrier to entry has been created. Rather than increase price competition, a barrier would serve to *decrease* it. In support of the view that there is price competition between new and old drugs, Peltzman finds that prescription drug prices have risen slightly faster than they would have in the absence of the amendments. He estimates the cost to consumers of this anticompetitive effect to be approximately $40 million a year, based on 1970 drug sales. [This estimate would be much higher if based on 1985 prices (58).]

Drug Lag

Drug controls over drug safety are almost completely based on premarket testing. Once a new drug has been approved by the FDA, there is relatively little postmarketing surveillance. In the premarket phase animal testing is required before the drug can be tested in human trials. This increase in premarket testing has led to a delay in the introduction of new drugs. Peltzman suggests that this delay is, at a minimum, two years (59).

The necessity of animal testing has been questioned by some experts. It has been criticized because of the limited relationship between the results of animal tests and subsequent results on humans. The effect of some drugs are observable only in humans (60); and some important drugs, such as penicillin, are lethal in animals.

Sir Alexander Fleming once remarked that the success of the penicillin project depended on the fact that, since he was not a pharmacologist, he had not tested the drug in animals at all and that, knowing in retrospect its animal toxicity, he would never have had the courage to try it on man! If even one new drug of the stature of penicillin or digitalis has been unjustifiably banished to a company's back shelf because of excessively stringent animal requirements, that event will have harmed more people than have been affected by all the toxicity that has occurred in the history of modern drug development. It is entirely conceivable that the losses from excessively conservative interpretation of animal toxicity tests are more harmful than the toxicity that would be experienced if drugs were tested in man, with appropriate safeguards, at an earlier stage. (61)

A related but no less important problem of the emphasis on premarket testing is that given the limited number of persons that can be tested in the premarket phase, only the most frequent harmful effects can be detected. Once a drug is marketed and used in a larger population, the less frequent adverse drug reactions begin to show up. It is in the postmarketing phase that drug tragedies can occur. Thus postmarketing surveillance should be an important concern of those empowered to protect the public safety. Unfortunately, although pre- and post-market testing may be viewed as substitutes, the emphasis is placed on the premarket phase.

Peltzman estimated the cost to the public of the drug lag. He did this by examining past drug innovations in drug therapy and calculated what the loss in benefits from these innovations would have been had they been introduced two years later than they had. It turns out that the losses would have been substantial and several times greater than the estimated value of the benefits of the legislation (62). Although such an exercise is conjectural, it does serve to indicate the immense importance in lives saved, decreased morbidity, and lower use of medical treatment from a more rapid introduction of important drug discoveries. When estimates are made to indicate the potential savings of drugs that would decrease heart disease and cancer by a small percentage, it is clear from Peltzman's calculations that the loss in potential payoffs are so great as to outweigh any possible benefits due to fewer ineffective drugs and decreased drug toxicity as a result of the new amendments.

A more recent study by Gieringer also calculated the cost of a delay in the introduction of new drugs in terms of lives that would have been saved, not in terms of monetary value. Assuming a delay of introduction of a new drug of only 8 months, Gieringer estimates that 21,000–51,000 lives per decade would have been saved. Using a delay factor of 19 months, it was estimated that 51,000–120,000 lives per decade could be saved. Compared to a worst case scenario of the number of lives saved as a result of the strict FDA regulations, Gieringer estimates the costs of the FDA Amendments to be greater than its benefits by a ratio of 4:1 (63). The estimates above are understated in that they consider only decreases in mortality, not decreased morbidity.

One means of documenting the drug lag is to compare how long important new drugs were available in England before they became available in this country. Wardell, a noted pharmacologist, claims that "in many therapeutic areas, useful and even uniquely effective or safe drugs have been introduced in Britain substantially earlier than in the United States, and at any given time the United States lacks a number of such drugs" (64). He concludes his cross-country comparison by saying: "In view of the clear benefits demonstrable from some of the drugs introduced in Britain, it appears that the United States has lost more than it has gained from adopting a more conservative approach than did Britain in the post-thalidomide era" (65).

As a specific example of the harmful effects of the drug lag Wardell cites the case of the beta-blocking agent propranolol:

"[It was] available in Britain in 1965 but was not available at all in the United States until 1968, and then it was approved only for relatively minor uses. It took another five years for the same drug to be approved for its major use, angina, and still another three years (until 1976) before it was approved for its other major use, hypertension. This, and the lack of availability of certain other beta blockers in the United States, resulted in a marked backwardness in American sophistication in the treatment of hypertension over much of the past ten years.

"Other beta blockers, such as practolol and alprenolol, have been shown abroad to produce a 40 percent reduction in the incidence of myocardial reinfarction and cardiac death in postcoronary patients. Although this effect could result in saving several thousand lives annually in the United States, these beta blockers are no long available in this country even for investigational purposes. *As a result of these interminable delays, American textbooks of pharmacology and medicine are in some fields so hopelessly out of date that when used abroad they are often irrelevant.* (66)"

Rate of Drug Innovation

The most controversial aspect of the 1962 Amendments has been its effect on the rate of drug innovation. Economists have suggested that the production of innovation can be explained within a traditional demand and supply framework. If drug companies anticipate a rising demand for drugs, the companies will respond with an increase in their supply of new products. Similarly, if the costs of innovation are increased, this should result in a decrease in the supply of new drugs. Within this framework, therefore, we would expect to observe a decrease in the rate of drug innovation as a result of the 1962 Amendments.

In the post-1962 period the cost of developing a new drug was greatly increased. These higher costs of development occurred for three reasons. There were more stringent testing procedures before a drug company could apply for a new drug approval from the FDA. Second, there was an increase in the number of years between the time the development of a new drug was initiated and its approval by the FDA. One economist has estimated that costs must be incurred for 10 years instead of five years before a company can begin to receive revenues from a new drug (67). A third reason is the greater risk and uncertainty of innovation. One such measure of risk is the attrition rate of new drugs. In the 1950s it was estimated that the attrition rate of new drugs was two out of three. Now less than one new drug out of 10 undergoing chemical testing is marketed (68).

It has been estimated by one analyst that the cost of developing a new drug has increased tenfold by 1971 compared to the pre-1962 period. (After allowing for inflation, the cost was still more than five times greater.) Another economist estimated the costs in 1974 to be more than 10 times greater than they were in 1960 (69). Hansen (cited earlier) concluded that the cost (in 1976 dollars) of each new chemical entity that is marketed represents a cost of approximately $61 million. (It is not surprising that new drugs that would serve potentially small markets are less likely to be developed. Even though such drugs may be badly needed, the increased costs of developing such drugs, given the size of the market, make such investments unprofitable.)

The increased development time, higher cost, and greater uncertainty of success resulted in a sharp decline in profitability of new drugs in the 1962–1971 period (70). We would therefore expect to observe a decline in the number of new drugs introduced in the post-1962 period. As anticipated, during the period 1957–1961 there were 233 new chemical entities. This declined to 93 during 1962–1966 and further to 76 in 1967–1971 (71). Peltzman attributes most of the reasons for this decline to the 1962 Amendments.

The FDA does not, of course, agree with this assessment. They have responded that the reasons for this decline are twofold. Ineffective new drugs were eliminated from the market, and second there has been a natural decline in drug innovation worldwide. It has become more difficult to develop new innovations as the opportunities for new research have declined. The latter reason is unrelated to the 1962 Amendments.

With respect to the FDA reply that the decline is a result of keeping ineffective drugs off the market, Peltzman refers to several studies to demonstrate that, at most, 10 percent of pre-1962 drugs were ineffective. Further, even though there is not agreement on what constitutes a significant new chemical entity, Peltzman used data from an unpublished FDA study to show that there was an annual average of 12.3 "important therapeutic advances" between 1950 and 1962 and only 9.1 per year between 1962 and 1970 (72). Thus the decline in the rate of innovation since 1962 is real.

In one study, Grabowski, Vernon, and Thomas undertook a cross country comparison to determine the reasons for the serious decline in drug innovation since 1962. To determine whether the 1962 Amendments contributed to this decline, they undertook a comparative study of the rate of innovation in this country and in the United Kingdom (UK). Until 1971, drug regulation in the UK was similar to regulation in this country in the period prior to 1962. If the reason for the decline in the rate of drug innovation was the worldwide phenomenon of a lack of research opportunities, the UK should have been similarly affected. Since the regulatory environment differed between the two countries, this comparison should help to isolate these separate effects. The authors state: "The data . . . clearly show that there has been a significant decline in the R&D productivities for the two countries over the post-amendment period. However, perhaps the most interesting result is the much stronger *relative* decline in R&D productivity that the United States experienced in the decade after 1962…Hence, over this period in which the United States shifted to a much more stringent regulatory environment than the United Kingdom, it also experienced a much more rapid decline in R&D productivity" (73).

It is difficult to determine whether the downward trend in innovation due to the nonregulatory effect in both countries is an adequate test of the depletion of research opportunities or whether it is due to other reasons. Another possible explanation is the thalidomide tragedy and scientific advances in the pharmacological sciences, both of which resulted in greater amounts being spent on research and development, and consequently resulted in fewer drug innovations. Under this explanation, the drug companies have been willing to incur higher development costs so as to preserve their reputations and to minimize their legal liabilities by forestalling any drug tragedies.

Thus the cross-country comparisons demonstrate that there has been an effect on new drug introductions as a result of the 1962 Amendments. The general downward trend in drug innovations in both countries, however, may be due to several reasons; to date it has not been possible to determine the contribution of each of these reasons to the decline.

The increased cost of development, as a result of the 1962 Amendments and by drug companies to minimize their liability, has been one factor leading to a decline in profitability from research and development. Adding to this decline in profitability has been the shortened "effective" life of a drug patent. Although a patent allows the drug firm to retain a monopoly of 17 years, the effective life of a patent is much less than 17 years. To protect their discoveries, drug companies file for a patent as soon as a new chemical entity is shown to have a promising therapeutic effect. The promising drug must still undergo years of testing. It has been estimated that in 1966, the effective life of a patent for a new drug coming on the market was 13.6 years, it declined to 9.5 years by 1979, and to only 6.8 years as of 1981 (74).

The profitability of research and development for drug companies has declined over time. As profitability has declined so have the number of new chemical entities. One study found that the average expected internal rate of return on new drugs fell from 22 percent in 1965 to 10 percent by 1978, which was lower than the industry's cost of capital (75). A more recent study also concludes that the industry's rate of return on research and development is insufficient. Joglekar and Paterson show that the performance of new chemical entities (NCE) is highly skewed. Only one out of every three NCEs offer a better return than an investment in a bond, "and the odds of exceeding it by an appreciable degree are small indeed . . . . The risk of investing in NCEs, created by the rarity of big sellers, is thus apparent. Given this risk, a 6.1% real IRR [internal rate of return] for the average NCE seems modest" (76).

A consequence of such risk in research and development is that a drug firm must be sufficiently large to be able to introduce a number of NCEs before it can achieve a few large successes; further, that these successes depend on foreign sales as well as sales over a large number of years (77).

Orphan Drugs

Indicative of the problem of increased cost of research and development and a consequently lower rate of return is the problem of orphan drugs. Orphan drugs are used to treat relatively rare diseases in the population. As the profitability of NCEs have decreased, drug companies have not found it worthwhile to devote their resources to research on orphan drugs. There was even evidence that potentially useful orphan drugs were not developed because their potential sales revenue was less than the costs of seeking FDA approval (78). To provide an incentive for drug companies to engage in research and development on orphan drugs, Congress passed legislation in 1983, which was amended in subsequent years, 1984 and 1985. The legislation provides for tax credits to defray part of the research costs of such drugs and exclusive marketing rights for seven years for unpatentable drugs. While the tax credits may stimulate the development of known orphan drugs, most of which are discovered by accident, it is too early to judge whether these incentives are sufficient to encourage research into orphan diseases.

Concluding Comments

All policies have trade-offs. It is not possible to receive benefits without also incurring costs. Policymakers should consider both aspects, the costs as well as the benefits of their decisions. Drug safety can be increased, that is, the risks of harmful side effects of a new drug can be lowered, by requiring still further testing and delaying for a greater number of years the marketing of new drugs. The cost of that policy, however, is to deny new drugs to people in need of them. Wardell cites the case of benzodiazepine hypnotic (nitrazapam), which was available in Europe five years before it was approved for marketing in this country in 1971. An advantage of this drug over other hypnotics is its safety in overdosage. Based on data in foreign markets and U.S. deaths due to overdosage of hypnotics, Wardell concluded that the five-year delay in availability in U.S. markets resulted in more than 1,200 deaths in this country (79). If a drug marketed in this country caused these many deaths, it would be considered a major drug disaster. But the fact that these were deaths that could have been prevented by earlier introduction of a new drug went unnoticed.

The difference between preventable deaths and deaths caused by drug toxicity are that the latter are visible; the victims have names and families, and their pictures may be in the paper. They are identifiable. Preventable deaths are statistical; as such they are anonymous. An agency such as the FDA is likely to place a greater emphasis on minimizing visible deaths rather than being as concerned with anonymous beneficiaries. In so doing, the FDA limits criticisms of its actions by the press and the public. Comprehensive premarket testing can also be viewed as a means by which the FDA protects itself.

From a societal perspective, however, criteria different from those used by the FDA should be considered. Given the enormous benefits from the early introduction of new drugs, greater emphasis should be given to the earlier introduction of new drugs rather than seeking to minimize the risks of drug toxicity through extensive premarket testing. Perhaps appropriate policy would be to encourage greater risk taking when introducing new drugs with a consequent strengthening of postmarketing surveillance to minimize the risk of drug toxicity.

PUBLIC POLICY TOWARD THE PHARMACEUTICAL INDUSTRY

Economic Performance of the Industry

The concern that critics of the pharmaceutical industry have had with respect to its economic performance has resulted in several proposals, each of which would result in lower drug prices and drug profitability. Several of these proposals, together with their effects, both direct and indirect, will be discussed.

The Effective Life of Drug Patents

An important source of monopoly power in the drug industry is patent protection. Critics believe that the length of time over which a patent protects a manufacturer is too long. If the patent were for a shorter period of time (it is currently for 17 years), the manufacturer would still be able to earn sufficient profits to provide incentives for research, without resulting in excessive profits. To lessen this source of monopoly power, it has been proposed (by various Senators) that after several years of exclusive patent rights, the manufacturer be required to license other drug firms to manufacture and market the patented drug, while paying the original manufacturer a "fair" royalty rate. Cross-licensing proposals have varied in their definition of how long the original patent holder is to have exclusive rights and what royalty rate should be paid to the original patent holder.

Cross-licensing would increase price competition among the various manufacturers and distributors of the drug. Drug prices would be reduced, as would profits to the original patent holder.

An important consequence of cross-licensing or of any proposal to decrease the effective life of a drug patent is that although it will not affect the supply of currently patented drugs, it would result in a decrease in the supplies of yet-undiscovered drugs. Not all research and development results in patented and profitable drugs. Only a small number of drugs eventually become profitable. Proposals that limit the profit on those that become successful will decrease the overall rate of return to research and development, which as discussed above is already quite low, and consequently lead to a decrease in drug innovation.

In 1984, the Drug Price Competition and Patent Term Restoration Act was enacted. Concern by academics (as well as the pharmaceutical industry) that the profitability of research and development had declined to where it adversely affected the number of NCEs led to legislative proposals by the drug companies to increase their profitability. Extension of the patent life of a drug was proposed as a means of compensating the drug companies for the lengthy delays caused by the regulatory review process. The Pharmaceutical Manufacturers' Association (PMA) was opposed by consumer groups, labor unions, and senior citizen groups. After several years of opposition, the Act was finally passed in 1984 and then it represented a compromise. The PMA received an extension of the effective life of a drug patent for five additional years (for NCEs approved after 1984), which was less than they had sought. The opponents of the patent term extension also received a change in policy so as to receive lower drug prices.

The first part of the Act enabled generic drugs to enter the market more rapidly. Generic drug manufacturers, who had lobbied strongly for the change, were able to bypass the lengthy and costly regulatory process, which was duplicative of that used by the company receiving the original patent. The PMA opposed permitting generic drugs to use an abbreviated drug application; the profitability of patented drugs would decline once their patent life expired. Previously, even though a patent expired, a drug would still retain its monopoly power since it took a number of years before generic drugs could complete the necessary regulatory requirements.

It is not clear whether the overall effect of the Act will be to increase the profitability of patented drugs. Will the increase in the effective life of a patent be offset by the more rapid increase in price competition from generics?

Generic Versus Brand Name Prescribing

Substitution of generic drugs for brand name drugs whose patents have expired is encouraged both through government policy as well as by those who must pay the bill for drug expenditures. Generic drugs are usually less expensive than brand name drugs and they are believed by many to be equally safe since the FDA is responsible for monitoring their quality. In addition to the 1984 Act described above, the issue of generic versus brand name prescribing has been manifested in two additional types of policies: repeal of antisubstitution laws in a state and the federal maximum allowable cost regulations.

Antisubstitution Laws. During the early 1950s, all the states enacted antisubstitution laws. Pharmacists were required by law to "dispense as written" all prescriptions that specified a particular brand name drug, even though an equivalent therapeutic drug was available at lower cost (80). The movement to repeal these laws was started by the government Maximum Allowable Cost Program (MAC). To reduce federal matching expenditures for Medicaid and increase price competition, Congress adopted regulations to require generic substitution. The MAC program, however, could not be effective unless the state antisubstitution laws were repealed. Under the maximum allowable cost (MAC) regulation, pharmacists are to substitute the chemically equivalent drug which is generally available at the lowest cost for any prescribed brand name drug. Pharmacists participating in the MAC program would, among multiple source drugs (comprising approximately 40 percent of ethical drugs), receive a dispensing fee plus the lowest cost of generic drugs that are "generally available." By use of the term "generally available," the drug manufacturer must reduce the price of their generic drugs to all buyers, not just to those on Medicaid. Thus, to be able to compete for Medicaid patients, drug manufacturers cannot maintain differential prices to Medicaid patients and private-pay patients.

In addition to the government, pharmacists and a number of consumer groups favored repeal of state laws that prohibit the pharmacist from substituting a generic drug for a brand name drug specified in a prescription without the prescribing physician's permission. More than 40 states have repealed their antisubstitution laws. The pharmacists claim that they are able to judge the quality of substitute drugs and that by substituting generic drugs they can save the consumer money.

Repeal of antisubstitution laws is opposed by the pharmaceutical industry and by many physicians. Their argument goes as follows. If a physician believed it was acceptable to substitute a generic drug for the brand name one prescribed, this could be indicated on the prescription form. To substitute without the physician's permission is to diminish the physician's role in caring for the patient. When prescribing for a patient, the physician should consider the patient's health history, whether the patient has any allergies, how the prescribed drug acts with other medications the patient may be taking, the price of that drug relative to others, and the quality of the drug, as indicated by the physician's confidence in certain manufacturers' products. Price is clearly a secondary consideration. It is generally difficult to monitor the drug response by an ambulatory patient, and this difficulty is increased when the drug taken by the patient is not the one prescribed by the physician.

Repeal of the antisubstitution laws would also clearly reduce drug firm profitability. One study indicated a significant decline on the internal rate of return earned on investment in drug research and development. Grabowski and Vernon estimate that with a 50 percent reduction in net income upon patent expiration as a result of generic substitution, the internal rate of return declines by 25 percent, from 7.5 to 5.6 (81).

Federal Maximum Allowable Cost Regulations. The effect of the MAC regulation is to lower the price of drugs for patients under the government-reimbursed program as well as to all other patients. The marginal cost of a drug is a small fraction of both the price and the average cost of a brand name drug. Thus substitution of generic drugs for brand name drugs should result in large reductions in both prices and profits of brand name drug manufacturers.

Two objections have been raised with the MAC regulation, which would also be applicable to repeal of antisubstitution laws. The first is with respect to the quality of generic drugs. It is assumed by many that the quality of all generic drugs is equal. Schwartzman, however, claims that with so many drug manufacturers [there were 757 drug manufacturing facilities in 1977 (82)] the FDA has, in the past, not been able to monitor adequately the quality of drugs produced by all manufacturers (83). Since the emphasis of the MAC regulation is on price competition according to chemically equivalent drugs, Schwartzman claims that the incentives for manufacturers to be concerned with quality is less than if they were producing drugs under their own brand name.

A second concern with the MAC regulation (and with other proposals that attempt to lower drug prices) is that it results in a decrease in drug industry profitability. A lower rate of return on drug firm research and development will result in a smaller quantity of product innovation. These long-run consequences of decreased profitability are less obvious to the public than the immediate savings to the government of lower drug prices. A lower rate of drug innovation is an important cost to society to which the government gives less weight when considering its own immediate needs for reduced health expenditures.

Federal Regulation of Drug Safety

Public policy should attempt to achieve an appropriate balance between minimizing the risk from early introduction of potentially hazardous drugs and providing ready access to therapeutically important drugs to patients who need them. It appears that the FDA has overemphasized the former while neglecting the latter. To achieve a more optimal mix between these two concerns, several policies have been suggested.

Postmarketing Surveillance

One way of permitting consumers to benefit from the early introduction of new drugs while helping to ensure that the public is adequately protected is to place a greater reliance on postmarketing surveillance. Present policy virtually neglects postmarketing surveillance and relies too heavily on premarket testing. Usually, it is not possible to detect widespread drug toxicity in the early stages of a drug's development. In that phase, its use is limited to a small number of people and it is prescribed under close supervision. Widespread toxicity can occur when a drug is used by a much larger number of people, over a long period of time, and in an unsupervised manner.[2] Thus surveillance is particularly necessary once a drug is widely marketed.

Up until four years ago, this country has had one of the lowest voluntary reporting rates of drug toxicity of all countries reporting to the World Health Organization's International Drug Monitoring Program. On a per capita basis, Britain's voluntary reporting rate was 10 times that of the United States. The lack of an effective post-

---

[2]The fast-tracking system of the FDA suffered a highly publicized setback in 1982 when an antiarthritic drug, Oraflex, was marketed after receiving fast-track approval, partially on the basis of foreign data. After the drug was marketed, there were allegations that the drug was implicated in 60 deaths in Britain and 12 in the United States. The drug company voluntarily withdrew the drug before the FDA took any action. Even though the drug had been tested, it is not possible to judge all the potential side effects of a drug until it is placed in wider use than when it is studied in clinical trials. There may have been a combined effect between Oraflex and other drugs. Sick elderly patients may have been taking several drugs simultaneously.

Speeding up the approval process by relying more on drug companies for information does not absolve the drug company from the economic liabilities of a drug tragedy. These economic consequences are likely to be the main determinant of how much information is necessary before a drug company is willing to market a new drug.

marketing surveillance system has also been criticized by the Government Accounting Office. Voluntary reporting has increased from 10,000 to 50,000 (1986) over the past four years (84).

Restricted Use of Drugs

It has been suggested that the restrictive regulations on use of drugs should not apply equally to all physicians. Currently, medical specialists in university hospitals are treated the same as general practitioners with respect to their access to drugs. To make certain drugs available that have not yet undergone their complete premarket testing, their distribution could be restricted to certain types of patients for whom the benefits of the drug would be particularly great. Earlier drug usage could be made available to those physicians who are expert in particular areas or who have undergone special training in their use.

These are just several of the ways in which patients can benefit from early availability of new drugs without permitting the widespread early release of powerful new drugs whose complete uses and effects are not yet fully known (85). Rather than placing stringent restrictions on the introduction of new drugs, a more flexible and responsive policy to patients' needs should be encouraged. In fact, the 1962 Amendments and their enforcement by the FDA should be held to the same standards that they would apply to new drugs. "Indeed, if judged by the same standards they themselves set for drugs, the 1962 laws could not be approved because no evidence of their safety or efficacy exists: They were implemented in a scientifically uncontrolled manner, and no measures of their effects were even sought. We are only now beginning to evaluate in retrospect the effects of the changes that began in 1962, and it is doubtful whether their full impact can ever be known" (86).

Additional Reforms

Other countries with less restrictive drug regulations are able to introduce new drugs more quickly than in this country. When these drugs are shown to be important therapeutic discoveries, the FDA should be willing to accept data based on foreign use of the drug. Prior to 1975 the FDA did not accept any foreign data for a new drug. The FDA has recently begun accepting such data; however, additional studies in this country must still be conducted. The drug lag could be greatly reduced if, for some drugs, greater reliance were placed on the experience of other countries with the drug.

Other countries place a greater reliance than the United States on expert advisory committees for decisions on approval of new drugs. If the FDA were required to act similarly, these advisory committees would not have the same reluctance as the FDA to delay approval of new drugs. The committees would, as in other countries, balance both the hidden and the visible costs and benefits of new drugs. The FDA would not bear the onus of visible deaths due to early introduction of new drugs.

The 1962 Amendments have resulted in such bizarre situations that drugs (such as benzodiazepine hypnotic) were kept off the market when they were safer than the drugs they were meant to replace.

In 1974 Congressional hearings were held on the FDA's performance with respect to the drug lag. In response to this criticism, the FDA gave greater priority to significant new drugs. This "fast track" clearance was supposed to permit significant new drugs to be introduced sooner than they would otherwise have been. Although this has been a move in the right direction, there is still a significant lag in the introduction of new drugs.

A Government Accounting Office (GAO) study (1981) on FDA procedures found that the FDA policy of giving priority to important new drugs has produced some progress. The GAO found that while approval times for new drug applications lengthened in four of the FDA's six reviewing divisions, they were reduced in the remaining two (87). Unless public and congressional pressures on the FDA for more rapid introduction of drugs persist, the main losers would once again be the anonymous beneficiaries: that large number of people who could benefit and yet are denied access to beneficial drugs.

Concluding Comments

An important imperfection in the pharmaceutical market is that whereas the physician prescribes drugs, he or she is not responsible for the cost of the prescription; it is paid for by the patient or a third-party payor. It is time consuming, hence costly, for the physician who desires to be well informed on the latest in drug therapy, new minor chemical modifications, side effects of various drugs, alternative dosage forms, and prices. Faced with high informational needs and an incentive system whereby someone else pays for the drug, it is not surprising that the current system of drug marketing is what it is.

The physician's role in the pharmaceutical market, however, is no different from the physician's role in the broader medical care delivery system. To change physician behavior, it is necessary to change the incentives facing the physician. As prepaid health plans increase their market shares and more physicians participate in these plans, both the incentives and information requirements facing physicians change. As drugs are included as a benefit in a prepaid health plan, there should be a change in the financial incentive facing the participating physician. Drug costs become one more component of care whose costs are to be minimized. Prepaid health plans are able to purchase drugs at volume discounts. The informational needs of physicians in a prepaid health plan are reduced. As physicians develop confidence in the organizations' pharmacists, they will be more willing to delegate some of the decisionmaking on drugs to them. In several health maintenance organizations (HMOs) today, physicians are able to indicate on their prescription form whether it is permissible for the pharmacist to substitute.

The pharmaceutical industry does not perform as well as many would prefer; it devotes more resources to promotion than its critics believe is necessary; the prices of drugs are higher than their costs of production; and low-income persons have difficulty paying for needed drugs. It is important, however, to retain a proper perspective on this industry. Many proposed policies to decrease promotion expenditures, prices, and profitability may result in greater long-term harm than their immediate benefits.

Drug costs represent a small percent of the costs of medical care and have been rising at a less rapid rate than medical care prices. The benefits of drug therapy are enormous. Drugs prolong life, alleviate pain, and are a very low-cost substitute for more expensive medical treatment; for example, Tagamet, an antiulcer drug, saves millions of dollars in hospital and surgical costs each year (88). A new class of heart drugs might eliminate coronary bypass surgery. Drugs are very cost effective. The main emphasis of public policy toward the pharmaceutical industry should therefore be to *increase* drug innovation. Too great an emphasis on correcting perceived monopoly abuses, such as requiring generic substitution, and policies to decrease drug prices and profits, will result in a lower rate of return on research and development and hence on product innovation. Further, the monopoly abuses may be more perceived than real. Profitability estimates are not as high as originally believed and promotional expenditures serve an important information function as well as being a means of entering new markets. There is also a greater degree of price competition than formerly believed. It would therefore be unfortunate if policies were instituted, based on incorrect perceptions, the net effect of which was to decrease drug innovation. Policies should instead be developed to provide greater incentives for research and development and to decrease the time required to bring new drugs to market. The benefits to society from increased drug innovation will far outweigh the immediate savings of lower drug prices. In this regard the FDA Amendments should be reevaluated with these objectives in mind.

REFERENCES

1. F. M. Scherer, *Industrial Market Structure and Economic Performance* (Boston: Houghton Mifflin, 1980), p. 67.

2. Henry G. Grabowski and John M. Vernon, "New Studies on Market Concentration, Theory of Supply, Entry and Promotion," in Robert I. Chien, ed., *Issues in Pharmaceutical Economics* (Lexington, Mass: Lexington Books, 1979), pp 31–32.

3. *Standard and Poors Industry Surveys*, Vol. I (New York: Standard and Poors Corporation, April 1986), p. H18.

4. Walter S. Measday, "The Pharmaceutical Industry," in Walter Adams, ed., *The Structure of American Industry*, 4th ed. (New York: Macmillan, 1971), p. 167.

5. George J. Stigler, "Introduction," in *Business Concentration and Price Policy*, National Bureau of Economic Research (Princeton, N.J.: Princeton University Press, 1955), p. 4.

6. Grabowski and Vernon, *op. cit.*, p. 32.

7. *Ibid.*, pp 33–35.

8. *Ibid.*, pp. 35–36.

9. The study by Douglas Cocks, "Product Innovation and the Dynamic Elements of Competition in the Ethical Pharmaceutical Industry," in Robert B. Helms, ed., *Drug Development and Marketing* (Washington, D.C.: American Enterprise Institute, 1975) used the Hymer-Pashigian instability index, which is calculated as follows:

$$I = \sum_{i=1}^{n} \left(\frac{S_{t,i}}{S_t} - \frac{S_{t-1,i}}{S_{t-1}} \right)$$

where I = index of instability
$S_{t,i}$ = sales of the ith firm at time t
S_t = total industry sales at time t

10. A. T. Kearney, *Study of Economics of Entry and Exit in the Pharmaceutical Industry* (Washington, D.C.: Pharmaceutical Manufacturers Association, April 30, 1974).

11. Grabowski and Vernon, *op. cit.* p. 39.

12. As reported in David Schwartzman, *Innovation in the Pharmaceutical Industry* (Baltimore: Johns Hopkins University Press, 1976), p. 76.

13. As reported in Schwartzman, *ibid.*, p. 79.

14. Grabowski and Vernon, *The Regulation of Pharmaceuticals: Balancing the Benefits and Risks* (Washington, D.C.: American Enterprise Institute, 1983), p. 19.

15. Schwartzman, *op. cit.*, p. 18.

16. *Standard and Poors Industry Survey*, Vol. 1, (New York: Standard and Poors Corporation, April 1986), p. H20.

17. *Ibid.*

18. Jerome E. Schnee and Erol Caglarcan, "Economic Structure and Performance of the Ethical Pharmaceutical Industry," in Cotton M. Lindsay, ed., *The Pharmaceutical Industry* (New York: Wiley, 1978), p. 32.

19. *Ibid.*, pp 32–33.

20. Grabowski and Vernon, "New Studies," p. 48.

21. Hansen estimates that when expenditures are capitalized to the date of marketing approval at a 10 percent interest rate, the estimated cost per marketed new chemical entity is $61.6 million (in 1976 dollars). Ronald W. Hansen, "The Pharmaceutical Development Process: Estimates of Development Costs and Times and the Effects of Proposed Regulatory Changes," in Chien, ed., *op. cit.*, p. 168.

22. An article discussing these two aspects of promotional expenditures is Keith B. Leffler, "Persuasion or Information? The Economics of Prescription Drug Advertising," *Journal of Law and Economics*, 24 (1), April 1981: 45–74.

23. Jerome Avorn et al., "Scientific Versus Commercial Sources of Influence on the Prescribing Behavior of Physicians," *American Journal of Medicine*, 73, July 1982: 4–8.

24. This was a survey conducted in 1966 by British physicians and reported in Schwartzman, *op. cit.*, pp 188–189.

25. *Ibid.*, p. 194.

26. Sam Peltzman, *Regulation of Pharmaceutical Innovation* (Washington, D.C.: American Enterprise Institute, 1974).

27. For a more extensive discussion of promotion expenses, its magnitude, and components, see Chapter 9 in Schwartzman, *op. cit.*

28. Grabowski and Vernon, "New Studies," p. 44.

29. *Ibid.*, p. 45.

30. Schwartzman, *op. cit.*, p. 202.

31. J. Fred Weston, "Pricing in the Pharmaceutical Industry," in Chien, ed., *op. cit.*, p. 77.

32. Schwartzman, "Pricing of Multiple Source Drugs," in Chien, ed., *op. cit.*, p. 97.

33. Schwartzman, "Pricing of Multiple Source Drugs," pp 99–100.

34. *Ibid.*, p. 99.

35. Bernard Bloom, David Wierz, and Mark Pauly, "Cost and Price of Comparable Branded and Generic Pharmaceuticals," *Journal of the American Medical Association*, 256, November 14, 1986: 2523–2530.

36. Schwartzman, "Pricing of Multiple Source Drugs," p. 99.

37. Weston, *op. cit.*, p. 94.

38. Walter J. Campbell and Rodney F. Smith, "Profitability and the Pharmaceutical Industry," in Cotton M. Lindsay, ed., *The Pharmaceutical Industry* (New York: Wiley, 1978), p. 114.

39. Kenneth W. Clarkson, "The Use of Pharmaceutical Profitability Measures for Public Policy Actions," in Robert I. Chien, ed., *Issues in Pharmaceutical Economics* (Lexington, Mass.: D.C. Health, 1979), p. 117.

40. As additional proof that corrected rates of return are a more accurate measure of profitability in the pharmaceutical industry, Clarkson finds that corrected rather than accounting rates of return are a more useful explanatory variable for explaining variations in stock prices of drug firms; *ibid.*, p. 118.

41. *Ibid.*, p. 113. In another part of his article, Clarkson presents a sensitivity analysis of the rate of return to different economic lives of various expenditure categories.

42. Schwartzman, *Innovation in the Pharmaceutical Industry* p. 156.

43. These studies are discussed in Schwartzman, *Innovation in the Pharmaceutical Industry* pp. 156–158; and in Campbell and Smith, *op. cit.*, pp. 113–115.

44. Schwartzman, *Innovation in the Pharmaceutical Industry* p. 159.

45. These studies are reported in Oswald H. Brownlee, "Rates of Return to Investment in the Pharmaceutical Industry: A Survey and Critical Appraisal," in Chien, ed., *op. cit.*, p. 139.

46. A brief history of federal drug regulation appears in Jerome E. Schnee, "Government Control of Therapeutic Drugs: Intent, Impact, and Issues," in Lindsay, ed., *op. cit.* For more detailed information, see the references in that chapter. A more recent history of drug regulation is Peter Temin, *Taking Your Medicine: Drug Regulation in the United States* (Cambridge, Mass.: Harvard University Press, 1981).

47. William M. Wardell, "The History of Drug Discovery, Development, and Regulation," in Chien, ed., *op. cit.*, p. 8.

48. A discussion of the Kefauver hearings and the congressional debate that preceded the 1962 Amendments was written by Richard Harris, *The Real Voice* (New York: Macmillan, 1964).

49. Wardell states: "The fact that thalidomide had not been approved for U.S. marketing was somehow irrelevant, as was the fact that the new requirements in the amendments, had they been in effect, would not have prevented a thalidomide-type tragedy." William M. Wardell and Louis Lasagna, *Regulation and Drug Development* (Washington, D.C.: American Enterprise Institute, 1975), p. 1.

50. Dale H. Gieringer, "The Safety and Efficacy of New Drug Approval," *Cato Journal*, Spring/Summer 1985: 5(1), 193–194.

51. Peltzman, *op. cit.*

52. *Ibid.*, pp. 37–38.

53. *Ibid.*, p. 45.

54. William M. Wardell, "Therapeutic Implications of the Drug Lag," *Clinical Pharmacology and Therapeutics*, 15(1), January 1974: 76.
55. *Ibid.*, p. 52.
56. The exact method by which Peltzman calculates the value of each of these benefits is described in Peltzman, *op. cit.*, Appendix.
57. Peltzman, *op. cit.*, p. 81.
58. *Ibid.*, pp. 47–48.
59. *Ibid.*, p. 57.
60. Wardell and Lasagna, *op. cit.*, p. 13.
61. *Ibid.*, pp. 138–139.
62. Peltzman, *op. cit.*, pp. 72–73.
63. Gieringer, *op. cit.*, p. 189.
64. Wardell and Lasagna, *op. cit.*, p. 97.
65. *Ibid.*, p. 105.
66. William M. Wardell, "The Impact of Regulation on New Drug Development," in Chien, ed., *op. cit.*, p. 147. (Italics in original quote.)
67. Oswald H. Brownlee, "The Economic Consequences of Regulating Without Regard to Economic Consequences," in Chien, ed., *op. cit.*, p. 216.
68. Henry G. Grabowski, John M. Vernon, and Lacy G. Thomas, "Estimating the Effects of Regulation on Innovation: An International Comparative Analysis of the Pharmaceutical Industry," *Journal of Law and Economics*, April 1978: 136.
69. Brownlee, *op. cit.*, p. 216. Additional cost estimates are cited in Wardell and Lasagna, *op. cit.*, p. 46.
70. Grabowski, Vernon, and Thomas, *op. cit.*, p. 158.
71. Grabowski and Vernon, "New Studies," p. 47.
72. Peltzman, *op. cit.*, pp. 86–87.
73. Grabowski, Vernon, and Thomas, *op. cit.*, p. 151.
74. Data for 1966 through 1979 are from Henry Grabowski, "Public Policy and Innovation: The Case of Pharmaceuticals," *Technovation*, 1, 1982: 174, Table 5. Data for 1981 are from Ronald W. Hansen, "The Relationship Between Regulation and R&D in the Pharmaceutical Industry" in *The Effectiveness of Medicines in Containing Health Care Costs: Impact of Innovation, Regulation and Quality*, Proceedings of a Symposium (Washington, D.C.: National Pharmaceutical Council, June 23, 1982) p. 17.
75. M. Statman, *Competition in the Pharmaceutical Industry: The Declining Profitability of Drug Innovation* (Washington, D.C.: American Enterprise Institute, 1983).
76. Prafulla Joglekar and Morton L. Paterson, "A Closer Look at the Returns and Risks of Pharmaceutical R&D," *Journal of Health Economics*, 5(2), June 1986: 175.
77. *Ibid.*
78. Louis Lasagna, "Who Will Adopt the Orphan Drugs?" *Regulation*, December 1979: 27–32.
79. As reported in Peltzman, *op. cit.*, p. 89.

80. Grabowski and Vernon, "Substitution Laws and Innovation in the Pharmaceutical Industry," *Law and Contemporary Problems*, 43(1), Spring 1979: 43–66.

81. *Ibid.*, p. 60.

82. A company may have more than one discrete manufacturing facility, *Fact Book* (Washington, D.C.: Pharmaceutical Manufacturers Association, 1980), p. 14. The General Accounting Office has estimated that the FDA must inspect 5,400 plants manufacturing drugs. Schwartzman, *Innovation in the Pharmaceutical Industry*, p. 24.

83. Schwartzman, *Innovation in the Pharmaceutical Industry*, p. 328.

84. Telephone conversation on February 5, 1987 with Dr. Charles Anello, Deputy Director, Office of Epidemiology and Biostatistics, Food and Drug Administration, Rockville, MD.

85. For a more complete set of suggestions for public policy in this area, see Wardell and Lasagna, *op. cit.*, Chapter 13. See also, Henry G. Grabowski and John M. Vernon, *The Regulation of Pharmaceuticals*, (Washington, D.C.: American Enterprise Institute, 1983), pp. 63–73.

86. Wardell and Lasagna, *op. cit.*, p. 164.

87. "FDA Approval of New Drugs Is Speedier, but More Progress Is Needed, GAO Says," *Wall Street Journal*, September 16, 1981.

88. John F. Geweke and Burton A. Weisbrod, "Some Economic Consequences of Technological Advance in Medical Care: The Case of the New Drug," in Robert B. Helms, ed., *Drugs and Health* (Washington, D.C.: American Enterprise Institute, 1981).

CHAPTER 18

The Political Economy of Health Care

INTRODUCTION (1)

A number of studies have been conducted to evaluate the effectiveness of federal subsidy programs in the medical care sector. An examination of federal manpower subsidies to increase the number of dentists found that an equivalent number of dental visits could have been produced, at less than one-tenth the cost, if the federal subsidies had been provided in a different manner, namely, if the wages of dental auxiliaries had been subsidized (2). Evaluations of the federal Nurse Training Act revealed that an increase in the number of employed registered nurses could have been achieved at between one-fifth and one-tenth the cost had an alternative approach been used; if a wage subsidy were provided to registered nurses, their participation rate would have increased (see Chapter 16). These analyses of federal manpower subsidy programs have questioned the justification offered for such programs, which were based on health manpower/population ratios to indicate a "need" or "shortage." The method used to distribute the subsidy funds (i.e., to educational institutions), was also questionable. A possible conclusion is that further economic analysis is needed if governmental programs are to be cost-effective. The assumption is that with additional information, policymakers would generate better legislation. However, another interpretation is that the resulting legislation is actually what was intended. Under this hypothesis the participants in the legislative process are assumed to be rational and to be aware of the effects of proposed legislation. If the resulting legislation is not cost effective, it is because it was not meant to be.

An examination of the beneficiaries of such legislation lends support to this hypothesis. The major beneficiaries of health manpower legislation were the health professional schools, since they were the recipients of the vast majority of the distributed funds.

If the outcome of legislation is the result intended, then to predict legislative outcomes it becomes necessary to have a model, not of the most cost-effective approach to achieving the stated objectives of the legislation, but rather of the supply and demand for legislation (see the references in Chapter 11). Within this economic framework of legislative outcomes, the supplier of legislation is the legislature, the particular legislative subcommittee with jurisdiction over the issue having the most influence. Legislators are willing to supply legislation in return for political support, that is, campaign funds, volunteers for helping in their reelection campaign, or simply votes. Legislators require political support if they are to be reelected, which is assumed to be their goal.

The demanders of legislative benefits are those organized groups, such as health associations, that seek legislative benefits for their members. Health interest organizations demand legislation because it benefits their members. The demand for legislation by these interest groups, which is an indication of how much a group would be willing to "pay" for those legislative benefits (in terms of campaign funds and so on), depends upon what benefits the legislation provides beyond the legislative benefits the members of the group already possess. The cost of obtaining these legislative benefits, as determined by the direct monetary and nonmonetary outlays necessary to achieve them, depends, among other things, on the action of other interested parties to that legislation. The greater the adverse effect of the legislation upon other interest groups, the greater will be their willingness to "pay" to forestall or defeat the proposed legislation, which in turn increases the cost of having such legislation passed. The cost of obtaining the legislation may well exceed the positive benefits to members of a group favoring the legislation, in which case they will be unsuccessful in achieving their legislative program.

There are a number of other participants in the legislative process; industry and unions may be demanders of health legislation, since they would be affected in their costs of production and in number of workers employed or wages paid. The executive branch of government proposes new programs to receive popular political support so as to increase its own reelection prospects. The executive branch also has responsibility for the government budget and therefore has a concentrated interest in legislation that increases the overall budget. Government agencies are also suppliers of legislative benefits; such agencies require political support so as to increase their budgets, thereby justifying larger salaries.

This chapter examines the legislative behavior of only one of the participants in the legislative process: the health interest groups (3). The reason for selecting them is that in the past much of the health legislation at both state and federal levels has been strongly influenced by these groups. In fact, the structure of our health care system is, in many respects, the result of legislative activity by these health associations. Health interest groups often provide the only testimony on legislation; their positions are well publicized and are presented as being synonymous with that of the public interest. All legislation is complex and requires knowledgeable persons to understand it. In the past the public has been inclined to believe that health legislation is best understood by health professionals and therefore has been willing to accept the politics of health as espoused by health professionals. A simple example of this point was President Ford's veto of the Nurse Training Act, which was overridden by Congress. Health professionals decried President Ford's action. Given the limited analysis in the media of the reasons for that veto, Congress believed that it was on safe political grounds in overriding it.

The impact of health interest groups has been enormous. One example is Medicare. Medicare was expected to cost $2 billion a year; it is now over $80 billion a year. Had Medicare and other health legislation been written in a different fashion—less to the liking of the health interest groups—health expenditures would undoubtedly have risen at a slower pace. The massive redistribution of income from patients and taxpayers to health professionals during this period is an indication of the legislative success of health professionals.

The belief that legislation can confer large monetary benefits to interest groups is not new. Nearly 200 years ago, in *The Federalist*, James Madison expressed this idea (4). The reason special-interest legislation is enacted is that the economic interests of producers are concentrated, while the interests of consumers are diffused over many areas of economic activity. The benefits to special-interest groups from legislation are potentially so large as to provide them with ample incentive to secure legislation on their behalf. The cost to each consumer from special-interest-group legislation is relatively small, since the costs are spread over a great many consumers. The proponents of such legislation are rarely so bold as to admit that their incomes will be increased by imposing what is the equivalent of a tax on all consumers of their products. Instead, such legislation is presented as being in the public's or country's interests.

Whereas producers often receive their entire incomes from the products they produce, consumers rarely spend more than a small portion of their income on any one product; thus their economic interests are considered diffuse. Further, for consumers to learn of the special-interest legislation that is being proposed, to ascertain the effects of such legislation on the prices they must pay for the affected products, and to inform other consumers and mobilize them against such legislation is clearly more costly to the consumer than any monetary benefits that would be derived from having the legislation defeated.

In the health services industry, as with other industries, consumers on the average spend a small portion of their incomes on medical care, approximately 10 percent. Because expenditures for medical care are a relatively small percentage of consumers' incomes, it is to their advantage to allocate their time and efforts to other activities that have a greater impact on their budgets and incomes. State practice acts, which define the tasks to be performed by different health professionals and set the requirements for licensure and state appropriations for medical, dental, and other health professional educational institutions are policy decisions that would appear to consumers to be too remote to affect their pocketbook. For health professionals, however, health legislation determines almost all of their income. Therefore, it is in their interests to be involved in the legislative process; they are willing to contribute money and time to political campaigns, testify at legislative hearings, and provide information to legislators and the public on their positions.

THE DEMAND FOR LEGISLATION BY HEALTH ASSOCIATIONS

To gain a better understanding of the type of health legislation that exists in this country, it is necessary to develop a model of the demand for legislation by health interest groups. Such a framework should indicate the type of legislation that different health associations would favor or oppose. If the framework presented is a fairly accurate predictor of the political behavior of different health associations, it should also be possible to anticipate future legislative changes and the form that such legislation might take. The political behavior of two types of health associations will be examined: first, those health associations that represent the interests of health manpower professions, namely the American Medical Association, the American Dental Association, and the American Nurses' Association, and second, those associations that represent nonprofit providers, namely, the American Hospital Association, the Blue Cross Association, the Association of American Medical Colleges, and the American Association of Dental Schools.

A framework of the demand for legislation will be presented to describe the specific types of health legislation that the various health associations desire. The necessity for having a framework is twofold: (a) it is not possible merely to state that health associations act in their own interests without first defining their interests, and (b) a model is required to indicate how particular legislation works to achieve those interests. Without such a framework it is not always obvious how legislation promotes the interests of the health associations. The test of the validity of the proposed approach is how accurately the proposed framework predicts the political positions of the health associations. Finally, the implications of such a framework for explaining the political behavior of health associations with regard to the structure, organization, and financing of medical care are presented.

DEFINITION OF HEALTH ASSOCIATION MEMBERS' SELF-INTEREST

The predictions made by the economic framework are based on the premise that the health association will demand legislation according to the self-interest of its members. It is thus necessary to define more precisely the self-interest of the different health associations to be analyzed.

Once the economic interests of health association members are defined it will be possible to demonstrate how particular legislation works to enhance their member's interests. The validity of the proposed framework can be tested by how well it predicts the political positions of the various health associations. Without a definition of interests and a legislative framework, it would not be obvious how specific legislation promotes the economic interest of the members of a health association. The final section of this chapter discusses the implications of the political behavior of health associations on the financing, quality, and organization of the health care delivery system.

Health professionals and health organizations, such as hospitals, have many goals. Even within the same profession, individuals place different weights on what they perceive to be their self-interest. The tendency, therefore, is to make the definition of self-interest complex. However, if the definition of self-interest is complex, encompassing this diversity, or if different motivations are specified for each piece of legislation, it is not possible to develop a good predictive model. Although it may seem more realistic to develop a complex goal statement, it is easier to evaluate the effects of legislation using a simple one. Besides, unless the membership easily understands the goal that its association is pursuing, the members may be distressed over the activities the association pursues with their dues. The true test of whether the simply defined goal accurately measures the member's self-interest is how well it predicts the association's legislative behavior.

The legislative goal of associations with individuals as members, such as physicians, dentists, nurses, optometrists, and so on, is assumed to be to *maximize the incomes of its current members*. Health professionals are no different from other individuals; they will say that they have many goals, of which income is only one.

However, income is the only goal that all the members have in common. (Goals such as increased autonomy and control over their practice are highly correlated with increased incomes. Income is thus a more general goal.)

The goals or "self-interest" of the associations representing nonprofit institutions, such as hospitals, Blue Cross, and medical and dental schools, are different from those of the health professional associations, since such institutions cannot retain profits. Medical and dental schools are assumed to be interested in maximizing the prestige of their institution. Prestige for a medical school is defined as having students who wish to become professors and researchers themselves, a faculty that is primarily interested in research, and a low student/faculty ratio. Little prestige accrues to a medical school that trains students to enter family practice or to practice in underserved areas.

In the past, hospitals were also interested in maximizing their prestige. Prestige for a hospital is its size and number of facilities and services. Hospitals were reimbursed according to their costs and patients had little incentive to shop for the least expensive hospital. Approximately 90 percent of hospital care was reimbursed, on behalf of the patient, by the government or by private insurance. Hospitals faced few constraints to achieving their goals. The availability of a full range of services made it easier for the hospital to attract physicians to its staff. Administrators of large prestigious hospitals were held in esteem by their peers; they were also able to earn higher incomes. Each hospital attempted to become a medical center.

Beginning in the early 1980s, hospital objectives began to change. The payment system for hospital care went from cost-based reimbursement to fixed prices; low-cost substitutes for hospitals, such as outpatient surgery centers, began to reduce hospital utilization, as did utilization control programs. As these changes occurred, hospitals became more concerned with survival than with emulating major teaching institutions. Even teaching hospitals began to act as though their future was in doubt. Hospitals began to minimize their costs, dropped money losing services and patients, and gave greater consideration to the profitability of their investments. To be successful in a more competitive environment, hospitals acted as though they were interested in maximizing their profits.

Blue Cross and Blue Shield plans were originally started by hospitals and physicians, respectively. Hospitals provided the initial capital to Blue Cross plans and controlled the organization. The same was true for medical societies and Blue Shield plans. It was not until the 1970s that these nonprofit organizations separated from the providers that controlled them. Until recently, therefore, the objectives of Blue Cross and Blue Shield plans were to serve their providers' interests.

During the period when Blue Cross and Blue Shield were controlled by their respective providers, their methods of provider payment and their benefit structure were in accordance with hospital and physician economic interests. These policies also coincided with these organizations' own interests. Nonprofit organizations want to grow. A larger organization provides management with greater responsibility, which justifies higher incomes for management. Like any nonprofit bureaucracy, these organizations also have some form of satisficing behavior as a goal: namely, extra personnel, larger facilities, and higher wages than if these organizations were in a very competitive industry.

As the health care sector became more competitive in the early 1980s, competition between Blue Cross and Blue Shield plans and commercial insurance companies increased. To survive in this new marketplace, Blue Cross and Blue Shield plans began to merge with one another (BCBS). Although these organizations remained nonprofit, their behavior became similar to for-profit insurance companies. By attempting to minimize costs, increase market share, and respond to employer demands on benefit design, BCBS acted as though they were attempting to maximize profits. An adversarial relationship began to replace BCBS's previously cooperative association with hospitals and physicians. In analyzing the legislative behavior of BCBS plans, it is important to keep in mind the periods when their objectives differed.

Although differences existed in the objectives of health associations representing health professionals, hospitals, medical and dental schools, and Blue Cross and Blue Shield plans, the members of these associations all tried to make as much money as possible. They would then retain it for themselves, as was the case with health professionals, or expend it to achieve prestige goals, as for hospitals and medical schools. The incomes of employees of prestigious institutions are likely to exceed those in less prestigious institutions. Thus the objective underlying the demand for legislation is the same for each of the health associations. Each health association attempts to achieve for its members through legislation what cannot be achieved through a competitive market, namely, a monopoly position. Increased monopoly power and the ability to price as a monopolist seller of services was, and is, the best way for them to achieve their goals.

A FRAMEWORK FOR ANALYZING LEGISLATIVE BEHAVIOR

There are five types of legislation that health associations demand on behalf of their members. Four of these increase revenues; the fifth decreases their members' costs. Legislation to increase revenues (a) increases the demand for the members' services, (b) enables the providers to charge the highest possible price for their services, (c) causes an increase in the price of services that substitute for those produced by the members, and (d) limits entry into the industry.

Legislative policies that lower the providers' cost of business are (a) subsidies (indirect) to reduce the providers' cost of producing their services, and (b) changes in state practice acts to allow for greater productivity of the inputs used in production. There are several caveats to this model. The model should predict an association's political position on legislation according to the earlier definition of its members' interests. However, it may occasionally be observed that the association takes a political position different than expected. Before concluding that the framework above is inaccurate, the following must be determined.

Is the association's preferred position no longer politically possible? No health association favors reexamination for licensure. Some of its members may not be able to pass the reexamination. If the examination is made sufficiently simple so that all members can pass, nonmembers would claim they should be allowed to enter the profession since they can pass the examination. If there is a great deal of pressure from the media, for example, for reexamination, the profession may propose a less costly alternative, continuing education. The association would not normally propose continuing education, since it imposes some costs on its members. However, to forestall a more costly policy, the association comes out in favor of continuing education. Thus the association's policy on continuing education, while it is not its preferred position, is consistent with the model's predictions.

Another example where it may appear that the political position of an association diverges from its members' interests occurs when the cost of taking a position exceeds its potential benefits. The American Hospital Association's position on the applicability of minimum wage laws to hospital employees is such an example. Minimum wage laws increase the cost of labor to hospitals. For many years the AHA was successful in exempting hospitals from such legislation. As hospital wages began increasing, most hospital employees were receiving wages in excess of the minimum wage. Thus its applicability to hospitals would have had a small effect. When the removal of hospitals' exemption was once again proposed, the AHA decided not to oppose it. Not only would the effect have been small, but the AHA determined that the legislation would have passed over its objections. The AHA decided that it would be a needless loss of political capital to oppose it. Similarly, in more recent years, the American Medical Association has been muted in its opposition to certain legislation because of its concern that its continually negative position may be of greater cost to its members than any possible benefits to be derived from opposing the legislation.

Except for the caveats mentioned above, health associations are expected to act in accordance with their members' economic interests. The five types of legislation each association is expected to favor and oppose are based on the economic framework above.

Demand Increasing Legislation

An association favors demand-increasing legislation since an increase in demand, with a given supply, will result in an increase in price, an increase in total revenue, and consequently, an increase in incomes or net revenues.

The most obvious way of increasing the demand for the services of an association's members is to have the government subsidize the purchase of insurance for the provider's services. No health provider, however, wishes the government to insure all persons in the population, like the British National Health Service. Instead, the demand for insurance subsidies is always discussed in relation to specific population groups in society: those persons with low incomes. The reason for selective government subsidies is twofold: first, those persons with higher incomes presumably have private insurance coverage or can afford to purchase the provider's services. The greatest increase in demand would result from extending coverage to those currently unable to pay for those services. Second, extending government subsidies to those currently able to pay for these services would greatly increase the cost of the program to the government. A greater commitment of government expenditures would result in the government developing a concentrated interest in controlling the provider's prices, utilization, and expenditures. Thus when demand subsidies are requested, they are always in relation to specific population groups or services rather than for the population at large.[1]

Two examples of the foregoing approach were the AMA's position on national health insurance and Blue Shield. The AMA successfully defeated President Truman's national health insurance proposal in 1948 because subsidies would have been provided to all persons regardless of their income levels. The AMA's opposition to Medicare was also based on the fact that all aged, regardless of their income levels, were to

---

[1]Even when demand subsidies are requested for a particular population group, it is proposed that such subsidies be phased in gradually. If the increase in demand is too large, this might create dissatisfaction among the patients when there is a limited supply; prices and waiting times would increase rapidly, possibly resulting in pressure on the government to enter the market. The government might then attempt to fix prices or permit other providers to serve the newly enfranchised recipients.

be subsidized. The approach favored by the AMA was a system of tax credits for the purchase of health insurance, which would decline as a person's income rose.

When medical societies developed (and controlled) Blue Shield, Blue Shield only provided coverage for physician services (not for physician substitutes) and paid the physician's bill in full only if the patient's income was below a certain level (originally, $7,500 a year). A low-income person purchasing Blue Shield would increase their use of physician services and not be concerned with which physician had a lower price. If the subscriber's income exceeded $7,500, the physician could charge the patient an amount in addition to the Blue Shield payment. Higher-income patients could afford to pay more.

The American Dental Association's major demand-increasing effort has been to expand insurance coverage for dental services. Insurance is generally purchased for events that are not likely to occur, but if they occur, are very expensive, such as for hospital care and in-hospital physician services. Dental expenditures are relatively small, expected, and not catastrophic. Dental care is therefore not insurable in the same sense as hospital or surgical services; in fact, it is not really insurance but a form of forced savings.

If there were no special incentive to purchase dental insurance, most people would just pay for dental care when they need it. The use of dental services is also highly related to income (5). Thus a major reason for the growth in dental insurance has been the favorable tax treatment of employer paid health insurance premiums. Such contributions are not considered as part of the employee's income; the employee does not have to pay taxes on employer paid health benefits. During the 1970s when the demand for dental insurance grew rapidly, the top tax bracket was 70 percent. For a person in a high tax bracket, $1,000 of extra income was worth only $300 after taxes. However, if the employer used that $1,000 to purchase health insurance for the employee, the employee could receive $1,000 worth of health benefits. The tax laws provided a discount on the purchase of health benefits to high-income employees. The demand for dental insurance grew as more persons moved into higher tax brackets.

The exclusion of employer-paid health benefits from the employee's taxable income results in a large revenue loss to the government. It has been estimated that the federal government will lose $45 billion from this tax exclusion in 1987 (6). The beneficiaries of this tax exclusion are clearly those in the upper-income groups.

President Reagan proposed placing a "cap" on the amount of employer paid health benefits that are excluded from taxable income. The ADA's major legislative strategy in the last several years has been to defeat any such tax cap. If a tax cap were passed, employees would want less comprehensive health benefits; they would have to pay for additional benefits with after-tax dollars. The ADA believes, and rightly so, that if the tax discount for purchasing dental insurance were eliminated, the incentive for employees to purchase such insurance would decline. With less dental insurance, consumers would have to pay the full price of dental care. The demand for such care would decline and consumers would be more inclined to "shop" among dentists for the lowest price.

Other approaches used by the American Dental Association (ADA) to increase the demand for dental care involves proposing that all costs incurred for dental and medical expenses be tax deductible, lobbying to include dental benefits in federal employee's health benefits, permitting dependents of military personnel to have free choice of civilian dentists even though military dental clinics are available, including dental benefits as part of Medicare Part B, as well as lobbying for increased funding of dental benefits as part of state Medicaid programs, and promoting the inclusion of dental care as part of the benefits of health maintenance organizations (HMOs) (7).

The American Nurses' Association (ANA) has favored three types of demand-increasing legislation. The first are proposals that increase the demand for those institutions in which registered nurses work; two-thirds of nurses work in hospitals. Increased demand for hospital care results in increased demand for registered nurses (RNs). An example of such a demand-increasing program was favoring proposals for national health insurance. Insurance coverage for hospital care, however, is more extensive than for any other delivery settings. Nurse associations have therefore also favored other demand-increasing proposals such as requiring (for certification purposes) a minimum number of RNs in the staffing of nursing homes and home health agencies.

A third type of demand proposal favored by nurse associations is one that widens the nurse's role, that is, increases the number of tasks that nurses are legally able to perform. As the number of tasks that RNs are permitted to perform increases, so does their value to the organization. Nurses will be able to perform more remunerative tasks. As the nurse's value increases, there will be an increase in the demand for nurses, with a consequent increase in their incomes. Also, nurses that can be used more flexibly can perform the tasks that might have required the hiring of two different types of health professionals. As nurses try to increase their roles, they wage a struggle in the legislative marketplace to prevent other health professionals, such as licensed practical nurses, or physician's assistants from performing tasks previously reserved to the RN.

The health professional association that is successful in enabling its members to increase their role, while preventing other health professionals from encroaching upon their own tasks, will be able to increase the demand, hence incomes, of its members. Examples of the legislative conflict over state practice acts are the attempts by optometrists to increase their role at the expense of ophthalmologists, psychologists versus psychiatrists, obstetricians versus nurse midwives, and podiatrists versus orthopedic surgeons.

The major approach used by hospitals to increase the demand for their services was the establishment and control of Blue Cross by hospitals. When Blue Cross was started, Blue Cross only paid the costs of hospital care. Once a subscriber had such coverage, there was no additional out-of-pocket cost for using the hospital. As the price of hospital care became free to the subscriber, use of the hospital increased. Blue Cross then paid the hospital generously for those services.

The American Hospital Association also favored government subsidies to stimulate the demand for hospital services by the aged and the poor. Medicare, which provided generous hospital coverage for the aged, increased the demand for hospitals by a high-user group with generally low incomes. Hospitals are currently in the forefront of lobbying efforts to receive federal subsidies for "uncompensated care," that is, the provision of hospital care to the poor for which they are not reimbursed.

Previously, Blue Cross and Blue Shield were supportive of the AHA's and the AMA's legislative proposals. It was in the interest of the AHA and AMA, as well as in Blue Cross and Blue Shield's own interest, that these organizations become the intermediaries under any government program to increase the demand for hospitals' and physicians' services. Hospitals and physicians preferred to be paid by Blue Cross and Blue Shield rather than directly by the government. The government was less likely to become directly involved with hospitals' costs. This legislative strategy was also favored by the Blues. Becoming an intermediary meant increased revenues, greater financial responsibility, larger staffs, and consequently higher salaries for the managers.

The Association of American Medical Colleges (AAMC) tactic to increase the demand for medical schools has been to demand legislation, at both the state and the federal levels, that would provide schools with unrestricted operating subsidies. Such subsidies would enable the schools to set tuition levels that are greatly below the actual costs of education. With artificially low tuition levels, the schools would experience an excess demand for their spaces by prospective applicants. The same is true for a dental education. As long as there is an excess demand for a medical education—and the schools do not willingly expand their spaces to satisfy this excess demand—the schools can determine the type of educational curriculum that comes closest to meeting their (and the AMA's or ADA's) preferences.

If there were no excess demand for a medical education, the schools would have to respond, that is, compete for applicants, as would any other supplier, by providing the type of service that demanders were willing to pay. Unless it was possible to maintain excess demand, the schools (and the health professional associations that originally controlled the schools) would not have been able to determine the type of educational system for medicine and dentistry in this country. These schools have a monopoly over the provision of medical and dental education. By charging tuition levels that were so low as to encourage excess demand for such an education, the schools are able to select the type of students they prefer. The schools are thereby able to establish the training times and educational requirements for entering the profession. These policies are also in the economic interest of physicians and dentists since their incomes are higher than they would be otherwise.

Securing the Highest Method of Reimbursement:

Regardless of whether the association member's goal is income, prestige, or growth, the method by which the provider is reimbursed is crucial to attainment of that goal. High prices, resulting in large net revenues, increase incomes and enable institutions to achieve their objectives through the expenditure of those revenues. The method of reimbursement, or the method by which the providers can charge for their services, has been crucial to understanding provider economic behavior.

Two basic approaches have been used by health associations to achieve the highest possible reimbursement for their members. The first has been to try and eliminate any price competition among their members. The ability to engage in price competition is more important to the new practitioner or firm entering an area. A new competitor must be able to let potential patients know they are available and must be able to offer them an incentive to attract them away from established providers.

To prevent price competition from occurring, health associations have termed the elements of price competition, such as advertising and fee splitting, as "unethical behavior" and have prohibited such behavior in their state practice acts (8). The medical and dental professions used strong sanctions against practitioners who engaged in unethical behavior. A physician could have his or her license suspended and be assessed financial penalties. Previously, medical societies were able to deny hospital privileges to physicians who advertised or engaged in price competition (9). Without hospital privileges a physician could not offer patients a complete medical service. Since new physicians in an area had the greatest incentive to engage in such "unethical" behavior, they were given probationary membership in the local medical society. They were thereby placed on notice that they could lose their hospital privileges if they engaged in such behavior.

A number of studies have shown that restrictions on advertising raise the price of optometric services from 20 to 50 percent (10). (Most of the studies on advertising in the health field have been conducted on prescription drugs and optometric services.) The American Optometric Association has claimed (without offering evidence) that higher prices reflect higher-quality services. The Federal Trade Commission (in 1980) attempted to resolve the issue of quality and advertising. The FTC used seven persons with similar visual conditions in their study, who were then trained at two optometric schools with regard to the components of an optometric exam. When these seven subjects went to specified optometrists, they recorded the price charged, the amount of time spent by the optometrist, and specific information on the tests and procedures performed by the optometrist. These subjects went to cities where advertising was prohibited as well as to cities permitting advertising. In cities that permitted advertising, they went to optometrists who advertised as well as to those who did not (11).

The conclusions of the study were that removal of advertising restrictions by the optometric societies would cause prices to decline by more than 20 percent; further, that nonadvertising optometrists *in markets where advertising occurs* provide service of superior quality than optometrists in nonadvertising markets. Optometrists who do not advertise (in markets where other optometrists advertise) compete by lowering their price—but not by as much as optometrists who advertise—and by spending more time with their patients. Thus optometric services are lower in price and, on average, higher in quality where advertising is permitted compared to where it is prohibited.

Price competition and advertising are not necessarily related to the provision of low-quality services. Defining such practices as unethical could only be interpreted as a means of preventing price competition.

As a result of the Federal Trade Commission's successful suit against the AMA (and upheld by the Supreme Court in 1982), state medical (and other professional) societies can no longer penalize and thereby prevent physicians from advertising. All professionals, such as dentists and lawyers, are now permitted to advertise. The AMA, ADA, and other professions that are regulated at the state level, tried to have Congress grant them an exception from the FTC's jurisdiction but were unsuccessful. Anticompetitive behavior in health care is now subject to antitrust laws.

The second approach used by health providers to secure the highest possible payment for their services is to engage in price discrimination. Price discrimination means charging different patients or payors different prices. These different prices are not a result of differences in costs (since it would be the same type of operation) but because the patients and/or their payors have different abilities to pay. Charging according to ability to pay results in greater revenues than a pricing system that charges everyone the same price.

The desire by organized medicine to maintain a system whereby physicians could price discriminate has influenced the financing and delivery of medical services for many years. Once medical insurance began being introduced, organized medicine attempted to retain the physician's ability to price discriminate. For example, when medical societies started Blue Shield plans, an income limit was included. Physicians were able to charge higher-income patients an amount in addition to the Blue Shield payment. The Blue Shield income limits were eventually eliminated as subscriber incomes rose. The Blue Shield benefit was not worth as much to a high-income person if they had to pay a significant amount each time they went to the physician, in addition to the annual premium. As Blue Shield organizations dropped the income limits so as to be able to enroll more high-income subscribers, some medical societies dropped their sponsorship of the Blue Shield plans.

To maintain their ability to price discriminate, physicians could decide when they wanted to participate in Blue Shield and when they wanted to charge the patient directly. In the latter case, the patient would then receive payment from Blue Shield for an amount less than the physician's charge. For persons with higher incomes, physicians would charge the patient directly, which would provide them with a higher payment than if the physician participated in Blue Shield.[2]

Payment of physicians under Medicare was based on the same principle. Physicians could decide to participate in Medicare on a case-by-case basis. If they thought they could make more money by charging the patient directly, they would do so. By having the option of participating when they want to, physicians are assured of payment from low-income persons, while still being able to charge a higher price to the higher-income patient. The method of pricing and flexibility of physician participation under Blue Shield and Medicare was crucial to their acceptance of these plans.[3]

The concern by physicians with their ability to price discriminate has limited the growth of prepaid health plans. Health maintenance organizations (HMOs) charge patients the same premium regardless of their income levels. If fee-for-service physicians charge higher-income patients a higher fee, then a plan that charges all persons the same premium is a form of price competition; it limits the physician's ability to price discriminate.

In his classic article, "Price Discrimination in Medicine," Kessel describes how county and state medical societies attempted to forestall the development of prepaid group plans (12). When physicians moved into an area with the intention of joining a prepaid plan, local medical societies prevented these physicians from receiving hospital privileges. Unless the plan had its own hospitals, which was unlikely, this medical society behavior effectively eliminated competition from the prepaid plan. There were several successful antitrust suits against medical societies for this behavior.[4] (Such suits are, however, costly to bring and take years to resolve.) Medical societies were subsequently successful in securing restrictive legislation at a state level that effectively limited the growth of these plans. For example, one such restrictive statute permitted only the medical profession to control and operate such plans. In 1976, Blue Shield of Spokane, Washington, agreed to discontinue their practice of discriminating against physicians who offered their services through a health maintenance organization. Blue Shield ended its boycott only after the FTC ordered it to do so on grounds that it was anticompetitive.

The federal government recently offered to pay HMOs a fixed price for Medicare patients. If HMOs sign up Medicare patients, they are reimbursed according to a per-

---

[2]Currently, Pennsylvania Blue Shield (PBS) is engaged in a lawsuit with the Pennsylvania Dental Association (PDA). PBS charges that the PDA has boycotted its dental plan because PBS will not allow dentists to "balance bill" its subscribers (i.e., charge patients an amount above the PBS payment).

[3]The physician's fee for Medicare, Blue Shield, and private-pay patients is supposed to be the same. The fee is based on the physician's "usual, customary, and reasonable" fee. Blue Shield and Medicare maintain the physician's fee schedules in their computers. However, Blue Shield pays physicians' fees if they are under a certain percentile limit and Medicare has for a number of years limited the annual increase in physicians' fees. Therefore, the physician's fee to a private patient is usually higher than the fee paid by Medicare and Blue Shield.

[4]Group Health Association in Washington, D.C., was one such case cited in the Kessel article.

centage of the average area cost of the combined amounts of Parts A and B of Medicare. If HMOs can provide care for less than that amount, they may keep the difference. This approach increases the choice available to the Medicare patient. To attract Medicare patients from the fee-for-service system, HMOs offer additional benefits. The AMA has opposed this approach and attempted to delay its implementation.

Dental societies have acted similarly with respect to advertising and price competition. Until the successful FTC suit, dental societies also included bans on advertising in their state practice acts. Since the FTC suit, a number of cases have been brought against dental societies for their failure to eliminate anticompetitive behavior. Certain dental societies have prohibited advertisements on quality, prohibited practice by a dentist under a trade name (which would adversely affect corporate dental chains), and placed restrictions on prepaid dental plans (13).

An important legislative activity of some dental societies has been to prohibit dentists from being included as part of any preferred provider organizations (PPOs). PPOs are organizations that offer services to employers, such as physicians, hospitals, or dentists, at a price that is generally below the prevailing price in the area. An employer or a union that agrees to use only the providers in the PPO hopes to achieve a savings on their health care costs. Providers that are not part of the PPO do not have access to the PPO's patient population. PPOs are a form of price competition. By legislatively attempting to limit PPOs from offering dental services, dental societies are attempting to limit price competition.

Dental societies have proposed other methods of limiting competition from PPOs and HMOs. The ADA's House of Delegates has proposed that legislation be sought to ensure that all patients have free choice of dentist and that any licensed dentist be allowed to participate in a prepayment plan. Such legislation, if enacted, would prevent PPOs and HMOs from selecting dentists according to their criteria; competition from these plans would be eliminated. If such plans are not in violation of the antitrust statutes, why is further legislation necessary to protect the public?

To protect dentists' ability to charge what the market would bear, the ADA has favored dental insurance but not the use of fee schedules by the insurer. The ADA has proposed that the dentist charge the patient and be reimbursed by the patient, with the patient in turn being reimbursed by the insurer. In this manner the dentist would be able to raise his or her price. There is currently an antitrust suit by Pennsylvania Blue Shield (PBS) against the Pennsylvania Dental Association (PDA) on a similar matter. PBS alleges a boycott by the PDA because PBA's dental plan pays the dentist according to their usual and customary fee. The PDA wants to be able to charge the patient an additional amount if they desire.

The ADA has also opposed the practice of insurance companies reimbursing a patient a lower amount if they go to a nonparticipating dentist. The ADA has called for legislation to prohibit insurance companies from this payment approach. (The dentist is not prohibited from participating with the insurance company. However, they would prefer not to participate, to receive the same amount as participating dentists, as well as to be able to charge the patient an additional amount.)

The American Nurses Association (ANA) is also attempting to use the fee-for-service approach, which has been used with such success by physicians, dentists, and other health professionals. Registered nurses are striving to become independent practitioners, such as nurse practitioners and nurse midwives, who will then be able to bill the patient on a fee-for-service basis. The ANA has attempted to secure such direct reimbursement for nurses through government programs, such as Medicare. Fee-for-service payment to a health professional, which in most cases is reimbursed by the government or private insurance, is the most direct route for health professionals to increase their income.

Another legislative approach being pursued by the ANA to raise the incomes of its members is to require the concept of "comparable worth" to be used for setting nurses' wages (14). Equal pay for equal work has already been enacted into law. Proponents of comparable worth go beyond that; they want equal pay for work of comparable value. If a registered nurse does work that is comparable in value to that of an electrician or a family physician, the nurse should receive a comparable (the same) income (15). Comparable-worth proponents seek to substitute fact-finding commissions for the marketplace, since the marketplace determines wages through the forces of supply and demand. The only way in which comparable worth can be implemented is to legislate it. The ANA is lobbying for the passage of comparable worth legislation at both the state and federal levels.

The American Hospital Association (AHA) has favored two concepts in the design of payment systems for its member hospitals. The first is to eliminate any incentive for hospitals to engage in price competition. When hospitals started Blue Cross, Blue Cross plans were required to offer a service benefit plan to their subscribers. A service benefit provides the hospitalized patient with services rather than dollars, which is characteristic of an indemnity plan. By guaranteeing payment to the hospital for the services used by the patient, the service benefit policy removes any incentive the patient (or the hospital) may have regarding the cost of the hospitalization. Since the patient does not have to make any out-of-pocket payments, the prospective patient has no disincentive to enter the most expensive hospital, which may or may not be the highest-quality hospital. Under a service benefit policy, hospitals cannot compete for patients on the basis of price. When Medicare was started, the method of Medicare reimbursement to hospitals (based on each hospital's costs plus 2 percent) also provided no incentive for patients to select less costly, more efficient, hospitals.

The second concept underlying hospitals' preferred method of payment is to be able to engage in price discrimination, that is, to be able to charge different payors different prices. Hospitals prefer several different payors rather than one major purchaser for their services. With multiple payors, hospitals can charge each payor a separate price, based on willingness to pay. An example of this strategy is hospital charges to Blue Cross patients as compared to what commercial insurers, government, and self-pay patients are charged. Hospitals gave Blue Cross a 20 percent discount. This discount enabled Blue Cross to offer a more expensive policy (a service benefit) that was in hospitals' interest. The discount was also a competitive advantage for Blue Cross and enabled them to increase their market share over the commercial companies.

Hospitals did very well financially under the initial Medicare payment policy. The government was very anxious for hospitals to participate in Medicare and therefore accepted much of the AHA's payment proposals. Not only were hospitals able to negotiate a 2 percent addition to their costs of serving Medicare patients and receive favorable treatment for depreciating their assets, but the manner in which hospital costs were calculated gave hospitals additional payment. Hospitals were not able to separate the actual costs of serving Medicare patients from their other patients. The method used to calculate Medicare costs was to use the ratio of what hospitals charge for Medicare patients to the charges for non-Medicare patients. That ratio was then used to determine the portion of the hospitals' total costs that should be paid for by Medicare. The effect of this policy was to provide hospitals with an incentive to raise charges on those services used predominately by the elderly, such as bed rails. By raising the proportion of their charges for the aged, a greater portion of the hospitals costs were paid for by the government. The hospital would then be able to make a higher profit on its charges to commercial insurance companies.

As Medicare began to reduce the amount it paid to hospitals over the years, the AHA proposed to the Congress (in 1982) that hospitals be able to decide each year whether or not they wanted to accept Medicare payment as payment in full for service provided to a Medicare patient. If a hospital decided that it did not want to take Medicare patients "on assignment," the hospital could charge the Medicare patient an additional amount. This approach would have enabled hospitals to price discriminate; higher-income aged could be charged more than lower-income aged. In rejecting this approach, the Congress was concerned with the political reaction of the elderly.

Another method by which hospitals were able to use price discrimination was to set a higher price/cost ratio for those services where there was a greater willingness to pay, that is, services that are less price elastic. Ancillary services, such as lab tests and x-rays, had higher price/cost ratios than the hospital's basic room charge. Once a patient was hospitalized, they had little choice as to the use or price of ancillary services. Patients who paid part of the hospital bill themselves could, before they entered a particular hospital, more easily compare charges for obstetric services and room rates to other hospitals. The charges for these services were much closer to their costs.

Medical and dental schools, as discussed above, seek unrestricted federal and state subsidies rather than charging their students the full cost of their education. Charging tuition that is below the actual costs of education and limiting the number of admissions results in an excess demand for an education.

The method by which medical and dental schools receive their subsidies is also very important. Subsidies go directly to the school, as do government funds to be distributed for loans and scholarships. Under this arrangement, the student receives a subsidy (tuition less than costs) only by attending a subsidized school. This method requires that students compete for medical and dental schools. If government subsidies went directly to the student for use at a medical or dental school, the schools would have to compete for students. As with subsidies, medical and dental schools prefer to distribute loans and scholarships themselves rather than having students apply directly to the government for such financial assistance. If the students received the subsidies and loans directly, they would have an incentive to shop among medical and dental schools according to their tuition rates and reputations. The current system provides a competitive advantage to schools receiving subsidies over other schools.

The methods used by health professionals and health institutions for pricing their services has enabled these providers to maximize their revenues. The health associations representing each of these provider groups have, in negotiating with the government, in establishing their own insurance organizations, and in proposing legislation, had a clear appreciation for which pricing strategies are in their members' economic interest. As a result, it is difficult to believe that the distinction between profit and not for profit has any meaning with regard to which group can provide its services at a lower price.

Legislation to Reduce the Price and/or Increase the Quantity of Complements

A registered nurse may be a substitute or a complement to the physician. It is difficult to determine when an input, such as a nurse, is a complement or a substitute based only on the task performed. A nurse may be as competent as a physician to perform certain tasks. If the nurse works for the physician and the physician receives the fee for the performance of that task, the nurse has increased the physician's productivity and is a complement. If, however, the nurse performs the same task and is a nurse practitioner billing independently of the physician, the nurse is a substitute for the physician providing that service. The essential element in determining whether an input is a complement or a substitute is who receives the payment for the services provided by that input. Whoever receives the payment controls the use of that input.

The state practice acts are the legal basis for determining which tasks each health profession can perform and under whose direction health professionals must work. A major legislative activity for each health association is to ensure that the state practice acts work to their members' interests. Health associations that represent complements (e.g., nurses, denturists, etc.) attempt to have their members become substitutes. Health associations whose members control complements seek to retain the status quo.

In the past, almost all of the health professions and health institutions were complements to the physician. That situation is now changing. The physician is no longer the sole entry point to the delivery of medical services. Hospitals and HMOs try and attract their own patients and subscribers. These organizations may then use nurse practitioners and salaried physicians to serve those patients. Other health professions (e.g., nurse midwives) are similarly seeking to be able to practice independently from physicians.

Providers can receive greater incomes if an increase in demand for their services is met through greater productivity than through an increase in the number of competing providers. The providers' income can be increased still further if their productivity increases are subsidized and they do not have to pay the full cost of increasing their productivity.

The following are several examples of legislation that subsidize providers' productivity. The American Hospital Association lobbied for passage of the Nurse Training Act in the belief that federal subsidies to increase the supply of RNs (through educational subsidies) would increase the supply of RNs available to hospitals. With a larger supply of nurses, nurses' wages would be lower than they would otherwise have been. For similar reasons, the AHA favored educational subsidies to increase the supply of allied health professionals. The AHA was a strong proponent of the Hill-Burton program, which provided capital subsidies to modernize hospitals. The AHA opposed legislation that would have increased the cost of inputs to hospitals. It opposed the extension of minimum-wage legislation to hospital employees and has called for a moratorium on the separate licensing of each health professional. (Separate licensing limits the hospital's ability to substitute different health professionals in the tasks they perform and to use such personnel in a more flexible manner.) Conversely, separate licensing is demanded by each health professional association so as to increase the demand for its members' services by restricting the tasks that other professions can perform.

More recently, the AHA has expressed opposition to proposals for a flat-rate income tax. A flat-rate tax would reduce marginal tax brackets by eliminating a number of deductions. The AHA was concerned that any elimination of the charitable contribution might affect hospitals adversely. The AHA was also concerned that lowering income tax brackets would make hospital's tax-exempt bond financing less attractive to investors.

The AMA also favored subsidies to hospitals. When a patient demands a treatment for a medical problem, the physician decides on the combination of resources and settings to use in the provision of that treatment. Hospital care was often the most costly component of that treatment. Before hospital insurance was so widespread, the physician was concerned over the cost of hospital care. The more the patient paid for hospital care, the less there would be available to pay for the physician's services. Similarly, the AMA favored subsidies to increase the supply of nurses, since it lowered the hospitals' costs of inputs. The AMA has, however, opposed the increased educational standards that the ANA wanted to impose on nursing institutions as a condition for receiving funds under the Nurse Training Act. Higher educational standards for nurses do not necessarily increase the productivity of nurses, but they do limit the supply of nurses and increase the nurses' qualifications to be a physician substitute for some tasks.

The AMA has favored internship and residency programs in hospitals. Interns and residents are excellent complements for physicians; they can take care of the physician's hospitalized patients and relieve the physician from serving in the hospital emergency room and from being on call at the hospital. The more advanced the resident is, the closer the resident is to being a potential substitute to the physician. Residents, however, are complements since it is the physician who bills for the service, not the resident. For this reason the AMA has favored the use of foreign medical graduates to serve as interns and residents. Once interns and residents graduate, however, they become substitutes to existing practitioners. The AMA has therefore favored the return of foreign medical graduates to their home country once their residencies are completed. [The AMA advocated a time limit on how long FMGs can remain in the United States as well as enforcement of the requirement that FMGs leave the country for two years before returning (16).] The AMA has also favored increased training times for U.S. medical graduates. Not only do longer training times increase the time each graduate serves as a complement but also delay the time when they become competitors.

A telling example of the AMA's attitude toward new health professionals was its position on the physician's assistant (PA). If PAs were to practice independently, they would be a substitute to some physicians (family practitioners). Thus the main concern of the AMA toward emerging health professionals was to ensure that these types of personnel become complements, not substitutes, to the physician. Thus whether there is direct or indirect supervision of the PA by the physician is less important to the AMA's political position than who gets the fee for their service.

Another important determinant of the AMA's position toward the introduction of PAs was whether or not PAs would create excess capacity among physicians in the community. Excess capacity causes increased competition among physicians for patients. If physicians faced insufficient demand for their services, then increased productivity, through the introduction of new types of personnel, would make it even more difficult for those physicians that would like to be busier. Indicative of this concern by its membership was the AMA's 1972 recommendation that all states enact legislation that would empower state boards of medical examiners to approve, *on an individual basis*, a given physician's request to employ a physician assistant and the proposed functions to be performed by that PA (17). Unless there was sufficient demand per physician in an area, permission to use a PA would not be granted, regardless of the PA's training.

Particularly during the late 1950s, 1960s, and early 1970s, when demand for physicians and dentists were increasing, state practice acts were relaxed to permit greater delegation of tasks. As excess capacity among physicians and dentists increased in the 1980s, medical and dental societies began to oppose further delegation of tasks (e.g., expanded function dental auxiliaries) and are likely to try and limit productivity increases. Growth in productivity among health professionals was related more to demand conditions facing physicians and dentists than to the competency of the new personnel to perform the tasks for which they were trained.

The latest legislative attempt by physicians and dentists to lower the cost of their inputs has been action at both the federal and state levels to limit increases in malpractice premiums. There are many reasons why malpractice premiums have risen in cost (18). One important reason, however, is incompetent physicians. "There have been estimates that as many as 5 to 15 per cent of doctors are not fully competent to practice medicine, either from a deficiency of medical skills or because of impairment from drugs, alcohol, or mental illness" (19). Professional associations have been more willing to seek legislation to place limits on the size of malpractice awards than to make a concerted effort to eliminate unqualified practitioners.

Blue Cross's premium consisted almost entirely of the costs of hospital care. Its main cost has therefore been the cost and quantity of hospital care used by its subscribers. Commercial insurance companies had broader coverage (although it included deductibles and cost sharing), and therefore hospital care was a smaller portion of the total premium. Thus to remain competitive against commercial insurance companies, Blue Cross had to keep the cost of hospital care (both hospital use and cost per unit) from rising so rapidly. Under the service benefit policy, however, neither patients, their physicians, nor the hospital had any incentive to be concerned with the cost or use of the hospital. In fact, it was in the hospital's interest to add facilities and services and pass these costs on to Blue Cross. As more hospitals added facilities and services in a race to determine who could be more prestigious, there was a great deal of duplication of costly facilities and services and therefore low use of many of these costly facilities. Blue Cross, however, was committed to paying for their costs. To limit the increase in these costly facilities, Blue Cross favored legislative restrictions on hospital investment.

Given its traditional relationship with hospitals, Blue Cross did not try to limit directly the rapid rise in hospital costs, either by instituting budget review or by setting a limit on what they would pay hospitals. Blue Cross and the major hospitals favored an indirect approach that prevented the development of new hospitals and smaller hospitals from expanding their beds and facilities. To receive Blue Cross (and Medicare) reimbursement for capital expenditures, a hospital had to receive the approval of a planning agency for its investment. Existing large hospitals either had the latest facilities or were the likeliest candidates to receive approval from the planning agency, whose criteria favored large, full-service, hospitals. These large institutions also favored the development and strengthening of planning agencies because it limited competition.

Blue Cross expected controls on investment to hold down hospital investment and rising Blue Cross premiums. Hospitals, however, had different objectives, and cost control was not one of them. To date, all studies have shown that controls on capital investment have not been effective in holding down either hospital investment or the rise in hospital costs (20). It was not until Blue Cross began to experience strong competitive pressures, sufficient to affect its survival, that it finally undertook more direct means of lowering the costs of their major input. Blue Cross finally began including lower-cost substitutes to hospitals as part of its benefits, instituting utilization control programs, and changing the method by which it pays hospitals.

(Another interest group that has recently formed is the Washington Business Group on Health. Comprised of representatives from major corporations, this group's common interest is in reducing the rise in their employee's health insurance premiums. The cost of labor is a significant part of these companies' business expense. The political positions of this group have this interest in mind. For example, they would be expected to oppose the shifting of Medicare costs of retired workers to the company rather than have Medicare remain as the primary payor of their retirees' medical costs. Similarly, proposals to save the Medicare Trust fund through increased social security taxes would be opposed since such taxes increase the cost of their labor inputs.)

Legislation to Decrease the Availability and/or Increase the Price of Substitutes:

All health associations try to increase the price of services that are substitutes to those provided by their members. (Similar to increasing the price of a substitute is decreasing its availability.) If the health association is successful in achieving the above, the demand for its members' services will be increased.

Health associations use three general approaches to increase the price of substitutes (or decrease their availability). The first is simply to have the substitute declared illegal. If substitute health professionals are not permitted to practice, or if substitutes are severely restricted in the tasks they are legally permitted to perform, there will be a shift in demand away from the substitute service. The second approach, used when the first approach is unsuccessful, is to exclude the substitute service from payment by any third party, including any government health programs. This approach raises the price of the substitute to a person with that payment coverage. The third approach is to try and raise the costs of that substitute provider. The substitute must then raise its own prices if they are to remain in business. The following examples illustrate the behavior of health associations for each of these approaches.

For many years the AMA regarded osteopaths as "cultists." It was considered "unethical" for physicians to teach in schools of osteopathy. Unable to prevent their licensure at a state level, the AMA tried to deny osteopaths hospital privileges. (A physician substitute is less than adequate if that substitute cannot provide a complete range of treatment.) As osteopaths developed their own hospitals and educational institutions, medical societies decided that the best approach to controlling the increase in supply of these physician substitutes was to merge with the osteopaths, make them physicians, and then eliminate any future increases in their supply. An example of this approach, which was used in California until it was overturned by the state supreme court, was to allow osteopaths to convert their D.O. degree to an M.D. degree on the basis of 12 Saturday refresher courses. (By 1966, 15 states had similar merger agreements between the medical and osteopathic societies.) After the merger between the two societies occurred in California, the Osteopathic Board of Examiners was no longer permitted to license osteopaths.

Optometrists and chiropractors are potential substitutes for ophthalmologists and family physicians. One approach used by the AMA toward such substitutes has been to raise their price relative to that of physicians. Medicare has been the vehicle for much legislative competition. An aged person with Medicare Part B pays less for physician services. The AMA has opposed including optometrists and chiropractors as providers under Part B, which would lower the out-of-pocket price to the aged of using such services. By including only physician services under Part B, the prices of substitute services to the aged are effectively increased relative to those of physicians. The AMA has also opposed direct payment of nurse anesthetists under Medicare (21).

In one case the intervention of the courts prevented physicians from artificially raising the price of a substitute. In Virginia, psychologists were not able to be reimbursed by Blue Shield as providers of psychotherapy services. Psychiatrists' services were therefore less expensive than a psychologists' services to a patient with Blue Shield coverage. The psychologists brought a successful antitrust case against Blue Shield (1980), claiming discrimination of nonphysician providers.

Other examples of the AMA's attempts to affect substitutes adversely was to oppose payment for chiropractic services under veterans' benefits and under the CHAMPUS program (health benefits for dependents of military personnel). The AMA has also opposed federal funding for advanced nurse training for fear that nurses will become independent nurse practitioners. The AMA's House of Delegates approved a resolution to recommend to all hospital staffs that only physicians perform histories and physicals. The floor debate indicated that the resolution was directed at physician assistants, registered nurses, and dentists.

One medical society effectively eliminated competition from two independent nurse midwives when the malpractice insurance of the backup obstetrician was canceled. The insurance company was controlled by the medical society. The backup obstetrician had to leave the state to get new insurance. (This antitrust case is pending.)

An example of the legislative behavior of dental societies toward substitute providers is illustrated by dentistry's actions toward denturists. "Denturism" is the term applied to the fitting and dispensing of dentures directly to patients by persons who are not licensed as dentists. Independently practicing denturists are a threat to dentist's incomes, since they offer to provide dentures at lower prices. Denturists are legal in seven of Canada's 10 provinces. As a result of their political success in Canada, denturists in the United States have become bolder by forcing referendums on the issue and by lobbying for changes in the state practice acts. Until recently, dental societies have been successful in having denturism declared illegal in each state. Since 1977, however, six states have passed laws legalizing denturism (22).

Occasionally, denturists have illegally sold dentures directly to patients. To eliminate this competition and to prevent it from increasing, local dental societies, such as in Texas, have responded in two ways: first, they offered to provide low-cost dentures to low-income persons; second, they pressured state officials to enforce the state laws against illegal denturists.

A special ADA commission set up to study the threat of denturists reported that the number of persons who are edentulous is much greater in the lower-income levels, and it is among these persons that the denturists have met with great success in selling low-cost dentures. An ADA editorial commenting on this special study commission's report proposed that:

> Organized dentistry should set up some system for supplying low-cost dentures
> to the indigent or the near indigent all over the country, but especially in those

states where the legislatures are considering bills that would allow dental mechanics to construct dentures and deliver them directly to the patient . . . this is
the type of program that would have a favorable impact on the public—not to
mention legislators . . . . The supplying of dentures to low income patients by
qualified dentists at a modest fee (or even at no fee in special cases) and in quantities meeting the public demands would go a long way toward heading off the
movement of legalized denturists. (23)

It is only the threat of competition that results in the dental profession's offer to
provide low-cost dentures to the indigent or the near-indigent. If the denturist's competitive threat is eliminated through dentistrys' successful use of the state's legal
authority, the net effect will be to cause the public, particularly the poor, to pay
higher prices for dentures.

The ADA is also concerned that dental hygienists remain complements, not become
substitutes, to dentists. In several states the dental hygienist association has attempted
to change the state practice act to permit hygienists to practice without dental supervision and become an independent practitioner. In 1986, the hygienists were successful
in achieving this goal in Colorado. The ADA views this activity by hygienists as a
"war" (24). The ADA has challenged the constitutionality of the Colorado legislation.
Further, the ADA has filed a friend of the court brief against individual hygienists
who challenged their state requirements that hygienists must be supervised by dentists.

One of the most important substitutes for registered nurses is foreign-trained registered nurses. Nurses' salaries are considerably higher in the United States than in other
countries, thereby providing a financial incentive for foreign nurses to enter the
United States. The American Nurses Association has been successful in decreasing the
availability of a low-cost substitute for U.S. registered nurses (their members) by making it more difficult for foreign-trained RNs to enter the United States. The ANA has
proposed that foreign RNs desiring to enter the United States be screened by examination in their home country before being allowed to enter the United States. Once a
foreign-trained RN enters the United States, they have to be screened again by having
to pass state board exams. Both the U.S. Department of Labor and the Immigration
Service require (as of 1978) that a foreign nurse graduate successfully pass a screening
exam, in English, that measures the nurse's proficiency in both language and nursing
before they will issue a work permit and a labor preference visa.

The ANA's position on screening prior to entering the United States is consistent
with a policy of reducing the inflow of foreign nurses. If the screening exam were
administered in the United States, foreign-trained RNs could still work in some nursing capacity in the United States even if they did not pass the exam. The foreign-
trained nurse could then retake the exam in the future. [In the 10-year period before
the exam was given, 82,000 foreign nurse graduates entered this country (25).] The
screening exam is an additional barrier for foreign nurses to pass before they can enter
the United States. If they do not pass the exam, they are unlikely to emigrate.

There are two additional legislative approaches that the ANA has used to raise the
cost of substitutes for RNs. The first is to favor increases in the wages of other health
professionals. A great deal of substitution of licensed practical nurses (LPNs) for RNs
has occurred. The larger the wage increases of RN substitutes, the less likely it is that
there will be substitution away from the RN. The disparity between RN wages and
those of other health professionals would be diminished.

The second legislative approach used by the ANA is to prevent other personnel from performing tasks performed by the RN. The ANA has opposed policies to permit physicians from having greater delegatory authority over which personnel can perform nursing tasks; the ANA has opposed permitting LPNs to be in charge of skilled nursing homes; otherwise, there would be substitution away from RNs (who receive higher wages) currently performing such functions. The California Nurses Association opposed a bill that would have authorized firemen with paramedic training to give medical and nursing care in hospital emergency departments. As a means of preventing physician's assistants from assuming a role that the RN would like, the ANA has favored a licensing moratorium. A moratorium would prevent any new health personnel from being licensed to perform RN tasks or tasks that RNs would like to perform.

The American Hospital Association has opposed the growth of freestanding ambulatory surgicenters (26). Surgicenters are low-cost substitutes to hospitals. Performing surgical procedures in a surgicenter decreases the use of the hospital. The hospital also loses the revenues from surgeries performed in these alternative settings. To limit the availability of these low-cost substitutes, hospital associations have argued that surgicenters should be permitted only when they are developed *in association* with hospitals. Hospitals would thereby be able to control the growth of a competitive source of care. As surgicenters increase, hospitals would be the ones to receive their revenues. Denying Blue Cross reimbursement to freestanding surgicenters and including surgicenters under Certificate of Need (CON) legislation have been the approaches favored by hospital associations. Hospitals have a great deal of influence in the CON process. If approvals are to be given for surgicenters, it is likely that it would be given to a hospital desiring to start one rather than a freestanding one. (Previously, when hospitals were reimbursed according to their costs by both Blue Cross and Medicare, they argued that surgicenters raise the cost of care since hospitals are left with excess capacity that third-party payors then have to cover.)

Health maintenance organizations were also included in state CON legislation for the same reason. HMOs decrease the use and revenues of hospitals. Several HMOs believed that CON legislation was inhibiting their ability to compete. They were able to persuade Congress to grant large HMOs an exemption from the federal CON legislation. In the 1979 CON Amendments, Congress also stated that CON should not be used in an anticompetitive manner. (Many states, however, still use CON to limit entry by new health facilities, even by home health agencies, which have virtually no economies of scale.)

[The value of CON legislation has not been lost on other groups. As occupancy rates have fallen, hospitals have tried to convert those empty beds into long-term care beds ("swing beds"). To do so usually requires either CON or state permission. Opposing the hospitals are nursing home associations, which are concerned that hospitals will take business away from them, particularly from private-pay rather than Medicaid patients.]

Hospital associations have used several methods to raise the price of their competitors, for-profit hospitals. They have opposed the granting of tax exempt status to for-profit hospitals, thereby raising their costs. They have lobbied successfully for reducing the return on equity of for-profit hospitals under Medicare reimbursement. Hospitals have opposed granting for-profit hospitals Blue Cross eligibility. Being ineligible for Blue Cross payment precludes the use of the hospital by patients with Blue Cross coverage.

Blue Cross competes against several substitutes. Commercial insurance companies are perhaps their most important competitor. To increase the cost of commercial insurers, Blue Cross has opposed granting them the same tax-exempt status that Blue Cross plans enjoy. Commercial insurance companies generally pay higher state taxes on their premiums than does Blue Cross. Blue Cross plans have also opposed state rate regulation of hospitals that enable all insurers to pay the same price for hospital care. Such policies remove Blue Cross's cost advantage since they receive a hospital discount. When Medicare was started Blue Cross was concerned that the Social Security Administration (SSA) would be the intermediary (i.e., pay the hospitals for Medicare patients). Together with the AHA, Blue Cross was successful in legislatively eliminating SSA from competing for this role.

Substitutes for American medical and dental schools are foreign schools whose graduates (who may be U.S. citizens) then want to practice in the United States. To reduce the likelihood that foreign medical schools will substitute for U.S. medical schools, the AAMC has favored strong restrictions on the number of foreign medical graduates who can enter the United States. In the past, the AAMC has had limited success. Many U.S. citizens attend a foreign medical school and then seek a residency in the United States. [In 1985 there were 13,451 graduates of foreign medical schools who were doing their residency training in the United States, representing 18 percent of all residents. Of these foreign-trained residents, 7,386 were U.S. citizens (27).] Until recently, Congress has been reluctant to limit residency opportunities for U.S. citizens trained overseas. Although the AMA has favored the return of alien FMGs to their home country once they have finished their U.S. residency, the AMA did not want to restrict residency opportunities for foreign-trained medical graduates, since residents increase physician productivity. Also important to the AMA's political position on this issue is the fact that approximately 20 percent of U.S. students studying abroad are the sons and daughters of U.S. physicians (28).

A number of factors are changing, making it likely that the AAMC will be more successful in decreasing the availability of a substitute supply of medical students. The increased supply of physicians has made the AMA concerned with the influx of foreign-trained U.S. graduates. The Congress is concerned with reducing expenditures under Medicare. (Medicare pays teaching hospitals for graduate medical education, and one method of reducing Medicare expenditures is to reduce the number of medical graduates that Medicare supports.) The AAMC has been a strong proponent for eliminating Medicare payments for residents trained in foreign medical schools. Eliminating Medicare payments to teaching hospitals for residents who received their degree from a foreign medical school would be a sufficient incentive for these hospitals not to accept such graduates. Given the large growth in U.S. medical school graduates, this policy should have little adverse effect on teaching hospitals.

The American Dental Association and the Association of American Dental Schools have been more successful in reducing the attractiveness of a foreign dental education. Practicing dentists do not use dental residents as do physicians. Therefore, their interest is solely with decreasing the supply of dentists. There are increased time requirements for a foreign-trained dentist desiring to practice in the United States. A minimum number of years of training in the foreign country is required as well as receiving a license to practice in that country. (For a U.S. citizen, this would mean learning a different language.) And once foreign-trained dentists enter the United States, additional requirements are imposed upon them; they are required to take the last two years of dental school in an accredited U.S. dental school. They may also be required to take additional examinations before the licensing exam (29). To date, such restrictive practices have raised the cost of a U.S. dental license for foreign trained dentists (for both U.S. and non-U.S. citizens). The consequence has been a decreased demand for a foreign dental education as a substitute for a U.S. dental education. The measure of how successful the dental profession and the dental schools have been is that less than 1 percent of all practicing dentists in the United States are foreign trained.[5]

Legislation to Limit Increases in Supply

Essential to the creation of a monopoly position are limits on the number of providers of a service. Health associations, however, have justified supply control policies on grounds of quality. Restrictions on entry, they maintain, ensure high quality of care to the public. These same health associations, however, oppose quality measures that would have an adverse economic effect upon existing providers (their members). *This apparent anomaly—stringent entry requirements and then virtually no quality assurance programs directed at existing providers—is only consistent with a policy that seeks to establish a monopoly for existing providers.*

If health associations were consistent in their desire to improve and maintain high-quality standards, they should favor all policies that ensure quality of care, regardless of the effect on their members. Quality control measures directed at existing providers, such as reexamination, relicensure, and monitoring the care actually provided would adversely affect the incomes of some providers. More important, such "outcome" measures of quality assurance would make entry or "process" measures less necessary, thereby permitting entry of a larger number of providers.

A test of the hypothesis that entry barriers are directed primarily toward developing a monopoly position rather than improving quality of care would be as follows: Does the health association favor quality measures, regardless of the effect on its member's incomes, or does it only favor those quality measures that enhance its members' incomes? If the health association favors only those quality measures that have a favorable impact on its members' economic position, it can be concluded that the real intent of those quality measures is the improvement of its members' competitive position rather than the assurance of quality of care in the most efficient manner.

The following examples illustrate health associations' positions on quality. Those quality programs that are in its members' interests are expected to be favored, while those that would have an adverse impact are expected to be opposed.

Health associations always favor state licensure. The profession is the group that lobbies for and demands licensure laws. The profession then controls the licensure process by having its own members appointed to the licensing board and by having them establish the requirements for licensure. Licensure, by itself, is not a sufficiently strong barrier to entry. Once licensure is achieved, the requirements for licensure are increased. The major requirement that is usually imposed is educational. Before any person can take a licensing exam, he or she must have had a specified education, usually for a minimum number of years. (The number of years are continually increased.) Further, the specified education must take place in an educational institution approved by the profession or by its representatives. The number of educational institu-

---

[5]As of March 1986, there were 7,336 dentists in Michigan. Of these, only 32 dentists were foreign trained, four-tenths of 1 percent. Telephone conversation with the Department of Licensing and Regulation, State of Michigan.

tions is kept limited so that, as in medicine and dentistry, there is a continual excess demand for admission. (Medical and dental schools, as well as optometric and veterinary, and so on, schools, favor such supply control policies since it provides them with monopoly power.) Placing limits on the number of educational spaces and specifying educational requirements in excess of the skills necessary to practice reduces the number of persons that can take the licensing exam.

If the licensure requirements merely specified passing an examination, potential applicants for the exam could receive the necessary knowledge in a number of ways, in different institutions, and in different lengths of time. Under such circumstances, the number of persons that could potentially take the exam and pass it would be much greater than if those applying to take the exam were limited by the number of approved educational spaces.

The approach to quality described above has been used by both the AMA and the ADA, as well as other health professions. In 1904 the AMA formed its Council on Medical Education. Its purpose was to upgrade the quality of medical education. To receive greater public acceptance of its work, the Council induced the Carnegie Foundation to survey existing medical schools. The result was the Flexner Report, which recommended closing many medical schools and upgrading educational standards. "Flexner forcefully argued that the country was suffering from an overproduction of doctors and that it was in the public interest to have fewer doctors who were better trained" (30).

As a result of the Flexner Report, state medical licensing boards imposed the requirement of graduation from an approved medical school before a person could take the licensure examination. Medical schools were to be approved by the AMA's own Council on Medical Education. The number of medical schools declined steadily, from 162 in 1906 to 69 in 1944. The graduates of schools that were closed continued to practice; they were not required to rectify their educational deficiencies. Whenever standards are raised, grandfather clauses protect the rights of existing practitioners, regardless of their abilities.

The American Dental Association has followed in the footsteps of organized medicine. A licensure requirement followed by an educational requirement still left dentistry with "too many" practitioners. Dental schools were effectively able to license their own graduates. The number of dental schools grew, from 10 in 1870 to 60 by 1902 (31). Many of these new schools were for-profit businesses. Limits were placed on the for-profit schools to control the growth in the supply of new graduates. State and local dental societies, as well as the nonprofit dental schools, lobbied state legislatures to change the dental practice acts. Under the new state practice acts, the state board of dental examiners mandated that all dental graduates would have to take a licensing examination and that only the graduates from approved schools would be permitted to take the exam.

The ADA had the Gies Report in 1926, its own version of the Flexner Report. Approval of dental schools as a requirement for licensure was to be determined by the ADA's Council on Dental Education. Indicative of the control the ADA has had on its Council on Dental Education is one of the duties of the Council, according to the ADA's bylaws: "to accredit on behalf of this association dental schools and schools in related fields of dental education in *accordance with requirements and standards approved by the House of Delegates*" Italics added (32). The result of this approach was similar; the number of schools and spaces declined and the educational requirements for becoming a dentist increased. Educational requirements became standardized and the for-profit dental schools went out of business. As with physicians, current dentists, whose interest the ADA served, were always grandfathered in as requirements were increased.

In the last five years there has been a growing concern among dentists (as well as among the other health professions) that there are too many practitioners. As would be expected, rather than relying on market forces to determine the number of dentists, the ADA approach is to reduce the number of dental school spaces. "Resolved, that public statements made by the American Dental Association . . . include the recognition that a surplus of dentists does exist to meet the current demand for dental services, . . . the ADA encourage and assist constituent societies in preparing legislation that may be used to petition state legislatures and governmental bodies with respect to private schools to adjust enrollment in dental schools" (33).

Optometrists have also followed the same supply control policies as medicine and dentistry. By the early 1900s, optometrists were able to secure licensure in all the states. However, there were many private schools for training optometrists. By the 1920s the American Optometric Association was successful in disqualifying 20 of the 30 optometric schools and in raising educational requirements. Today, optometry requires six years of education in an approved optometric school and at least two years (most applicants have completed four years) of traditional undergraduate college education (34). Increasing educational requirements for a profession involve not just increasing the number of years of professional training but also requiring more years of undergraduate training. (It is not intuitively obvious why a professional must also have a traditional college education.)

Nursing is also moving in the direction of requiring more stringent educational requirements. Previously, most nurses graduated from diploma schools of nursing. In 1955, 90 percent of nurse graduates were from diploma schools. These programs were operated in conjunction with hospitals and generally lasted two years. By 1980, most nurse graduates received an associate degree (A.A.) from a two-year college (48 percent graduated with an A.A. degree, 19 percent from a diploma school and 33 percent with a four-year B.A. degree; see Table 16–6). The growth in demand for an A.A. degree was related to their high rate of return, whereas a nurse with a B.A. degree received a similar income but was required to take an additional two years of education. The marketplace did not place a sufficiently high return on the additional two years of education to make it worthwhile for most nurses to seek a four-year degree. Since the four-year degree did not meet the market test, the profession decided to impose it.

The ANA has proposed that nursing education take place only in colleges that offer a B.A. degree (35). Only four-year nurse graduates would be referred to as professional nurses; otherwise, the nurse would be a technical nurse. Nurse associations are lobbying their state legislatures for these increased educational requirements. By proposing an increase in the educational requirement of two-thirds of the nurse graduates, the ANA must be well aware that the result will be a decrease in the number of nurse graduates. Any increase in an educational requirement increases the tuition that the student must pay as well as the foregone income a student could have earned during those additional years. The consequence of this policy, however, will be a much smaller increase in the supply of registered nurses, increased wages for RNs, and higher costs of health care. With an increased educational requirement, the ANA will also try to justify an increase in tasks that nurses are able to perform. The effect of increased education and an increase in nursing tasks would be an increase in incomes of existing nurses, who would be grandfathered in as professional nurses.

It is unlikely that one would ever observe a situation where a health association proposes increased educational requirements which are then applicable to its existing members. A health association would favor additional training requirements for its existing members only to forestall more stringent requirements proposed by others. Health associations do not favor relicensure or reexamination requirements for their current members, even though increased knowledge is the basis for requiring additional training for those entering the profession. Reexamination and relicensure would lower the incomes of their members, since they would have to take the time to study for the exam. They may also not be able to pass the exam. No health association proposes that the time required to prepare a person to enter their profession be reduced. It has been suggested that one way to reduce the rising cost of a medical and dental education is to reduce the number of years required, for example, one less year of college or of professional school. A person should be willing to pay much higher tuition levels for the years they are in school if they could enter practice one year earlier. However, the only direction with regard to the number of years of education required is the ADA's recent proposal that each dental graduate take an *additional* one year postdoctoral program, which includes a hospital experience (36).

As medical and dental knowledge have increased and educational requirements for new graduates lengthen, the public is led to believe that all persons in a profession are equally (or at least minimally) qualified. This is unlikely to be the case, particularly for those practitioners who were trained 30 years ago and have not maintained their knowledge.

At times the profession imposes requirements on new entrants into the profession that are blatantly barriers to entry. For example, foreign medical and dental graduates were required to be U.S. citizens before they were allowed to practice in some states (37). Further, a dentist desiring to practice in Hawaii, for example, no matter how well trained he or she was or how long in practice in another state, is required to live in that state for one year before they are permitted to practice (38). Such requirements cannot be remotely related to the profession's concern with quality.

If the members of a profession are concerned with quality, then they should favor the monitoring of quality among themselves. Yet associations have opposed any attempts by others to review the quality of care practiced by their members. Health associations that have proposed continuing education for their members have done so in response to demands by those *outside* the profession for stronger continuing education requirements. These requirements are made easy to achieve and at low cost to the members of the profession.

An indication of the lack of quality control in the health professions is provided by evidence over time on the number of disciplinary actions taken against physicians by state licensing boards. One such study, conducted in 1969, found that in the preceding *five* years a total of 938 formal actions had been taken. These disciplinary actions varied from revocation of licenses to simple reprimands. Given the number of physicians involved in patient care during those years, these disciplinary actions amount to .69 per 1,000 physicians per year. Another study through 1972 resulted in an annual disciplinary rate of .74 per 1,000 physicians. These numbers include a number of states that had taken no disciplinary actions. Over the period 1980–1982, the disciplinary rate rose slightly to 1.3 per 1,000 physicians. The author of these studies, Dr. Derbyshire, asks the question: "Does organized medicine adequately discipline unethical physicians? The answer is no" (39).

The Florida Board of Medical Examiners was reorganized in 1979 and a lay person was appointed as director. The impetus for this change was a belief that the Florida medical licensing board was not performing its function. There was widespread media coverage on Florida physicians who had harmed their patients, violated the law, and were found to be still practicing. As a result, Florida strengthened the regulatory process. (A new governor was elected at that time and the state's Medical Practice Act came up for renewal under the state's sunset law provisions.) In 1982, there were 147 disciplinary actions against physicians in Florida. This included revoking and suspending physicians' licenses. These actions represented a threefold increase from a prior period. Since there were over 20,000 physicians in Florida, these disciplinary actions represented 7.4 per 1,000 physicians.

Other states had widely varying rates of disciplinary actions. In 1982, Pennsylvania recorded only .5 disciplinary actions per 1,000 physicians; New York had 1.1, California had 2.8. Seventeen states reported 3.0 or greater. The author of the study above states: "It is difficult to believe that in any given year any state or territory would not have at least one physician per thousand who posed a threat to the health and safety of its citizens, and yet in 1982, 14 states reported less than that number of disciplinary actions. Has the balance of interests in these states tipped too far in the direction of protecting the profession to the detriment of its citizens?" (40).

It is also unfortunate that physicians who lose their license in one state can then move to another state and practice again. Only 15 states (as of 1984) permit their licensing boards to take action solely on another state's findings. Also, the U.S. Government Accounting Office has recommended that physicians losing their license in one state not be able to collect from Medicare and Medicaid as they move from state to state (41).

The AMA has recently (1986) acknowledged that physician peer review programs have not been performing as well as they should. "Because of the fear of personal liability, physicians are reluctant to report colleagues to state medical boards, and adverse hospital review determinations too often stay within the hospital. Peer review can be more careful, vigorous, and uniform . . ." (42). A likely reason for this new report by the AMA's Board of Trustees on its plans to improve self-regulation among its members is that both government and business are demanding an accounting on quality assurance. Dr. Nelson, Chairman of the AMA's Board of Trustees, stated "Some big businesses, as payors for care, are realizing that they cannot only look at cost. They have to look at quality and they are demanding that the information be available to them" (43).

The current method of quality assurance for health professionals is aimed solely at entry into the profession rather than with monitoring the quality of care practiced. The inadequate performance of state licensing boards in disciplining their members is evidence of this practice. Further, little communication exists between state licensing boards to check the credentials and status of a physician moving from a different state. The public is less protected against unethical and incompetent practitioners than it has been led to believe. The public will become better protected, not as a result of the good intentions of the profession, but when the health professions are forced to respond to the demands for quality from those outside the professions.

Hospitals and Blue Cross plans have also been advocates of supply control policies. These institutions have also realized that the first step in achieving monopoly control is to limit entry. Large hospitals have favored Certificate of Need (CON) legislation and bed-reduction programs. CON was used by these institutions to limit investment by smaller hospitals and to prevent entry by potential competitors, such as for-profit hospitals. More recently, as hospital occupancy rates have fallen, large hospitals have favored bed reduction programs. Eliminating excess beds reduces incentives for hospitals to compete among themselves. It is also proposed that the excess beds to be eliminated come from the smaller hospitals, which are often lower in cost. CON and bed reduction programs increase the chances of survival for the large nonprofit hospital. Such restrictive policies, however, have not limited hospital investment or the increase in hospital costs. The public, however, has had less choice of hospitals and has had to travel further, as when they must go from the suburbs and use the larger hospitals in the center of the city.

Blue Cross plans were established so as not to compete with one another. Blue Cross plans were required to sign up 75 percent of the hospitals and beds in an area. This requirement precluded more than one Blue Cross plan from being established within any one market. Blue Cross had a virtual monopoly over the type of product it was selling since no other insurance plan offered a service benefit policy for hospitalization. (No other insurance company could have competed with Blue Cross on a similar product since they would not have received the hospital discount given to Blue Cross.)

To compete with Blue Cross, commercial insurance companies had to offer a different type of product, such as payment of a fixed dollar amount for hospital care. To offset Blue Cross's hospital discount, the commercials also had to include lower-cost substitutes to hospital care. The result was that commercial insurance companies innovated with the concept of major medical insurance. Major medical did not cover all the costs of hospital care, but it provided medical insurance against larger expenditures both in and outside the hospital.

In more recent years, the health insurance market has become more competitive. The market for health insurance has not been growing as it had in the past. In fact, in some areas the market has been declining. Many businesses decided to insure their own employees. Other types of insurance plans, such as health maintenance organizations, have taken market share away from the traditional health insurers. Blue Cross plans have had to adapt to this new environment in a number of ways. They have changed their product, offering care in other settings than in the hospital, they have established their own HMOs, and some Blue Cross plans are now beginning to compete with other Blue Cross plans.

There are now several good substitutes to Blue Cross, a company's own health insurance plan, commercial insurance, and HMOs. If Blue Cross plans begin entering one another's markets, the monopoly that a Blue Cross plan has over the use of the Blue Cross name will be eroded. Such a trend would present great problems for the Blue Cross Association.

IMPLICATIONS OF THE LEGISLATIVE SUCCESS OF HEALTH ASSOCIATIONS

Health professionals and health institutions do not exhibit characteristics of a natural monopoly, that is, large economies of scale sufficient to preclude entry of competitors in their market. Because these professionals and institutions cannot achieve a monopoly position through the normal competitive process, they seek to achieve it through legislation. The first step toward increasing their monopoly power is to erect barriers to entry. The next is to limit competition among their members. They then attempt to improve their monopoly position by further demanding legislation that will increase the demand for their services, permit them to price as would a price-discriminating monopolist, lower their costs of doing business, and disadvantage their competitors either by causing them to become illegal providers or by forcing them to raise their prices.

Health professionals, particularly physicians and dentists, have been successful in the legislative marketplace, as evidenced by the design of public programs to pay for their services and by their relatively high incomes. There are, however, "costs" to the rest of society as a result of the redistribution of wealth to members of health associations that have achieved legislative success. Although it is difficult to quantify these costs, it is likely that the costs of restrictive policies in medical care are greatly in excess of the benefits received by members of the successful health associations.

There are three types of costs that are imposed on the rest of society as a result of the restrictions discussed above. The first is higher prices. The more successful health associations are in achieving their members' goals, the higher will be the price of their members' services. The greater the price competition between members of different health associations, the lower will be the prices of both groups' services. The establishment of low-cost denture clinics by state dental societies is an example. When competition is reduced, as is the case when state dental societies apply pressure to have the laws against denturists enforced, the price of dentures will once again increase. Allowing freestanding surgicenters to compete with hospitals lowers the cost to the patient for minor surgical procedures (through reduced insurance premiums). Other tactics used by health associations to prevent price competition among their members included prohibitions against advertising, limiting productivity increases to prevent excess capacity, preventing physicians in HMOs from having hospital privileges, and requiring "free choice" of provider under both public and private insurance plans. These restrictions have resulted in health care prices being higher than they would otherwise be.

The beneficiaries of restrictive policies that maintain high health care prices are, of course, the health care professionals themselves. These higher prices are borne by patients and by taxpayers who finance government programs.

The second implication of successful legislative behavior by health associations is that the public is provided with a false assurance with respect to the quality of the medical care it receives. The state has delegated its responsibility for protecting the public to the individual licensing boards, which in turn have been controlled and operated in the interests of the providers themselves. The approach toward quality assurance used by both the profession and by licensing boards is needlessly costly and inefficient; and it has not been concerned with removing incompetent or unethical providers (e.g., those that perform unnecessary surgery). The emphasis on quality has been on entry into the profession. There has been virtually no oversight of practitioners on the quality of the care they provide. State licensing boards too rarely take disciplinary action against their members.

Measures to monitor the quality of care provided by practitioners have been proposed by outsiders. A revamped licensing board system as was undertaken by Florida is one approach. Utilization review programs and second opinions for surgery are examples of specific types of programs. Reexamination for relicensure is another. Health associations have not been proponents of such programs. Granting control over quality to the profession has increased the costs of their services and has not resolved the original concern of protecting the public from incompetent or unethical providers. The public is not as well protected as they have been led to believe.

The third effect of legislative success by a health association is that innovation in the delivery of medical care has been inhibited. Innovation provides benefits to consumers; they have greater choice, higher quality, and lower costs. Innovation, however, threatens the monopoly power of a protected provider group; it is therefore opposed. Medical and dental societies have been protectors of the fee-for-service delivery system. These organizations have delayed the introduction of alternative delivery systems, such as prepaid health plans and preferred provider organizations. Rather than being procompetitive, "free choice" of provider has been used by the professions to eliminate competition from alternative delivery systems. HMOs and PPOs cannot offer their subscribers free choice of any provider if they are to be able to select providers according to price and quality criteria. Compared to HMO and PPO premiums, traditional insurance premiums become relatively expensive once they allow their subscribers to go to any provider. Restrictions against "contract" medicine or dentistry and requiring free choice of provider prevents these alternative delivery systems from competing successfully against traditional insurance plans.

Medical and dental societies have inhibited the development of new types of health personnel, such as nurse midwives and expanded function dental auxiliaries, because they might become potential substitutes. The determination of which tasks a health profession is able to perform is related more to their economic effects on another health profession rather than their qualifications and training.

Hospital associations have sought, through certificate of need legislation, to stifle innovations such as the growth of freestanding surgicenters. It was the commercial insurance companies that introduced major medical insurance, a distinct innovation that also increased their share of the health insurance market. The process of a professional education (medical, dental, and optometric) has changed little over time (except for an increase in years) because it has remained under the auspices of accredited schools and their professions. It is quite possible that the necessary knowledge could be provided to students in a shorter period of time, thereby decreasing the total cost of such an education.

Innovation offers the hope of greater productivity, lower costs, and an increase in quality. The political activities of health associations should be viewed in their proper perspective, namely, to benefit their members while imposing a cost on the rest of society. Past reliance on professional regulation to protect the patient has reduced incentives for innovation. However, the movement toward market competition in the delivery of health services does not negate the need to be concerned with quality. In fact, since there is concern over the quality of care that will be provided under a competitive system, explicit quality mechanisms should be developed, publicized, and monitored by state authorities, who have, in the past, delegated this authority to the professions themselves. These quality measures, however, should be concerned with the provision of care itself rather than just with the process of becoming a professional.

REFERENCES

1. In 1975, the Federal Trade Commission (FTC) charged that the American Medical Association (AMA), the Connecticut State Medical Society, and the New Haven County Medical Association restricted the ability of their members to advertise. The AMA claimed that the FTC did not have jurisdiction over them because they were a not-for-profit organization. The approach used in this chapter and in an earlier book by the author, *Health Associations and the Demand for Legislation: The Political Economy of Health* (Lexington, Mass.: Ballinger, 1977), with its applications to the AMA, was the basis for testimony by the author, on the jurisdictional issue, to demonstrate that the AMA acted in the economic interests of its members. The administrative law judge found in favor of the FTC on both the advertising and jurisdictional issues. These decisions were upheld on appeal and in 1982 the U.S. Supreme Court, by a tie vote, upheld the lower court rulings.

2. Paul J. Feldstein, "A Preliminary Evaluation of Federal Dental Manpower Subsidy Programs," *Inquiry*, 11(3), September 1974.

3. For a more complete discussion of the participants and their goals, see Chapter 2, "An Economic Version of the Interest Group Theory of Government," in Paul J. Feldstein, *The Politics of Health Legislation: An Economic Perspective* (Ann Arbor, Mich.: Health Administration Press, 1988).

4. James Madison, *Federalist*, 10, 1787.

5. It has been estimated that the income elasticity of demand for dental services is approximately 2.; that is, a 10 percent increase in income would lead to a 20 percent increase in expenditures on dental services. Charles Upton and William Silverman, "The Demand for Dental Services," *Journal of Human Resources*, 7, Spring 1972: p. 250.

6. *Containing Medical Care Costs Through Market Forces* (Washington, D.C.: Congressional Budget Office, Congress of the United States, May 1982), p. 26.

7. One demand-increasing proposal is reputed to have had an adverse effect on patients' oral health. In 1974 the Federal Social Court in Germany ruled that false teeth should be included in the country's compulsory health insurance programs. "Fillings went out of fashion and prevention was ignored as vast quantities of teeth were pulled and replaced. By 1980, German dentists were using 28 tons of tooth gold a year, one third of the world total." Dentists incomes soared, exceeding those of physicians by 30 percent. The sickness funds reported a huge deficit, forcing them to raise the level of compulsory contributions. "Dentists Gnashing Teeth in West Germany," *Wall Street Journal*, December 26, 1985: p. 11.

8. Fee splitting occurs when a physician refers a patient to a surgeon and in return receives part of the surgeon's fee. Fee splitting is an indication that the surgeon's fee is in excess of his or her cost; the surgeon can still make a profit by rebating part of the fee. If the surgeon's fee was not in excess of the surgeon's cost (including the opportunity cost of the surgeon's time), the surgeon would be unwilling to split the fee. If all surgeons can act as a cartel (through the use of the state practice acts) to prevent any one surgeon from rebating part of a fee, their incomes are higher than if fee splitting were permitted. Fee splitting is a way of eroding the surgeons' monopoly power. Surgeons opposed to fee splitting consider it to be unethical because the referring physician has a monetary incentive to select the sur-

geon. Any concern the medical profession has with the quality of surgeons or with the ethical behavior of physicians should be addressed directly through examination and monitoring procedures, not by prohibiting price competition. Unfortunately, as will be discussed, the medical profession has not favored reexamination or monitoring the quality of care provided by its members. For a more complete discussion of fee splitting, see Mark V. Pauly, "The Ethics and Economics of Kickbacks and Fee Splitting," *Bell Journal of Economics*, 10(1), Spring 1979: 344–352.

9. Reuben Kessel, "Price Discrimination in Medicine," *Journal of Law and Economics*, October 1958.

10. See, for example, Lee Benham and Alexandra Benham, "Regulating Through the Professions: A Perspective on Information Control," *Journal of Law and Economics*, October 1975: 421–447.

11. John E. Kwoka, Jr., "Advertising and the Price and Quality of Optometric Services," *American Economic Review*, 74(1), March 1984: 211–216.

12. Reuben Kessel, *op. cit.*

13. The FTC brought a case against the Indiana Federation of Dentists on grounds of boycotting an insurer for requiring submission of radiographs by dentists. The U.S. Supreme Court in 1986 upheld the FTC by an unanimous decision, thereby agreeing with the FTC that the Indiana Federation of Dentists had engaged in an illegal conspiracy. Other state dental boards have undergone similar FTC review. "The Federation argued that if insurers are allowed to determine whether they will pay a claim for dental treatment on the basis of x-rays, they might decline erroneously to pay for necessary treatment and deprive the patient of fully adequate care. The court strongly objected to this argument, likening it to the argument, also rejected in a separate case, 'that an unrestrained market in which consumers are given access to the information they believe to be relevant to their choices will lead them to make unwise and even dangerous choices.' "U.S. Supreme Court Upholds FTC Order," *ADA News*, June 16, 1986: p. 2.

14. *1985 Health Legislation Fact Sheets*, (Kansas City, Mo.: American Nurses Association, Division of Governmental Affairs, undated), p. 2.

15. For a discussion of comparable worth as it applies to nursing, see Joanne Disch and Paul Feldstein, "An Economic Analysis of Comparable Worth," *Journal of Nursing Administration*, 16(6), June 1986.

16. For a review of immigration policies toward the FMG, see Alfonso Mejia, Helena Pizurki, and Erica Royston, *Foreign Medical Graduates* (Lexington, Mass.: Lexington Books, 1980), Appendix, "Immigration and Licensure Policies."

17. *AMA House of Delegates Proceedings*, 121st Annual Convention, June 20–24, 1972, Report Z (Chicago: American Medical Association), p. 115. For an excellent study of state legislation authorizing and regulating the practice of physician assistants, see Stephen C. Crane, *The Legislative Marketplace: A Model of Political Exchange to Explain State Health Regulatory Policy*, doctoral dissertation, School of Public Health, University of Michigan, 1981. In his extensive study of the determinants of state PA policy, Crane states: "It is clear that the single variable that best accounts for PA policy restrictiveness is the policy preferences of special interest groups" (p. 332).

18. Patricia M. Danzon *Medical Malpractice: Theory, Evidence and Public Policy* (Cambridge, Mass.: Harvard University Press, 1985).

19. Richard J. Feinstein, "The Ethics of Professional Regulation," *New England Journal of Medicine*, 312(12), March 21, 1985: 801–804.

20. David S. Salkever and Thomas W. Bice, *Hospital Certificate-of-Need Controls: Impact on Investment, Costs, and Use* (Washington, D.C.: American Enterprise Institute, 1979).

21. *Statements of the American Medical Association*, Compendium of Statements to the Congress and Administrative Agencies, Department of Federal Legislation (Chicago: American Medical Association, 1983, 1984).

22. The six states are: Maine (1977), Arizona (1978), Colorado (1979), Oregon (1980), Idaho (1982), and Montana (1984). Colorado just passed a bill permitting the independent practice of hygienists. This unprecedented action was attributed, by the Colorado Dental Association's Executive Director, to the state's sunset laws, which gave an opportunity for the bill's proponents to lobby for it. The proponents were feminists (since most hygienists are women), consumer advocates, and a large number of deregulators in the state legislature. The political influence of these groups also changed the composition of the state dental board, making dentists a minority; *ADA News*, May 19, 1986: p. 5.

23. "Action Urgently Needed on 'Denturist' Movement," editorial, *Journal of the American Dental Association*, 92, 1976: p. 665.

24. Dale F. Redig, "Which Side of This War Are You On?" *ADA News*, November 17, 1986: p.4.

25. *The CGFNS Story: Screening Foreign Nurses for Professional Careers in the United States*, (Philadelphia: Commission on Graduates of Foreign Nursing Schools, 1985).

26. AHA Board of Trustees policy statement reported in *"Hospitals," Journal of the American Hospital Association*, 47(15), August 1, 1973: p. 132.

27. John K. Iglehart, "Reducing Residency Opportunities for Graduates of Foreign Medical Schools," *New England Journal of Medicine*, 313(13), September 25, 1985: p. 832.

28. *Ibid.*, p. 835.

29. "In the Association's [ADA's] view, testing alone cannot provide adequate assurance of competence. Therefore the Association recommends that a foreign-trained dentist be required to complete supplementary education programs in an accredited dental school of at least two-years duration as a precondition to licensure." *Dentistry in the United States*, Information on Education and Licensure (Chicago: American Dental Association, 1985), p. 27.

30. Kessel, *op. cit.*, p. 27.

31. Kenneth C. Fraundorf, "Organized Dentistry and the Pursuit of Entry Control," *Journal of Health Politics, Policy and Law*, 8(4), Winter 1984: 759–781.

32. *Constitution and Bylaws*, revised to January 1, 1963 Bylaws, Section 1110B, p. 29 (Chicago: American Dental Association, 1963).

33. 1984 House of Delegates Resolutions, October 25 p. 537. This resolution follows a previous one (124H-1981) where the ADA was to encourage their "constituent dental societies to utilize these reports [on dentist supply] in petitioning their legislative bodies to consider by lawful means the number of dentists that should be

trained." *Transactions*, 125th Annual Session, October 20–25, 1984 (Chicago: American Dental Association, 1984).

34. James W. Begun, *Professionalism and the Public Interest: Price and Quality in Optometry* (Cambridge, Mass.: MIT Press, 1981). See also James W. Begun and Ronald C. Lippincott, "A Case Study in the Politics of Free-Market Health Care," *Journal of Health Politics, Policy and Law*, 7(3), Fall 1982: 667–685.

35. For a more complete discussion of this proposal, see Andrew K. Dolan, "The New York State Nurses Association 1985 Proposal: Who Needs It?" *Journal of Health Politics, Policy and Law*, 2(4), Winter 1978: 508–530.

36. "Dentistry's Blueprint for the Future," *JADA*, 108(1), January 1984: 20–30.

37. Many states adopted the citizenship requirement for FMGs after the AMA's House of Delegates passed such a resolution in 1938. Five states have continued such a requirement as late as 1975. Mejia, Pizurki, and Royston, *op. cit.*, p. 189.

38. Another entry barrier used in dentistry is restrictions on interstate mobility of dentists. Various studies have shown that dentists graduating from a dental school within a state have a greater chance of passing that state's licensing exam than do dentists from other states. Unlike medicine, most states do not permit reciprocal licensing for dentists. See, for example, Lawrence Shepard, "Licensing Restrictions and the Cost of Dental Care," *Journal of Law and Economics*, 21, April 1978.

39. Robert C. Derbyshire, "Medical Ethics and Discipline," *JAMA*, 228(1), April 1, 1974: 59–62, p. 60. See also Robert C. Derbyshire, *Medical Licensure and Discipline in the United States* (Baltimore: Johns Hopkins University Press, 1969); and Robert C. Derbyshire, "Medical Discipline in Disarray: Offenders and Offenses," *Hospital Practice*, March 1984: 98a–98v.

40. Richard J. Feinstein, *op. cit.*, p. 803. In view of the poor record of state medical boards in disciplining physicians, the comments by Dr. James Sammons, Executive Vice President of the AMA, are all the more revealing. In opposing mandatory reevaluations for relicensing, Dr. Sammons stated: "There are better ways to measure competency. [Reviews in hospitals and state medical boards] are best able to weed out incompetent physicians." "Cuomo's Plan for Testing Doctors Is Part of Growing National Effort," *New York Times*, June 9, 1986: 1, 19.

41. Sharon McIlrath, "Physician Licensure Crackdown Sought," *American Medical News*, 27, May 11, 1984: p. 1.

42. "AMA Adopts New Self-Regulation Plan for MD Profession," *ADA News*, November 17, 1986: p. 18. See also "AMA Initiative on Quality of Medical Care and Professional Self-Regulation," Board of Trustees, American Medical Association, *Journal of the American Medical Association*, 256, August 22, 1986: 1036–1037.

43. *Ibid.*

CHAPTER 19

The Role of Government in Health and Medical Care

The involvement of government in the health and medical sector in the United States has increased very rapidly. Federal expenditures for personal medical services have risen sharply since the passage of Medicare and Medicaid in the mid-1960s. Various levels of government are also suppliers of medical services: the Veterans Administration's system of hospitals, and medical services supplied to military dependents in military facilities under the auspices of the Department of Defense. Different levels of government also provide indirect subsidies for medical services in the form of subsidies for medical research, for hospital construction (under the Hill-Burton Act), and for health manpower under federally supported programs, and subsidies by states for health professional education. At least as important as this financial involvement of government in medical service is the less obvious role of government in setting the rules under which medical services are paid for, organized, and produced, and the protection provided to patients through mechanisms such as licensing. Although government has long been involved in establishing the rules of the game for medical care, its role in financing medical care, particularly with regard to national health insurance, has been more controversial.

Some people view this increasing involvement of government in the medical sector as inevitable and beneficial; to others it is improper and the cause of inefficiencies. To clarify the debate over the increasing involvement of government in medical care, it is useful to review the traditional criteria for the role of government in a market system and to apply these criteria to medical care. Differences in opinion over the role of government in medical care can then be separated into differences regarding (1) whether the traditional criteria for government involvement are appropriate, and (2) given the appropriateness of the criteria, whether such criteria warrant government involvement in medical care. The first set of differences involve value judgments over the role of government. The sooner these differences are recognized as such, the sooner the participants will be able to focus the debate on whether there are more appropriate alternatives to the traditional criteria for government involvement. Given a set of criteria for government involvement, whether or not government involvement is warranted is more easily resolved because the existence of certain situations in medical care can be determined empirically. The evaluation of government programs in medical care, therefore, depends both upon appropriate criteria for government involvement and upon the applicability of such criteria to medical care.

There are two traditional areas where government is acknowledged to have a role in a market-oriented system (1). Each of these areas will be discussed briefly.

MARKET IMPERFECTIONS

In a competitive market, economic efficiency on the demand and supply sides typically cannot be achieved when the assumptions underlying competitive markets are violated. The most important assumptions that are not fulfilled in medical care are: consumers have perfect information, there is complete mobility of resources,[1] and patients and providers have an incentive to minimize their costs of purchasing and providing medical treatment. Although advertising has recently been permitted, consumers still lack information concerning their medical diagnosis, treatment needs, the quality of different providers, and the prices charged by different providers. Barriers to the mobility of resources exist as a result of restrictions placed on the tasks that various personnel are permitted to perform, entry into health manpower professions, and entry by institutions into various institutional markets. The incentives of patients and providers to be concerned with the costs of medical care were lessened by the purchase of excess insurance coverage as a consequence of the tax deductibility of health insurance premiums, the purchase of insurance by employers as a nontaxable fringe benefit to their employees, and the use, in the past, by third-party payors, including government, of cost-based payment to providers.

Empirical evidence of inadequate price information is the wide dispersion of prices for a given service within an area and significantly lower prices (e.g., optometric services) in states that permitted advertising. Patients' ignorance as to their medical need, diagnosis, treatment requirements, and the quality of their provider has given rise to the belief that physicians have some leeway in inducing their own demand; studies show different surgery rates for similar patient populations depending upon the method of physician reimbursement. One approach for overcoming the patient's lack of knowledge has been second opinions for surgery.

Examples of the widespread existence of barriers in medical delivery are the continual excess demands by applicants for a medical (and dental) education, continually high rates of return to the medical profession, and the willingness of U.S. citizens to bear higher costs and study for a longer period in foreign medical schools in order to become a U.S. physician. In the institutional sector, lack of consumer information and barriers to entry resulted in prices that exceed average costs. For example, for many

---

[1]Another imperfection would be with respect to the capital markets. If full-cost tuition were charged to medical students, students would not be able to borrow from banks based just upon their prospective earnings and without collateral. This type of market imperfection exists for all forms of higher education and is not peculiar to medical or dental education. At present, however, other market imperfections in the health education market, such as barriers to entry, are of greater overriding concern, since they prevent full-cost tuition from being instituted.

years Blue Cross was able to use community rating to price its hospital coverage. Hospitals were able to price their services so as to cross-subsidize different services and patients; their ability to price according to the patient's elasticity of demand (as the physician did) was indicative of a lack of price competition. Excess insurance for patients and cost-based reimbursement to providers resulted in inappropriate utilization, excessive duplication of facilities, rapidly rising medical costs, and a consequent concern for the efficiency with which medical care was produced.

The effect of barriers to entry and the lack of price competition was that patients paid a price for medical care that did not reflect their marginal valuation of using those services. Utilization of medical services by patients whose insurance is subsidized (either by the government or through tax deductions) exceeds what they would be willing to pay for that care if they had to pay the full price. Similarly, the price paid for medical care by third-party payors, the government, and patients (both through their out-of-pocket expenditures and through their taxes) exceeded the minimum costs of providing that care.

Thus it is apparent that there were (and still are) imperfections in the market for medical services. Many have been created by the government itself. To discuss the appropriate role of government in the face of these imperfections, it is first necessary to understand why these imperfections were originally instituted. The *ostensible* reason for placing restrictions on entry, information, and price competition was to provide consumer protection. Given the technical nature of medical services and the potential harm that may be inflicted upon an uninformed patient by an incompetent provider, the government, working through the health professions and health institutions, placed its emphasis for consumer protection on nonprofit providers. Training requirements in nonprofit institutions were specified; licensure, which was to be carried out by the health professions, placed strong restrictions on who was permitted to practice and on who was responsible for performing medical services; information on prices, quality, and accessibility was prohibited to prevent unethical providers from misleading the sick. Thus the very imperfections that prevented the medical sector from performing more efficiently were instituted under government auspices.

How can the demand for consumer protection [2] be satisfied while eliminating imperfections that cause inefficiencies in the medical sector? An alternative approach to the current system of quality assurance would be to rely more on outcome, rather than process, measures of quality. Relying more on examinations rather than standardized educational requirements and monitoring the quality of care provided by HMOs rather than restricting the tasks performed by health professions are examples of such outcome approaches. Private mechanisms, such as malpractice and improved consumer choice, would also ensure that the goals of consumer protection are achieved. Consumer protection could be achieved more directly and more efficiently by an approach that actually monitored the quality of care provided. It would no longer be necessary to rely solely on proxy methods to accomplish this objective.

---

[2]A demand for consumer protection might be considered an externality; namely, if the government or some agency were to ensure that all providers are competent, all consumers would benefit from the lower risks and lower search costs when seeking a provider. The reason for including a discussion of consumer protection in this section rather than in the following one, which discusses externalities, is that whether or not externalities are in fact the real reason for the market imperfections mentioned, the proposed policy prescriptions are similar to what would be the situation if such imperfections were simply a result of monopoly behavior on the part of the providers.

Eliminating restrictions that cause market imperfections would enable the market mechanism to allocate medical resources more efficiently. Providing government subsidies to alleviate the consequences of such imperfections, rather than eliminating the imperfections themselves, cannot be justified on theoretical grounds. If entry and practice barriers limit the availability of medical care by increasing its price, a system of government construction or manpower subsidies, which have as their stated goal an increase in availability of medical resources, cannot be justified on grounds of economic efficiency. Such subsidies merely mask the effects of the market imperfections. These subsidies would have to be justified on grounds other than as a means of improving market efficiency. The appropriate role of government, when faced with imperfections in the marketplace, should be to eliminate restrictive practices and directly address the need that the restrictions were ostensibly imposed to meet (i.e., consumer protection). Government subsidies cannot be justified as a means of improving market efficiency when there are imperfections of the type discussed.

Many people, however, oppose the elimination of restrictions on information and on medical practice. The elimination of market imperfections would not be, in their opinion, an improvement over the current system. Such persons oppose a market approach for determining the quantity and quality of medical care to be provided. Their opposition to competition under a market approach is not based on grounds of greater economic efficiency, but instead, is a result of a value judgment that such criteria are inappropriate in medical care. Patients, in their opinion, do not have sufficient information, nor are they rational enough to make competent choices as to the appropriate providers and correct amounts of medical care when they are ill. Indeed, they feel, such a decision should not involve the consumer at all but should be determined professionally; the professional determination, or allocation, of medical care should be based on medical need and not on consumer choice.

One of the criteria for economic efficiency in the demand for a service is that consumers will use a service until the price they pay for the last unit purchased equals the additional value they receive from it. When the marginal utility of the last unit consumed equals the price paid, consumers are maximizing their utility. Since the price they must pay represents forgone utility that could be received from other goods and services, consumers adjust their utilization when prices change so that the marginal value of their last unit equals the new price. Consumers use different quantities of services, even though they face the same prices, because the marginal utilities to them of additional units differ. Each consumer, however, is assumed to match the marginal utility of that last unit to the forgone utility of other goods and services. Further, when the consumer is the sole beneficiary of his or her purchases, it is said that his or her marginal private benefit is equivalent to marginal social benefit.

If consumers are assumed not to be rational, or if persons do not believe that consumer choice should prevail, the traditional demand curve does not represent marginal social utility. Under such circumstances, traditional economic policy, which favors removing imperfections so as to satisfy consumer wants, will not achieve the goals of those persons who do not believe in consumer choice and sovereignty in determining the amount of medical care to be provided.

What criteria do those who oppose consumer sovereignty in medical care suggest for determining the quantity of medical services? Determination of need or establishment of health priorities for consumers, which they favor, is difficult to operationalize. Government bureaus would presumably be required to establish resource levels. The criteria that such agencies would use for placing a marginal value on services so as to allocate resources have not been developed. Nor would everyone agree with the value judgment that a person should be prohibited from consuming something that he or she is willing to pay for (as long as it does not have any negative effects on other persons). Based on their own valuation of their time, some people may prefer to pay a higher price rather than wait longer for the receipt of a service. Substituting collective judgment for an individual's judgment to determine how much medical care is to be available represents a difference in values and is unrelated to whether a market system will be more efficient than an alternative system for achieving the same set of values.

This difference in values regarding the criteria for determining how much medical care should be available, and to whom, is also related to another set of values. Those opposed to the use of consumer sovereignty in the demand for medical care are also opposed to the use of competition on the supply side. The proponents of market competition assume that when providers compete for consumers, they will minimize their costs (enabling them to sell their service at a lower price) and provide those services that consumers desire. Persons who do not believe that consumers should determine what providers should produce often express similar disbelief in the ability of suppliers to compete with one another without harming patients. We often find that such persons want to substitute regulation and monopolization for competition on the supply side. Regardless of differences in values regarding who should determine the quantity and quality of medical services, it should be possible to allow different delivery systems to compete on the supply side. Although there may be a distrust of competition in its ability to achieve efficiency without harming patients, allowing such competition to exist and to be an alternative to a more controlled delivery system (e.g., a system of VA hospitals) would provide a fairer test of which approach is more efficient at achieving a level of output, whether it is established by government agencies or by consumers.

The reason for this discussion of differences in values in medical care is because the appropriate role of government is continually debated with regard to the values and criteria that underlie a market system. Much of the criticism of a market approach is not based upon the market's ability to achieve the specified economic criteria. Instead, the disagreement is a result of differences in values and unspecified criteria, thus the discussion on the role of government and public policy alternatives would be sharpened if these distinctions were defined more explicitly .

MARKET FAILURE

There are certain situations where markets, with no imperfections, will still not produce the optimal amount of output, which is defined as price equaling marginal cost. One such situation would be a "natural" monopoly in the provision of a particular service. In a natural monopoly the economies of scale are so large that given the size of the market, it would be less expensive to have one firm produce that service. If competition prevailed, one of the firms would be able to lower its costs by increasing its scale of production, thereby driving other firms out of business. In a situation of natural monopoly, competition cannot exist; because of the monopolists' pricing strategy, the output is likely to be less than optimal. The situations in which natural monopolies exist in the health field are rare. Relatively good substitutes exist for most medical services at a local level. Economies of scale in hospitals are slight; individual hospital

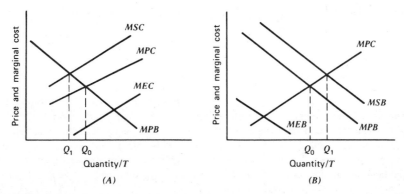

Figure 19-1. Externalities in production and consumption: (*A*) a case of external costs, (*B*) a case of external benefits.

services such as cobalt therapy units may be subject to relatively large economies. Such services, however, serve a much larger market than is served by the hospital in which they are located. Thus the market served by such specialized facilities and services is large enough for competition to exist between several of them. Because few services in medical care appear to have the characteristics of a natural monopoly, the natural-monopoly argument has not been an important justification for government intervention or subsidies in medical care.

Another possible reason for market failure in medical care is the existence of externalities. Externalities occur when an action undertaken by an individual (or firm) has secondary effects on others, which may be favorable or unfavorable. Externalities result in a nonoptimal amount of output being produced, because an individual or firm considers only their own benefits and costs when making a production or consumption decision. If costs or benefits are received by others as a result of someone's private decision, the level of output produced in the market will be based upon either too small a level of benefits (i.e., positive external benefits) or too small a level of costs of production (i.e., positive external costs). For example, as shown in Figure 19-1*B*, when there are external benefits (*MEB*), the result of an individual's considering only the (marginal private) benefits (*MPB*) which he or she expects to derive from that purchase would be a level of output determined by the intersection of the marginal-private-benefit (*MPB*) schedule and the marginal private costs (*MPC*) of producing that service. The resulting level of output, Q_0, would be smaller than if the external benefits to others (*MEB*) were also included. If the marginal private benefits and the marginal external benefits were added together (to result in the marginal-social-benefits (*MSB*) curve), the resulting level of output would be Q_1, which is greater than Q_0.

A situation where external costs are imposed on others would be similar in approach, although opposite in effect, for purposes of determining the optimal level of output. A firm deciding how much output to produce would consider only the marginal private benefits and marginal private costs; it would not take into account any costs imposed on others, such as through air pollution. If the marginal costs imposed on others (*MEC*) were added to the firm's costs of production, the resulting costs of producing that output, the marginal-social-cost curve (*MSC*), would represent the full costs of production. The level of output that would be produced in the latter case would be smaller, Q_1, than when the external costs were not considered, Q_0.

Individual consumers and producers in a competitive market do not normally take into consideration the external benefits or costs imposed on others as a result of their decisions. When such external costs and benefits are not incorporated into the private decisionmaking process, the resultant output level is not optimal. Some persons receive benefits for which they would be willing to pay but do not, whereas others bear additional costs for which they did not receive any benefits. (In the latter case, the persons purchasing the good or service that results in an external cost are paying a price that is less than the full cost of producing that service.) Externalities therefore have two effects. The first is the effect on economic efficiency: it is only when all the marginal benefits (MSB) equal all the marginal costs (MSC) that the optimal level of output is determined. The second effect is redistribution: some persons receive an external benefit for which they do not compensate those providing it, or a cost is imposed on them for which they are not reimbursed.

To incorporate external costs and benefits into the private decisionmaking calculus when large numbers of individuals are involved requires some form of collective, nonmarket decisionmaking.[3] When large numbers of persons are involved, it becomes difficult to make voluntary arrangements that are satisfactory to all concerned. Group or collective decisionmaking, in which all persons must abide by the decision, is required to determine both the optimal level of output and to whom the compensation is to be paid (and on whom the taxes should be assessed). It is a legitimate role for government to serve as the group's agent in a nonmarket situation.

The existence of externalities legitimizes a role for government in health care, but of what should that role consist? It is not sufficient merely to claim that externalities exist and then justify all types of government intervention and financing of health and medical care. The proper role of government is twofold. First, it must determine the exact nature and size of external benefits and costs, if externalities are believed to exist. The measurement of externalities is a difficult task, both conceptually and empirically, as will be discussed below. Nonmarket studies, referred to as cost-benefit analysis, are important for determining the optimal level of output in situations where externalities exist (2). A problem with cost-benefit studies that have been undertaken in the health field is that they suggest it is appropriate for the government to undertake *any* program that has "favorable' cost-benefit ratios. It is important to determine whether such programs have any external effects; if there are no external effects, then the role of government, if any, must be justified on other grounds. An example of inappropriate cost-benefit analysis is its application to personal health programs that have no external effects. The analyst may propose a system of government subsidies based solely on a finding of a favorable cost-benefit ratio. If there are no external effects and the individuals involved do not wish to spend their own funds on the program, it would not be appropriate to have the government intervene, unless one is willing to declare that the individuals making the decision are not rational or, as is more likely, that the individuals do not share the same values as the analyst.

The second proper role of government when externalities exist is to determine how the externalities will be financed—who will be compensated and who will be taxed. To use the air pollution mentioned previously as an example of a situation where external costs are imposed on others. The government should determine the magnitude of the external costs and then place a unit tax (equivalent to the size of the external

---

[3]When few individuals are involved, it is possible that they will reach agreement among themselves as to the proper levels of compensation, and the resulting level of output will be optimal.

costs) on those who are producing the particular product that is causing the pollution. The per unit tax will cause an increase in the polluters' costs of production and a consequent decrease in production and pollution (as shown in Figure 19–1A). The proceeds of the tax can then be used to reimburse those who bear these external costs. Similarly, when there are external benefits, as in the case of medical research, then those receiving the external benefits should be similarly taxed and the proceeds used to subsidize an increase in medical research. The financing principles should attempt to affix the taxes and subsidies to those who generate the external costs and benefits. A system of financing based on ability to pay would be inappropriate unless such a system reflected the extent of the external benefits and costs. Not all nonmarket decisionmaking should be based at a federal level, however. For some health programs, the benefits and costs are purely local in character (e.g., water fluoridation); the appropriate level of financing, therefore, is local.

Situations involving externalities do not necessarily require government production or provision of particular services. If a particular service does not have the characteristics of a natural monopoly, there is no reason why there could not be competition in the provision of that service. Medical schools and other research institutions could compete for research grants. Research is not necessarily produced more efficiently if undertaken solely by federally employed researchers. The criterion for whether the service should be governmentally or privately provided should be efficiency; there is nothing inherent in the nature of externalities which suggests that services should be publicly provided.[4]

Several types of situations in the health and medical fields give rise to externalities. The first type may be referred to as the "consumer protection" argument, which was discussed previously. Given the technical nature of medical care and the patient's lack of knowledge regarding diagnosis, treatment needs, and the provider's competence, consumers might benefit from the establishment of certain minimum standards and the provision of information. If the private market did not provide minimum standards (possibly through malpractice actions) or the necessary information required by consumers, or if all consumers desired the government to ensure some minimum standards, consumer protection would become an externality and hence a legitimate role for the government. The methods by which the government could fulfill this public demand for protection would be similar to those discussed previously.

Another externality with regard to personal medical services is what may be referred to as "externalities in consumption." If healthier and wealthier individuals do not want to see persons less fortunate than themselves go without necessary medical care and are willing to contribute to their medical care, an externality in consumption is said to exist. This is because the utility of individuals depends not only upon the

---

[4]Using the criterion of efficiency, is there any reason for allowing the federal government to have a monopoly on the provision of medical care for veterans? Presumably, the government could determine how much it was willing to spend on medical care for a specific class of veterans (those with a service-connected disability) and then allow them a choice as to whether they wished to purchase care in the private medical sector or in the government's Veterans Administration hospitals. Such potential competition would be threatening to the Veterans Administration bureaucracy. Prohibiting competition for the provision of governmentally financed services often has less to do with efficiency and choice considerations than with the survival of an entrenched government bureaucracy. It would also reduce the size of the VA organization, since 85 percent of its beds are filled with veterans who do not have a service-connected disability. (Instead of reducing the size of its bureaucracy and budget as the number of veterans of the type for whom it was originally established to provide medical care decreases, the VA would prefer to maintain its institutions and budget by expanding the eligible class of veterans.)

quantity of goods and services they themselves purchase, but also upon the amount of certain goods and services (such as medical care) purchased by others. Under such circumstances, if some contribute to the medical services of the less fortunate, then other persons, who similarly would have been willing to contribute, receive an external benefit; everybody receives the benefit of seeing the less fortunate receive medical care, even though everybody did not necessarily contribute. Theoretically, each person who receives an external benefit should contribute according to the size of the external benefit. Unless there is some form of nonmarket decisionmaking, it will not be possible to collect from all the persons who receive an external benefit.

The implications from the preceding discussion are twofold. First, government, acting as the agent for the collective desires of those wishing to contribute, should tax those persons (assuming the government knows the utility functions of each individual exactly) the amount they would be willing to contribute and should provide a subsidy to the desired recipients equivalent to the magnitude of the collected tax. Second, the form of that subsidy (e.g., medical services) and the determination of its method of distribution (possibly an income-related determination of recipients), should represent the desires of the *donors*, not those of the recipients (3). This is because some donors may be willing to contribute, and thereby receive an external benefit, only if their contributions go to a particular income group, for a particular type of service, and are distributed in a certain manner. There are a number of ways in which subsidies could be provided to help those who are ill or who have low incomes. These persons could be given an income supplement rather than just an increase in their medical services; with an increase in their incomes, they could spend those funds on housing, nutritional foods, or medical services. If it is a lack of access to medical services that the more fortunate wish to redress, it would be inappropriate, from the donor's perspective, to allow those funds to be spent on goods and services other than medical care. Under circumstances of externalities in consumption, in-kind subsidies are efficient.

The justification for national health insurance and other forms of in-kind subsidies (to be discussed more completely in subsequent sections) is presumably based on the assumption that there are externalities in consumption; otherwise, proposed in-kind subsidies would not be efficient. If the objective of the subsidies were the redistribution of income, direct cash supplements would be a more efficient means to this end. The recipients of the subsidy would always prefer cash, which can be used to satisfy their most important needs, rather than a subsidy that can be used for only one of their needs, a need which may not represent their highest priority (4). For in-kind subsidies to be efficient, therefore, the intent must be to satisfy the preferences of the *donors* rather than the recipients. When an in-kind subsidy is called for, as in the case of externalities in consumption, the type of person the donors are willing to subsidize and the amount of subsidy to be provided to each person are probably inversely related to the recipient's income: the lower the recipient's income, the greater will be the donor's willingness to provide a subsidy. It is unlikely that a person will receive an external benefit from seeing a person with a possibly higher income than his own receive a subsidy. These aspects of in-kind subsidies should be kept in mind when national health insurance and other in-kind subsidies are discussed subsequently.

Requiring everyone to purchase minimum health insurance that includes catastrophic coverage might also be justified on grounds of externalities. If a person decides to self-insure, then other persons are bearing part of the cost of that decision. If the person who self-insures is unfortunate enough to incur catastrophic medical expense that he or she is unable to pay, the community (through welfare payments) will have to reimburse the medical providers for that person's medical services. The rest of the community will have to bear part of the cost (in terms of higher taxes) of that individual's decision to self-insure (or purchase less than catastrophic insurance). It would be more equitable, therefore, if these costs were borne in full by individuals at risk, similar to an uninsured motorists fund.

The third type of externality that occurs in the health field is usually associated with public health programs rather than with personal medical services. Vaccination programs, clean water supplies, air pollution abatement, and medical research are examples of goods that result in large external benefits. It has generally been with respect to these types of programs that a great many cost-benefit studies have been undertaken.

REDISTRIBUTION USING IN-KIND SUBSIDIES

There are many types of in-kind subsidies in medical care. Some of these are demand subsidies, others are supply subsidies; some are indirect with regard to the beneficiary groups they hope to affect, others are direct. National health insurance would be classified as a direct demand subsidy. Before discussing national health insurance, it would be instructive to discuss the different types of in-kind subsidies in medical care, their magnitude, their probable effects, and their probable beneficiaries. When we develop a better understanding of in-kind subsidies, their actual as compared with their stated purposes becomes clearer, and a context within which national health insurance can be analyzed is provided. If national health insurance is enacted, it is then questionable whether current in-kind subsidies should be continued. If national health insurance is a more efficient in-kind subsidy, then perhaps current in-kind subsidies should be used to help fund a national health insurance program.[5]

The major in-kind subsidies on the demand side are Medicare and Medicaid. Expenditures under these programs (and other direct subsidies on the demand side such as maternal and child health care) were $120.7 billion in 1985 (5). The other demand-side subsidies are indirect; there is the current tax deductibility of medical expenses in excess of 7.5 percent of adjusted gross income and the provision of employer-paid health insurance premiums as a fringe benefit, which is excluded from the employee's taxable income. These indirect subsidies were estimated to cost approximately $20 billion a year (6).

On the supply side there are subsidy programs for health manpower education at both federal and state levels, federal subsidies for hospital construction, and federal and state provision of medical services through the Veterans Administration and state

---

[5]Regardless of their stated intent, in-kind medical care subsidies do not have as their actual objective an increase in health status. Instead, their goal appears to be an increase in use of medical services. For example, total public spending on medical services for those 65 years of age and older were $2,823 per person in 1984; for the nonaged the equivalent figure was $242. If the actual purpose of government medical care expenditures were to achieve an increase in health levels, these expenditures might well have been allocated to different population groups, disease categories, and to non-medical-care programs. Even if it were agreed that the in-kind subsidy was to be provided to the aged alone, a different allocation of funds for non-medical-care services would be called for. An equivalent cash supplement to the aged to enable them to increase their consumption of food, housing, and heating would probably contribute more to their health than a subsidy restricted to medical services alone. Personal communication with Helen Lazenby June 3, 1987.

and local government hospitals. There are also numerous indirect supply subsidy programs, for example, which grant tax-exempt status to nonprofit providers such as nonprofit hospitals and Blue Cross plans, and state assistance in financing hospital bond issues.

The size of these demand and supply subsidies, both direct and indirect, is very large: roughly $216 billion in 1985.[6] Since expenditures for personal medical care totaled approximately $371 billion in 1985, it is clear that the role of government in the financing and provision of personal medical services is large and increasing.

Given the significant role of government in personal medical services, it is important to determine who are the beneficiaries of these subsidies and the efficiency with which these subsidies are being distributed. These two issues are interrelated; as discussed previously, the argument for in-kind subsidies is based upon externalities in consumption. As such, the primary recipients should be those persons with low incomes and/or poor health. If the subsidies are distributed in such a way as to benefit higher-income groups or provide them with a greater proportionate share of the subsidy, then the distribution of the subsidy is inefficient; that is, the desired beneficiary group (low-income persons) could receive a greater amount of the subsidy if it were provided in a different, presumably more direct manner.[7]

It is generally easier to calculate the beneficiary groups under demand rather than supply subsidies. Under the Medicaid program, for example, the designated beneficiaries are the medically indigent. Since Medicaid is a federal-state matching program, the definition of medical indigency and the benefits provided under the program vary by state. However, as shown in Table 19–1, expenditures under Medicaid go predominantly to the poor and near-poor. This relationship between income level and Medicaid expenditure holds for both per capita and total Medicaid expenditures. When one examines indirect demand subsidy programs, it becomes even less obvious that the subsidies are going to those persons with the lowest incomes and/or greatest medical needs. Under Medicare, because the beneficiary group is defined by age rather than income level, the subsidy is more evenly distributed than Medicaid across income levels. Not all aged persons have lower incomes than nonaged persons or are of poorer health. Although per capita Medicare expenditures decrease with higher income levels, the percent of total Medicare expenditures going to each income level is more evenly distributed. The poor and near-poor received 28 percent of total Medicare expenditures as compared to the high-income group, who received 21 percent.

When tax subsidy programs, such as the exclusion of employer-provided health insurance premiums from taxable income and the deduction of medical expenses are examined, higher-income groups are the major beneficiaries. Middle-income and high-income groups together receive 94 percent of those subsidy dollars.

When government expenditures for all three programs are combined, the total benefits are very evenly divided across the different income groups: the biggest losers, however, appear to be the other-low-income group, with 16 percent of total government expenditures; this group receives few Medicaid benefits and their incomes are too low to benefit from the tax subsidy programs. The poor and near-poor, middle-income, and high-income groups received 29, 27, and 28 percent, respectively. Medi-

[6]Forty-three percent was used as the percentage of government expenditures in total health spending to derive the estimates for 1985.

[7]This assumes that the method of distribution is not prescribed by the same externalities argument that gave rise to the subsidy in the first place.

TABLE 19-1. Major Federal Government Expenditures on Health Services, 1977

All Persons	Income Tax Savings	Medicare[a]	Medicaid	Total Federal[b]
Per Capita Government Expenditures				
Poor and near-poor	$ 2	$141	$184	$327
Other low-income	16	99	63	178
Middle-income	43	57	16	116
High-income	90	48	4	142

Total Government Expenditures (Billions of Dollars)

	$	%	$	%	$	%	$	%
Poor and near-poor	0.1	1	4.3	28	5.6	62	10.0	29
Other low-income	0.5	5	3.1	20	2.0	22	5.6	16
Middle-income	3.5	34	4.7	31	1.3	14	9.5	27
High-income	6.2	60	3.3	21	0.2	2	9.7	28
Total expenditures	10.3	100	15.4	100	9.1	100	34.8	100

Sources: This table is from Gail R. Wilensky, "Government and the Financing of Health Care," *American Economic Review* (May 1982): 205, Table 2.

[a] Less Part B premiums.

[b] Excludes expenditures from veterans programs and small federal programs. The definition of income groups are as follows: The "poor" include those whose family income was less than or equal to the 1977 poverty level as well as those whose income was between 101 and 125 percent of that level. "Other low income" includes those whose income is 1.26 to two times the poverty level, "middle income" is 2.01 to four times the poverty level, and "high income" is 4.01 times the poverty level or more. For a family of four in 1977, these four groups distribute as follows: less than $8,000 to $9,999, $10,000 to $15,999, $16,000 to $31,999, and greater than $32,000. The percent of the population in each group is 14, 15, 39, and 32 percent, respectively.

caid expenditures, which heavily favor the low-income groups, are offset by the tax subsidy programs. The redistributional effects of Medicare are small.

The government is attempting to reduce its expenditures on Medicare and Medicaid. As it does so, the redistributional effects of government health expenditures will go more to the higher-income groups, unless changes are also made in the tax subsidy programs.

It would thus appear that the more directly the demand subsidy is aimed at a designated population group, the more likely it is that the intended recipients will receive a larger proportion of that subsidy. Direct subsidy programs of this sort would be more in accordance with the stated goals of the legislation. Indirect demand subsidy programs are a less efficient way of subsidizing a particular beneficiary group. If in-kind medical subsidies are justified on grounds of externalities, the beneficiaries should presumably be those with lower incomes and/or greater needs for medical care than the persons favoring such subsidies. Direct demand subsidies would be both a more obvious and a more direct means of assuring that this objective is achieved. It is perhaps an indication of the true, as compared to the stated, intent of the legislation that in-kind subsidies are indirect, such as the tax subsidy programs.

There are two ways in which demand subsidies impose costs on those persons not receiving them. First, those persons must pay increased taxes to pay for the subsidy program. Second, an increase in demand by the recipients of the subsidies leads to an increase in the cost of medical services. These higher prices for medical services both increase the cost and decrease the use (depending upon the price elasticity of demand) for those persons not being subsidized. After Medicare and Medicaid were introduced, prices in the medical sector more than doubled, as shown previously in Table 10–4.

The demand subsidy will have secondary effects throughout the entire medical sector. A demand subsidy will cause an increase in demand in the different institutional markets: hospitals, physician services, and so on. How large the increase in demand will be in each of the separate institutional markets will depend, in part, upon the type of demand subsidy-(i.e., how much price is reduced to the beneficiaries)-in each of the institutional settings and the elasticity of supply in that market. A more inelastic supply will result in greater price increases, which will tend to reduce demand in both the beneficiary and nonbeneficiary groups. As demand increases in each of the institutional settings, there will be an increase in the derived demand for the inputs (different types of health manpower and nonlabor inputs) used in that setting. With increased demands for health manpower, wages and incomes in the manpower markets will increase, together with participation rates. In the long run, an increase in the incomes of health personnel will result in increased demands for a health professional education, and if the health education market responds, there will be an increase in the stock of trained health manpower. How much of the demand subsidy will end up in higher prices rather than in increased services will depend upon the elasticity of supply in the various medical markets. The greater the number of restrictions on entry into the health professions, and on the tasks that different health personnel can perform, and the greater the lack of efficiency incentives in methods of provider payment, the greater the inelasticity of supply and the higher will be the increases in medical prices.

Supply subsidies may also be classified according to whether they are directly targeted to a beneficiary group or whether their benefits are diffused among many population groups. An example of a supply subsidy that is directed at a designated beneficiary group is the provision of funds to establish a clinic in a low-income neighborhood. Even if there is no corresponding demand subsidy, the new clinic will result in an increased use of medical services by those with low incomes because it will decrease the patients' cost of travel to the facility. Most direct supply subsidies are not of this type; the major direct supply subsidies are the Veterans Administration hospitals and state and local government hospitals.

The Veterans Administration medical system is fairly extensive, consisting of 120 general hospitals, 50 mental hospitals, and numerous clinics and rehabilitation centers. Although the major stated role of the VA is to provide medical care to veterans with a service-connected disability, only 15 percent of the veterans in VA hospitals are there for that purpose. The remaining 85 percent have low incomes and receive care for illnesses unrelated to their military service (7).

State and local government hospitals account for approximately 20 percent of all admissions to short-term general hospitals and approximately 25 percent of all hospital outpatient visits. These hospitals have served as important sources of medical care for the indigent and have relieved the private hospitals and physicians of the financial risk of caring for these patients.

In view of the increase in Medicare and Medicaid, and the possibility of enacting national health insurance, all of which are targeted to the same population groups served by the VA and other government hospital systems, what is the likely and proper role for these providers? If the medically indigent were to receive a demand subsidy with benefits at least as complete as those presently available to them in the VA and other government hospitals, the demand for care in these institutions is likely to decline sharply. State and local government hospitals have had a reputation for providing care of lower quality or of less satisfaction to patients than is provided by community nonprofit hospitals. VA hospitals are inconveniently located in relation to their beneficiary population (there are only 120 VA hospitals as opposed to more than 3,500 community hospitals), and it is unlikely that the advantages of being in a VA hospital are sufficient to offset the patient's considerable travel costs. If the benefits (i.e., price) under national health insurance for the 85 percent of the VA patient population who are medically indigent were the same as the benefits for the community's medically indigent, it is likely that the VA patient population would choose care in a community hospital.

If all providers, including the VA and the other government hospitals, had to compete for patients under a demand subsidy arrangement, the VA and governmental hospitals would either have to change or they would not be able to survive in a competitive environment. For the VA system to compete for the 85 percent of its population who use the VA because they are medically indigent, it would have to provide ambulatory services, change its organizational and reimbursement arrangements with its physicians, increase its relative efficiency by lowering length of stay and using less costly substitutes for inpatient care, and compete on a more local basis for patients, since patient travel costs and time are likely to be significant determinants in choosing medical delivery systems.

The VA hospital system has been able to survive since the passage of Medicare and Medicaid because the VA was able to fill the gaps in that coverage for the medically indigent veteran. Will there be a role for the VA if the benefits under national health insurance are more complete for the medically indigent? It is unlikely that a bureaucracy as large as the VA will accept the market's judgment of an 80 percent reduction in its budget, but it is equally unlikely that such a large, centrally controlled bureaucracy will be able to undertake the drastic changes in its role, organization, and delivery system that would be necessary for them to compete on an equal basis with the private medical system. If the VA cannot survive under these conditions, what economic justification is there for providing additional large subsidies to enable the VA to maintain its current expanded role?

The role of state and local governmental hospitals under national health insurance is also uncertain. With the passage of Medicare and Medicaid, these hospitals were able to bill for their services and increase their source of revenues. Patients also came to these hospitals because there were gaps in their Medicare coverage. The hospitals became less dependent upon local governments for financial support. With additional funds, these hospitals were able to increase their staffing (from 234 employees per 100 patients in 1965 to 385 in 1985; this compared with 252 and 386, respectively, in community hospitals) and to improve their plant and equipment. It has been hypothesized that because these governmental hospitals were controlled on a local basis and operated with more decentralized management than the VA hospital system, it was easier for them to adapt and to compete with community hospitals (8). If the medically indigent served by these hospitals were to be provided with more comprehensive benefits under national health insurance, it is possible that these hospitals would be able to adapt and survive without additional subsidies. It would be questionable that direct supply subsidies would still be necessary if the population group originally served by these institutions were provided with a direct demand subsidy and chose to exercise those benefits in a different medical care delivery system. (The existence of public hospitals is usually an indication that the size of the direct demand subsidies is insufficient for the private sector to serve these population groups.)

Indirect supply subsidies, the other major type of in-kind supply subsidies, are exemplified by funds for training additional health manpower and capital grants to hospitals. These indirect supply subsidies have their initial effects on a particular medical market. For the subsidy to result in increased medical services, its effect must eventually be transmitted through several medical markets. For example, when a subsidy is given to medical schools to increase the number of physicians, several years pass before there is an increase in the number of additional graduates. These graduates will then work in a number of settings, ranging from hospitals to physicians' offices. The increase in the amount of services eventually received by the members of a particular beneficiary group will depend upon their elasticity of demand for those services. (The increased supply of services is a downward shift along a patient's demand curve for that service.) If demand by members of the beneficiary group is relatively inelastic (i.e., not very responsive to changes in the price of the service), there will be relatively little increase in their use of medical services. Since indirect supply subsidies are not generally targeted to particular beneficiary groups, the beneficiaries will be all those persons using the service; they will be paying a lower price than before the subsidy. Because low-income persons do not use medical services as much as those with high incomes, they may receive less benefit than high users from such subsidies; the high users may also have relatively higher incomes.

In addition to their being inefficient, in that the highest proportion of the subsidy does not go to low-income persons, general supply subsidies present further problems. When only one input into the process of producing medical care is subsidized, a manager who is attempting to use the lowest-cost combination of inputs will tend to use more of the subsidized input because its cost has been artificially reduced. For example, a subsidy to train additional registered nurses will, if it is successful, result in a greater increase in the supply of nurses and a relatively lower wage for them. Because the wage of nurses is lowered, hospitals will substitute away from other nursing personnel toward more registered nurses in providing patient care. This is a more costly approach to providing patient care than if the hospital were merely awarded an equivalent unrestricted subsidy. In the latter case, the hospital would use a combination of registered and nonregistered nurses and other inputs based on their relative prices and productivities. Consequently, the hospital would use fewer registered nurses than if only RN wages were artificially reduced through a subsidy. Subsidies that increase the supply of a particular input are therefore less efficient (more costly) than an equivalent dollar subsidy.

It is also often difficult to determine what additional services have been produced as a result of a supply subsidy. Although one might be able to count the number of additional persons trained as a result of the subsidy (which is not as easy as it might appear), it is more difficult to calculate the net increase in services resulting from the additional health manpower. Without additional nurses, the wage rate of existing nurses would have risen more rapidly, which in turn would have caused a greater increase in the participation rate of trained nurses not currently employed. In the long run, with higher wages in the profession, there would be an increase in the number of persons seeking a career in nursing. Similarly, without a subsidy to increase the number of physicians, the productivity of existing physicians might be greater. Thus, to assume that the additional services provided by the subsidized manpower are the net benefits of the supply subsidy program is to greatly overstate its benefits.

To understand exactly what impact supply subsidies have on increased utilization of services, and for which beneficiary groups, it is necessary to use a complex econometric model of the medical sector. For example, a subsidy to increase the number of registered nurses will have its initial impact on the nursing education market. How many additional nurses will be graduated as a result of that subsidy will depend, in part, on the objectives of the different types of nursing schools and on which schools receive the subsidies. The number of nurses will also depend upon the elasticity of demand for a nursing education by prospective nurses, since the subsidy will reduce their educational costs. The impact of additional nurses on the market for nurses will affect nurses' wages, participation rates, and nurse employment. How many additional nurses will be employed in the various institutional settings will depend upon the elasticity of demand for nurses in each of the different settings and the new wage for nurses. (The determination of wages and employment will, of course, be a simultaneous process.) The greater the substitutability of registered nurses for other types of nursing personnel, the higher will be the elasticity of demand and the greater will be the decrease in demand for nonregistered nurses. Each of the institutional settings that employs registered nurses will have a slightly lower cost for its nursing personnel; the cost of care in each institutional setting will also be lower. How much lower will depend upon how many registered nurses are employed and the elasticity of the demand for nurses (i.e., whether many more nurses are hired as a result of their relatively lower wage). The effect of the nurse subsidy on cost of care will vary for each institutional setting; hospitals, which hire the majority of nurses, would receive the largest cost reduction. Since the relative cost of the different institutional settings has changed, how much the price of care will be reduced in each of the institutional settings as a result of a lowering of costs will depend upon the elasticity of demand for services and the environment in which an institution competes. If there are no competitive pressures on the institution, if the institution attempts to maximize its prestige, and if the institution is reimbursed on a cost basis, it is less likely that the cost savings will be passed on to patients and other third-party payors. Thus, the final impact of supply subsidies on supply of medical services as compared with the impact of demand subsidies is much more difficult to determine. It is equally difficult to determine which consumer or payor group receives the major benefit of the subsidy, if any of them receives any benefit at all.

Supply subsidies in medical care have generally been direct in their impact on low-income persons when the government itself has served as the supplier. When supply subsidies have been indirect, in-kind subsidies have provided benefits to all those persons who use medical services; but as with the Hill-Burton program for hospital construction, nothing was done to help those who could not afford to use the hospital. A demand subsidy was still required for the medically indigent. In-kind supply subsidies take longer than direct demand subsidies to provide greater access to medical services to a beneficiary group. They are also economically inefficient, either because patients have no choice as to which provider they must go to, as under the VA system, or because the relative cost of inputs is distorted. Finally, the benefits of indirect supply subsidies are overstated, since employee participation rates and productivity increases are, in fact, likely to be lower than what they would otherwise have been.

Although direct demand subsidies would appear to be a more efficient method of providing an in-kind subsidy, supply subsidies are legislatively popular. The probable reason is not that legislators are necessarily unaware of which is the more efficient subsidy method, but rather that the providers of medical care and manpower education are important beneficiaries of such proposals. Such supply subsidies are generally the direct result of lobbying by these interest groups.

The intent of the preceding discussion on existing in-kind subsidies in medical care was to provide both an indication of the current magnitude of their support and some criteria by which to judge the efficiency of alternative types of in-kind subsidies. If national health insurance is to be undertaken, then one should specifically determine which of the many demand and supply (direct and indirect) subsidies should remain; any funds saved might be used to bear part of the cost of national health insurance.

REFERENCES

1. For a complete discussion of the role of government, see Richard A. Musgrave and Peggy B. Musgrave, *Public Finance in Theory and Practice* (New York: McGraw-Hill, 1984). Musgrave categorizes government programs into those that affect the allocation of resources, those that alter the distribution of incomes, and stabilization programs (i.e., those that regulate the level of economic activity).

2. For an extensive discussion of cost-benefit analysis, see Edward M. Gramlich, *Benefit-Cost Analysis of Government Programs* (Englewood Cliffs, N.J.: Prentice-Hall, 1981).

3. For a more extended discussion of this proposition see Paul Feldman, "Efficiency, Distribution, and the Role of Government in a Market Economy," *Journal of Political Economy* 79(3), May-June 1971: 508–526.

4. A proof of this statement may be found in a number of texts on microeconomics. See, for example, Richard H. Leftwich and Ross D. Eckert, *The Price System and Resource Allocation*, (Hinsdale, Ill.: Dryden Press, 1985), pp. 127–129.

5. Daniel R. Waldo, Katherine R. Levit, and Helen Lazenby, "National Health Expenditures, 1985," *Health Care Financing Review*, 8(1) Fall 1986: 19.

6. Previously, one-half of the health insurance premium, up to a maximum of $150, was deductible, as was medical expenses in excess of 3 percent of adjusted gross income. Including the exclusion from the employee's taxable income of employer paid health insurance premiums, these indirect subsidies were estimated to have cost approximately $20 billion a year. Charles E. Phelps, "Public Sector Medicine: History and Analysis," in *New Directions in Public Health Care* (San Francisco: Institute for Contemporary Studies, 1980), pp. 130–131.

7. Phelps *op. cit.*, p. 153.

8. *Ibid.*, p. 162.

CHAPTER 20

National Health Insurance: An Approach to the Redistribution of Medical Care

This discussion on national health insurance (NHI) begins with a theoretical framework that can be used to analyze various proposals in terms of the efficiency with which they achieve the different values that underlie proposals for NHI. No attempt will be made to select one set of values over another; instead, the analysis will be concerned with the most efficient means for achieving a given set of values. Some empirical evidence based on Medicare will be used to support the theoretical conclusions. This theoretical discussion will then be used as a basis for developing a set of criteria for evaluating alternative health insurance proposals. The current system of financing medical care and several suggested proposals for NHI will then be discussed according to the criteria developed. No attempt will be made to provide a detailed discussion of current legislative proposals, inasmuch as a number of other publications have provided such detailed analyses (1). Also, since new legislative proposals are constantly being made, a basic understanding of the concepts underlying such proposals should be more useful for understanding both current and future proposals.

ACHIEVING EFFICIENCY FOR DIFFERENT VALUES UNDERLYING NATIONAL HEALTH INSURANCE

A Theoretical Discussion

National health insurance (NHI) may be viewed as an in-kind demand subsidy based on the argument that there are externalities in consumption. If the nonpoor wish to subsidize the poor, this will result in a demand for government subsidies. The degree

527

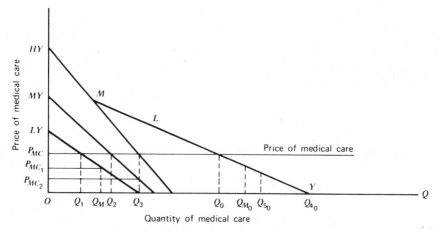

Figure 20-1. Demand curves of different income groups.

of subsidization will differ depending upon the values held by the nonpoor with respect to redistribution of medical care services. One set of values may be termed minimum provision, meaning that no person in society should receive less than a certain quantity of medical care in case of illness. A second set of values might be called equal financial access to medical care. If these values were the basis for the externalities in consumption, they would suggest an NHI plan that would equalize the financial barriers to all persons; in other words, the price of medical services would be the same for everyone. The third set of values that people may share with respect to redistribution of medical care services goes beyond equal financial access to require equal treatment for equal needs—in other words, equal consumption of medical services regardless of economic or other factors affecting utilization. The different demands for government subsidies reflect varying sets of values that are believed to exist in the population. The first set of values would require the smallest level of subsidization; the third set of values would be the most expensive to achieve.

It is not possible to state which set of values is most appropriate; whichever set of values the population selects would be the proper basis for the level of government subsidies under NHI. Although it is not possible to determine a priori the set of values that is likely to be chosen by the population, it is possible to determine the most efficient approach for achieving each of the three sets of values. It should be possible to state which types of national health insurance are likely to be more efficient than others, regardless of the set of values that one holds.

Minimum provision may be achieved in one of two ways: those persons whose consumption of medical care is below the minimum may be subsidized to bring their consumption up to the minimum, or, alternatively, a subsidy can be provided to *everyone* so that at the resulting new, lower price, no one person's consumption would be below the minimum specified by society. These two alternatives are shown in Figure 20-1. Assuming that there are three different income groups—high incomes (HY), middle incomes (MY), and low incomes (LY)—their demands for medical care would be shown by the three demand curves, HY, MY, and LY, respectively. The aggregate demand curve of all three income groups is shown by $HYMLY$. The reason the three demand curves do not result in the same consumption of medical care at zero price is that there are factors, other than financial ones, that result in differences in demand between different income groups. For example, low-income groups may incur greater costs in traveling to providers than do higher-income groups; differences in attitudes may also affect their utilization. Provider preferences in dealing with different income groups may also play a role. If the current price of medical care is P_{mc}, the utilization of the three income groups would be Q_1, Q_2, and Q_3, and their aggregate utilization would be Q_0, which is the intersection of the aggregate demand curve and the supply of medical care (assuming, for simplicity, perfect elasticity).

If society wanted to assure that no one received less than a minimum amount of medical care, Q_m, a national health insurance system that either reduced the price of medical care to everyone or that set the price to zero for everyone would achieve this goal. A system of subsidies that lowers the price of medical care just to those whose consumption is less than the minimum would also achieve this goal. If medical care were free, everyone's consumption would increase, with the total going from Q_0 to Q_{40}. If, instead, a subsidy were provided to just those persons whose consumption was below the minimum (i.e., by lowering the price to lower-income persons to P_{mc1}), the aggregate increase in use of medical care would be from Q_0 to Q_{m0}. The cost to society of this approach to achieving minimum provision would be the subsidy required to increase the low-income group's utilization, which is $P_{mc} - P_{mc1}$, multiplied by that group's utilization, Q_m. The cost of making medical care free to all persons would be the price of medical care multiplied by the new and greater quantity that would result when the price was reduced to everyone, which is P_{mc} multiplied by Q_{40}. Since both approaches would achieve the goal of minimum provision, the approach that provided a subsidy to the lower-income group only would be less costly, hence more efficient, than a scheme that reduced the price to everyone.[1]

If society's values with respect to redistribution of medical care were that all persons should have equal financial access to medical care, then this could be achieved by establishing a free medical care system (or a low price to all persons), as in the previous illustration, or through a system of subsidies that varied according to income levels. Equal financial access could be achieved through a subsidy system that reduced the price of medical care to low-income persons to zero; their consumption would thereby increase to Q_3. A subsidy to middle-income groups equal to $P_{mc} - P_{mc2}$ would also increase their consumption to Q_3. At consumption level Q_3, the utilization of medical care for the three income groups would be equal. The aggregate increase in medical care use would go from Q_0 to Q_{50}. Equal financial access would require a more expensive subsidy ($Q_3 \times P_{mc}$ for the low-income group, plus $Q_3 \times (P_{mc} - P_{mc2})$ for the middle-income group) than would be required for achieving minimum provision, but it would still be less costly than a medical care system that eliminated all financial barriers for everyone.

It is unlikely that the external demand for subsidization, based on the value that there should be equal financial access, would include the value judgment that the demands of higher-income persons should be increased beyond levels that they currently spend, and that this increase should be financed through higher taxes. If such persons are currently purchasing Q_3 amount of medical care, then the value to them of additional units of care is less than the price they would have to pay to consume it. It would be illogical for people to vote for an additional tax on themselves to purchase addi-

---

[1] For simplicity's sake it is assumed that the different proposals do not differ in their administrative costs nor in the response by suppliers to those proposals.

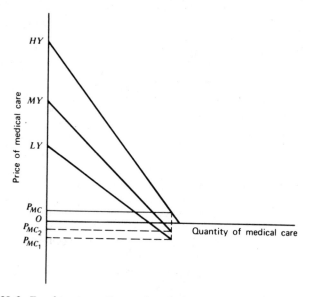

Figure 20-2. Equal treatment for equal needs through a system of negative prices.

tional units of medical care when they were previously not willing to pay the equivalent amount of money to purchase those same units.

Equal treatment for equal needs expresses the third set of values that give rise to a demand for medical care subsidies. Since demands for medical care vary for more reasons than just financial ones, merely making the price of medical care free to all will not result in equal consumption. As shown in Figure 20-1, high-income groups would still consume more medical care at zero price than would the middle- and lower-income groups. Thus a free medical care system would not be able to achieve that set of values defined as equal treatment for equal needs. The value likely to be achieved through a free medical care system would be equal financial access, which, as we have shown, could be achieved at lower cost by a system of subsidies that varied by income level.

The only way in which equal treatment for equal needs could be achieved would be by differential subsidies, varying according to income level. For example, as shown in Figure 20-2, lowering the price of medical care to zero for both low- and middle-income groups would still not increase their utilization to where it equaled that of the high-income group. Only if the low- and middle-income groups were subsidized further, through a system of negative prices, could their utilization be equal. (Negative prices mean that such groups are paid to increase their use.) How large the negative prices would have to be would depend, in part, upon the consumption levels of the high-income groups. If high-income groups do not vote to increase their own consumption through subsidies which they will then have to repay in higher taxes, the size of the subsidy required to increase the other groups' consumption to the point where it equals the higher income group's will be less.

It is unlikely that legislation would be passed that would actually pay people to increase their use of medical care. Instead, a negative price would be paid by means of a direct in-kind supply subsidy to low-income groups. For example, although the price

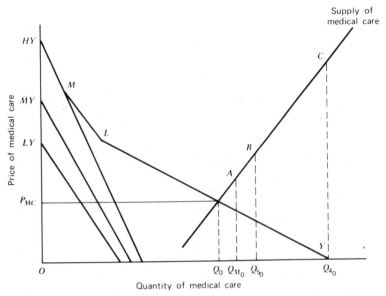

Figure 20–3. The cost of different demand subsidies when supply of medical care is relatively inelastic.

of medical care to a low-income person would be zero, substantial travel and access costs might deter that person from using more medical services. Establishing clinics and neighborhood health centers in low-income areas and providing incentives for health personnel to practice there would increase access and decrease travel costs, thereby increasing use.

The cost in resources and the consequent increase in taxes required to achieve each of the three sets of values are even greater when the more realistic assumption is made that supply is not perfectly elastic but is, instead, relatively inelastic. Figure 20–3 is similar to Figure 20–1, except that the supply of medical care is less elastic. The consequence of a rising supply curve is that as demand is subsidized, the cost of a subsidy will be greater than if supply were more elastic. The cost of the subsidy necessary to achieve minimum provision is the utilization of the low-income group multiplied by the higher price of medical care (point A on the supply curve). This higher price will also be borne by those persons in society who favor medical care subsidies to low-income groups.[2] The taxes required to fund equal financial access will be greater than those required to achieve minimum provision. The price paid by the government will continue to increase, as will the price paid by those not receiving subsidies. As might be expected, as the price to those who are not being subsidized rises, and the cost of achieving a given set of values increases, the amount that they are willing to subsidize others will decline.

For national health insurance to have the redistributive effects that are desired by society, increased utilization must occur; it will most easily occur when the price elas-

---

[2]Because the supply of medical care is not elastic, it is necessary to think in terms of the postsubsidy market price that an income group will face when the price of medical care is subsidized. National health insurance based on a tax credit is one way of achieving this.

ticity of demand for medical services by those persons receiving subsidies is high. The greater the price elasticities of demand, the greater the increase in demand along an inelastic supply will be; therefore, rapidly increasing prices and total expenditures for the subsidy program will be the consequences.

It is precisely because of these expected higher costs that proposals for national health insurance have included approaches for changing the delivery system as well. In evaluating alternative national health insurance proposals, the demand proposals should be analyzed separately from the supply proposals. Presumably, proposals to enhance efficiency on the supply side, which were discussed in a previous chapter, can be incorporated into any NHI plan. A supply proposal becomes an integral part of the demand proposal only when its proponents are not willing to accept the criterion of economic efficiency in supply. Under one previous proposal for NHI, the Kennedy-Corman Health Security Act, which would have made medical care free to all, a great deal of emphasis is placed upon how the supply side will be financed and organized. Expenditure limits by region and by type of provider would be established. As shown in Figure 20–3, total expenditures and prices would increase sharply under a free medical care system. Arbitrary establishment of dollar limits is an outgrowth of a political process and is unrelated to underlying supply and demand conditions. Expenditure limits would serve as a cost-control mechanism, but if cost control is the consequence of this approach, either intended or otherwise, the proponents of a free medical care system should be more explicit in defining the set of values that underlie this approach. They should also demonstrate how arbitrarily determined expenditure limits on the supply side would achieve these values.

The advocates of a free medical system might argue that it would still be possible to achieve, through greater efficiency, the program's stated goals at a lower expenditure level than indicated by the supply curve in Figure 20–3. Since the advocates of a free medical system are opposed to competition as a way of determining the most efficient system and set of providers, reliance would have to be placed upon government to manage the medical system and to bring about greater efficiency in supply. Previous attempts by government to regulate or manage the supply of a good or service, both outside and within the medical care field, lend little credibility to the belief that the government will become an efficient and innovative manager in the near future. It is more likely that the current medical care system would be frozen in existing patterns. The government has not been able to close the Veterans Administration, Public Health Service, or any municipal hospitals, when it wanted to do so on grounds of efficiency (similar to its difficulty in closing military bases), because of political pressure from employee groups and the constituencies of these facilities. It is likely that each provider group within each region would attempt to protect its expenditure allocation each year; such actions would prevent changes in methods of delivery when dollar allocations to providers would be affected.

The ability of government to bring about greater efficiency is not borne out by the evidence, even in the health field. Lengths of stay in Veterans Administration hospitals are much longer than in nongovernment hospitals (for similar diagnoses), and there has been little substitution away from hospitals, when medically possible, to less expensive services, such as ambulatory care. It is unlikely that the quality of managers in a medical system controlled by government would be improved. It is more likely that the quality of management would decline because such an all-inclusive system would preclude a point of reference outside itself by which managers could be evaluated. There also would be no incentives for managers to seek to change the system, and the financial rewards to good management would be greater in nongovernment-controlled sectors. Evidence to support this contention may be found not only in VA hospitals, but also in AMTRAK and the postal service. In the medical system, too, unions would become more powerful in the decisionmaking process, and as in the postal service, might inhibit the introduction of laborsaving innovations.

For each of the set of values examined—minimum provision, equal financial access, and equal treatment for equal needs—it was shown that these values can be achieved more efficiently if the subsidy varies by income level rather than if changes are sought through a system that either results in an equal price reduction to all or makes medical care free to everyone, regardless of income level. Although this analysis was theoretical, empirical data support these conclusions.

Some Empirical Evidence from the Medicare Program

Medicare is an existing in-kind demand subsidy to the aged. (Part A of Medicare provides hospital coverage, while Part B is a voluntary program primarily for physician services, whose premium is subsidized by the government.) The benefits available to all the aged under Medicare are similar, as is the reduced price they must pay for the use of medical care. To use physician services (Part B of Medicare), an aged person was initially required to pay a $50 deductible and 20 percent copayment above and beyond that deductible.[3] It would appear that the pricing mechanism was designed to ensure either equal financial access to medical care or equal treatment for equal medical needs for the aged.

As long as demand for medical care among the aged differs according to income and accessibility, then, as shown in Figure 20–1, a similar price to all persons, such as the aged under Medicare, would result in differences in utilization. Guaranteeing the same price to high-income aged would result in a greater utilization level for them in comparison with the low-income aged because it would represent a smaller financial burden to them and because their travel costs are lower, owing to their location in areas where they are closer to medical providers.

According to data shown in Table 20–1, the aged with higher incomes were more likely to pay the deductible and use the Part B supplementary coverage under Medicare: 552.3 persons per 1,000 Medicare enrollees with incomes in excess of $15,000, 431.7 persons per 1,000 among those aged with incomes less than $5,000. Services used by the higher-income aged also cost the government more: $10.40 compared with $7.02 per reimbursable service. (These higher prices represent higher prices for the same services as well as possibly higher-quality services, as when specialists are used.) The Medicare reimbursement per person enrolled was more than twice as high for the higher-income aged, $160.30 compared with $78.77. By 1977 the difference between the income groups lessened.

When Medicare utilization is examined for differences according to race, large disparities persist, as shown in Table 20–2. Whites are more likely than non whites to use physician services; one reason is that nonwhites receive more of their ambulatory services from hospital outpatient departments than do whites. The Medicare reimbursement is also on the average higher for whites than for nonwhites.

---

[3]The deductible has been increased several times; it was raised to $60 in 1973 and is currently $75. The inflation-adjusted value of the deductible declined to $27 in 1982.

TABLE 20-1. Medicare Reimbursements for Covered Services Under the Supplementary Medical Insurance Program and Persons Served, by Income, 1968 and 1977

Income Group	Persons Receiving Reimbursable Services Per 1,000 Medicare Enrollees	Medicare Reimbursement Per Reimbursable Service	Medicare Reimbursement Per Person Enrolled
	1968		
Under $5,000	431.7	$ 7.02	$ 78.77
Over $15,000	552.3	10.40	160.30
Ratio, over $15,000 to under $5,000 incomes	1.28	1.48	2.04
	1977		
At or near poverty line	773.4	6.43	60.32
High-income	801.7	5.82	57.72
Ratio, high-income to at or near poverty line	1.04	.91	.96

Source: For 1968 data: Karen Davis, "Equal Treatment and Unequal Benefits: The Medicare Program." *Milbank Memorial Fund Quarterly/Health and Society* 53(4): 457. Copyright Milbank Memorial Fund. Table 1. For 1977 data: G. Wilensky, L. Rossiter, and L. Finney, "The Medicare Subsidy of Private Health Insurance," Rockville, Md.: National Center for Health Services Research, National Health Care Expenditure Survey, 1983.

If Medicare were based upon the assumption that there should be equal treatment for equal needs, than one would expect to observe an equal number of physician visits according to level of medical need. This is unlikely to occur when all aged recipients face the same price but differ according to income, race, and accessibility, as shown in Table 20–3. Regardless of health status, aged persons with higher incomes had more physician visits than did aged with lesser incomes. Of those aged who are classified as being in poor health, in 1969 the low-income aged (less than $5,000 in income) had 10.47 physician visits per year compared to 16.98 visits per aged person with a high income (greater than $15,000 per year). When the 1977 data were examined, differences still existed according to income level, although they were less. Those aged on Medicaid generally show high visit rates, presumably because of their low out-of-pocket price. Visit rates for the high-income aged have declined since 1969.

The smaller differences in visit rates among aged in different income groups and the decrease in visit rates among the high-income aged over time may be explained as follows. Between 1969 and 1977 the "real" price (adjusted for inflation) has gone down for the low-income aged, hence increasing their visit rates, while the "real" price faced by the high-income aged increased, thereby decreasing their visit rates. Physicians serving low-income aged are likely to accept Medicare assignment; that is, they are willing to accept the Medicare fee as the price for their services. Medicare fee increases have been limited by the Medicare Economic Index, which has increased much more slowly than the rate of inflation. Thus, to low-income aged, the "real"

TABLE 20-2. Persons Served and Medicare Reimbursement per Person Served, by Race, 1968 and 1977

	Persons Served Per 1,000 Enrollees		Reimbursement Per Person Served		Medicare Reimbursement per Person Enrolled
	Physician Services	Hospital Outpatient Services	Physician Services	Hospital Outpatient Services	
1968					
Whites	394.9	71.6	$199.44	$39.02	$82.70
Blacks and other races	279.4	89.9	173.37	50.43	54.20
Ratio, white to other	1.413	.796	1.150	.774	1.526
1977					
Whites	770.	227.	60.01	70.46	62.23
Blacks	652.	315.	42.99	47.57	43.04
Ratio, whites to blacks	1.18	.72	1.40	1.48	1.45

Source: Davis, Karen. 1975. Equal Treatment and Unequal Benefits: The Medicare Program. *Milbank Memorial Fund Quarterly/Health and Society* 53:468, 469. The 1977 data are from G. Wilensky, L. Rossiter, and L. Finney, "The Medicare Subsidy of Private Health Insurance," National Center for Health Services Research, National Health Care Expenditure Survey, 1983.

TABLE 20-3. Average Physician Visits for the Elderly, by Health Status and Family Income, Adjusted for Other Determinants, 1969 and 1977

	Health Status[a]		
	Good	Average	Poor
	1969		
Family income:			
Under $5,000			
No aid[b]	2.78	5.64	10.47
Aid	3.86	7.52	13.42
$5,000–9,999	3.14	6.60	11.70
$10,000–14,999	3.75	7.27	12.98
$15,000 and over	5.35	9.53	16.98
	1977[c]		
At or near poverty line			
No Medicaid	3.72	6.56	9.06
Medicaid	5.89	7.36	10.43
Middle-income	4.21	7.31	10.66
High-income	4.34	7.30	—[d]

Source: 1969 data are from Karen Davis, *National Health Insurance: Benefits , Costs and Consequences* (Washington, D.C.: Brookings Institution, 1975), p. 85. The 1977 data are from G. Wilensky, L. Rossiter, and L. Finney, "The Medicare Subsidy of Private Health Insurance," National Center for Health Services Research, National Health Care Expenditure Survey, 1983.

[a]Good health status is defined as absence of any chronic conditions, limitations of activity, or restricted activity days. Average and poor health are defined as at the mean and twice the mean level, respectively, of the three morbidity indicators used.

[b]Aid indicates public assistant recipients.

[c]For 1977 data, respondents were asked to characterize their own health status relative to people of the same age.

[d]Cell size too small to estimate.

price of a physician visit has declined. The physician assignment rate, those physicians participating in Medicare, declined after Medicare started, reaching a low of 50.5 percent in 1977. Physicians are also less likely to take assignment for those aged who have higher incomes. All aged are required to pay a deductible and a copayment. However, the high-income aged person going to a nonparticipating physician must also pay the full difference between what Medicare reimburses as the physician's fee and the physician's actual fee. Physicians not accepting assignment were also able to raise their fees more rapidly than the increases permitted under the Medicare Economic Index. Thus high-income aged, using nonparticipating physicians, have experienced an increase in the "real" prices they pay for physician visits.

The 1969 data are therefore consistent with the expectation that visit rates will differ when different income groups face the *same* price. The 1977 data (and the change from 1969) are also consistent with what would be expected when different income groups pay *different* prices for physician visits.

Based on our experience with Medicare, it is obvious that a lower but similar price to all aged persons will achieve neither equal financial access nor equal treatment for equal needs. As could have been hypothesized based on the earlier theoretical discussion, Medicare is an inefficient approach for achieving either of the foregoing sets of values, because higher-income persons use a greater number of services than do lower-income persons, and the services they use are more costly. If the Medicare subsidy varied according to income level, the same services could have been provided to the low-income aged at a lower total cost. Not only would the overall level of utilization under Medicare be less if the subsidy varied by income, but the rise in medical prices would also have been less, since there would have been a smaller overall increase in demand. The record of the Medicare program should be kept in mind when specific proposals for national health insurance are analyzed in the following section.

SPECIFIC CRITERIA FOR EVALUATING NATIONAL HEALTH INSURANCE PLANS

Before discussing specific proposals for national health insurance, it would be useful to have a common set of criteria by which these alternative plans may be evaluated.

The Beneficiaries

Based on the previous discussion of the different sets of values held by society regarding redistribution of medical care, it may be said that the primary recipients of national health insurance should be those who are or might become medically indigent. The medically indigent are those persons who have low incomes and cannot buy as much medical care as society would prefer them to have; those persons whose medical expenses are large in relation to their incomes are potentially medically indigent. A person in the latter category may not necessarily have a low income, however, in the event of a serious illness even persons with middle incomes might be hard pressed to pay their medical bills.

Subsidies under national health insurance, therefore, should vary according to income (they should be larger for low-income persons and decline as income increases) and subsidies should be available so that an upper limit on liability for medical expenses could be set to protect even higher-income persons from suffering an undue financial hardship. Since what constitutes a financial hardship depends upon a person's income, the maximum medical liability for a person should be related to one's income in the form of a fraction of that income. (An alternative approach to eliminating potential financial hardship would be to require everyone to have major-medical or catastrophic insurance coverage. Because what is catastrophic for a low-income person may not be for a high-income person, a uniform definition may set the level too low for high-income persons, thereby encouraging greater use on their part once the limit is reached.)

The primary beneficiary groups included under national health insurance should be categorized according to both income and the size of the medical bill in relation to income. Categorizing population groups by age is a less direct approach for determining current medical need and potential financial hardship. Although many of the aged are low-income, not all of them require the same degree of financial subsidy; many younger persons have greater medical and financial needs than do some of the aged.

As discussed in Chapter 6, it would not be efficient for the government to provide subsidies to higher-income persons for a large fraction of their medical expenses. As long as there is moral hazard, the cost of subsidies to higher-income families will be greater than the value of the additional care received by these persons. Subsidies for medical care under national health insurance should be decreased with increased incomes.

How large the medical subsidies for low-income persons should be is basically a value judgment. Some persons would prefer that the poor receive all their medical care, including preventive care, without any charge; others would prefer a less generous subsidy. Any plan for national health insurance should be able to incorporate either of these conflicting values by varying the degree of subsidization in relation to income levels.

Incentives for Efficiency

A second criterion by which alternative health insurance plans should be judged is whether there are any incentives to encourage the efficient use of medical resources. The efficient use of resources may be accomplished in several ways. First, the combination of medical services that is least costly for providing a medical treatment should be used. If the benefit coverage is restricted to hospital care, excluding ambulatory and other nonhospital services, more of the care will be provided in the hospital even though it would be less costly to substitute ambulatory, nursing home, and home care services. Second, consumers (particularly the nonpoor) should be provided with some incentives to seek out less costly providers and not to overutilize. An approach that has been suggested for providing consumers with both of these incentives is to include deductibles and copayments: deductibles, in addition to reducing the administrative cost of handling many small bills and thereby reduce the overall cost of national health insurance, would, together with copayments, provide consumers with a monetary incentive to be aware of the provider's prices. In this way, cost savings could be achieved at the "front end", instead of having to exclude coverage for costly but necessary procedures and, as under Medicare, set an upper limit on the number of hospital days for which an aged person is covered.

The providers of medical services should also have incentives for efficiency under any national health insurance plan. Ideally, physicians should bear some fiscal responsibility for their use of medical resources. Suggestions for improving provider efficiency are varied and include allowing the providers to compete for patients, as HMOs do currently.

Equitable Financing

A third criterion for evaluating alternative NHI plans is the equitability of their financing. If NHI is based on the desire by those who are not poor to provide more medical services to those who have lower incomes, then the most equitable method of financing would be to have the nonpoor bear a higher proportion of the costs of NHI.[4] An equitable method of financing would be one in which the contribution was greater for those with higher incomes. Greater reliance on the income tax would be more equitable than relying on a social security tax; income taxes generally rise with increased incomes, but social security taxes are a fixed percentage of income up to a specified level of income. Social security taxes are therefore regressive, because they constitute a larger fraction of income for a low-income person than for a high-income person.

Medicare (Part A, Hospital Services) was financed by an increase in the Social Security tax. In 1965 the social security tax paid by both employee and employer was 3.625 percent (for a total of 7.25 percent) of the employee's wage up to a maximum annual wage of $4,800. To finance Medicare, the social security tax was increased to 4.2 percent (a total of 8.4 percent) on an increased wage base of $6,600. By 1988 the social security tax on both the employee and employer had risen to 7.51 percent (a total of 15.2) up to a maximum wage base of $45,000. The Medicare portion of the social security tax is currently 1.45 percent (a total of 2.9 percent). The social security tax is legislated to reach 7.65 percent by 1990.

Any financing mechanism should be analyzed in terms of its economic effects. It is first necessary, however, to determine who actually pays the social security tax, that is, who bears its burden. Although the employee and employer each pay one-half of the social security tax, the actual incidence of the tax is determined by the elasticity of the demand and supply curves for labor.

Assume that the initial wage rate is $10 an hour, as shown in Figure 20-4A. If the government were to impose a $2 an hour tax on the employee, the new labor supply curve would be ST, which is equal to the initial labor supply curve, S, plus the tax of $2 an hour. The new equilibrium wage will rise to $10.50 an hour. However, the employee would have to pay $2. of the $10.50 an hour to the government. The employees net wage is $8.50 an hour, $1.50 less per hour than their previous earnings. The employer pays $.50 an hour more than previously. Thus in the example above , the employee pays 75 percent of the $2 an hour tax, while the employer pays 25 percent.

Assume that instead of placing the tax on the employee, the $2 an hour tax is placed on the employer. As shown in Figure 20-4B, the size of the tax is indicated by the vertical distance between the two equilibrium points. (The employer's demand for labor shifts down with a per unit tax because the initial demand represents the maximum amount of labor the firm will hire at any given wage.) The burden of the tax when it is imposed on the employer is the same as when it was imposed on the employee. The employee receives $8.50 an hour, the employer pays the government $2 per hour, and the employer ends up paying $10.50 an hour, $.50 an hour more than previously. In both cases less labor is hired.

Figure 20-5 shows who bears the burden of a tax on labor when the demand for labor is less elastic (Figure 20-5A) and more elastic (Figure 20-5B). The elasticity of labor supply is the same in both cases.

---

[4]Compulsory catastrophic coverage is justified on different grounds. If someone does not have catastrophic coverage and suffers a large medical expense that has to be subsidized by the community, that person, who may not have a low income, is shifting the risk, hence the cost of catastrophic coverage to the rest of the community. If all persons have an equal chance of incurring a catastrophic illness of equal cost, they should make an equal contribution.

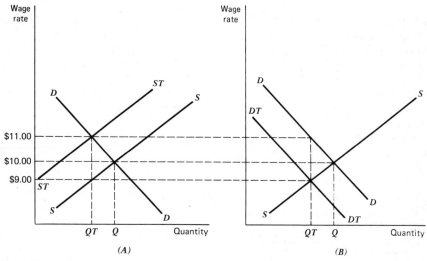

Figure 20–4. The burden of a tax on labor is the same regardless of who pays the tax: (A) employees pay the tax, (B) employers pay the tax.

When the demand for labor is less elastic (Figure 20–5A) a greater portion of the tax is borne by the employer. The greater the elasticity of demand for labor (Figure 20–5B), the greater will be the burden of the tax on the employee. The demand for unskilled labor is believed to be more elastic than the demand for skilled labor.

Figure 20–6 describes the situation under different elasticities of labor supply. When the tax is imposed on business, as shown by a downward shift of $2 an hour in the demand for labor, and the labor supply is completely inelastic with regard to the wage (Figure 20–6A), a tax on labor is shifted entirely onto labor. As the labor supply becomes more elastic (Figure 20–6B), the employer pays a portion of the tax.

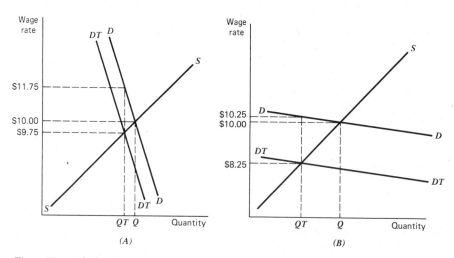

Figure 20–5. The burden of a tax on labor according to different elasticities of demand for labor: (A) less elastic demand for labor, (B) more elastic demand for labor.

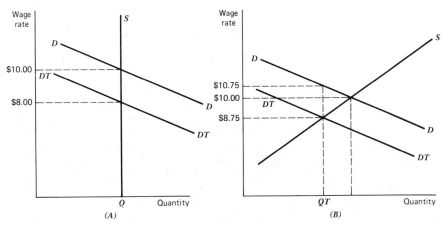

Figure 20-6. The burden of a tax on labor according to different elasticities of labor supply: (*A*) inelastic supply of labor, (*B*) more elastic supply of labor.

As shown in the diagrams, the burden of the social security tax is determined by the elasticity of the demand and supply for labor and not on who is obligated by the government to pay the tax. (Although the net wage received by labor is shown to decrease as a result of the tax, in a dynamic economy increases in the social security tax may result in wages not rising as much as they would have otherwise). Most people are not aware that only one-half of the social security tax is imposed on labor. Thus the size of the tax on labor appears smaller than it is. The main advantage of placing half of the social security tax on the employer is political. It is not obvious to the employee who bears the true burden of the entire tax.

There are two additional effects of the social security tax that should be considered. When business bears a portion of the tax, as shown in Figure 20-4, the prices of the firm's goods and services are increased. (An increase in the wage results in an increase in the firm's marginal and average total cost curves.) Those industries most adversely affected by the tax on labor are those that are more labor intensive and those that face increased price competition from foreign competitors. Second, when the price of labor is increased, employers will hire fewer employees. The decline in the demand for labor is greater, the greater is the employer's elasticity of demand for labor; this is shown in Figure 20-5. The lower the skill level of labor, the greater is their elasticity of demand.

An increase in the income tax (to raise an equivalent amount of money as a social security tax) will not affect the price of goods and services or the demand for labor.

One other issue to be considered in evaluating the social security tax as a method for financing medical services is which income groups will bear the greatest burden of the tax. If all employees must pay 7.51 percent of their wages, up to a maximum of $45,000., then a person with $45,000 of income as well as a person with $80,000 of income each pays $3,379.50 a year (plus the employer's contribution). The $3,379.50 payment represents a greater proportionate tax on a low income than on a high income employee. For this reason the social security tax is referred to as a "regressive" tax. As the social security wage base has increased over time, the social security tax has become more of a proportionate tax. Low-income individuals, however, may have too low an income to pay any income taxes but they still have to pay social security taxes on their earnings.

As the prices of goods and services increase, as a result of increases in the social security tax, these price increases are also regressive in their effects. The percentage increase in prices is greater for low-income groups.

An analysis of the social security tax is important for understanding more than just the financing of the original Medicare legislation. To assure the continued financial stability of Medicare, social security taxes have been increased. Current policies continue to rely on the social security approach and proposals to expand Medicare coverage, such as including long-term care, also propose social security as the financing mechanism. Similarly, proposals to mandate employer coverage of employees' health benefits is equivalent to a tax on labor. It is generally low-wage employees, having less than the specified level of benefits, that would be most affected by such a tax on labor.

In addition to these three criteria—the population group to be covered, incentives for efficiency, and the method of financing—two other supplementary goals are usually mentioned. First, the national health insurance plan should not be very costly to administer, so that as much of the money as possible goes to pay medical rather than administrative expenses. Second, it should be politically acceptable to the public, the providers, and the government. Political acceptability includes such issues as methods of reimbursing providers, whether there is a role for insurance companies and Blue Cross-Blue Shield, how large a tax increase would be necessitated by the program, and the impact on the federal budget. These aspects are discussed subsequently in more detail.

Alternative Proposals for National Health Insurance

Using the criteria that have been presented, a brief evaluation will be undertaken of the current system for financing care and of several types of proposals that either are popular or appear to have legislative support.

The Current System for Financing Medical Expenses

Tax Subsidies for the Purchase of Health Insurance

In the past, the federal government financed the purchase of medical care and insurance for the nonpoor by allowing as a tax deduction one-half of health insurance premiums up to $150 (eliminated after 1983), by permitting deductions on the income tax return of medical expenses in excess of 3 percent of income (rising to 5 percent after 1983 and to 7.5 percent in 1987), and by excluding from taxable income insurance premiums paid by the employer on behalf of the employee (still in effect). It has been estimated that the cost, in terms of lost federal taxes, of these subsidies was between $30 and $40 billion dollars a year in 1985 (2). The beneficiaries of these subsidies are all persons who are employed and who file tax returns, but as shown earlier, the major beneficiaries are those in higher-income groups. A deduction from income is worth more to a person in a higher-income bracket than to a person with a lower income. For example, employer-paid premiums for health insurance totaling $1,000 will cost the person in a 15 percent tax bracket $850, whereas they will cost a person in the 33 percent bracket only $666. If the true actuarial value of that premium is $900 (the remaining $100 going for administrative cost), the person in the 33 percent bracket will demand more insurance because it costs him or her much *less* than the actuarial value of that insurance.

Up until the 1980s, tax brackets were much higher, up to 70 percent. Thus the incentive for high-income persons to have their employers purchase their health insurance was even greater in the past.

The consequences of these tax subsidies were (and are) that higher-income persons receive greater benefits than do lower-income persons and "too much" health insurance coverage is purchased by the higher-income person. It becomes worthwhile for higher-income persons to insure (through their employer) against small, routine medical expenses. This is because the cost of the insurance is less than the cost of those services if high-income persons were to pay for it themselves. The coverage that existed for many years, and still does, has generally been shallow, covering many small and moderate bills, but not covering catastrophic illnesses. Coverage for hospital and surgical expense has been more complete (particularly the front-end expenses) than coverage for nonhospital expenses, thereby discouraging the use of less costly substitutes for hospital care. Efficiency in the use of resources has not been encouraged. As discussed earlier, however, employers and unions have become more concerned with the rise in health insurance premiums, and this is leading to changes in insurance packages to cover less costly substitutes as well as provide for increased patient sensitivity to costs.

Medicare

Medicare, a federal program to cover the medical expenses of the aged, was started in 1966. It was extended in 1974 to all persons with chronic renal disease. Although the aged have obviously benefited from this program, a number of its aspects could certainly be improved. All aged, regardless of their income levels, are presently included. The benefits and the prices the aged must pay, the deductibles and copayments for both hospital and physician services, are the same for each aged person. The deductible for hospital care has risen to $520 in 1987, for physician services it is now $75, and the monthly premium for Part B (physician services) has also risen to $17.90 month, prices which all the aged, regardless of their incomes, must pay. Those aged with higher incomes can afford to purchase more medical services and to buy supplementary coverage for those gaps not covered by Medicare. The catastrophic coverage under Medicare has not, until 1987, been complete and the services covered are not comprehensive. There are limited benefits for posthospital care, such as skilled nursing and home care, and outpatient prescription drugs.

Before Medicare, in 1966, the average out-of-pocket medical expense, including private insurance, for an aged person was $313 ($237 plus $76 for private insurance premiums); this amount represented 70 percent of the average expenditure by an aged person for medical care. The remainder was paid for by government. As a percent of income, the out-of-pocket expense was 15 percent of aged incomes, on average. By 1984, the average out-of-pocket expense had increased to $1,379 ($1,059 plus $320 for insurance); this represented 33 percent of average medical expenditures for the aged. Surprisingly, these out-of-pocket expenditures again represent, in 1984, 15 percent of aged incomes (3). These averages, however, mask large differences in out-of-pocket outlays as a percent of income. Low-income aged spend a greater percent of their incomes on medical care than do higher-income aged. Because Medicare benefits are not income-related, many aged find it difficult to pay the necessary out-of-pocket expenses. What occurs, in fact, is that because of large out-of-pocket expenses and gaps in benefit coverage, approximately 20 percent of the aged must rely on Medicaid.

Medicare is financed by a social security tax.

Hospitals used to be reimbursed according to their costs, which did not provide any incentives for efficiency. In 1983, the federal government started to phase in payment according to a classification system, DRGs, and an inflation factor. Hospitals' incentives have since changed. The method of reimbursement for physician services was the physicians' "usual, customary, and reasonable" fee, but as physician expenditures under Medicare began to exceed the government's estimates, a fee index was developed and limits were placed on physician fee increases. It is likely that a fixed fee schedule will be implemented for physicians serving Medicare patients.

Medicaid

Medicaid, which also began in 1966, is a federal-state matching program whose designated beneficiary group is the poor. The role of the federal government is primarily one of sharing the costs of the program with the states, who are themselves responsible for defining the eligibility requirements and determining the benefit coverage. As in the case with Medicare, although the direct beneficiaries of Medicaid have been helped, there are equity and efficiency concerns with the current program.

Because Medicaid is administered by each state, there are wide variations in eligibility requirements and in services covered. In some states, people may lose all of their eligibility if their income rises so that it is slightly above the cutoff level; in other words, eligibility is not graduated according to income level. Although the beneficiary group is the poor, it was estimated that approximately one-third to one-half of the population below the poverty level were not eligible for Medicaid benefits because of differences in eligibility among states (4). Even within a state there are variations in access and use of services between white and nonwhite persons and between urban and rural dwellers.

Medicaid is financed through general tax revenues from the states and from federal income taxes. This is a more equitable method of financing than a social security tax. · Because the increases in Medicaid costs have risen so rapidly—from $3.45 billion from federal and state governments in 1968 to $39.8 billion in 1985—states have found themselves under pressure to reduce their share of the rising Medicaid costs. The methods used have been to limit eligibility, reduce benefits, and pay medical providers less. This latter approach has, in a number of places, resulted in different systems of medical care; lower levels of state reimbursement have limited the willingness of many providers to serve Medicaid patients. With the difficulties that some states have in meeting the increases in Medicaid expenditures, the gaps in Medicaid are unlikely to be resolved unless there is additional financing from sources other than the states.

Proposals for Financing Medical Expenses

The Committee for National Health Insurance

The most comprehensive of all the proposals for NHI is the plan developed by the Committee for National Health Insurance (CNHI); in legislative form it has been sponsored by Senator Kennedy. Under this proposal the entire population would be covered and the benefits would be uniform for all. An important characteristic of this plan is that there are no out-of-pocket expenses for basic medical services. Covered

¶ not fluctuating w/ economy

services under this plan are generally more inclusive than those currently provided in many high-option insurance packages.

Greater comprehensiveness of benefit coverage is desirable in that it provides an incentive to the patient and the physician to prescribe less costly services. Increased benefit coverage is also advantageous in that it will increase the coverage of low-income persons. However, some benefits are included, such as vision and dental care, that are not substitutes to costly institutional services but that have very high price elasticities of their own. For those who purchase individual insurance coverage (approximately 15 percent of the insured population), where the premium represents a much smaller fraction of the actuarial value of the coverage, the administrative costs of insurance for such persons should be lower.

There are several difficulties with the broad coverage proposed in this bill. Since the price of medical care is the same for all income groups (zero), differences will still exist in utilization of services, owing to the value of waiting time, the location of the provider, and the race of the patient. As discussed previously , to increase the use of services by the poor will require "negative" prices, although this has not been proposed. Equal financial access or equal treatment for equal needs could be more efficiently achieved with a system of differential subsidies. Another problem is encountered with regard to the high-income group: currently, many persons do not purchase coverage for drugs or dental services because of the relatively high transaction costs involved and the problem of moral hazard. Including such services among the benefits to be covered in effect requires these persons to purchase such services. They are clearly worse off, since they now have to purchase services they previously chose not to purchase when they had a choice.

Under a medical care system with no out-of-pocket expenses, patients will have an incentive to overutilize services and to demand the highest-quality care from specialists and hospitals. Hospitals, on their part, will try to oblige patients and their physicians. To prevent medical expenditures under such a system from rapidly escalating, cost controls would have to be imposed on the providers. It is likely, therefore, that a medical system with no out- of-pocket expenses will be subject to arbitrary expenditure limits. It is unlikely that these limits will be related to changes in consumer demands or to input price increases that result from economywide price increases. If the resources provided are less than what is demanded by consumers, some form of rationing will have to occur. One such method is through increased waiting times. Allocation by time costs is inefficient, both because those who have lower time costs may not have greater medical needs and because the value of time spent in waiting is lost. An allocation process similar to waiting times would be allocating according to the patient's elasticity of demand for the particular services. Those services with more elastic demands are less likely to be provided than those services with less elastic demands. Emergency, acute, and catastrophic care are more likely to be provided than health education and preventive care for children and adults, although both the proponents and opponents of such a system would like to see more of the latter provided. The current system's emphasis on the acutely sick patient is unlikely to be changed.

The proposed method of financing is a combination of social security taxes and income taxes; the inequitable nature of social security financing and its adverse impact on employment has been discussed previously.

The medical system proposed by the CNHI is to be administered by a single federal agency. Part of the increase in administrative costs under the new system will be offset by the decrease in administrative costs inherent in the current insurance system. The creation of a new agency to allocate resources and to control inflation throughout the entire medical system is likely to result in large administrative costs. The steady growth of bureaucratic agencies in government can rarely, if ever, be justified on grounds of achieving greater efficiency in production. There would also be no yardstick by which to evaluate the performance of such an agency.

As to its political feasibility, the CNHI proposal has received a great deal of opposition from various provider interest groups. Physicians have opposed it because it would change their method of reimbursement and method of practice. Hospitals would receive predetermined allocations from a single source, which would limit their ability to grow and add services. Insurance companies and Blue Cross-Blue Shield would be eliminated. An additional aspect of the question of political feasibility is the fear on the part of the executive branch of the federal government that the federal budget would require either additional taxes or cutbacks in other programs (and fewer new programs) if medical costs continue to increase as they have in the recent past. As a result of this opposition, it is considered unlikely that such a comprehensive proposal will be enacted in the near future.

Mandating National Health Insurance Through Employers (5)

Requiring employers to provide health insurance benefits to their employees and families offers a number of political advantages to an administration. First, it offers the illusion that federal expenditures are unaffected. For those population groups that are not employed, additional federal expenditures would be required. However, for the vast majority of the population who are employed, and their families, additional federal revenues would not be needed. Congress would not have to pass a special tax to raise revenues for the program and other federal programs would be seemingly unaffected by a mandated NHI program. Second, a mandated program does not disturb the current medical delivery system nor does it change the role of private insurance companies. A mandated program would have the effect of increasing the demand for insurance and, consequently, for medical services. Important interest groups, the health insurance companies and provider groups, should be expected to support it. Third, mandating a minimum set of insurance benefits permits unions and higher-income employees to retain their current negotiated benefits, which are generally greater than the mandated benefits.

Although an employer-mandated NHI does not have the political drawbacks that other NHI programs have, there are still problems with such an approach. To start with, federal revenues, hence expenditures, are affected by a mandated NHI program. Employer-purchased health insurance is not considered as taxable income to the employee; instead, it is a business expense. Increased business expenses reduce the firm's taxable revenues. Mandated employer premiums are an additional cost for each of the firm's employees, whose current benefits are below the mandated level. This cost is eventually borne by those workers in terms of lower wages. For those firms whose employees' insurance coverage is less than the mandated amount, it is equivalent to requiring the workers to trade some of their taxable income for nontaxable health insurance coverage. The federal government will lose revenue as taxable income is used to purchase health benefits. For those firms whose employees currently have insurance coverage in excess of the mandated amount, there should be no change in federal revenues. To estimate the lost federal revenues of mandated insurance, it is necessary to determine the number of employees whose current insurance coverage is below the mandated amount, and by how much.

Firms with large numbers of employees generally have health insurance coverage greater than that which would be mandated. Firms with 100 or more employees constitute approximately 50 percent of all employees, while firms with fewer than 20 employees and firms with 20–99 employees account for 24 and 25 percent of employees, respectively (6). Thus the firms most likely to be affected by a mandated program would be the smaller firms. Phelps estimates that, as of 1980, an "intermediate" plan, one in which the employer contribution is $430 for an individual employee and $1,100 for an employee with a family, would result in an increase of $20 billion in new insurance premiums (7). The loss in federal revenues as a result of an intermediate mandated NHI program was estimated to be approximately $7 billion in 1980.

There are also important indirect effects of a mandated employer program. A mandated program increases the cost of labor to the firm, thereby decreasing the firm's demand for labor. The decrease in demand for labor should be greater among unskilled workers, whose wages may be close to the minimum wage. Skilled labor is less likely to be affected since they are likely to have health benefits close to or in excess of the mandated benefits, and the additional cost, if any, of the mandated program is likely to be a small percentage of their wages. Substitution toward skilled labor and capital, away from unskilled labor, is likely to occur. An increase in unemployment among unskilled labor is also likely to occur. These effects, which are not obvious consequences of the legislation, are also costs that should be considered.

Mandated employer insurance programs have no effect on the problem of "overinsurance"; that is, employees have more comprehensive insurance than they otherwise would have because health insurance is a nontaxable fringe benefit. Increased health insurance coverage will only serve to exacerbate current concerns with utilization and rising medical prices.

Neither the benefits nor financing mechanisms of a mandated employer program are income related. The financing requirement is similar to a flat tax per worker, which more closely approximates a payroll tax, rather than an income tax, which would be more redistributive.

Mandated employer health benefits, proposed by both Presidents Nixon and Carter as an approach for national health insurance, is slowly being implemented at both the state and federal levels. For example, in 1986, as part of the Consolidated Omnibus Budget Reconciliation Act (COBRA), employers were required to continue their health insurance coverage for terminated employees and their dependents. (The terminated employees were able to pay for that coverage at the employer's group rates.) Further, after 1983, employers were required to pay the medical expenses for an employee or their spouse if either of them had employer-paid health insurance, *even though the employee or spouse was eligible for Medicare*. By making the employer the first payor rather than Medicare, Medicare expenditures are reduced. Medicare then pays what the employer's insurance coverage does not pay.

As the Medicare deductible and Part B premiums are increased, those employer health plans that supplement Medicare for their retirees incur increased costs. When Congress eliminated the mandatory retirement age for all but a few occupations, employers became the primary payor for employees desiring to continue working who are Medicare eligible. A concern of employers is that Medicare will eventually require the employer rather than Medicare to become the first payor of their retirees' health benefits.

There are now approximately 640 state mandated coverages (8). These coverages generally require employers to include coverage for specific diseases (e.g., Alzheimer's) or require reimbursement for certain health providers, such as audiologists and chiropractors, or coverage for certain dependents (e.g., divorced spouses). It has been estimated that the cost of mandated benefits in Maryland in 1985 was $533 per employee, 17 percent of the total premium (9).

The intent behind much of the employer-mandated coverage appears to be to reduce either Medicare or Medicaid expenditures by shifting those costs onto the employer. Other interest groups lobbying for mandated coverage are specific provider organizations to require payment for their members' services or to mandate coverage of the services provided by their members.

Employers who have self-insured plans are exempt from state laws on mandated coverage. Thus as the cost of mandated coverage increases, insurance companies are concerned that employers will drop their coverage and move to a self-insured status. The likely result of this will be federal legislation eliminating the advantage of self-insurance.

The effects of mandated coverage are particularly large on companies that employ a greater number of Medicare-eligible employees, on companies (and consequently the employees) whose employees receive low wages, and on companies whose employer coverage is less than the mandated coverage.

Changes in the Tax Treatment of Employment-Based Health Insurance (10)

Employer contributions to their employee's health insurance plans are not included as part of the employee's taxable income. This exclusion is equivalent to a discount on the purchase of insurance equal to the employee's marginal tax rate. The consequences of this policy is a demand for more comprehensive insurance coverage.

To rectify the foregoing situation it has been proposed that either employers' contributions toward their employees' insurance become completely taxable or that a dollar limit be established, such as $150 a month for a family, above which employer contributions become taxable. The proponents of such a change in the tax laws see a number of advantages, not least of which is that it will increase federal tax revenues. In 1982, the Congressional Budget Office estimated that the loss in federal revenues from this tax exclusion was $23 billion and would reach $45 billion by 1987 (11). Eliminating the exclusion (or reducing it, which is politically more feasible) results in taxing income that would be used to purchase more comprehensive insurance coverage.

Under the current tax system, those receiving the highest benefits from employer contributions also have the highest incomes. As shown in Table 20-4, both the percentage of households receiving employer contributions and the average employer contribution increase with higher household incomes. Placing a dollar limit on the size of the employer contribution that is nontaxable would have two effects; equity would be improved, those with the highest incomes would receive less of a tax subsidy for the purchase of health insurance, and employees would either join managed care plans or they would purchase less health insurance, namely, policies with more deductibles and copayment features. Providers in managed care systems and increased patient sensitivity to medical prices would lead to greater efficiency in the provision of medical services. There would be greater concern with the benefits and costs of medical use as well as with the selection of medical providers.

TABLE 20-4. Employer Contributions to Health Benefit Plans and Employee Tax Benefits, 1983

Annual Household Income	Households Receiving Contributions		
	Percentage Receiving Employer Contribution	Average Employer Contribution	Average Tax Benefit[a]
$ 0– 10,000	13	$ 636	$129
10,001– 15,000	31	972	269
15,001– 20,000	47	1,029	307
20,001– 30,000	59	1,375	460
30,001– 50,000	73	1,798	683
50,001–100,000	73	2,025	857
Over 100,000	62	1,761	886

Source: *Containing Medical Care Costs Through Market Forces* (Washington, D.C.: Congressional Budget Office, 1982), p. 27, Table 2, which is based on CBO estimates.

[a] Tax benefits include both federal tax reductions and the employer's and employee's share of federal payroll taxes. About three-quarters of the tax benefits are income tax reductions. State and local income tax reductions are excluded.

There are, however, political as well as technical difficulties in placing a limit on the employer's contribution. Unions that have bargained for and received health benefits greater than the dollar limit have opposed such proposals. A dollar limit below their current negotiated benefit level would increase taxes on their member's wages and make them worse off. Health insurance companies have also opposed such proposals. Placing a dollar limit on the employer's contribution that is tax free would decrease the demand for health insurance. Provider interest groups, such as the American Dental Association, have also opposed tax caps since they believe that insurance coverage for their members' services would be eliminated. There are also certain technical difficulties with such an approach; however, these are not insurmountable.

Since health care costs vary across the country, a dollar limit will enable employees in one part of the country to buy more health insurance than could those located in areas with high medical prices. For example, the average tax benefit of households receiving contributions is estimated to be $633 in the west and north central regions and only $462 in the south (12). Although this problem can be resolved by indexing the dollar exclusion to an area's medical prices, it increases the administrative cost of the proposal. Further, employees belonging to large groups would still have a cost advantage in the purchase of insurance over the self-employed and those in small groups.

Placing a limit on the tax exclusion would decrease the demand for insurance by those with high incomes. Thus these proposals have a different objective than other NHI proposals; their purpose is to reduce the extent of overinsurance. Such a proposal would not, by itself, reform the current system of financing nor would it increase the demand for medical services by those receiving less than the taxable dollar limit. These tax limit proposals must be combined with proposals that increase the availability of insurance if lower-income populations are to have increased coverage. It is the latter proposals which are examined next.

Income-Related NHI Proposals

Tax Credit Proposals. Legislative proposals favoring the use of a tax credit have frequently been introduced into Congress. Although such proposals differ in a number of respects, it might work in the following way. A taxpayer would be allowed to subtract from the amount of the tax he or she would otherwise be required to pay a given dollar amount that would be used to purchase health insurance (proof of purchase would be required). The dollar amount that the taxpayer would be allowed to deduct would depend upon the person's income. The maximum dollar amount that may be deducted against taxes would be related to an insurance premium for a given set of benefits. These benefits could be comprehensive, thereby resulting in a greater dollar deduction, or they could be for catastrophic care. Individuals whose tax credit exceeded their tax liabilities would receive a refund for the difference. Currently, a taxpayer can only deduct those medical expenses if they exceed a certain percent of adjusted gross income. A tax credit approach would channel greater benefits to lower-income taxpayers than does the current medical expense deduction.

Some tax credit proposals are voluntary, others are compulsory. If a program is voluntary, then there is the problem of people not participating and possibly having to go on welfare if they are unable to meet a catastrophic expense. Under certain tax credit proposals Medicare and Medicaid would be continued, others proposals would incorporate them into a single tax credit system for everyone. If Medicare and Medicaid are to be retained separate from the tax credit system, then the gaps and problems in these programs would have to be remedied. Some people have suggested that tax credits be used solely for the purchase of insurance; others have suggested that the credit be applied directly against medical expenses. Proposals that favor a credit against medical expenses would mean that the person could deduct a certain percentage of those expenses from his or her tax liability, depending upon their income level.

Tax credit proposals could provide an incentive for increased efficiency in the provision of medical services. If the tax credit deduction is based upon an average premium for providing a given set of benefits in an area, insurance companies would presumably compete among themselves for those premiums. The successful insurance companies would then face a fixed premium for providing a given set of benefits; they would have an incentive to minimize the cost of providing those benefits.

A tax credit approach could also be used in conjunction with employer- purchased health insurance. As long as the employer-purchased health insurance met the minimum government benefits, employees would be able to take a deduction against their taxes, depending upon their taxable income.

Tax credit proposals for the purchase of a minimum set of government established benefits would be financed in an equitable manner, since the tax credit would be related to the taxpayer's income. Use of the tax credit to require the purchase of an insurance premium or enrollment in an HMO would also serve to provide such organizations with an incentive to minimize the cost of the services they provide.

Catastrophic Proposals. Proposals that emphasize catastrophic health insurance have been introduced in various sessions of Congress. In 1987, President Reagan introduced a catastrophic plan for Medicare beneficiaries, however, long-term care services were excluded. Different definitions are often used for defining catastrophic health expenditures. In some legislation, income-related definitions, such as expenditures exceeding 10 percent of a family's income, are used. In other proposals, absolute dollar amounts such as $2,000 are used. Any definition based on an absolute dollar amount would not be as progressive in its distribution of benefits as would an income- related definition. What might be considered catastrophic to low-income families may be an average expenditure to high-income groups (13).

Examining out-of-pocket medical expenditures in relation to family incomes, Berki finds that in 1977 there were 7.5 million families, representing 9.6 percent of all families, that spent more than 10 percent of their incomes on medical care (14). Of these families, 80 percent spent less than $2,000. Thus what caused these families to have a catastrophic medical expense (i.e., more than 10 percent of their family income), was not the size of the expenditure but their low incomes and poor insurance coverage. This finding becomes even more obvious when families are classified as being above or below the poverty level, and the size of their medical expenditure. Of those families spending 10 percent or more of their incomes on medical care, only 6 percent of those above the poverty level were in this category, while 29.8 percent of those below the poverty level incurred such an expense. The average expense was more than twice as large for those above the poverty level than for those below it ($1,834. versus $828). Catastrophic proposals that rely solely on dollar limits would not be as equitable as those that are income related.

The advantage of federal catastrophic coverage is that federal dollars would be spent for a relatively small, although important portion of total expenditures. Proponents of federal catastrophic coverage maintain that such insurance protection would be more equitable than the current medical expense deduction, which permits taxpayers who itemize to deduct from their income out-of-pocket medical expenses in excess of 7.5 percent of their adjusted gross income. (Until 1983 the deduction was 3 percent of adjusted gross income, rising to 5 percent until the current 7.5 percent for 1987.) Generally, low- and moderate-income persons do not itemize. Second, deductions are worth more to persons in higher tax brackets. Thus it is not surprising that the benefits of this tax provision have gone predominantly to those with higher incomes. Another difficulty with the deduction is that the tax refunds would not be available until after the tax returns are filed.

Catastrophic insurance proposals based upon a dollar limit, such as that proposed for Medicare beneficiaries, are often combined with separate proposals for aiding low-income persons. An example of such a proposal is having the federal government become responsible for Medicaid, thereby providing for uniform eligibility and benefits to low-income persons. This would be an improvement over the current Medicaid program, which varies by state and excludes a large part of the population classified as poor. However, eligibility for public programs often has sharp cutoff points. Once a person's income exceeds the eligibility requirements, his or her medical benefits are completely eliminated. Thus, with a certain income limit, there may be a disincentive to earn more money because the loss in benefits would be greater than the increase in income. To rectify this situation, assistance for low-income persons should be gradually reduced as their income rises.

Persons who do not qualify for the low-income coverage, which includes the majority of the population, would have to rely on the current system. Since the demand for insurance is related to income and place of employment, low- and middle-income persons would continue to have less coverage and would be more likely to suffer financial hardship as a result of moderate medical expenses that do not enable them to qualify for catastrophic coverage. High- income persons would continue to have more insurance coverage, including coverage for those medical expenses that are considered small and routine. Thus this proposal might also be combined with one which places a limit on the amount of employer-paid contributions that are tax deductible.

One example of a catastrophic-type NHI proposal that has been proposed by several economists is the following. Each family would be responsible for its own medical bills up to a certain percentage (e.g., 15 percent), of its income. Based upon the adjusted gross income on a family's tax return, the government would reimburse them for medical expenses in excess of that percent. There are many variations on this basic approach. For example, the maximum liability as a percent of income could be increased with higher family incomes. Further, in place of what is basically a large deductible for anything below the maximum percentage, there could be a copayment up to the maximum percentage. For low-income families, there could be a small deductible and copayment that would not exceed a relatively small percentage of their income. The deductibles, copayments, and maximum liability could all increase with income (15). The possible combinations are shown in Table 20–5.

Depending upon the extent to which society wishes to subsidize medical care, the deductible levels, copayments, and maximum limits can be set higher or lower than those shown in Table 20–5, which is merely illustrative. It is not necessary to require low-income groups to pay any deductibles or copayments. If a family incurred an expense in excess of its maximum limit, government-guaranteed loans could be used to pay that expense until the family filed its tax return and was reimbursed by the government. An example of how an income-related catastrophic plan would work, using Table 20–5 as a source for discussion, is as follows. If a person with an income of $30,000 incurred medical expenses totaling $3,000 during a year, then the family would be liable for the first $400 and 25 percent of the remainder up to a limit of 15 percent of its income, which in this case would be $4,500. Thus the family would pay $400 as a deductible and then 25 percent of the remaining $2,600, which is $650, for a total of $1,050. On its income tax return, the family would file for a refund of the difference between $4,000 and $1,050. The family in question may have a cash-flow problem until it is reimbursed from the government, making a government loan program necessary (16).

With this type of insurance program, there may be a demand for supplementary insurance to cover all or part of what the consumer would have to pay. Consumers should be able to purchase such supplementary insurance. Because there currently are tax subsidies for the purchase of health insurance and for payment of medical expenses (in excess of 5 percent of one's income), it would be a necessary part of this and other income-related insurance plans to take away such subsidies to prevent a situation wherein "too much" health insurance would be purchased.[5] (With the tax subsidies, the after-tax cost of the insurance to the higher-income consumer could be less than the actuarial value of the insurance. In this case, the consumer would demand too much insurance, because the actuarial value would be greater than the amount that he or she had to pay for it.)

The advantages of an income-related insurance plan as just described would be as follows:

1. Those who receive the largest subsidies would be those with the lowest incomes and those whose medical bills represent the greatest financial hardship. A means test is necessary, but it would be no harder to administer than the current method of filing for deductions on one's income tax form.

---

[5]It has been argued that under NHI plans containing a deductible, the demand for supplementary insurance would be negligible if the favorable tax treatment of supplementary insurance were removed. It is unlikely that there would be any demand for supplementary insurance if the NHI plan covered only unreimbursed expenditures. See Emmett B. Keeler, Daniel T. Morrow, and Joseph P. Newhouse, "The Demand for Supplementary Health Insurance, or Do Deductibles Matter?" *Journal of Political Economy*, 85(4), August 1977.

TABLE 20-5. An Income-Related National Health Insurance Plan with Varying Deductibles, Copayments, and Maximum Liabilities

Adjusted Gross Income	Deductible	Copayment	Maximum Liability as a Percent of Income
Income level 1 (low)	$ 50	10%	5%
Income level 2	75	10	7
Income level 3	100	15	9
.	.	.	.
.	.	.	.
.	.	.	.
Income level N (high)	400	25	15

2. <u>Since all medical services would be included under the expense limits, there is unlikely to be greater use of more costly services,</u> as would be the case if certain services were covered whereas others are not. Instead, the services would be likely to be used with consideration given to both their price and effectiveness in treatment.

3. Since families with higher incomes would have to pay part of the cost of medical services, NHI would provide these families with an incentive to be concerned with the prices they paid.

4. By providing government protection against large medical expenses instead of insuring for small claims, not only would the administrative cost be reduced, but the NHI plan would also be providing coverage for those expenses that are generally more insurable. Consumers are more willing to pay an amount above the pure premium for large and unexpected expenses than they are for those that are small and routine.

To increase the use of medical care by low-income persons beyond what they would demand at a zero price, this type of income-related insurance plan would have to be supplemented with supply subsidies to low-income and rural areas in the form of neighborhood health centers and special incentives for health personnel to locate in these areas.

There are several ways in which this system could be implemented. One is to use the current system of filing income tax returns. Another is to have the Internal Revenue Service issue each family a health care credit card that would have the appropriate cost-sharing and maximum liabilities information precoded. Using the patient's credit card, the provider would bill fees and charges to the IRS and to a fiscal intermediary. The IRS, in turn, would then bill the patient for the portion of the bill for which he or she would be responsible.

There are, however, several drawbacks to such an income-related insurance plan. There would be only a minimal role for health insurance carriers. This would lessen its chances for political acceptance. There is also no role for the government beyond the reimbursement of medical expenses by the Internal Revenue Service. It is politically unlikely that Congress and the government bureaucracy would go along with such a passive role for the government. A further problem is that once the maximum liability limit has been reached, the consumer and the provider have no incentive to limit the amount of care to what is just medically required. Similarly, if low-income persons were to have all, or a large part, of their medical expenses reimbursed, there would need to be some means for outside limits to be placed on their total medical expenses. Otherwise, providers would be able to prescribe unlimited and unnecessary services at high prices just because they will be reimbursed by the government.

Lending support to the idea that cost constraints are still needed once a patient has reached a catastrophic level of medical expenses are the findings from a study by Zook et al.:

> In any given year, about half of the resources in a typical hospital are consumed by only 13 percent of the patients. The most expensive one-fifth of patients accounts for nearly 70 percent of total resources. Since one person in ten is hospitalized each year, this implies that 1.3 percent of the nation's population may account for half of all charges in short-stay hospitals. This skewness is not primarily a function of patient age. Though the aged account for nearly 40 percent of high-cost patients, there is a similar pattern of concentration within each age cohort. (In fact, some of the most expensive patients begin their "careers" at birth with non-lethal congenital abnormalities.) (17)

The authors further state, "A reassessment of high-cost illness also makes it clear that catastrophic plans seldom give appropriate incentives to hospitals and insurers to control costs. By tempting hospitals to get the patient's bill up to $3,500 whenever possible (to reach a range in which there is full federal payment) it may exert a further inflationary impact on medical costs" (18).

Income Related Vouchers. As a way of resolving some of these concerns while still retaining the basic features of an income-related insurance plan, a voucher system might be used. Under such an approach, Congress might specify a standard package of medical services that would become compulsory for everyone to purchase. Alternatively, there could be several standard packages, with the intermediate packages including deductibles and copayments, while the minimum package would be a catastrophic policy. The most generous standard package could be based on the medical needs of a low-income family. Everyone would receive a voucher, including the high-income family which may decide to purchase just the minimum standard catastrophic coverage. The percentage of the premium that would be paid for by the government would again be inversely related to income and paid for by a tax credit on the income tax return. The vouchers would be good only for a health plan approved by the government; the plans, which might be managed care plans such as those offered by health maintenance organizations (HMOs), would have to offer each of the standard benefit packages. Everyone would have to register once a year with his or her voucher at one approved plan. Persons who had minimum standard benefit packages could purchase additional care from any provider; however, if they ever required care for what could be a catastrophic expense, that would be provided by the approved health plan at which they had previously registered.

Approved health plans would compete for consumers and for their vouchers. If a voucher for a low-income family included a very generous set of benefits, then in order to attract consumers possessing such a voucher, a plan might choose to provide additional services. To prevent unscrupulous providers from taking advantage of a group of consumers, the government's responsibility for a plan's approval status might be exercised by placing limits on the number of consumers from any income or age group to be served by a given plan.[6]

Voucher proposals can also be combined with other proposals, such as a change in the tax treatment of employer-paid health benefits. For example, a dollar limit may be placed on the employer contribution that is considered tax free to the employee. Employees choosing an insurance or health plan whose premium is less than the amount of the tax exclusion would be entitled to receive a tax-free rebate of the difference.

In some respects, a voucher system is more complicated than an income related proposal that simply works through the patient's tax return. Under a voucher system, the government would have to determine annually the value of its standard premiums for each actuarial category. Offsetting such higher administrative costs, however, are the incentives in a voucher plan that would exist for both consumers and providers. Because the voucher system is a form of prepayment, the consumer only has to choose which plan to join. They should find it easier to evaluate competing health plans than a set of individual providers. Under a voucher system, which would reimburse the health plan a predetermined amount, the provider would have no incentive to prescribe unnecessarily or to increase the cost of catastrophic medical care. A voucher system that is based on approved prepaid health plans would also encourage changes in the delivery of medical care (19).

An income-related voucher plan, based on a minimum set of specified benefits, can be used as a substitute for Medicaid. Also, the working poor could participate in such a proposal. Employers who provide health benefits to their employees, either through insurance companies or their own self- insured plan, could be exempt from any federal program as long as the benefits were at least equal to the government's minimum requirements. Others, such as the self-employed, could purchase their health insurance with the minimum requirements; whether or not the government would provide them with a subsidy would depend upon their taxable income. It should thus be possible to introduce a national health insurance scheme by permitting flexibility in health insurance benefits, while providing income-related federal subsidies to those most in need of such subsidies. Income-related vouchers would achieve both increased equity and economic efficiency in the use of medical services.

The goals underlying NHI have changed over time. Earlier discussions of NHI assumed that there must be an increase in benefit coverage and in eligible population groups. NHI proposals are now viewed differently. Given its concern over the size of its budget, the federal government is more concerned with limiting its budgetary commitments under Medicare and Medicaid. Each president since Nixon has tried to shift the costs of proposed NHI programs off the federal budget onto employers and employees. Proponents of comprehensive NHI now seek support for their program as being a means for *controlling* health expenditures. Setting expenditure limits for each provider group is a means of limiting the annual increase in medical expenditures.

There is, however, growing concern over what providers refer to as "uncompensated care": those unable to pay their hospital and other medical expenses. Within this category are the uninsured, consisting of the poor and low-income wage earners and

---

[6]Pauly also discusses the use of a voucher system, but the voucher would have a flexible price. The advantage would be in avoiding having too many people who must make out-of-pocket payments, which would be the result if a voucher with a single price were set in the low range of potential costs. The disadvantage of a flexible-price voucher is that it would tend to discourage the seeking out of low-price plans. Mark V. Pauly, *National Health Insurance Policies: An Analysis* (Washington, D.C.: American Enterprise Institute, 1971.)

their dependents. There are also large numbers of low-income aged who cannot pay their Medicare deductibles. There are thus demands by both providers and others in society to enact legislation to assist those that are without coverage and to fill the gaps in Medicare coverage. There is continual debate as to where the necessary funds will come from. The various methods of financing, such as federal general taxes, employer-mandated insurance, payroll taxes, and excise taxes on cigarettes and alcohol, vary in their progressivity, impact on employment, visibility, and whether they are on or off the federal budget.

The eventual outcome on NHI, if ever, will be a political compromise. Each of the interest groups involved will seek to protect its members' interests. The federal and state governments will seek to limit their budgetary commitments, insurance companies and the Blues will attempt to retain as large a role as possible, health care providers will attempt to secure reimbursement for the uninsured, associations for retired persons will seek greater governmental protection against the aged's growing out-of-pocket and catastrophic expenses, and business and labor will attempt to prevent the costs of mandated programs containing additional benefits from being shifted onto them. Given the need for political compromise if any NHI bill is to pass, it is difficult to predict whether the goals of such legislation will be clearly specified or that equity or economic efficiency will be achieved.

This is not to imply that economic analysis is of limited use in the political process. Economic analysis can be a powerful tool in that it can sharpen the debate, provide information as to the equity and efficiency consequences of alternative proposals, and thereby influence the final outcome. Economists will have served this purpose with regard to NHI if they can clarify the issues by separating those that involve differences in the values underlying various goals of NHI from issues of efficiency with regard to achieving a given set of NHI goals.

REFERENCES

1. Following is a selected list of such references: Karen Davis, *National Health Insurance: Benefits, Costs, and Consequences* (Washington, D.C.: Brookings Institution, 1975). Robert D. Eilers and Sue S. Moyerman, eds., *National Health Insurance: Conference Proceedings* (Homewood, Ill.: Richard D. Irwin, 1971). Bridger M. Mitchell and William B. Schwartz, *The Financing of National Health Insurance*, Rand Publication R-1711 (Washington, D.C.: U.S. Department of Health, Education, and Welfare, 1976); Mark V. Pauly, ed., *National Health Insurance: What Now, What Later, What Never* (Washington, D.C.: American Enterprise Institute for Public Policy Research, 1980); *Catastrophic Health Insurance* (Washington, D.C.: Congressional Budget Office, Congress of the United States, 1977). *Tax Subsidies for Medical Care: Current Policies and Possible Alternatives* (Washington, D.C.: Congressional Budget Office, Congress of the United States, 1980). *Containing Medical Care Costs Through Market Forces* (Washington, D.C.: Congressional Budget Office, Congress of the United States, May 1982). For an analysis of the redistributive effects of both current and proposed methods of financing medical care using a microsimulation model, see Stephen Long, Margaret Cooke, and Jay Crozier, "Income Redistribution Under National Health Insurance Financing Alternatives," in J. van der Gaag, W.

Neenan, and T. Tsukahara, eds., *Economics of Health Care* (New York: Praeger, 1982).

2. Charles E. Phelps, "Large Scale Tax Reform: The Case of Employer Paid Health Insurance Premiums," Workshop Paper 20, Applied Economics Workshop, University of Rochester, Rochester, N.Y., September 1985.

3. Marion Gornick, et al., "Twenty Years of Medicare and Medicaid: Covered Populations, Use of Benefits, and Program Expenditures," *Health Care Financing Review*, Annual Supplement, 1985: 52–53.

4. John K. Iglehart, "The Political Contest over Health Care Resumes," *New England Journal of Medicine*, 316(10), March 5, 1987: 642; "less than half the people whose incomes fall below the official poverty line (an annual income of $8,800 for a family of three in 1986) meet the program's arbitrary and often confusing Medicaid eligibility standards."

5. For a more complete discussion of this subject, upon which this section is based, see Charles E. Phelps, "National Health Insurance by Regulation: Mandated Employee Benefits," in Mark Pauly, ed., *op. cit.*

6. *Ibid.*, p. 54.

7. Phelps provides tables that show the estimated increases in 1980 employer payments for different premium levels and employer share required; *ibid.*, pp 69–70.

8. Brian Rasmussen, "Mandated Coverage: An Employer Debate," *Business and Health*, April 1987: 12.

9. Ibid.

10. For a more complete discussion of this and related proposals, see *Tax Subsidies for Medical Care: Current Policies and Possible Alternatives* (Washington, D.C.: Congressional Budget Office, Congress of the United States, 1980). See also *Containing Medical Care Costs Through Market Forces*.

11. *Containing Medical Care Costs Through Market Forces*, p.26.

12. *Ibid.*, p. 27.

13. For a more complete discussion of catastrophic insurance, alternative proposals, and their estimated costs, see *Catastrophic Health Insurance*.

14. S. E. Berki, "A Look at Catastrophic Medical Expenses and the Poor," *Health Affairs*, 5(4) Winter 1986.

15. Examples of income-related national health insurance plans similar to that described here have been proposed by the following: Jacob Meerman and Millard Long, "Aid for the Medically Indigent," *Vanderbilt Law Review*, December 1962: 173–191; Mark V. Pauly, *Medical Care at Public Expense* (New York: Praeger, 1971); Charles Baird, "A Proposal for Financing the Purchase of Health Services," *Journal of Human Resources*, Winter 1970: 89–105; and Martin S. Feldstein, "A New Approach to National Health Insurance," *Public Interest*, Spring 1971: 93–105.

16. For a discussion of loans for medical services see Robert Eilers, "Postpayment Medical Expense Coverage: A Proposed Salvation for Insured and Insurer," *Medical Care*, May–June 1969.

17. Christopher Zook, Francis Moore, and Richard Zeckhauser, "Catastrophic Health Insurance—A Misguided Prescription?" *The Public Interest*, Winter 1981: 68.

18. *Ibid.*, pp 74–75.

19. Various people have proposed vouchers and competing health plans. One such proposal, which combines a voucher system and competition between qualified health plans, is the Consumer Choice Health Plan. Alain Enthoven, *Health Plan* (Reading, Mass.: Addison-Wesley, 1980).

CHAPTER 21

The Market for Long Term Care Services

INTRODUCTION

The population of this country is becoming older. These demographic trends have profound implications for society. As the proportion of retirees to the working age population increases, there are concerns regarding economic growth. There is also the fiscal burden of an aging population. Political conflict between age groups also becomes more likely as public financing of services to the aged impose greater per capita burdens on the working population. The two largest redistribution programs for the aged are social security and Medicare. The programmatic nature of these programs ensures that they will continue to increase; these programs are entitlements, which means that all aged are eligible, the benefits are adjusted for inflation, as well as for higher earnings of retirees in the case of social security, and legislative changes over the years have made these programs increasingly more generous. The increasing dependency ratio between the number of retired persons and the working population suggests that it will become even more difficult to provide additional benefits to the aged. Yet long term care is in the forefront of public policy for the aged. How this issue is resolved affects not only the aged with such needs, but whether additional burdens will be placed on the working age population to finance these additional benefits.

This Chapter discusses a number of long-term care issues; the growing needs for long-term care, the likely demands for such services over time, the provision of long-term care services, the financing of such services, and current government policies with respect to long-term care. To achieve an increased understanding of the public policy implications of this emerging market, the concept of economic efficiency is used for evaluating the performance of this market. Since public policy also results in redistributional consequences, the equity aspects of the financing and provision of long-term care services are also discussed.

THE DEMAND FOR LONG-TERM CARE SERVICES

Long-term care is more than nursing home services. The nursing home is the end of a continuum of services to assist an impaired person to function in activities necessary for daily living. When viewed in this manner, nursing homes are substitutes for independent living. The nursing home provides a limited amount of medically related services, as well as housing, food, and socialization services. Long-term care services include housing, socialization, food, in-home chore and personal care, transportation, and medical care, services that are all found in nursing homes. Long-term care is generally not the result of a specific medical problem but instead, is the care required to assist those whose physical and mental disabilities impair their functioning in those activities necessary for daily living. Thus long-term care refers broadly to the medical, residential, and social services that are provided to chronically disabled persons over an extended period of time, either in their own home or in a separate facility.

The demand for long-term care services is related to the need in the population for such services as well as economic factors. Need for long-term care services is indicated by the aging of the population. Important economic factors are the prices of institutional and noninstitutional services, government and private insurance programs, income and assets of the recipients, and "nonmarket" care giving by family members and relatives. The extent of consumer knowledge (or lack thereof) also has an important effect on demands for long-term care services. Each of these will be briefly discussed.

Determinants of Demand for Long-Term Care Services

Demographic Profile of the Population

The need for long-term care services increases with age. This can be seen by examining the need for personal care assistance, which is the largest component of the need for long-term care. As shown in Table 21–1, less than .03 percent of the population under 45 years of age needs personal care assistance. Between the ages 45 and 64, 1.1 percent of the population requires such assistance. The percent of the population requiring personal care services steadily rises for age groups 65 and over. While only 2.6 percent of the 65–69 age group needs such services, 16.8 percent of those 80–84 and 31.6 percent of those 85 and over need personal care services.

Just as personal care dependency increases with age, so does the proportion of older persons institutionalized at any point in time. Only .1 percent of the population under the age 65 was institutionalized in 1977 compared to 4.8 percent of the population 65 and over; this varied from 2 percent of those 65 to 74, 6 percent of those 75 to 84, and 23 percent of those over 85 years of age. The major characteristics of those institutionalized are mental disorders, severe functional dependencies, and weak social support systems (1). Since older people have the highest dependency and institutionalization rates, and since nursing home expenditures are by far the largest commonly accepted long-term care expense, analysts examining the use of long-term care services have tended to focus on those 65 and over.

The major sources of long-term care are nursing homes, which care for 29 percent of the long-term care population, and the community, in which the remaining 71 per-

TABLE 21-1. Percent of the U.S. Population Needing Personal Care, 1977

Age Group	Percent of Population
Under 45	.3
45–64	1.1
65–69	2.6
70–74	5.1
75–79	9.7
80–84	16.8
85+	31.6

SOURCES: Tabulated from data on persons needing personal care in the National Nursing Home Survey and the Health Interview Survey collected by the National Center for Health Statistics and from data on population from the U.S. Bureau of Census and published in William J. Scanlon and Judith Fedor, "The Long-Term Care Market Place: An Overview," *Health Care Financing Review*, 38(1), January 1984: 20.

Note: Persons needing personal care are those requiring assistance with activities of daily living—bathing, dressing, transferring, toileting, and eating.

cent reside. While the dependent elderly in nursing homes are generally more disabled than those in the community, it has been estimated that for every aged person in a nursing home, there are twice as many aged in the community requiring a similar level of care (2).

In addition to differences in need for long-term care services by age, there are differences according to gender. Women live longer and have a higher disability rate than do men of the same age. This has important implications for substitute sources of care. Disabled males are more likely than females to have a spouse to assist them and to remain in their own homes rather than be institutionalized.

Demographic trends will cause a huge expansion in the long-term care population and in the demand for long-term care services. In 1950, there were 12.4 million aged, representing 8.1 percent of the population. By 1985 the number of aged had increased to 28.6 million and were more than 12 percent of the population. The aged are expected to become an increasing portion of the population, reaching 15.5 percent, or 45 million, by the year 2020.

The fastest-growing portion of the aged are those over 85 years of age. As shown in Table 21-2, the age group 85 and over increased by 44.6 percent between 1970 to 1980, while those 65 to 74 increased by 23.4 percent. Between 1990 and 2000, those 85 years and older are expected to increase by 29.4 percent compared to -2.6 percent for those 65 to 74 and 15.6 percent for those 75 to 84.

Assuming the same dependency and institutionalization rates in the year 2000 as in 1980, the number of dependent older persons would grow by 56 percent in the two decades, while the number of institutionalized persons would grow by 73 percent. Again the fastest rate of growth is in the oldest age groups which are more likely to require long-term care. The implication of this changing age structure is clear: demographic trends will cause a steady increase in the numbers of very dependent older persons needing long-term care services.

TABLE 21-2. Percent Increases in U.S. Population for 10-Year
Intervals by Age Groups: Selected Years and Projections,
1950–2010

Year	65–74 Years	75–84 Years	85 Years or Over
1950–1960	30.1	41.2	59.3
1960–1970	13.0	31.7	52.3
1970–1980	23.4	14.2	44.6
1980–1990	13.8	26.6	20.1
1990–2000	– 2.6	15.6	29.4
2000–2010	13.3	– 2.4	19.4

SOURCE: U.S. Bureau of the Census, *Current Population Reports*, Series P-25,
and publshed in Pamela Doty, Korfin Liu, and Joshua Weiner, "Special Report: An Overview of Long Term Care," *Health Care Financing Review*, 6(3),
Spring 1985: 70.

Economic Factors Affecting Demand

Price. The out-of-pocket price to a patient without any insurance coverage is highest
for nursing home care. Nursing home prices vary greatly both within a state and from
state to state. These price differences reflect different levels of services, quality of service, levels of efficiency, and profitability. Prices are generally higher for skilled nursing facilities (SNFs) than for intermediate-care facilities (ICFs), which is consistent
with the expected higher levels of service in SNFs. Private-pay prices for nursing home
care ranged from $12,000 to $50,000 a year in 1985. The most commonly quoted private-pay rate for SNFs in Massachusetts in 1985 was $27,000.

The price for home services varies according to the type of service. A home nurse
visit may be $60, while that of an unskilled personal care attendant is much less per
hour and would depend upon whether the consumer purchases the service directly
from the worker or contracts for the service through an agency. There are also high-
technology home therapies that can be as high as $4,000 a month. It is difficult to
compare prices for long-term services in an institutional and home setting since the
quantity of services needed in the home can vary greatly.

The demand for marketed long-term care services depends substantially on the
supply of nonmarket or "informal" long-term care services. Everything else held constant, the higher the level of nonmarket care giving, the lower the demand for marketed long-term care services. As shown in Table 21–3, family members provide most
of the long-term care services outside of the marketplace. For all persons 65 years and
over requiring personal care services, the spouse provides 53 percent of the care days to
the husband; children provide 19 percent and relatives provide 18 percent of the care
days. Only 11 percent of the care days are provided through a formal arrangement. As
shown in Table 21–3, when the recipient is female, male spouses (who are less likely to
be alive) provide only 17 percent of the care days and the largest burden falls on the
children and relatives, 37 and 30 percent respectively. The cost of nonmarket long-
term care services is not easily measured. For example, the burden of an older woman
caring for a still-older dependent husband can have significant emotional, physical

TABLE 21-3. Percent Distribution of Helper Days, by Sex and Relationship to Individuals 65 Years of Age or Over with Limitations to Activities of Daily Living

Age and Relationship	Helper Days	
	Male	Female
All persons 65 years or over		
Spouse	53	17
Offspring	19	37
Other relative	18	30
Formal	11	16
65–74 years		
Spouse	61	31
Offspring	15	27
Other relative	15	28
Formal	9	14
75–84 years		
Spouse	53	14
Offspring	18	38
Other relative	18	32
Formal	11	15
85 years or over		
Spouse	31	3
Offspring	31	47
Other relative	22	30
Formal	16	19

SOURCE: Preliminary data from the 1982 National Long-Term Care Survey, Department of Health and Human Services, 1982, and published in Pamela Doty, Korfin Liu, and Joshua Weiner, "Special Report: An Overview of Long-Term Care," *Health Care Financing Review*, 6(3), Spring 1985: 70.

health, and economic consequences on the caregiver. There are also the jobs that are given up by children of the dependent adult, lost efforts in their own homes, as well as forgone leisure to perform their care-giving tasks.

Although there are important noneconomic motivations for nonmarket care giving, there are also powerful economic incentives to do so. Nursing homes and private insurance coverage are very expensive, and relying on Medicaid requires impoverishment. As a result, a long stay in a nursing home for a husband can mean financial ruin for a wife. It can also mean the depletion of assets that can be bequeathed to children or to relatives.

Incomes of the Elderly. The biggest consumers of long-term care services are the elderly, who pay a large portion of their expenses out of pocket. As shown in Table 21–4, the elderly pay only 3.1 percent and 26.1 percent, respectively, of hospital and physician expenditures themselves, since the remainder are in large part paid for by Medicare. For nonacute care, however, the aged pay most of it themselves. The aged pay

TABLE 21-4. Percent Distribution of Personal Health Care Expenditures Per Capita for People 65 Years of Age or Over, by Sources of Funds and Type of Service: United States, 1984

Source of Funds	Total Care	Type of Service			
		Hospital	Physician	Nursing Home	Other Care
		Percent			
Total per capita	100.0	100.0	100.0	100.0	100.0
Private	32.8	11.4	39.7	51.9	65.3
Consumer	32.4	11.0	39.6	51.2	64.8
Out-of-pocket	25.2	3.1	26.1	50.1	59.9
Insurance	7.2	7.9	13.5	1.1	4.9
Other private	.4	.4	.0	.7	.5
Government	67.2	88.6	60.3	48.1	34.7
Medicare	48.8	74.8	57.8	2.1	19.9
Medicaid	12.8	4.8	1.9	41.5	11.4
Other government	5.6	9.1	0.7	4.4	3.4
		Amount			
Total	$4,202	$1,900	$868	$880	$554
Private	1,379	216	344	457	362
Consumer	1,363	209	344	451	359
Out-of-pocket	1,059	59	227	441	332
Insurance	304	150	117	10	27
Other private	16	7	1	6	3
Government	2,823	1,684	524	423	192
Medicare	2,051	1,420	502	19	110
Medicaid	536	91	16	365	63
Other government	236	172	6	39	19

SOURCE: Daniel Waldo and Helen Lazenby, "Demographic Characteristics and Health Care Use and Expenditures by the Aged in the U.S., 1977–1984," *Health Care Financing Review*, 6(1), Fall 1984: 10–11.

out-of-pocket 50.1 percent of nursing home expenditures (Medicaid pays 41.5 percent) and 59.9 percent of other care, which consists primarily of services in the home. Medicare and Medicaid also pay for some home health care, but the total from all government sources was less than 35 percent (3). Examining the income of the elderly therefore can shed light on their current and potential demand for marketed long-term care services and for insurance against those expenses.

The income of the elderly relative to the nonelderly has been generally underestimated. The aged pay, on average, only 13 percent of their income in taxes, compared to 23 percent for all ages (4). About two-thirds of all houses without a mortgage in 1980 were owned by elderly people (5); some form of imputed rent on these homes would substantially increase the incomes of the elderly, on average. The elderly receive many in-kind subsidies, the value of which is not shown as part of their reported income on surveys: housing subsidies ($10 billion in 1984), food stamps ($630 million), social services ($370 million), subsidized meal programs, as well as medical care services (i.e., Medicare and Medicaid) (6). The aged also earn a disproportionate share of the types of income, such as pensions, interest, and dividends, that are the most systematically underreported in income surveys (7). One study that attempted to adjust the income of the elderly for just differential tax rates and for underreporting of income found that the after-tax average household income of the aged in 1983 would rise

TABLE 21-5. Estimates of Disposable Income for Elderly Families and Individuals in 1984 (1984 Dollars)

	Quintile					
	Bottom	Second	Third	Fourth	Top	Mean
Families						
1984 average disposable income for quintile	$6,436	$11,263	$16,001	$22,437	$40,277	$19,283
Percent of families	6.7	11.7	16.6	23.2	41.8	
Unrelated Individuals						
1984 average disposable income for quintile	$3,076	$4,901	$6,612	$9,918	$21,050	$9,115
Percent of individuals	6.8	10.8	14.5	21.8	46.2	

SOURCE: Marilyn Moon, "Impact of the Reagan Years on the Distribution of Income of the Elderly," *Gerontologist*, 26(1), February 1986: 36, Table 3.

to .93 of the nonaged compared to .71 without these adjustments (8). Further adjustments for differences in household size, the value of in-kind subsidies, and imputed rent would place the average income of the elderly above that of the nonelderly population.

Table 21–5 is a comparison of incomes among the aged. The distribution of incomes for both aged families as well as individuals are shown. These data are not adjusted for the factors discussed above; they therefore understate the income of the aged.

The stereotype of the elderly as a poor group is clearly wrong, although there are certainly many poor elderly. However, the distribution of income among the elderly, not just the average level, affects the demand for long term care services. The top 20 percent of elderly families has 41.8 percent of all elderly disposable income (averaging $40,277 per family), while the bottom 20 percent has only 6.7 percent (averaging $6,436 per family). While many of the elderly in the top 20 percent of the income distribution could pay for long-term care services and catastrophic nursing home expenses without impoverishing their spouse, this is inconceivable for those in the bottom (60 percent or greater) part of the income distribution. The distribution of income for elderly individuals is even more unequal than for elderly families. Only a small fraction of elderly individuals could purchase long-term care services without exhausting their assets. Elderly individuals comprise 30 percent of all the elderly and 80 percent of elderly individuals are women (9). This income disparity between sexes is important when considering the potential demand for long-term care services; elderly women represent 75 percent of the institutionalized elderly (10).

The ability to purchase long-term care services also varies by race and by disability level. The black elderly have lower incomes than do the white elderly, particularly black elderly women. The disabled noninstitutionalized elderly, on average, have lower incomes than those with fewer disabilities (11).

Important for any discussions of long-term care policies is the fact that the elderly vary greatly in their incomes and that many elderly, particularly women, blacks, the disabled, and those living alone, are least able to afford long-term care services.

Government and Private Insurance Coverage. Also affecting the demand for long-term care services is the extent of third-party coverage. To date, private insurance for long-term care is negligible, covering less than 1 percent of nursing home expenditures. (The reasons for such a small private insurance market are discussed below.) The major payor for nursing home care is Medicaid. To become Medicaid eligible, a couple must spend down their assets to $2,400 (an individual to $1,600), excluding such assets such as a house and some personal items. The institutionalized elderly under Medicaid must also turn over almost all of their income. While Medicaid also pays for some noninstitutional long-term care services, it is small in comparison with its expenditures on nursing home care. There are currently a number of Medicaid demonstration projects to determine whether paying for community-based long-term care services, using case managers, would reduce nursing home use and expenditures. Noninstitutional services, however, are a small part of total long-term care expenditures under Medicaid. Medicaid subsidization of nursing home care, but not of alternatives to such care, creates a distortion in prices facing the elderly person which favors institutionalization.

Other sources of government funding for long-term care services are the Veterans Administration ($700 million in 1984) and Medicare (12). Medicare, however, does not cover chronic long-term care services. The $600 million spent by Medicare in 1984 for nursing homes was for post-acute nursing home services in skilled nursing facilities. Similarly, Medicare spent $1.9 billion in 1984 for post-acute home care visits. The Medicare home health benefit is for short-term, part-time, or intermittent skilled care, and is to enable patients to regain their independent functioning.

The extent of third-party coverage for long-term care, other than Medicaid, is minimal.

Preadmission Screening for Medicaid Nursing Homes Preadmission screening is yet another factor affecting the demand for long term care and its components. As an attempt to reduce its expenditures for nursing home care, Medicaid limits the number of nursing home beds in the state and then rations access to those beds. Thus this regulatory program, used in approximately one-half of the states, affects not only the demand for nursing home beds but also the demands for noninstitutional care, both marketed and nonmarketed long-term care services. Preadmission screening programs can also increase equity among Medicaid recipients; a more disabled patient would have a better chance of entering a nursing home than would a less disabled Medicaid recipient. Screening programs may counteract, in part, the tendency of nursing home operators to choose light-care over heavy-care Medicaid-eligible patients. Nursing home operators, however, cannot be forced to admit heavy-care patients. One additional problem with such preadmission programs is that they are not effective in screening all Medicaid nursing home patients since many private-pay patients in a nursing home eventually spend down to become Medicaid eligible.

Consumer Ignorance, Search Costs, and Uncertainty

The demand side of the market for long-term care services is characterized by a uniquely large amount of consumer ignorance and uncertainty. The ignorance is due to a variety of factors. An elderly person's cognitive or affective functioning may be impaired, thereby reducing his or her capacity to make utility-maximizing decisions. At times decisions must be made by someone other than the person involved, usually a family member or a friend, and periodically by a physician. A person's functioning level, or degree of dependence, may change quickly or their support system may alter drastically due to the changed functioning level of the spouse. As a result, a whole new set of consumption choices have to be evaluated. The financing and delivery of services provided by government agencies compounds the problem—it is often difficult to figure out what services are available at what subsidy. All of this increases search costs, as a decision made by a relative for another person consumes the relative's time; each change in condition requires new learning, assessing of needs, and searching for competing providers of possible services; the fragmented social services system can make arranging services extremely difficult. In addition, the instability of the elderly person's condition creates uncertainty about what to do over a period of time.

All these problems can lead consumers to choose institutional over noninstitutional services.

The market response, both private and public, to high search costs and uncertainty has been case management. The case manager improves efficiency on the demand side by helping elderly people and their families understand what services can be purchased to deal with a disability, how services can substitute for or complement other services, what prices the consumer has to pay, who is eligible for subsidized services, where or how services can be found, how to combine formal services with informal care, and how better to use informal care. To the extent that the case manager is familiar with the probable course of the disability, future consumption of services can be predicted. The net result of case management is that noninstitutional care for an older person can become, and be perceived as being, more feasible than was previously the case.

Unfortunately, case management is not yet widely available, and where it does exist, most people do not know of its availability. Hopefully, case management as a market response to high search costs will develop more rapidly in coming years.

Currently, however, problems of consumer ignorance, search costs, and uncertainty are very powerful factors in the market for long-term care. The presence of these factors violates in a significant way the conditions for efficiency in this market.

Empirical Estimates of the Determinants of Nursing Home Utilization and Demand

Demand for nursing home care, which is related to the factors cited above, such as price, income, age, and disability, is likely to be different from *use* of nursing homes, which refers to the amount actually purchased or consumed. Although demand and use are usually the same, the distinction is relevant in the nursing home market because there are shortages of beds at the prevailing Medicaid price; the demand for beds by Medicaid eligibles exceeds the supply of beds at the Medicaid price. The implications of demand being greater than observed utilization are twofold. For private-pay patients an increase in demand is likely to lead to an increase in observed use, since supply will increase in response to an increase in the private-pay price. Second, liberalized Medicaid eligibility policies would lead to an increase in demand by those newly eligible, but would not affect utilization either because the supply of beds would still be limited by Medicaid or the Medicaid price to nursing homes would not be increased. Thus there is likely to be a divergence in demand and utilization between private-pay and Medicaid patients.

Several studies have attempted to estimate the demand for and utilization of nurs-ing homes (13). These studies differ in their methodology, data used, whether in-comes, out-of pocket prices, and disability levels were used, and whether it was possi-ble to distinguish the behavior of private-pay patients who spend down their assets and become Medicaid eligible from other patients.

Price of Nursing Home Care

Chiswick (14) found a high price elasticity of demand − 2.3, suggesting that there were good community substitutes for institutionalization. Scanlon (15), analyzing the private demand for nursing home care, found that the private-pay price had a sizable and negative effect on demand by private-pay patients, the price elasticity of demand was approximately − 1.0.

Price of Alternatives to Nursing Home Care

Previous studies found that these prices had no impact on utilization, although data limitations may have importantly affected these results.

Income

Scanlon found a very large and positive effect of per capita income for private-pay patients (16); the income elasticity of demand was between 2.27 and 2.83, indicating that for private-pay patients, nursing home care is a normal good. Other studies found that low income increases the chances of institutionalization (17). Thus for Medicaid-eligible people, nursing home care is an inferior good; the amount of noninstitutional services that can be bought by an elderly person rises as income rises, while the amount of Medicaid nursing home care that is used does not rise.

Age and Disability

As an older person ages, on average, disability increases, assets decline (as assets are used for consumption needs), and the chance of having a living spouse declines. The studies show a positive elasticity of utilization for the age variable. Weissert and Scanlon (18) found that personal care dependencies and mental disorders had the greatest impact on the likelihood of institutionalization, followed by a variety of phys-ical disorders and age. Branch and Jette (19), examining the likelihood that a group of elderly people would be institutionalized over a six-year period, found variables mea-suring advancing age, living alone, and disability to be important predictors. Nocks et al. (20) found that variables representing disability and dependency in personal care were positively related to nursing home utilization.

Informal Support

Chiswick concluded that the higher the opportunity cost of informal support care to the providers of that care (as indicated by the labor force participation by adult mar-ried women), the greater the demand for institutional care. Weissert and Scanlon found that being married with an informal living arrangement support variable had a negative impact on the likelihood of institutionalization.

Race

Blacks are a much smaller proportion of the nursing home population than they are of the general population. Explanations include discrimination, greater family support, and greater concentration of blacks in states with restrictive nursing home policies. Scanlon found a positive effect of blacks on nursing home utilization, probably due to blacks having higher levels of disabilities and lower incomes than whites.

Based on the above, it would be expected that both private-pay and Medicaid pay patient demand for institutional services would increase with an increase in disability level and the price of noninstitutional substitutes, and would decrease with an increase in the level of informal support.

Efficiency and Equity in Demand for Long-Term Care

A number of factors cause inefficiencies to occur on the demand side. For example, when Medicaid subsidizes the price of nursing homes but not the prices of other long-term care services, a greater-than-optimal amount of nursing home care is demanded. Further, given the excess demand for nursing homes by Medicaid eligibles, those patients selected by the nursing homes may not be those most in need of nursing home care; Medicaid nursing home expenditures may therefore be allocated inefficiently . Perhaps the most important cause of inefficiency for both private-pay and Medicaid patients is their lack of knowledge of alternative suppliers, their relevant prices, and how the different types of care can be substituted for, or complemented with, each other. Without this information, consumers are not in a position to evaluate marginal benefits or relative prices; perceived benefits and prices differ from the actual benefits and prices. The development of case management systems would be a means of enhancing efficiency on the demand side.

As a result of current financing systems, people who were never poor can become impoverished quickly if they require care in a nursing home. Sixty-three percent of older persons who live alone would be impoverished within 13 weeks of entering a nursing home; 83 percent would be impoverished after a year. For married couples, 37 percent would be impoverished within the 13-week period if one spouse entered a nursing home; 57 percent would be impoverished after a year and 80 percent after two years (21). As a consequence, couples married for many years may divorce so that the partner entering the nursing home will not impoverish the other partner. Covert transfers of assets to children occur when a parent has to enter a nursing home.

A two-class system of nursing home patients exists. Private-pay patients have easier access to nursing homes than do Medicaid patients, and private-pay patients in predominately private-pay nursing homes receive a higher quality of care. Heavy-care Medicaid patients have more difficulty in gaining access to nursing homes than do light-duty Medicaid patients because of Medicaid's method of paying for such patients. Further, access to nursing homes varies greatly depending upon which state a person lives in. Like people are not treated similarly.

Medicaid was meant to serve the medical needs of the poor. Its use as a catastrophic long-term care program was unexpected, and its eligibility requirements for that purpose are harsh—the impoverishment of the elderly person and their spouse. Problems associated with changes in financing long-term care are discussed below.

The demand for long-term care services is expected to increase in coming years. However, the composition of that demand is likely to change. The aged population is increasing, particularly those most likely to demand long-term care, namely the old-elderly. The incomes of the aged are also increasing, which is likely to lead to an increase in demand for noninstitutional services since the aged prefer to remain in their own homes as long as possible. Higher-income elderly are also likely to increase the demand for private-pay nursing homes. If limits continue to be placed on the number of nursing home beds in a state there should be a shift in nursing home beds toward private-pay patients and away from those serving Medicaid patients. The divergence among the elderly in their ability to pay for long-term care services is likely to become greater. As the number of elderly and their ability to pay increases, we would expect the supply side to respond, both in terms of quantity of services and in innovative methods of delivering those services. The case management approach is likely to become more prevalent as the ability of the elderly to pay for such services increases and as Medicaid views it as an approach to decreasing their nursing home expenditures.

THE SUPPLY OF LONG-TERM CARE SERVICES

Background

The supply of long-term care services consists of marketed and nonmarketed services. The provision of nonmarketed services depends on noneconomic reasons, such as the desire to care for a spouse or a parent, as well as economic factors, such as the price of marketed long-term care services, which is a substitute for nonmarketed services. The supply of marketed long-term care services depends upon the price paid for such services, the cost of inputs for producing such services, and government regulation. (Technology is assumed to be held constant.) As the price paid for long-term care services increases, so does its supply; an increase in the price of inputs used in producing long-term care will lead to a smaller supply of such services, holding constant the price of long-term care and government regulation limiting the number of nursing home beds will limit the supply of nursing home services.

The supply of marketed long-term care services consists of institutional care (i.e., nursing homes), and noninstitutional care that is generally provided in the recipient's home. Medicare reimburses for services provided in the home; however, these services are *not* considered to be long-term care services; a physician is responsible for establishing and periodically reviewing the services provided, and the services are generally provided for a short duration. Medicaid provides for home-based services that include nonnursing care, such as homemaker-type services. Medicare-certified home health agencies have expanded rapidly and now exceed 5,000. Agencies providing homemaker-type services, meals, adult day care, and congregate housing for the elderly have also been growing.

The following analysis of the supply of long-term care services, however, emphasizes nursing homes. Between 80 and 90 percent of all long-term care expenditures are for nursing home care. Further, the nursing home industry is subject to a great deal of government regulation; state agencies establish limits on the number of nursing home beds, establish standards of care in those facilities, and determine reimbursement for nursing home services. Nursing homes are also the most expensive element of long-term care, to the government as a payor under Medicaid and to private-pay patients. The rise in expenditures for nursing homes has also been very rapid, from $2.1 billion in 1965 to $10.1 billion in 1975 to $30.0 billion in 1985. The rapid growth in this industry makes it suitable for analysis in terms of its efficiency and equity.

As of 1982 there were 17,819 nursing homes which contained 1.5 million beds. Occupancy rates for nursing homes are high, generally 90 percent, and there were almost 1.4 million nursing home residents in 1982. In addition to nursing homes, there were over 8,000 residential facilities with approximately 133,000 beds (22), Within the category of nursing homes, 75 percent are proprietary (for-profit), the remainder are nonprofit (20 percent) and government controlled (5 percent). The West had half as many nursing homes (2,636) as either the north central region (5,894) or the south (5,423); the northeast had 3,866 nursing homes. Forty percent of the nursing homes are certified by Medicare and Medicaid as skilled nursing facilities (SNF), another 31 percent are certified by Medicaid as intermediate care facilities (ICF), and the remainder, 29 percent, are not certified. SNFs generally provide a higher level of care than do ICFs. The average bed size of a nursing home in 1982 was 84 beds, with proprietary homes being smaller (80 beds) than nonprofit homes (95 beds). SNFs were also much larger (122 beds) than ICFs (80 beds) or uncertified homes (31 beds).

The picture that emerges from this description of the nursing home industry is that it is predominately for-profit, operates at high occupancy rates, and is heavily dependent upon Medicaid for payment as either skilled or intermediate care facilities.

Determinants of Nursing Home Costs

Since government is a monopsonist in the market for nursing home care, researchers have attempted to estimate the determinants of nursing home average costs, which governments could use as a basis for reimbursing nursing home firms. If factors that determine nursing home costs can be identified, it is possible to establish appropriate nursing home reimbursement incentives to achieve state and federal government efficiency and equity objectives.

For example, a key government objective is cost containment, and governments want to know if larger-scale facilities have lower average costs than those of smaller-scale facilities. If this were the case, governments could consider nursing home reimbursement incentives that would encourage larger and discourage smaller facility size. If a key government objective is easier access to nursing home care by the most disabled Medicaid patient, and if cost function studies determine that the more disabled patients cost nursing homes more to care for, governments could establish reimbursement incentives that reward firms for caring for the more disabled elderly.

The major limitation to cost function studies is the ability to separate the nursing home's product (i.e., the type of patient it serves and the quality of care provided), from other factors affecting the cost of care in that home. For example, if nonprofit facilities treat higher cost, more disabled patients than those treated by for-profit facilities, then ownership status also becomes a proxy for disability status. Yet facilities may also differ as to their efficiency; the incentives for cost minimization facing a for-profit and a nonprofit facility are different. Thus ownership status may also be a proxy for efficiency incentives. Determining the most efficient average cost curve for each type of patient for purposes of government reimbursement is difficult when each of the factors affecting costs cannot be estimated separately. The public policy usefulness of the results is thereby reduced.

Most studies have relied on secondary data sources; that is, researchers used predictor variables based on their availability rather than desirability. Yet both patient characteristics and quality of care are crucial to an analysis of the determinants of nursing home costs because the product produced by a firm with low quality and a lightly disabled patient population is very different from that produced by a firm with high quality and a severely disabled patient population. Each firm would be on a separate average cost curve, reflecting product differences.

The consequences of these data limitations in measuring product characteristics has important policy consequences. It becomes more difficult to set reimbursement rates that help control (or encourage) provider behavior to achieve two potentially important government policy goals: adequate access to nursing home care by heavy-care Medicaid-pay patients, and a desired level of quality—that is, the desired supply volume of a nursing home product of a particular type.

Researchers have made more advances in measuring patient characteristics that are related to cost than in measuring quality characteristics related to cost. Measuring and estimating the impact on costs of quality care has proven to be quite difficult.

Following is a brief summary of the results of nursing home cost studies (23).

1. *Size.* No study shows more than a small effect of size (holding occupancy rates constant) on costs.

2. *Occupancy rates.* Most studies show that average costs per patient day decline as occupancy rates increase (holding size and other variables constant). This indicates that marginal costs per patient day tend to be below average costs until all beds are either filled or almost completely filled.

3. *Ownership type.* Virtually every study has shown that proprietary (for-profit) facilities have lower average costs per patient day than do nonprofit or government facilities. There are several possible explanations for these findings: (a) proprietary firms are more efficient; (b) nonprofit facilities have a higher cost casemix and/or higher quality, and case-mix and quality measures do not sufficiently adjust for product differences; (c) nonprofit facilities have a philanthropic wage policy, paying higher wage rates to their employees and/or to family members of the managers than are paid by proprietaries; and (d) nonprofit homes may purchase services from manager-owned suppliers.

   Studies have shown that hospital-based nursing home facilities have substantially greater average costs than those of free-standing (not hospital-related) nursing homes. However, if the type of patient found in a hospital-based facility is qualitatively different (on average) than in a freestanding facility and if patient characteristics were not adequately controlled for, these results might be measuring the effects of patient characteristics.

4. *Nursing home location.* Nursing homes that face higher input prices because of their location (rather than incentives for efficiency) are expected to be on higher average cost curves. Most studies that include location or input prices as a market characteristic conclude that either location of the facility or level of wages in the area or both significantly affect average cost per patient day.

5. *Patient characteristics and quality.* Most studies have used at least one indicator of patient condition, although some of the measures were very inadequate. Most but not all of these studies showed a positive, significant relationship between severity of patient condition and costs.

6. *Level of care.* This variable has been included in many analyses even though the distinction between a skilled nursing facility (SNF) and an intermediate care facility (ICF) is often obscure in practice. In theory, patients requiring more nursing care are treated in SNFs rather than ICFs, although many ICFs in some states have more disabled patients than SNFs in another state, and even in the same state, ICF patients can be more disabled than SNF patients. At best, the SNF/ICF distinction is a proxy for patient disability within a state. At worst, it simply reflects the effects of past reimbursement groupings, whereby states reimbursed SNFs at a higher rate than ICFs. While most studies show that SNFs have higher costs than ICFs, in the absence of strong patient characteristics and quality data, it is impossible to conclude that this difference reflects appropriate, efficient resource use.

7. *Percent of Medicaid-pay patients.* This variable has the defect of possibly representing simultaneously very different determinants of costs. (a) If case-mix variables are inadequate, it can serve as a proxy for case-mix differences between Medicaid and non-Medicaid patients. (b) If quality measures are inadequate, it can be a proxy for quality differences; if facilities with a high proportion of Medicaid-pay patients have lower facility quality, they could have lower costs. Since these homes do not have to compete for private patients on the basis of amenities, they could cut quality as they react to the lower Medicaid rate. In general, these results may be subject to different interpretations.

A few recent studies have used much improved primary, or a combination of primary and secondary, patient-level data and have shed substantial light on the relationship of patient characteristics on nursing home costs, and so have important public policy implications.

Schlenker et al. (24) were able to overcome limitations due to secondary data imposed on many of the previous nursing home cost studies by designing their own patient characteristics and quality measures in their studies of Colorado nursing homes.

The authors selected case-mix variables from 18 major medical diagnostic groupings, 27 long-term care problems, and several "activities of daily living" (ADL) indicators of dependence/independence in such activities as bathing and toileting. They aggregated patient-level results to the facility level. The authors concluded that case-mix measures are powerful predictors of costs. Case-mix measures alone explained one-third of nursing cost variation in freestanding facilities, and 43 percent of the variation variable for all facilities, including those which are hospital based, in their study group. While case-mix variables alone accounted for 25 percent of the variation in total cost for freestanding facilities, they accounted for a dramatically higher 45 percent of variation in total cost when the 10 additional hospital-based facilities were included.

Quality, as measured by "process" and not "outcome" indicators, was a much less powerful predictor of cost than was casemix. When used alone as a predictor variable, quality measures explained only 6 to 13 percent of the variation in nursing home costs. In a later study, quality measures proved to be only somewhat more important.

One public policy implication of these studies is clear: since casemix is an important determinant of cost, reimbursement systems should adjust payment to providers to account for case-mix differences, to avoid nursing home discrimination against heavy-care patients. There are less clear public policy implications for the issue of quality. If quality is a less important determinant of cost, it may be possible to achieve quality changes with relatively minor reimbursement incentives. The latter conclusion is tempered by recognition of the need for better measures of quality, including outcome measures.

A second approach used in estimating costs based on primary data representing patient characteristics are the studies using resource utilization groups (RUGs) (25). These researchers have created a patient classification system based on 16 patient groups. They based the patient groups on an initial hierarchy of five distinct clinical categories statistically different from each other in resource use: special care, rehabilitation, clinically complex, severe behavioral problem, and reduced physical function. For example, the special care group included very heavy care patients who have a very low functional level.

The RUGs researchers used criteria to group patients that consciously avoided negative incentives for nursing home operators, or that encouraged gaming and assessment manipulation that could harm the patient and be expensive to the state.

Cost function studies have had a variety of limitations which have reduced their public policy usefulness. The studies have not had very good measures of quality. Since government still cannot base reimbursement for quality on research results, it does not have an adequate control over the type of product produced.

Conclusions about the relative efficiency of nonprofits and proprietary nursing home firms must be tempered until researchers include good measures of quality. Hospital-based nursing homes treat a more severely impaired patient than do freestanding facilities, making payment on the basis of patient characteristics very important. Further research is needed into the differences between patient characteristics and resource utilization. The measurement of quality, its relationship to cost, along with methods of quality validation and reimbursement, remain important issues on the health services research agenda.

Analysis of the Supply of Nursing Home Services

To predict nursing home behavior in response to changes in the market and to government policies, a model of the nursing home as a firm is necessary (26). Nursing homes are assumed to act as though they were profit maximizers. This model of the nursing home is shown in Figure 21-1. There are two types of patients, private pay and Medicaid pay; further, the Medicaid reimbursement price is below the private-pay price and is a flat-rate price; nursing homes can have as many Medicaid patients as they want at the flat-rate price, shown by the horizontal line MP. The nursing home faces a demand curve DD for private-pay patients which is downward sloping since each firm differs somewhat from other nursing homes in terms of its location, level of care, and/ or its quality. [Location is a particularly important factor to consumers of nursing homes since five of six nursing home residents lived in a nursing home located less than 25 miles from their home (27).] Associated with the demand curve is a marginal revenue curve MR, which shows the marginal revenue received by the firm for each bed day supplied. The average costs of the typical firm is shown by AC and the marginal costs of producing an additional bed day is shown by MC.

If the nursing home were to accept only private-pay patients, the firm's profit-maximizing strategy would be to set price at that point where its marginal cost equals its marginal revenue; that point would also determine the number of private-pay patients the firm will accept. A firm that accepts both private-pay and Medicaid-pay patients faces a demand curve that has three segments: DL, ZM, and ND. For seg-

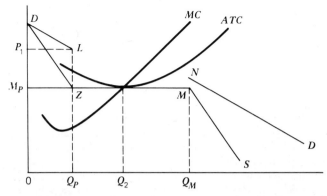

Figure 21-1. A model of pricing and output for private pay and Medicaid patients by a proprietary nursing home.

ments DL and ND the firm is a price setter; for ZM, which is the Medicaid price, the firm is a price taker. At Q_p, where the Medicaid price equals marginal revenue from private-pay patients, the original private-pay demand curve is shifted to the right by the amount ZM or by the Q_pQ_m Medicaid patients who demand care. At each point along ZM, marginal revenue from Medicaid patients exceeds that which can be obtained from more than Q_p private-pay patients. To the right of Q_m, private-pay demand is once again relevant, since marginal revenue from Medicaid-pay patients becomes zero to the right of Q_m. For the profit-maximizing firm the relevant marginal revenue curve becomes $DZMS$.

The typical nursing home faces the situation shown in Figure 21-1; the firm's marginal revenue equals its marginal cost at a point to the right of Z and to the left of M. The profit-maximizing firm will produce OQ_2 units of output. The firm acts as a price discriminator. It sets marginal cost equal to marginal revenue for each type of patient, and sells different quantities at different prices in each market. The firms sells OQ_p bed days for private-pay patients at price P_1 and Q_pQ_m at the Medicaid price M_p. Unless the marginal revenues for each type of patient were equal, the firm could increase profits by reducing output in the market where marginal revenue was lower and increasing output where marginal revenue was higher.

At the Medicaid price of M_p, Q_2Q_m Medicaid patients who demand nursing home care do not receive it. Thus excess demand by Medicaid patients can exist in an equilibrium situation. The consequence is a waiting list for Medicaid patients and difficulty by hospitals in discharging their Medicaid patients to a nursing home.

In a situation of excess demand by Medicaid patients, the firm is also able to discriminate according to the type of Medicaid patient it will accept. If the Medicaid price is the same for all types of Medicaid patients, the firm has an incentive to choose less costly patients, those requiring the fewest services. Given excess demand at the single Medicaid price, even if it is profitable at the existing reimbursement price to accept a heavy-care person on Medicaid, it is more profitable for the firm to accept a light-care person. With a larger bed supply, firms would serve both types of persons. But faced with excess demand in equilibrium, profit-maximizing firms would discriminate against heavy-care patients if they are to maximize their profits.

Government Policy Toward Nursing Homes

Since state governments purchase the majority of nursing home services on behalf of Medicaid patients, it is a monopsonist; the government is a large buyer in a market with many small suppliers. The government's monopsony power allows it to set nursing home rates that are different from private-pay prices. The government's potential power is enormous since it is also the regulator of nursing home services. Since the government is both the largest purchaser and chief regulator of nursing homes, its policies will affect the performance of this industry. To understand the performance of this industry, it is therefore important to understand the government's objectives.

Ideally, the government should be interested in setting prices so that each nursing home will attempt to be internally efficient as well as to take advantage of economies of scale, that is, the home should be of a size that is at the lowest point on the long-run average-cost curve. Annual rates of increase in the government's price should reflect relative increases in input prices. Further, government payment should reflect both the quality level desired by government and the type of patient cared for in the home (i.e., light or heavy care patients). Finally, since nursing homes are but one input in the production of long-term care services, government payment should attempt to minimize the cost of producing long-term care services; that is, lower-cost substitutes, such as home care services, should be used whenever it is both medically and socially possible.

Observed government behavior is such as to question whether government payment and regulatory policies are intended to achieve the objectives noted above. (Except for a few experiments, state governments do not coordinate payment for long-term care services so as to minimize the cost of long-term care services.) By examining actual government reimbursement and regulatory policies, it may be possible to infer intended rather than stated government objectives with respect to nursing homes.

By 1979 almost all states enacted Certificate of Need (CON) regulations affecting nursing homes. By controlling the number of nursing home beds in the state, the government can indirectly control the number of Medicaid patients and therefore Medicaid expenditures. Since CON limits entry into the nursing home industry, existing nursing homes can charge higher prices to private-pay patients (and have the option of providing lower-quality care) than would be the case without CON regulations. From the earlier discussion on the demand for nursing home care, it was shown that demand for nursing home beds is increasing over time. With a limited supply of beds, an increased demand, both by private-pay and Medicaid-pay patients, will result in the proprietary nursing home increasing prices to private-pay patients and admitting more private-pay patients relative to Medicaid-pay patients. With reference to Figure 21–2, an increase in demand by private-pay patients will shift their demand to the right, causing the new marginal revenue line, $D'Z'$, to intersect the horizontal Medicaid price at some point to the right of its current location (Z' instead of Z). When the nursing home operator again equates marginal revenue in each of the two separate markets to marginal cost, the number of private-pay bed days will increase (from Q_p to Q'_p), fewer bed days will be available for Medicaid patients, and the private-pay price will increase (from P_1 to P'_1) to that point on the new demand curve above the intersection of the new marginal revenue curve and the Medicaid price.

The impact on efficiency and equity is not hard to determine. Because nursing homes can charge higher prices to private-pay patients, nursing homes that are internally inefficient or that have obsolete facilities can survive and even prosper. Access

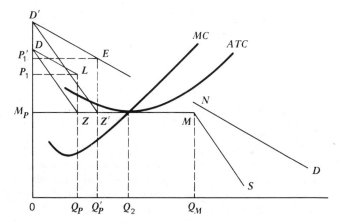

Figure 21-2. An increase in private pay demand in a nursing home serving private pay and Medicaid patients.

for Medicaid patients has been reduced, particularly for heavy-care Medicaid patients, and excess Medicaid demand has increased, since total Medicaid demand is also growing over time.

The cost to the government for Medicaid nursing home care falls as it purchases fewer Medicaid bed days. Although the government may spend somewhat more on home services to those unable to be admitted to the nursing home, there should be a net savings to the government. (This savings could be offset, however, if the patient has to reenter the acute care system). An additional burden, however, is imposed on the Medicaid patient unable to enter the nursing home and/or on family and friends to care for that person.

Economic profits to the nursing home are increased (the difference between the private-pay price and the firm's average total cost curve multiplied by its number of private-pay patients). There is thus a redistribution of income from private-pay patients to nursing homes. These additional profits are unable to induce entry into the industry since entry is restricted by CON. As would be expected, anecdotal evidence suggests that nursing homes favor CON restrictions. After conducting interviews in eight states, Feder and Scanlon concluded: "In every state we visited, they [the nursing home operators] recognized the advantages of restricting entry . . . In California, for example, a spokesman for the nursing home association described his members as 'happy as clams' with entry restrictions, and anxious to ensure that they covered all possible competitive threats, including reclassification of hospital beds to nursing home status" (28).

As a monopsonist, the reimbursement system can also be used by government to achieve certain policy objectives. States have substantial discretion in the design of their nursing home reimbursement systems. The different reimbursement systems that states can choose between are retrospective, prospective, or a flat rate. Under retrospective systems, states give each nursing home an interim rate based on the home's previous costs and then pay the home a final amount after the firm's actual costs have been incurred and reported. A ceiling is usually set at some dollar amount or at some percentile (e.g., 75th), of all the nursing home's costs. If a state uses a prospective payment system, a rate is set in advance for each facility based on that facility's previous costs. Again, a ceiling may or may not be used. A flat-rate payment system pays all facilities one rate regardless of their individual facility's costs. The flat rate may be determined through negotiation with the nursing home association or be based on the cost experience of a grouping of nursing homes. The payment systems noted above may be modified by adjusting payment for characteristics of the nursing home's patient population; attempts to do so, however, are limited by appropriate patient classification systems (29). Unless adjustments for patient care requirements are made, there is a disincentive for proprietary homes to admit heavy care patients, particularly under a prospective or flat-rate payment system.

According to one survey of state payment systems for SNFs, it was found that 29 states used prospective rates by facility, 10 states used retrospective payment, 7 states used a prospective flat rate, and 4 states used some combination of the above (30).

The various payment systems provide differing incentives for efficiency and for the type of patient to be admitted. Nursing homes are able to react to payment policies by becoming more efficient, changing their size, selecting a different case mix of Medicaid patients, changing the level of quality provided to Medicaid patients, and varying the number of Medicaid patients admitted. Any payment system must evaluate its effects on each of the outcomes noted above. For example, under a retrospective system, as long as a home is under a ceiling, there is no incentive to be efficient, since they will collect whatever costs they report. Prospective and flat rate systems, if the home can keep the difference between its costs and the payment, provide efficiency incentives. However, under a prospective system based on a facility's specific costs the incentive for efficiency may be less if the state tightens the prospective rate because the home has done well in the previous year. Except for the flat-rate system, the payment systems have little effect on scale efficiency. This is of less concern since there appear to be very small economies of scale for nursing homes (31). Further, under CON regulations, a home may be unable to expand its size to take advantage of any scale economies. To the extent there are any budget constraints placed on the home by any of the payment systems, an incentive is provided to the homes to select a lighter-care mix of patients.

One additional concern of policymakers is the extent to which a payment system creates fraud incentives. A retrospective system with a high ceiling offers the greatest fraud incentives. Rather than necessarily admitting heavy-care patients, a firm could produce efficiently and achieve economic profits by buying overpriced services from a firm owned by the owner or by hiring and paying high salaries to family members or friends.

There have been several studies that have attempted to determine the effects on nursing home costs of different payment systems (32). These studies generally find that flat-rate payment systems have the lowest rate of change in costs, followed by prospective and by retrospective systems. The authors note, however, that all the features of the reimbursement system must be considered, rather than just the general approach, to determine the effect of the payment system on cost increases.

To understand government policies toward nursing homes it is important to determine whether the government itself has a particular interest in the outcome rather than considering the government's role as merely trying to achieve the ideal objectives of economic efficiency and increased equity. Attributing a motivation to the government beyond that of an ideal regulator provides a more accurate explanation as to why the ideal objectives of efficiency and equity in the provision of nursing home services are rarely, if ever, achieved.

Limiting the increase in Medicaid expenditures has become an overriding concern of government Medicaid agencies. The state's portion of Medicaid, which has been increasing rapidly in the past 15 years, is funded from state income taxes. There are many competing constituencies within a state for these state taxes, for example, educational institutions. State legislators, desiring reelection, are reluctant to vote for increased state taxes, yet to be able to respond to competing demands (and receive political support) from various constituencies for state funding, legislators must make trade-offs as to how the limited state funds are allocated. The cost to the legislators of increased Medicaid funding is the forgone political support they would receive by allocating those funds to other constituencies. Thus constraining the increase in Medicaid expenditures becomes one objective of government policy.

When attempting to limit Medicaid expenditures, however, government agencies (who are assumed to adhere to the preferences of the legislature) face another constraint. Too little funding for nursing home care would result in nursing homes refusing to provide such services and threatening to transfer patients, or that the level of quality would be so low that there would be a major scandal, with adverse publicity on the regulatory agency. Thus the regulatory agency must also consider the preferences of the nursing home association, which also has a concentrated interest in funding for nursing homes. As a monopsonist, state government payment and regulatory policies have a major affect on the profitability of nursing homes. It is therefore in the interest of the nursing home industry to represent their interests (and provide political support) to legislators so as to receive favorable payment and regulatory policies.

A third group with an interest in Medicaid funding and regulatory policies are the patients and their families. Unfortunately, this group has not been successful in organizing themselves, representing their interests before the legislature, and providing political support (votes).

Thus the outcome of Medicaid policy within a state appears to be a compromise between the interests of the government, seeking to constrain its expenditures, and the nursing home industry, seeking increased profitability. The resulting policy has usually been for the government to constrain Medicaid expenditures by limiting the rise in payments to nursing homes, limiting the number of nursing home beds, and providing minimal regulation of the quality of care provided by the nursing home. The net effect of these policies is to create both inefficiencies and inequities in the supply of nursing home care.

These government policies are also satisfactory to the nursing home industry. By limiting entry, CON regulations reduce competition among firms, allowing firms to raise private-pay prices, and permit the firms to be more selective in the Medicaid patients they admit, decreasing access to heavy care patients. Payment systems are generally acceptable to the industry, although they would prefer higher rates, and the lax government regulation of quality enable the firms to increase their profitability.

Based on the objectives of government hypothesized above, the quality of nursing home care is examined. Government nursing home policies are unlikely to result in quality levels for Medicaid patients that are equivalent to those provided to private-pay patients.

The Regulation of Quality in the Nursing Home Industry

While quality is a concern for noninstitutional long-term care, almost all past attention has focused on nursing homes. Quality in nursing home care is multidimensional. However, two major areas can be identified—quality of care and quality of life.

Quality-of-care issues include how well a nursing home assesses the care needs of the resident patient, develops a care plan for the resident, and implements that plan.

Quality-of-life issues are quite varied; they include the degree to which residents have privacy, independence, personal control over daily activities, the ability to keep personal belongings, input into care planning, and personal safety and security of possessions. They also include the ability to eat decent food, and to engage in varied social activities. On a more basic level, they include protection from physical and psychological abuse.

Quality-of-life issues are relevant because, unlike an acute care setting, a nursing home is a total living situation for a long-term patient—a home as well as a place to receive medical and personal care services.

Quality in the nursing home industry is very heterogeneous. While there are many firms that provide good or very good quality nursing home services, other firms provide care that a 1986 Institute of Medicine report has called "shockingly deficient." Reflecting on the regulatory system and the persistence of serious problems in the quality of nursing home services, the same report observed: "There is broad consensus that government regulation of nursing homes, as it now functions, is not satisfactory because it allows too many marginal or substandard facilities to continue in operation. . . . The apparent inability of the current regulatory system either to force substandard facilities to improve their performance or to eliminate them is the underlying circumstance that prompted this study" (33).

These observations are certainly not new. Why has the regulatory system allowed substandard facilities to continue to operate despite the eruption of periodically highly publicized scandals on nursing home quality?

There are two groups that have a concentrated interest in nursing home reimbursement and in the quality of care provided: the government and the nursing home industry. Although these two groups differ with respect to reimbursement, neither has an economic interest in improving the quality of nursing home services for Medicaid-pay patients.

The demand side of the market for nursing homes is imperfect because consumers are ill informed as to both the type of care needed and the quality of nursing homes. Problems of consumer choice are compounded by the cognitive impairment of substantial numbers of prospective patients. Given the limits placed on the number of nursing home beds in most states, the difficulties of finding a nursing home bed are particularly troublesome when finding a bed is medically urgent. Moreover, once in a nursing home, patients are often restricted from moving, both because of the difficulty of finding another bed and because of the trauma often associated with transfer. The regulation of quality by government agencies developed because of these limited abilities of prospective patients to make appropriate choices. Why, then, has government regulation of quality consistently failed?

Government's primary objective with respect to nursing homes has been containment of the growth of its Medicaid payments. Certificate of Need regulation and Medicaid rate-setting policies have been able to limit the rise in government expenditures, but they have had a negative impact on quality. In a market where there is competition among firms, a firm producing a poor quality product runs the risk of losing market share to other firms producing higher-quality services for the same price. Limits on the number of nursing home beds, however, have created excess demand for those beds by Medicaid patients. The nursing homes are able to get all the Medicaid patients they want without having to raise quality. Why should they incur the additional expense of improving quality if it is not necessary for them to use it to attract additional Medicaid patients? Nursing homes can set their own prices for private-pay patients. Since these patients are more remunerative than Medicaid patients, the nursing homes will compete for private-pay patients—on the basis of price and quality. Nursing homes will provide high quality services either because it increases their demand by private-pay patients, hence increases their profitability, or because it helps achieve the firm's noneconomic goals. However, since quality costs money, firms serving Medicaid patients see improved quality adding to production costs but not to revenues. The incentive for nursing homes to provide poor quality to Medicaid patients remains as long as government policies encourage excess demand for Medicaid beds (34). Even if the Medicaid rate is increased so as to enable the homes to increase quality, it is not necessary for the nursing homes to do so as long as they have excess demand for their beds.

Given government's primary goal of limiting its Medicaid expenditures, it is not surprising that regulatory agencies would be less than rigorous in setting, monitoring, and enforcing high standards of quality. Regulation of quality of care can be quite costly to the government. Further, uniformly higher levels of quality standards would be used by the industry to press for higher reimbursement rates for Medicaid-pay patients, which would undermine the cost-control effort. Since the government is interested primarily in limiting its expenditures, it has followed the easiest path—accepting lax regulation of the quality of nursing home services.

Since quality assurance is not a priority of a regulatory agency, the quality criteria for licensure and certification of facilities permits firms great latitude in the quality of care they could provide. Quality criteria can be divided into those that pertain to structure, process, and outcomes (35) of the provision of nursing home services. Structural criteria include the resources available to provide care—the credentials or training of the staff, the ratio of staff to patients, the safety features in the facility, the equipment available to be used. Process criteria include the type and method of provision, as well as quantity of services actually delivered to the residents. Outcome criteria include changes in the functional, physical, and mental status of the residents.

Government regulations have tended to focus on structural criteria of quality, despite the fact that they simply measure the capacity to deliver appropriate services—not whether the services were actually delivered or whether they had any impact on the outcomes of residents. As Kurowski and Shaughnessy (36) observe, while these criteria have in the past been objective, reliable, and easy to measure relative to other criteria, there is little evidence of consistent associations between these measures and process of care or outcomes measures. Even though process measures indicate what services were in fact provided, regulatory quality criteria focused much less attention on them. Even less used are outcome measures of quality, despite the fact that these criteria can provide a summary of the net effect of the nursing home services on the health and well-being of the resident.

Even the best quality criteria are useless without active monitoring and enforcement of sanctions (or incentives) to promote desired firm behavior. The only federal enforcement sanction available has been decertification—denying a facility the ability to receive Medicaid or Medicare-pay patients. This is a drastic action, both for the firm and for the residents of the facility, who may have great difficulty finding another bed in another home, and who can suffer from "transfer trauma." It has seldom been used. Recently, many states have used their capacity to license facilities in their state to institute "intermediate" or less drastic sanctions. These sanctions include fines, suspension of admissions, and receiverships. The extent of available sanctions and the degree to which they are used varies greatly from state to state. Referring to this interstate variation, the Institute of Medicine report concludes that "Despite extensive government regulation for more than 10 years, some nursing homes can be found in every state that provide seriously inadequate quality of care and quality of life. . . . Tolerance of inadequate care also appears to be widespread (37).

There are several factors that could tend to improve the quality of nursing home services over time. The Institute of Medicine report emphasizes improved regulatory quality criteria focusing on residents and outcomes, more federal involvement in quality issues, improved state monitoring and enforcement procedures, enhanced provisions for civil and legal rights of residents, and greater resident, consumer advocate, and community involvement in quality of care and quality of life issues.

It is worthwhile to keep in mind that *the problem is not coming up with ways to improve regulatory efforts—the problem is getting regulatory agencies actually to do something to improve the quality of care.* According to the economic theory of regulation, public policy changes will occur only if nursing home residents and their advocates can form a more effective concentrated interest—to raise the political costs of inaction to the regulatory agency and legislators to the point where it is worth their while to pursue more rigorously the elimination of substandard nursing home care.

With this caveat, we outline possible changes that rely more on improving the efficiency of the market:

1. *Remove CON restrictions.* Entry of new firms into the marketplace would create the conditions for greater nonprice (quality) competition. Producers of low-quality Medicaid-pay nursing home care would be forced either to upgrade their care or to lose market share to producers of higher-quality care. This would be compatible with government cost control if strict, mandatory pre-nursing home screening programs were instituted, not only for people eligible for Medicaid at the point of entry into a nursing home, but also for people likely to spend down to Medicaid status while in the nursing home. No longer would an inefficient or low-quality home be protected by excess demand.

2. *Increase noninstitutional alternatives to nursing home care.* The federal government has taken steps in this direction by permitting Medicaid to experiment with case management approaches and the funding of noninstitutional long-term care services for persons eligible to enter nursing homes. The net effect would be similar to that of removing CON regulations: more competition could force firms producing inadequate care either to upgrade their care or lose business and profits. To control costs a mandatory pre-nursing home screening program would be necessary. To promote quality of long term care services in noninstitutional settings, outcome-based reimbursement could also be instituted.

3. *Create cash incentives for quality care through outcomes-based reimbursement.* A central conclusion of the Institute of Medicine report was the need to shift from the current regulatory emphasis on structural quality criteria to "resident-centered and outcome-oriented" criteria. If pressures to control costs were to ease and pressures to improve quality were to increase, governments could raise overall reimbursement levels for Medicaid-pay patients via this method of tying increased payments to improved resident outcomes.

Two research projects have investigated the possibility of rewarding (or penalizing) firms for outcomes over time achieved by residents in their nursing homes. Kane et al. (38) surveyed residents in four Los Angeles nursing homes recognized as providing good quality care for predominantly Medicaid-pay patients. The team developed a scaling system that would adjust nursing home reimbursement for the outcomes achieved. Weissert et al. (39) studied the impact on nursing home behavior of a variety of incentives, including outcomes-based reimbursement, in a demonstration project involving 18 nursing homes in San Diego. Results of this project are not yet available.

Similar to positive cash incentives for improved quality, there should be negative financial incentives for poor quality. Closure of a home is too drastic a measure and is therefore seldom used. Graduated financial penalties and placing the home in receivership would be less harmful to the home's residents. A receiver could operate the home until the deficiencies are improved or until the home is sold.

4. *Develop alternative financing sources for long-term care.* The development of the market for private long-term care insurance and "lifecare" communities would reduce government's role in financing long-term care, and so reduce its interest in restricting bed supply. With greater competition among providers, and with more people able to pay a private-pay price, more people would be able to purchase a good-quality product.

Quality is more likely to improve once there is greater market competition for patients. Similar to other areas of the economy, such as hotel services, universities, and automobiles, improved quality results from market competition, not government regulation. Relying solely on government agencies to improve the quality of nursing home services would be to repeat our past mistakes and we should expect to be shocked again and again at revelations of the poor quality of our nursing homes.

FINANCING LONG-TERM CARE

Government financing of long-term care is a growing political issue. Nursing home services and home care are currently paid for under Medicaid; Medicare provides short-term coverage for skilled nursing care and for limited services in the home. Private insurance (referred to as "Medigap") also provides limited coverage for those areas not covered by Medicare. Private insurance pays for less than 1 percent of nursing home expenditures, and Medicare pays for less than 2 percent of such expenditures (40). Important gaps in coverage exist for chronic-care services. These gaps in coverage have caused many of the elderly to deplete their assets so as to qualify for Medicaid.

To evaluate government policies for financing long-term care, it is necessary to determine both the effects on equity and economic efficiency of each of the various proposals. Equity considerations are of concern when the government, state or federal, assists in financing long-term care; do lower income groups receive proportionately more benefits relative to their costs than those in higher-income groups? To determine the equity of various proposals it becomes important to determine which elderly receive government benefits and the method used to finance those benefits. Economic efficiency involves two considerations: are the benefits greater than (or at least equal to) the costs of producing those benefits, and is the least cost combination of benefits provided?

To determine whether or not a role for government is necessary, first the market for private long-term care insurance is examined. The current efforts of government financing of long-term care are then evaluated. The section concludes with an examination of alternative policies and their implications in terms of equity and efficiency of alternative government policies for financing long-term care for the aged.

Private Long-Term Care Insurance

A well-functioning market for long term care insurance would permit the aged to insure against the uncertain catastrophic costs of long-term care. Government financing could then be used to assist those aged who are unable to buy private insurance. However, given the concern by the aged with their potential long-term care costs, we observe that private insurance covers only 1 percent of total nursing home expenditures ($300 million out of a total of $35 billion in 1985) (41). Are there imperfections in the long-term care insurance market to cause private insurance to be such a small percent of the total market?

The aged may be considered to be as risk averse as other population groups; thus they should be willing to buy long-term care insurance if sold at its pure premium. Evidence of the aged's risk aversion is indicated by the fact that approximately two-thirds of the aged purchase private supplemental (to Medicare) insurance. The average annual premiums for these policies ranged from $234 to $473 in 1982 (42).

The probability of using a nursing home, as discussed earlier, depends upon the person's health status, their age, whether someone can care for them in their own home, and so on. The cost of a stay in a nursing home can be expensive if required; the magnitude of the loss can be $30,000 a year, and 10 percent of the elderly stay more than 90 days in a nursing home. Since long-term care can be a financially catastrophic event, the aged should be willing to pay a price for such insurance greatly in excess of the pure premium. However, one reason why there is such a small demand for long-term care insurance is that many aged believe that the magnitude of a possible long-term care loss is smaller than it would actually be. The aged *incorrectly* believe that Medicare covers long-term nursing care. A 1985 national survey by the American Association of Retired Persons found that 70 percent of the aged believed that Medicare provides coverage for long stays in a nursing home, regardless of the type of care required (43). In fact, Medicare pays for a limited amount of care in a skilled nursing facility *after* the patient has been in a hospital. And skilled care is for those patients that can benefit from therapy, as after a stroke. Medigap policies are also mistakenly believed to cover long-term care services; instead, such policies often cover the deductibles and cost sharing of a stay in a skilled nursing facility. Those aged who believe that their current coverage provides benefits for long-term care are unlikely to purchase insurance against those events.

Another important reason for the small demand for long term care insurance is the high price of such insurance relative to its pure premium. There are two important reasons for this. First, there are the high marketing and sales costs of signing up the aged. The aged are not part of a large employee group and must be signed up on an individual basis. Second, there is the problem of adverse selection. Those aged who are most in need of expensive chronic care and nursing home services are more likely to purchase such insurance. To protect themselves against adverse selection, insurance companies base their premiums on a higher risk group of the aged rather than on all the aged.

A third reason for the small demand for long-term care insurance is that the pure premium can be large relative to the income of an elderly person. Prototype policies providing a daily indemnity payment are relatively expensive for many elderly, particularly the old-elderly (44). Contributing to a high actuarially fair premium is the problem of moral hazard, particularly with regard to home care; if the price of such a service is reduced as a result of insurance coverage, a person is likely to increase his or her use. The insured family is likely to substitute marketed services for care currently provided by family members and friends.

Uncertainty as to the ageds' utilization rates of chronic care services and rates of inflation have led insurance companies to increase their premiums so as to hedge against future losses. The range of activities of daily living—bathing, dressing, feeding, companionship, and other social support services—are "custodial" types of care and it is difficult for insurance companies to estimate the use and cost of these programs.

Also contributing to a high pure premium is the delivery system for long term care. Services provided in the home, which are a low-cost substitute for extended care in a nursing home, are not well developed. Further, the availability of case managers to search out the appropriate settings to provide chronic long-term services, to contract with different providers, and to monitor the quality of care provided are relatively rare. Instead, when long term care is required, it is often provided in the most expensive setting, the nursing home.

Insurance companies have developed several mechanisms to protect themselves against the problems of adverse selection and moral hazard. A large deductible is often included or the insurance takes effect after the person has been in a nursing home for a certain period of time (e.g., 45 days). Delaying the time until a person may be eligible to use the nursing home (e.g., 2 years), is another method used to decrease adverse selection. Cost sharing is often used to decrease moral hazard; indemnity payments, such as a flat rate per day, with the amounts being less than the price per unit, are also used by insurance companies. Other common features of private insurance plans are limiting insurance coverage to services in a nursing home (to limit the moral hazard of home services), limiting coverage in a nursing home for a certain number of years, excluding preexisting conditions, and providing reimbursement only after some prior event, such as hospitalization.

Large deductibles and cost sharing are more acceptable to those aged with higher incomes. Low-income aged are unlikely to be able to afford such large out-of-pocket payments; they are therefore less likely to purchase long-term care insurance. Their catastrophic insurance program is Medicaid. Thus most private insurance is directed at the middle-income aged.

In addition to indemnity long-term care insurance, there are a limited number of long-term care programs for the middle- and high-income elderly. Life-Care Communities charge a large admission fee, from $50,000 to $150,000, which the aged person can pay by selling his or her home. In return for the initial fee plus a monthly payment, from $250 to $2,500, the person moves into a community that promises to provide care for the rest of his or her life. As long as the person is able to, they live independently in a home or an apartment. When they can no longer do so, they move into an on-site nursing facility. The advantage of such communities is that they offer protection against depletion of a person's assets and access to good-quality nursing facilities for its members. The approximately 300 such communities in existence vary in their policies and in their financial soundness. Many provide partial refunds of their member's assets on withdrawal or death, and some communities do not offer unlimited chronic or custodial care. The disadvantage of Life-Care Communities is that many aged do not want to leave their communities and move into a new community. Further, because of the high initial investment and significant monthly fees, such communities are applicable to only a small percent of the aged.

Social HMOs (S/HMOs) are HMOs that are financed by an aged person's Medicare payment (Parts A and B) plus an additional amount to provide long-term care benefits. S/HMOs coordinate acute and long-term care needs of their elderly members. Demonstrations of S/HMOs are currently being conducted at four sites to determine their feasibility. The long-term care benefits currently being examined in these demonstrations are limited and do not guarantee a subscriber lifetime care should he or she require it.

Home equity conversion is another proposal to enable the elderly to pay for their long-term care needs; the aged mortgage their home and receive monthly payments. Approximately two-thirds of the elderly own their own homes. This proposal is more attractive to the single old-elderly (generally, women) who are at highest risk for a nursing home. The disadvantages of this approach are that it is psychologically difficult for the aged to mortgage their homes. Should they do so, their incentive to maintain the home declines (which is a problem for the bank), the person may outlive the mortgage payments or the payments may be insufficient for the person's long-term care needs, and since Medicaid treats a home as a protected asset for the spouse, why should the family deplete the asset? Home equity conversion is more applicable for meeting the elderly's daily living needs rather than long-term care requirements.

The aged have several concerns that they hope to alleviate by participating in long-term care programs. First, most aged would prefer to stay out of a nursing home and be treated in their own home as long as possible. Thus long-term care benefits should be able to provide the aged with coverage for services in their home. Second, if a person has to enter a nursing home, it should be a good-quality facility. Given the shortage of nursing homes as a result of regulations limiting their supply, access to a good-quality nursing home is a major reason why the elderly join Life-Care Communities. Third, those aged that have assets desire to protect their estates, either for spouses or for children. Related to this concern is the desire not to impoverish a spouse by entering a nursing home or to spend down assets to go on Medicaid. There are a number of instances where the aged have had to be divorced to protect the financial security of the spouse when one member had to qualify for Medicaid.

The current long-term care programs available in the private sector, Life-Care Communities, are able to alleviate these concerns for only a small percent of the elderly, those of high income. Lack of knowledge as to their current long-term care coverage, high marketing costs for long-term care insurance, limited incomes in relation to the pure premium, and adverse selection have resulted in a limited long-term care insurance market.

Public Financing of Long-Term Care Services

The demand for public financing of long-term care for the elderly has two motivations. The first is based on a desire to help the aged who are too poor to receive care in a nursing home or to pay for services in their own home. Currently, low-income aged must fall back onto Medicaid when they can no longer be cared for in their homes; it is difficult for these aged to gain entry into a nursing home (because of supply controls) and, when they do, the quality of their care is suspect. The second motivation underlying government intervention in long-term care is to assist the middle-class elderly. As discussed above, the elderly do not want to deplete their assets if they require long-term care in a home. They want to retain funds for their spouse and they want to be able to leave their assets to their children. It is with regard to the latter group of the aged that government intervention becomes controversial. Should the middle- and upper-income aged be subsidized so as to be able to retain their assets?

To the extent that the nonpoor aged are subsidized in their use of long term care services, their costs must be financed by imposing a tax on other population groups. Medicare and Social Security are financed by a tax on labor, up to a maximum annual amount. This tax is borne by both low- as well as high-income employees. It is inequitable for a low-income employee to be taxed to provide a subsidy to an aged person of higher income with greater assets. The effect of such a subsidy is a redistribution of wealth from low-wage employees to higher-income aged and their children who will inherit their assets.

The Reagan administration has proposed (1987) a catastrophic health insurance benefit for the elderly to be funded by an increase in the Medicare Part B premium. The proposed benefit would have a large deductible ($2,000) and exclude the most important catastrophic illness for which the aged lack coverage, namely, long-term care. Currently, only 3 percent of the aged exceed the $2,000 out-of-pocket expenses for Medicare-covered services. Once the proposal was introduced, political pressure began for expanding the proposal to include long-term care services. If long-term care is included (e.g., as Medicare Part C), the premium would have to be increased substantially; otherwise, subsidies would have to be provided. If the premium were increased to reflect the pure premium and administrative costs of such a plan, many low income elderly would not be able to afford the premium. The beneficiaries would be those aged able to pay the premium; if the premium does not rise over time to reflect the full costs of that benefit, then net subsidies would be provided to those aged buying into the program. (The premium for Part B of Medicare is subsidized so that the size of the subsidy has increased as use and fees for physician services has risen. It is likely that the same political pressures will hold down the increase in long-term care premiums.)

A more equitable proposal would be to make any premium for a new government-financed long-term care benefit income-related.

Although nursing home care is potentially catastrophic financially, to minimize the cost of long-term care, it is necessary to treat the elderly in their own homes. Thus any long-term care program should also provide coverage for services in the home. The demand for home services, however, is likely to be very price elastic. To ensure that home health services are used as a substitute for nursing home care, a case management system, used in conjunction with long-term care coverage, would provide incentives for minimizing the cost of long-term care to the elderly. Demonstration projects are being conducted that add case management services to the existing set of services provided by Medicaid.

To conclude this section on financing of long-term care, there appears to be economic inefficiency in consumption; that is, those aged desiring to purchase long-term care insurance have not been able to do so, thereby preventing them from equating the marginal benefits of long-term care insurance to its marginal costs. The market for long-term insurance is imperfect; however, this market is expected to improve as insurance companies develop information on the costs of such policies and as the aged gain more knowledge of what their current insurance does and does not cover. Further, current approaches for financing long-term care, particularly Medicaid, create a distortion in demand for nursing home care. To a Medicaid-eligible person the price of nursing home services is reduced but noninstitutional services are not similarly subsidized.

As insurance companies gain additional information on the costs of providing long-term care insurance, new types of policies will be developed. They will probably contain large deductibles and consist of indemnity payments. Premiums will vary by age. Protection against long term care expenses are also likely to be developed in conjunction with HMOs for an additional premium; case managers will act as informed purchasers, and will decide upon the appropriate level of care required by the subscriber and the particular provider to be used. Low-income elderly unable to afford long-term care insurance will either have to resort to Medicaid or state governments may decide to contract with HMOs and S/HMOs to provide such care. The extent to which long-term care premiums for the aged will be subsidized by the federal government, and who should bear the cost of such subsidies, are likely to be part of a continuing political controversy.

CONCLUDING COMMENTS

The age structure of the population is changing. The number of persons 65 years of age and older is increasing, in both absolute and relative terms, particularly the old-aged. The need for long-term care is directly related to the aging of the population, particularly for those in the 85 and older age group, which is also the fastest-growing age group. The increasing number of dependent elderly will demand both institutional and noninstitutional services long-term services.

There is a growing disparity among the aged in their ability to pay for long-term care. Those aged least able to pay for long-term care are also those who will be in the oldest age groups and who are more likely to need such services. For those aged able to afford long-term care, we are likely to observe an increasing private market ready to provide both community and institutional services. Private long-term care insurance is also likely to evolve for those aged with greater assets and incomes. To protect themselves against the problems of adverse selection and moral hazard, insurance companies will use deductibles, cost sharing, and/or indemnity policies. Increased reliance on case management programs will also be used. Medicaid is likely to remain as the long-term care insurance for the low-income aged.

As more of the aged become private-pay patients, nursing homes will shift more of their beds away from Medicaid-pay patients. With continued CON limits on the number of nursing home beds, fewer beds will be available to Medicaid patients. Medicaid agencies will be forced to decide whether to ease limits on construction of new nursing homes as the waiting lists for Medicaid patients increase. Medicaid agencies are also likely to increase their use of case management to limit nursing home care to only the most severely disabled aged. Medicaid funds are likely to be reallocated to pay for community services as institutional use becomes more limited.

The private market for long-term care is likely to improve as insurance companies and new providers develop information on the costs and methods of providing noninstitutional services. Many aged will continue to lack information on their long-term care treatment alternatives and on the performance of different providers. However, the integration by large health providers, such as HMOs, of their long-term care and acute services may resolve some of the concerns by those who are less well informed.

The growth of the aged, in addition to increasing the demand for long term care, is important for another reason. The aged are becoming an increasing proportion of the population, thus they are becoming a more important bloc of voters. The aged also share a common desire to achieve protection against the costs of long-term care. To the extent that the aged can achieve legislation that provides them with protection against long term care, they will achieve an economic benefit. The cost of this redistribution of wealth toward the aged will be borne by others—different age groups. The political influence of the aged is not just a result of their increased numbers; they have among the highest voting participation rates of all age groups. The youngest age groups have the lowest; the near aged, those 55 and over, also vote in favor of policies for the aged, since they will soon receive the same benefits without having to pay the full costs of such programs; and the children of the aged vote in favor of policies to relieve themselves of the financial burden of caring for their parents (45). To the extent that legislation is enacted to protect the aged, *regardless of their income levels*, against the costs of long-term care, the redistribution of incomes resulting from government programs will be worsened. Low-income workers would bear an increased burden for providing new health benefits to the aged, some of whom have greater incomes and assets than themselves.

Government policy to assure access to long-term care for the aged should be evaluated in terms of efficiency—whether the cost of achieving that objective is least costly—and equity—are the benefits directed toward those with low incomes and financed by those with higher incomes, regardless of age level?

REFERENCES

1. Pamela Doty, Korbin Liu, and Joshua Wiener, "Special Report: An Overview of Long-Term Care," *Health Care Financing Review*, 6(3), Spring 1985: p. 70.

2. *Ibid.*

3. Daniel R. Waldo and Helen C. Lazenby, "Demographic Characteristics and Health Care Use and Expenditures by the Aged in the United States: 1977–1984," *Health Care Financing Review*, 6(1), Fall 1984: 1.

4. Stephen Crystal, "Measuring Income and Inequality Among the Elderly," *The Gerontologist*, 26(1), February 1986: 56.

5. U.S. Senate, Special Committee on Aging, *Developments in Aging: 1983*, Vol. 1 (Washington, D.C.: U.S. Government Printing Office, March 1984).

6. U.S. Senate, Special Committee on Aging, *America in Transition: An Aging Society*, 1984–85 edition (Washington, D.C.: U.S. Government Printing Office, February 1985).

7. Crystal, *op. cit.*

8. *Ibid.*

9. *Ibid.*

10. Kenneth G. Manton and Beth J. Soldo, "Dynamics of Health Changes in the Oldest Old: New Perspectives and Evidence," *Milbank Memorial Fund Quarterly*, 63(2), 1985: 206.

11. Robyn Stone, "The Feminization of Poverty and Older Women: An Update," paper presented at the 113th Annual Meeting of the American Public Health Association, Washington, D.C., November 17–21, 1985.

12. Katherine R. Levit et al., "National Health Expenditures, 1984," *Health Care Financing Review*, 7(1), Fall 1985:1

13. See Burton Dunlop, "Determinants of Long-Term Care Facility Utilization by the Elderly: An Empirical Analysis", Working paper (Washington, D.C.: Urban Institute, March 1976); B. Chiswick, "The Demand for Nursing Home Care: An Analysis of the Substitution Between Institutional and Noninstitution Care," *Journal of Human Resources*, 11, Summer 1976: 295; and William J. Scanlon, "A Theory of the Nursing Home Market," *Inquiry* 17(1), Spring 1980: 25.

14. Chiswick, *op. cit.*

15. Scanlon, *op. cit.*

16. *Ibid.*.

17. See U.S. General Accounting Office, *Medicaid and Nursing Home Care: Cost Increases and the Need for Services Are Creating Problems for the States and the Elderly* (Washington, D.C.: U.S. Government Printing Office, October 21, 1983).

18. William G. Weissert and William Scanlon, *Determinants of Institutionalization of the Aged* (Washington, D.C.: Urban Institute, July 1983).

19. Larry G. Branch and Alan M. Jette, "A Prospective Study of Long-Term Care Institutionalization Among the Aged," *American Journal of Public Health* 72(12), December 1982: 1373.

20. Barry C. Nocks et al., "The Effects of a Community-Based Long-Term Care Project on Nursing Home Utilization", *The Gerontologist*, 26(2), April 1986: 150.

21. U.S. House of Representatives, Select Committee on Aging, *America's Elderly at Risk* (Washington, D.C.: U.S. Government Printing Office, July 1985).

22. *Advancedata*, National Center for Health Statistics, U.S. Department of Health and Human Services no. 111, September 20, 1985.

23. The following are a partial list of nursing home cost studies: Howard Birnbaum, Christine Bishop, James A. Lee, Gail Jensen, "Why Do Nursing Home Costs Vary? The Determinants of Nursing Home Costs," *Medical Care*, 19(11), November 1981, 1095–1107; H. E. Frech III and Paul B. Ginsburg, "The Cost of Nursing Home Care in the United States: Government Financing, Ownership and Efficiency," in J. van der Gaag and M. Perlman, eds. *Health, Economics and Health Economics* (Amsterdam: North-Holland, 1981); James A. Lee and Howard Birnbaum, "The Determinants of Nursing Home Operating Costs in New York State," *Health Services Research*, 18(2), Summer 1983 Part II: 285–308; Hans C. Palmer and Phillip G. Cotterill, "Studies of Nursing Home Costs," in Ronald J. Vogel and Hans C. Palmer, eds., *Long-Term Care. Perspectives from Research and Demonstrations* (Washington, D.C.: Health Care Financing Administration 1982); William Scanlon and William Weissert, "Nursing Home Cost Function Analysis: A Critique," *Health Services Research*, 18(3), Fall 1983 pp. 387–391; Helen L. Smits, "Incentives in Case-Mix Measures for Long-Term Care," *Health Care Financing Review*, 6(2), Winter 1984: 53–59; and Steven G. Ullman, "The Impact

of Quality on Cost in the Provision of Long-Term Care," *Inquiry*, 22, Fall 1985: 293–302.

24. Robert E. Schlenker and Peter W. Shaughnessy, "Case Mix, Quality, and Cost Relationships in Colorado Nursing Homes," *Health Care Financing Review*, 6(2), Winter 1984 61–71; Robert E. Schlenker, Peter W. Shaughnessy, and Inez Yslas, "Estimating Patient-Level Nursing Home Costs," *Health Services Research*, 20(1), April 1985: 103–128.

25. Leo M. Cooney and Brant E. Fries, "Validation and Use of Resource Utilization Groups as a Case-Mix Measure for Long-Term Care," *Medical Care*, 23(2), February 1985: 123–132; James N. Cameron, "Case-Mix and Resource Use in Long-Term Care," *Medical Care*, 23(4), April 1985: 296–309.

26. This discussion is based on William J. Scanlon, "A Theory of the Nursing Home Market," *Inquiry*, 17 Spring 1980: 25–41.

27. Ronald J. Vogel, "The Industrial Organization of the Nursing Home Industry," in Ronald Vogel and Hans C. Palmer, eds., *Long Term Care: Perspectives From Research and Demonstrations*, (Washington, D.C.: Health Care Financing Administration, 1983).

28. Judith Feder and William Scanlon, "Regulating the Bed Supply in Nursing Homes," *Milbank Memorial Fund Quarterly*, 58(1), 1980: p. 54.

29. For example, in New York reimbursement is based on resource utilization groups (RUGs). Brant Fries and Leo Cooney, "Resource Utilization Groups: A Patient Classification System for Long Term Care," *Medical Care*, 23(2), February 1985: 110–122.

30. Judith Lave, "Cost Containment Policies in Long Term Care," *Inquiry*, 22(1), Spring 1985: 7–23.

31. Howard Birnbaum, Christine Bishop, James Lee, and Gail Jensen, "Why Do Nursing Home Costs Vary? The Determinants of Nursing Home Costs," *Medical Care*, 19(11), November 1981: 1095–1107.

32. John Holahan, "State Rate Setting and Its Effect on the Cost of Nursing Home Care," *Journal of Health Politics, Policy and Law*, 9, Winter 1985: 647–667; Charlene Harrington and James Swan, "Medicaid Nursing Home Reimbursement Policies, Rates, and Expenditures," *Health Care Financing Review*, 6(1), Fall 1984: 39–49.

33. Institute of Medicine, Committee on Nursing Home Regulation, *Improving the Quality of Care in Nursing Homes* (Washington, D.C.: National Academy Press, 1986), 2–3.

34. For a more complete discussion of the effect of excess demand on quality of care, see John A. Nyman, "Prospective and 'Cost-Plus' Medicaid Reimbursement, Excess Medicaid Demand and the Quality of Nursing Home Care", *Journal of Health Economics*, 4, 1985: 237–259.

35. Avedis Donabedian, "Evaluating the Quality of Medical Care," *Milbank Memorial Fund Quarterly*, 44, 1966: 166–206; Avedis Donabedian, *Exploration in Quality Assessment and Monitoring*, Vol. I: *The Definition of Quality and Approaches to Its Assessment* (Ann Arbor, Mich.: Health Administration Press, 1980).

36. Bettina D. Kurowski and Peter W. Shaughnessy, "The Measurement and Assurance of Quality," Chapter 6 in Vogel and Palmer, eds., *op. cit.*

37. Institute of Medicine, *op. cit.*, p. 13.

38. Robert L. Kane et al. "Assessing the Outcomes of Nursing Home Patients," *Journal of Gerontology*, 38(4), 1983: 385–393; Robert L. Kane et al., "Predicting the Outcomes of Nursing Home Patients," *The Gerontologist*, 23(2), 1983: 200–206; Robert L. Kane et al., *Outcome-Based Reimbursement for Nursing-Home Care* (Santa Monica, Calif.: Rand Corporation, December 1983).

39. William G. Weissert et al., "Care for the Chronically Ill: Nursing Home Incentive Experiment," *Health Care Financing Review*, 5(1), Winter 1983.

40. Waldo and Lazenby, *op. cit.*

41. Daniel R. Waldo et al., "National Health Expenditures, 1985," *Health Care Financing Review*, 8(1), Fall 1986: p. 1.

42. Nelda McCall, Thomas Rice, and Judith Sangl, "Consumer Knowledge of Medicare and Supplemental Health Insurance Benefits," *Health Services Research*, 20(6), February 1986: 633–634.

43. Jay N. Greenberg, Don S. Westwater, and Walter N. Leutz, "Long-Term Care Insurance: How Will It Sell?," *Business and Health*, November 1986: p. 21.

44. Mark Meiners and Gordon Trapnell, "Long Term Care Insurance: Premium Estimates for Prototype Policies," *Medical Care*, 22(10), October 1984: 901–910.

45. For a more complete discussion of politics as a means of redistributing wealth from those with less political influence to those with more, and with particular reference to Medicare, see Paul J. Feldstein, *The Politics of Health Legislation: An Economic Perspective*, (Ann Arbor, Mich.: Health Administration Press, 1988) Chapter 9.

CHAPTER 22

Concluding Comments on the Economics of Medical Care

The purpose of this book has been to demonstrate how the tools of economics can be applied to the study of medical care issues. Economic concepts define and clarify the different aspects of medical care, making them more susceptible to analysis. Differences in values among persons on particular issues can be separated from differences in the efficiency with which various approaches can achieve a specified set of values. In addition, economics offers criteria for determining whether particular policies increase or decrease *efficiency* and *equity* in medical care. Of course, economic analysis cannot resolve all the concerns that health professionals and the public have with regard to medical care—different problems require different training and analytical expertise. Particularly suited to economic analysis are problems that relate to issues of scarcity. Economics can illustrate the choices a society can make when its resources are insufficient to achieve everything it desires.

The two economic tools used throughout this book are marginal analysis, which underlies all optimization problems, and supply and demand analysis, which is used for predicting new equilibrium situations. These two tools are interrelated in that supply and demand analysis assumes that individuals or firms are attempting to maximize some goal (e.g., utility or profits) subject to certain budget constraints. The welfare criteria we have been concerned with are the effects on equity as a result of different policies, both government and private, and the implications of different market structures, such as competitive and monopolistic markets.

The use of our economic tools may lead to predictions that turn out to be different than what we observe. One such example is that high rates of return to a medical education should have led to an increase in the supply of physicians during the 1960s. When predictions differ from what we observe (there were very small increases in the supply of physicians during the 1960s), it does not mean that the theory is wrong or not useful. Instead, it is an indication that one or more of the assumptions underlying the theory have been violated. In the physician example cited above, the assumption of free entry in medical education was incorrect. When the underlying assumptions are different from what is expected, there is a possible role for public policy.

There are a number of assumptions with respect to medical care that cause it to be different from other industries. Lack of consumer information, uncertainty of a medical expense and the outcome of a treatment, the dual role of the physician as the patient's agent and the supplier of a service, the large number of not-for-profit firms, payment of providers (in the past) on a cost basis, limitations on entry into the professions and on tasks that different professionals may perform, and the desire by society to provide all its members with a minimum level of medical care are some of the characteristics of this market. Although many of these characteristics may exist in other sectors, together they result in a certain amount of uniqueness to medical care.

Important policy differences occur with respect to these set of unique characteristics. Should the medical care sector be made to conform to more traditional economic markets (e.g., change payment methods so as to change incentives, permit advertising to increase information, etc.), or should medical care be insulated from traditional market forces? In the past, public policy was different than it is today.

Public policy has been directed at three types of issues. These issues are the three basic questions that any economic system or industry must resolve.

One decision that any society must make is how much of its limited resources to spend on medical care. It should be recognized that the choice in question is *not* how much to spend on health, but how much to spend on medical services. People do not desire increased health at any cost, as evidenced by their refusal to stop smoking, wear seat belts, and change their personal health habits. Medical services expenditures serve, to some extent, as a substitute for undertaking other activities to enhance health; part of the costs of neglecting these activities are borne by the population at large through taxes and higher medical care prices. While the decision of how much to spend on health may be more relevant, the emphasis of our medical care system and government financing is to provide more medical services. Increasing medical services is only one approach, and perhaps one of the most costly, for improving health.

Before it can be determined how much should be spent on medical care, it must be decided whether consumers or government will make the necessary decisions. It should again be recognized that this basic decision, which will determine the size and growth of the medical sector, depends upon resolving the issue of whose values are to dominate medical care. Are consumers to determine how much of their income is to be allocated to medical care, or is that decision to be made by a government agency? The answer will determine whether the consumer's or agency's preferences will dominate.

A market approach for allocating resources to different goods and services maximizes the consumer's preferences. Opponents of consumer decisionmaking in medical care argue that medical care is a special case in which a market approach may not be applicable: first, because consumers may not be aware of their medical needs; second, because they may not spend as much as some persons believe they should on their medical needs; and third, because they do not have sufficient information to judge different providers. Under such circumstances, opponents of a market approach propose substituting another mechanism for making the necessary allocation choices in medical care, but they do not explicitly state the criteria by which such a system of decisionmaking should be judged. The proponents of relying on consumer preferences recognize the limitations of the current medical system and how it affects consumer ability to make choices, and seek to improve the consumer's decisionmaking process.

The amount, type, and quality of medical services provided have not represented either consumer or third-party preferences. Consumers' demands for medical care have been distorted both by their excess health coverage resulting from tax subsidies for the purchase of health insurance and by the lack of information on which to base their choices. The most knowledgeable purchaser in the medical market—the patient's physician—lacked the fiscal responsibility to be concerned with medical costs and also had a financial interest in the service that he or she provides. These distortions in the medical care market resulted in the provision of either too many or too few of certain types of services. Public and private policy in the last several years sought to improve the consumers' ability to make choices and change the incentives facing the providers. In the private sector there is increased use of deductibles and cost sharing. Both Medicare and Medicaid are increasing their use of managed care programs. Consumers are being given financial incentives to limit their use of medical services.

Offsetting these policies to limit expenditures are advances in medical technology. The technical feasibility of, for example, organ transplants means that public and private insurance programs will now provide coverage for these activities. It would be very difficult for public programs to deny the aged and the poor access to lifesaving technology.

Thus, while greater financial constraints are being placed on the consumer, the decision of how much to spend on medical services and on which types of services is being left to private decisionmaking, with the government continuing to expand benefit coverages. As government and business expenditures for medical services continue to increase, there may be a change in values as to how this decision should be made.

The second basic decision to be made in any medical system is how medical services should be produced to ensure that output is provided at lowest cost. Rapidly increasing medical costs, duplication of expensive facilities and services, provision of unnecessary services, excessive testing, and unnecessary use of expensive settings all suggested that the efficiency with which medical care was provided could have been improved. The alternatives were to rely on greater regulation and controls implemented by government agencies, or to rely on competitive market pressures to achieve greater efficiency.

Many people have a basic distrust of a market system; many are also concerned that the patient would not be adequately protected if providers have a profit incentive. This concern for consumer protection resulted in the development, at a state level, of a great many restrictions, which health professions and health institutions have actively participated in developing. However, restrictions on who can perform certain tasks, who may enter the health professions, and who may be reimbursed for providing medical services have not eliminated the public's concern that unnecessary services are being performed and that unethical health providers still practice. What many of these restrictions accomplished, however, was the reduction of competition in the provision of medical services.

The movement to a market competitive medical system started in the early 1980s. The Supreme Court ruled in 1982 that the antitrust laws were applicable to the health professions. Business and government began searching for ways to reduce their health expenditures. As restrictions began to be reduced and incentives for efficiency increased, the health sector has undergone a major restructuring. Providers began to take advantage of economies of scale in the provision of services. Hospitals merged and the number of hospital beds in large multihospital systems increased. More physicians are joining group practices so as to be able to market their services as PPOs to businesses and to bargain with insurance companies. Managed care systems are increasing, as insurance companies and the government find that providers have better incentives to minimize the cost of care when they are paid an annual fee.

A great deal of regulation still exists in medical care. Many states still rely on CON laws. DRGs are a system of regulated prices. And there are still many state restrictions on tasks that different professionals may perform. The current trend, however, is away from a regulatory approach for organizing the delivery system and toward a more price-competitive system. As the incentives facing the providers change, so will the structure of the medical system. The organization of medical services will begin to reflect the most efficient methods of delivery. Large, vertically integrated, health care corporations are likely to become the preferred delivery system in large urban areas.

The concern with efficiency in supply and with containment of rapidly escalating medical expenditures has been an important public policy issue. Current programs and beneficiaries would have had to be reduced unless the increase in governmental expenditures could be limited. The alternative to cost containment was either increased taxes or reductions in other politically popular programs. Further, unless ways were found to reduce medical cost increases, new programs could not be started. Thus efficiency issues, how to provide medical services, affect concerns about equity and access, which is the third basic decision that must be made in medical care.

Equity issues, namely, how much medical care should be redistributed to different population groups and by what mechanisms, is at the forefront of public policy in health care today. The choice of how much medical care to provide to particular population groups is affected by the costs of such programs. Proposals to restructure medical care or to change Medicare and Medicaid are often justified as much by their ability to contain costs as for their success in redistributing medical services.

All public policy has certain redistributive effects. However, explicit redistributive programs, such as Medicare, Medicaid, care for the uninsured, tax subsidies for the purchase of health insurance, and financing medical (and other health professional) education, involve raising funds and distributing benefits. However, some types of taxes and some methods of distributing benefits result in greater equity than others. If low-income persons pay more in taxes than they receive in benefits, they are worse off as a result of that policy. Similarly, when high-income groups receive more in benefits than they pay in taxes, they are made better off. Both types of situations exist in medical care. Unless the costs and benefits of public programs, including tax policies, by income group can be directly measured, such perverse redistributive situations are likely to continue.

Redistributive issues are the driving force behind public policy in health care today. Hospitals are seeking reimbursement for care provided to the uninsured. The aged are seeking relief from the potential burden of catastrophic long-term care expenses. The federal government is seeking to lessen its expenditure commitment by shifting more of the retirees' health costs to the employer. The federal and state governments are seeking to lessen their expenditures under Medicaid by mandating employers to provide coverage for all their employees. A large unknown in the coming years is the cost of AIDs and how it will be financed.

How efficiently each of our current (and proposed) subsidy programs redistributes medical services to those least able to afford them is questionable. Tax subsidy programs generally benefit those with higher incomes. Given a choice, many of those who receive care in government hospitals would prefer to receive their care in community hospitals. The large majority of the subsidies to health professional education are received by those who come from families with higher incomes and who subsequently enter those professions whose incomes are among the highest in the country. Recognizing that these huge subsidy programs provide redistributive benefits to different population groups is a first step in deciding whether the resulting redistributive effects are desirable. Second, it should be determined whether such subsidies could be provided more efficiently so that they are received by those in greatest financial need.

Implementing redistributive programs involves providing benefits (in excess of their costs) to one group by imposing costs (in excess of the benefits they receive) on other groups. To anticipate which groups will receive net benefits and which groups are likely to bear those costs requires a theory of legislation. According to the economic theory of legislation discussed in Chapter 11, legislation is provided in return for political support. Within such a framework, it is unlikely that redistributive legislation will be provided or financed in as equitable a manner as possible unless those groups willing to offer the greatest amount of political support desire it to be that way.

Funding for redistributive programs could be reduced if government subsidies were targeted more directly to desired beneficiary groups. However, the political feasibility of achieving an efficient strategy for redistribution is questionable. Each subsidy program has created a distinct constituency. Attempts to change the current distribution of subsidies encounters strong political opposition from all those with an interest in continuing the specific subsidies. The potential beneficiaries of a more direct subsidy system, namely the poor, are not as well organized to engage in the political process, as is indicated by the very fact of their need for such subsidies. Economic analysis of current, as well as of proposed, subsidy programs can indicate who is likely to receive such subsidies and whether the stated objectives of such subsidies can be provided in a more efficient manner. Although such information may not determine the outcome of legislation, it is an input into the political process and raises the political costs to those who might otherwise benefit from less efficient subsidy schemes.

Medical care is different from other industries. Yet economic analysis can be of use in several respects; it offers a perspective within which medical care issues can be viewed and analyzed; economics can be used to analyze the effects of legislation, both current and proposed, that affects the demand and supply sides of the medical markets; and economics can be put to the more traditional tasks required in any industry, such as planning and forecasting. In addition to its tools—the prediction of changes in prices, quantities, and total expenditures, and the formulation of rules for cost minimization—economics provides a set of criteria for evaluating whether or not various policies achieve greater efficiency and equity in medical care. The application of those tools and criteria should result in an increased understanding of medical care issues, should enable a person to separate differences in values from differences in approaches to achieving a given set of values, and should evaluate all the costs and benefits of different choices in medical care.

APPENDIX

Review Questions

CHAPTER 1

1. Every economy, as well as the medical care sector, must decide the following: what should be produced, how it should be produced, how it should be distributed, and how to allow for growth and innovation. With respect to the medical care sector, how are these choices currently made? How have they changed over time? What are the assumptions and value judgments underlying each of these choices?

2. What are the two basic tools of economics? Give an example of each with respect to health, medical services, and hospitals.

3. Prices serve various purposes. For each purpose, give an application of the use of prices, or its lack thereof, in the medical care industry.

4. What are the economic criteria for an optimal rate of output? How well are these criteria met with respect to the medical care sector?

CHAPTER 2

1. Explain why one would or would not use the total contribution of health services as compared to the marginal contribution of health services for decisionmaking, if the objective were to determine how to allocate a limited budget for increasing health levels.

2. If you were employed as a consultant to determine how we should spend our resources to maximize the health level of the population, what kinds of information would you need to know?

3. What is a production function for health? How might it be used for allocating resources to health? How would you use it to explain changes in health status over time?

4. As an economist for an agency whose objective is to improve the health level of a community, what type of information would you want to enable you to suggest to

the agency director what programs to support, and how much should be requested in total by the agency in order to achieve its objective?

CHAPTER 3

1. With an increase in demand for medical care, how will different supply elasticities affect total medical expenditures?

2. Economics is concerned with questions of efficiency and equity. Assume that the price of a specific input (e.g., registered nurses) were subsidized.

   A. Trace through the effect of such a policy in all the medical markets and evaluate this policy in terms of its effect on the goal of increasing the level of the population's health.

   B. Evaluate this policy in terms of economic efficiency.

   C. Evaluate this policy in terms of equity.

CHAPTER 4

1. Evaluate the present Medical Care Price Index. What should the MCPI conceptually measure? What are its limitations?

2. Contrast the Scitovsky and MCPI approaches for measuring changes in the price of medical care.

3. Why do you think, as Scitovsky found, that the costs of episodes of illnesses have increased faster than the prices of the medical care goods and services used in treating the illnesses?

4. It has been proposed that the change in insurance premiums for a given package of benefits be used as an alternative to the current medical care price index. Evaluate this proposal.

CHAPTER 5

1. If the price of medical care were set to zero for everyone, then would individual demands for medical care still differ? Why and why not? Under what conditions would you favor a "negative" price for medical care?

2. Why do economists tend to reject the concept of need as the sole determinant of use in favor of the concept of the demand for medical care?

3. Distinguish between and/or relate the concepts need and demand.

4. What are the various consequences if hospital planning in the United States is done according to need rather than demand?

5. What variables should be included in a comprehensive measure of the price a person pays to consume medical care?

6. Define cross-price elasticity of demand. What is the meaning (in words) of a cross-price elasticity of demand of + 6.5? Would you expect the goods to be substitutes or complements?

7. Anderson and Benham found that the income elasticity of demand for medical care *expenditures* exceeded the income elasticity of demand for medical care *services*. Why do you suppose they obtained this result?

8. Discuss the determinants of the demand for medical care. Select *one* of the determinants and *briefly* outline what we know about its influence.

9. **A.** If you were to raise the fees charged for outpatient care in your hospital, would you expect total revenue from the OPD to increase or decrease? Why?

   B. If you were to raise the fees for inpatient care, would you expect total revenues from inpatient care to increase or decrease? Why?

   C. Do you think the change in revenues would be relatively larger for inpatient care or outpatient care? Why?

   D. Would you expect outpatient revenues to be affected more by inpatient price than inpatient revenues are affected by outpatient price? Why?

   E. How is the effect of outpatient fees on outpatient use (and hence outpatient revenues) influenced by the magnitude of the time and travel costs borne by people in your service area?

10. Justify your answers to both parts of this question with the theoretical or empirical material with which you are familiar.

   A. Why would you expect the relationship between income and medical care utilization to be stronger in 1960 than in 1975?

   B. Why might the estimate of the income elasticity of demand for medical care be higher if one adjusts for health status than if one does not?

   C. If you do not adjust for insurance coverage, would you expect to overestimate or underestimate the income elasticity of demand for medical care?

11. The assessment of the relationship between income and medical care utilization is complicated by the influence of several related variables. Select three of these variables and indicate how they affect the observed relationship between income and use.

12. What are the various methods that can be used to ration utilization of health services, and what are the implications of using each approach?

13. Evaluate the statement, "Medical care is never free, although the individual recipient may pay nothing."

14. How can a model of demand for hospital care be used to explain changes in hospital utilization over time?

15. How can a model of demand for medical care be used to explain the rise in medical expenditures over time?

16. How could you use a model of demand for medical care for purposes of policy (e.g., improving equity)? For example, as a national health policy analyst, you desire to increase the utilization of ambulatory medical care of low-income peo-

ple. How would you use the results for demand analysis to suggest recommendations?

17. What are the differences between forecasting the demand for hospital services and the demand for a particular hospital's services? What types of analyses would you undertake to determine the demand for *your* hospital's services? Be explicit regarding the factors that would be included in the analyses, including the reasons for their inclusion.

18. The physician has a dual role in medical care, as the patient's agent and as a supplier of a service. Under what circumstances would these roles be in conflict? What empirical evidence supports each of these different roles?

19. What was the expected effect on the demand for county, municipal, and VA hospitals of the introduction of Medicare and Medicaid?

20. What was the expected effect (define) on Blue Shield, MDs, and medical care of Titles 18 and 19 (Medicare and Medicaid)?

21. Evaluate the use of bed population ratios as a basis for planning hospital facilities. How might an economist go about the same task?

22. What factors might cause physicians to experience an increase in the number of requests for annual physical examinations even though they do not change their fees for this service?

23. It has been said that there is economic inefficiency on the demand side of the medical care market. What are both the reasons for and effects of this economic inefficiency?

CHAPTER 6

1. How would you use utility analysis to analyze the following statement? Consumers should purchase health insurance policies that cover 100 percent of all medical care expenses. Anything less than 100 percent coverage reflects either irrational consumer behavior or market failure in the insurance industry. (Organize your discussion around diagrams.)

2. Explain why health insurance is more common for hospital expenses than for ambulatory care expenses.

3. How will a change in the price of medical care affect the demand for health insurance?

4. What is meant by an "actuarially fair" premium?

5. What are the characteristics of an insurable risk?

6. Discuss each of the factors affecting the demand for health insurance. Indicate the effect that each has on demand.

7. What are the welfare implications of having everyone purchase the same (very comprehensive) health insurance coverage?

8. What is "moral hazard," and how does its existence affect the demand for health insurance? What alternative approaches are used by insurance companies to control it?

9. What is adverse selection? How does its existence affect the market for health insurance? What are some ways in which insurance companies try to protect themselves from adverse selection?

10. What information would you need to know (and how would you use it) to determine whether expanding benefit coverage (e.g., covering hospice services), would lower the cost of an insurance premium?

11. How and under what circumstances might the inclusion of coinsurance and deductibles make an insurance policy more attractive to some people?

12. It has been proposed that a limit be placed on the amount of employer paid health insurance that is not taxed. What are the reasons for this argument in terms of:

    A. Economic efficiency.
    B. Equity. (Be sure to define efficiency and equity in your answer.)
    C. Who do you think would be likely to favor and oppose this proposal?

13. Evaluate Blue Cross's hospital service benefit policy in terms of economic efficiency. Why did hospitals favor it?

14. It has been said that extensive (both public and private) insurance coverage resulted in an "erosion of the medical marketplace." Explain this statement.

CHAPTER 7

1. **The following will affect the supply of medical care:**
    A. Price of medical care.
    B. The prices of inputs.
    C. Technological or scientific knowledge.
       Changes in any of the above will result in changes in the supply of medical care. Explain how an increase and a decrease in each of the above, while the effect of the other two are held constant, will cause changes in supply, and what the direction of that change will be.

2. Contrast the differences in technical versus economic efficiency with respect to the field of medical care.

3. Different combinations of physician and hospital services can be used to produce a medical treatment. If hospital services were essentially "free" to the physician and to the patient (Blue Cross's service benefit policy), what combination of hospital and physicians' services would be used by the physician to provide a medical treatment?

4. Apply the concept of a production function and the idea of "marginal rate of substitution" to an HMO. Show how this knowledge may be used for decisionmaking.

5. If hospitals and physicians are part of an HMO, what would determine their relative proportions in providing a medical treatment?

6. What is the effect likely to be on the combination of hospital and physician services used in treatment as a result of the large increase in the supply of physicians?

CHAPTER 8

1. Blue Cross has several cost advantages over commercial insurance companies. Blue Cross receives a discount from hospitals, does not have to pay taxes, and does not have to earn and distribute profits to shareholders. Conceptually, what effect should these cost advantages have on Blue Cross's market share? What hypotheses have been suggested to explain the lack of such an expected effect on market share?

2. Outline the structure of the insurance industry. How does the structure above deviate from the purely competitive model? What changes, if any, would you suggest to change the performance of this industry?

3. What are the possible consequences of community rating on economic efficiency and equity?

CHAPTER 9

1. Explain the "target-income" hypothesis of physician behavior. What empirical evidence has been used to support this theory? What are alternative explanations to support the observed data?

2. What are the policy implications with respect to the supply of physicians of alternative theories on physician-induced demand?

3. What are different methods for constructing a relative value scale for physician fees? What are the advantages and disadvantages of each of these methods? Why is it claimed that relative value scales will improve equity among physicians?

4. What similarities can you see between the physician industry and the industry that provides legal advice?

5. Contrast medical care to other repair industries (e.g., auto, TV repair). What are the similarities and differences between medical care and these other industries? How have these differences (or similarities) affected the structure of the medical care market?

6. Outline the structure of the physician services market. How does the structure above deviate from the purely competitive model? What changes, if any, would you suggest to change the performance of this industry?

7. The following statement appeared in the Wall Street Journal: "Most people who provide services say they're sorry that they have to raise prices, but they say they have no choice. Doctors say their fees have gone up because of whopping increases in malpractice insurance premiums." How would you use economic analysis to analyze this statement? Be explicit regarding any of your assumptions. (Hint: Are malpractice premiums a variable or a fixed cost?)

8. What are different reasons for observing variations in physician fees? Which reasons are compatible with a competitive model? Which reasons are compatible with a monopoly model?

9. One indication that physicians engage in price discrimination is the degree to which they accept Medicare patients on assignment. Explain how physicians decide how many patients on assignment, the price they charge their nonassigned patients, and the effect on both of the above of an increase in the price Medicare pays physicians.

CHAPTER 10

1. What are the difficulties with empirical studies that attempt to measure the extent of economies of scale in hospitals?

2. Contrast and evaluate the different theories of hospital cost inflation that occurred during the 1960s and 1970s.

3. Two models of hospital behavior are the profit-maximizing and utility or prestige-maximizing models. Describe each and contrast their predictions.

4. Of what use to an administrator or planner is knowledge of his or her cost curves?

5. A great many changes have occurred in the hospital industry over the last 10 years. Distinguish between vertical and horizontal integration. Explain under what circumstances you would expect to observe more of one than the other. Predict what changes you expect to witness in the structure of the hospital sector in the next five years.

6. The economic forces affecting hospitals are changing. Within an economic framework, discuss the changing economic outlook for hospitals. What are some strategies that hospitals might undertake to ensure their ability to survive in the years ahead?

7. Using an economic framework, analyze the rise that has occurred in medical care prices, and using the same framework, what would you forecast for the next several years? Be explicit regarding any assumptions underlying your analysis.

8. The past two decades have displayed a large increase in the demand for medical care. However, the various components of the medical care sector (e.g., physician's services, hospital services, etc.) have displayed widely differing price behavior. How would you account for these differences?

9. In planning the location of health facilities, what type of data are needed, and how would this information be used for determining the number, size, and location of such facilities?

10. You have just been appointed economic consultant to the Veterans Administration (Hospitals). How would you use economic analysis to improve or evaluate the efficiency of the VA system? State as many economic concepts that you think are relevant, and for each concept stated give as many specific examples of it as applied to the Veterans Administration. (It is assumed that the VA will generally remain a provider of care.)

11. It has often been suggested that hospitals are public utilities and therefore should be subject to the same type of regulation as public utilities. What are the economic characteristics of a public utility? In what respects does or does not the structure of the hospital industry resemble that of a public utility?

CHAPTER 11

1. Describe the economic theory of regulation. Contrast its predictions to the public interest theory of regulation with respect to certificate of need legislation. What evidence leads you to select one theory over the other?

2. What are alternative (theoretical) methods for a hospital (or any firm or agency) to set its prices? What are the effects of these alternative methods of pricing on (A) the allocation of resources, and (B) income redistribution of different categories of patients?

3. Blue Cross is interested in controlling (limiting) hospital utilization. For example, they worked with planning councils to control the number of beds built in any area, and they favored using criteria for admission and length of stay in the hospital. Why was this the case? What are alternative approaches the Blues could have used to achieve reduced utilization? Why were they reluctant to use these alternative approaches?

4. The move from cost-based payment for hospital services to payment based on DRGs was expected to change hospital behavior. discuss what you would expect to observe as the payment method changed. What are the advantages and disadvantages of the DRG payment approach?

5. Economists claim that there are several causes of economic inefficiency in medical care. List three basic causes, and for each describe why it results in economic inefficiency.

6. How has the lack of information affected the structure of the medical care market?

CHAPTER 12

1. Why did the health field become a market-competitive industry over the last several years?

2. Why was the introduction of advertising in the health field expected to lower the prices charged by physicians and dentists? What studies support this hypothesis?

3. If advertising in the health field is expected to result in lower prices, why do firms producing breakfast cereals, soaps, and so on, undertake such extensive advertising campaigns?

4. Choose two different methods of reducing the rising price of medical care and explain what their intended effect (both direct and indirect) will be. What change, if any, will occur as a result of each of your two proposals?

5. What alternative approaches have been proposed for increasing the role of market competition in medical care?

6. If HMOs are such a good idea, why has it taken them so long to increase their market share?

7. "Free choice" of physician has been interpreted by organized medicine (and dentistry) to mean that a patient's choice of physician should not be restricted to those physicians participating in a particular delivery system. Under what circumstances has this interpretation of "free choice" resulted in anticompetitive behavior by organized medicine?

8. How can the existence of adverse selection and preferred risk selection by HMOs increase the cost to the government of Medicare voucher proposal?

9. What type of information would you need to estimate a premium for an HMO population and how would you use it?

10. Why are HMOs expected to be a less costly method of providing medical care than the fee-for-service system? In your answer, be explicit regarding the necessary assumptions that should prevail in HMOs for this to occur.

CHAPTER 13

1. What are the different types of personnel shortage? How is each measured, what are the weaknesses of the various methods of measurement, and what are the various ways of alleviating such shortages?

2. How is it possible for wastage and shortage to coexist in the same market?

3. What are the problems of using health manpower ratios to project health manpower "requirements"?

4. What are the major types of labor market imperfections in the health field that cause wages to be either higher or lower than if such restrictions did not exist?

5. Through the 1970s, it had been claimed that there was a shortage of physicians. A proposal to remedy this problem was to provide subsidies to prospective M.D.s (tuition, interest-free loans, etc.). Comment on the effect this proposal would have had on reducing the shortage of physicians. Be explicit regarding your assumptions.

6. "Trying to prove that there is a shortage of doctors by comparing their incomes to the incomes of lawyers only results in proving that there is a surplus of lawyers."

   A. How do you evaluate this statement?

   B. What does the relative income approach tell you about the supply of physicians?

7. There are economic and noneconomic definitions of shortages with respect to health manpower markets. For physicians, distinguish between the different economic definitions of shortage (e.g., dynamic versus static shortages), and describe

the data you would need to differentiate between these different definitions. What might be appropriate public policies for each type of shortage?

8. GMNEC has predicted a surplus of physicians by 1990. Discuss the expected effects of this surplus on physician incomes, on the prices of physician services, and on the structural characteristics of the delivery of medical care.

9. Assume that a particular physician specialty association decides to limit the number of residencies in that specialty. Using diagrams, what would be the expected effect on that specialty and on other physician specialties? Should the physician specialty association be concerned about Federal Trade Commission scrutiny?

10. You have just been appointed as staff economist to the minister of health for XYW country. Next week, you are to submit a proposal on the number of physicians needed in your country. How would you organize (outline) your economic analysis? How would your analysis and proposals differ under the following assumptions?

   A. The medical care sector is predominantly a private market.

   B. The medical care sector is predominantly public, as the Veterans Administration or the national health service.

CHAPTER 14

1. Why have physicians wanted to price discriminate? What are the necessary conditions for price discrimination? How well have the conditions for price discrimination been satisfied in the case of surgeons? In the case of primary care physicians?

CHAPTER 15

1. Describe the economic factors that affect the demand for a medical education. How are each of these factors likely to change in the coming years?

2. In what ways does the U.S. medical education market differ from a competitive industry? What would you hypothesize the consequences would be if medical education were to become more like business administration schools?

3. What are the reasons for and against subsidizing medical education? How would you evaluate these reasons according to the criteria of economic efficiency and equity?

4. Evaluate in terms of both equity and economic efficiency: The Carnegie Commission Report on Medical Education (1970) recommends federal subsidies to medical schools and students in order to achieve a uniform level of tuition of $1,000 at all schools. (The subsidy would go to the schools.)

CHAPTER 16

1. You are an economic consultant to the American Nurses Association. What would you expect the effects of changes in the health care markets, such as prospective payment for hospitals, growth in HMOs, the increased supply of physicians, and so on, to be on the employment and earnings of RNs? In your answer trace through the effects you expect on both the product and factor markets.

2. Various measures have been used to indicate that there has been a shortage of nurses.

    A. Evaluate the use of such measures to indicate the existence of a shortage.

    B. What information would you use to indicate whether or not a shortage exists?

    C. As part of (B), distinguish between a dynamic and a static shortage.

3. Nurses are restricted in the tasks they are permitted to perform. Certain nurse specialties (e.g., nurse–midwives) would like to bill for their services on a fee-for-service basis rather than work for obstetricians. Using the theory of the demand for labor, explain how changes in each of the above would affect the demand for registered nurses.

4. "Comparable worth" proponents seek equal pay for work of comparable value. What are the consequences of setting nurses' wages according to the concept of comparable worth? Describe the factors that determine wages in a competitive market (including those factors that cause shifts in the demand for labor). What are noncompetitive situations that have resulted in lower wages nurses?

5. Nursing associations have proposed increasing the educational requirements to a four-year B.A. degree for all persons desiring to become professional nurses. What are the economic consequences of instituting such a change? Who would be expected to favor it, and who would be expected to oppose it?

6. Contrast the market for registered nurses during the periods before and after Medicare. How well did the market for hospital-employed nurses perform in each of these two periods?

7. How would unionization in a monopsony market for nurses' services increase both nurses' wages and hospital employment?

CHAPTER 17

1. One of the goals of the 1962 Drug Amendments is increased drug safety. Why, then, do some economists assert that these amendments were more harmful to the public than beneficial?

2. What are alternative explanations for the decline in new drugs since the 1960s?

CHAPTER 18

1. Select some health legislation (or an aspect of it) and describe how two different groups in the health field (e.g., AMA, AAMC, AHA, ANA, etc.) would be in favor

and (the other) opposed to the same legislation based on some objective function of that group.

2. There are a number of restrictions in the methods by which medical care is organized and provided. With regard to restrictions on entry, on tasks performed, and (previously) on information, contrast the reasons for such restrictions in terms of improved quality versus enhancement of provider incomes.

3. Apply the theoretical model of the demand for legislation to predict legislation demanded by the American Medical Association (AMA) or the American Dental Association (ADA). Be explicit regarding the objective of the AMA or ADA, and justify the choice of that objective.

4. A profession would be expected to be in favor of proposals that increase the demand for their services. The extension of Blue Shield (insurance for physician visits) would be one method by which the demand for physician services would be increased. However, physicians would not be in favor of extending Blue Shield coverage to everyone in the population. How can you explain this apparent anomaly?

5. What are some practices in medical care that are purported to result in higher standards of quality that are in effect restrictive devices intended to confer monopoly power on the practitioners of the profession? What are alternative ways of achieving the goal of higher quality without the restrictive element?

CHAPTER 19

1. What are economic rationales for government intervention in health care?

2. The case for a public role in the medical care sector is often made on noneconomic grounds. It is also often made by allusion to the *unique* characteristics of health and medical care from the economic point of view. What case would you make for a public role in the medical care sector within the framework of traditional economic analysis? Be as complete as possible and draw your examples from the health and medical care field.

3. A great deal of time and energy is being devoted by researchers, celebrities, and government to support the effort to find a cure for AIDS.

   A. Why is there such a demand for a cure for AIDS?

   B. Money to support AIDS research is coming from several sources. What are the most economically efficient ways of financing this research?

4. Define externalities. Why do they occur? What are examples of externalities in the health field? Explain why the presence of externalities will, in the absence of some collective action, lead to a suboptimal rate of output. what type of collective action is called for?

5. If a cost-benefit analysis is "favorable," does this suggest that the government should always undertake such an expenditure? In your answer, discuss the criteria that should be used or who should undertake such projects, and how they should be financed.

6. Critically evaluate the application of cost-benefit analysis as it has been applied to the health field.

7. Although there may be economic justification for government intervention in the health and medical sectors, what are the bases upon which government should provide subsidies, impose taxes, regulate, or become a producer themselves of the service? Provide examples of and evaluate government intervention in each of these roles.

8. Assume that in country X, where medical care was privately paid for, a new government was elected, with one of its policies being free medical care for all. As the new minister of health, what are the various actions you would have to undertake to ensure that at a zero price for all medical care services, an adequate supply will be available in the future?

9. What economic arguments support government financing of personal health services?

10. If the objective is one of redistribution, what are the welfare implications of achieving this redistribution by providing cash supplements versus medical care to the desired beneficiary group?

11. What are the reasons for having public provision (e.g., operation) of a service versus private provision, or private provision with government regulation?

CHAPTER 20

1. What criteria are most appropriate for evaluating a government's health insurance scheme?

2. The social security tax is imposed on both the employer and the employee. Using supply and demand diagrams for labor, show how the elasticity of demand for labor determines who (either the employer or the employee) actually bears the burden of the social security tax.

3. If society were to establish as a principle for national health insurance that everyone should have equal consumption of medical care for equal needs, explain why a policy that established the same price to everyone for medical care (or makes medical care free to all, i.e., zero price) will not achieve society's goal.

4. Suppose that uniform, comprehensive, national health insurance were implemented. Trace the effects of this action on the medical care system. Consider demand and supply in each of the different medical care markets (e.g., institutional, manpower, and educational markets, prices, quantities, wages, employment, and total expenditures). What assumptions become crucial to your analysis?

5. Both Presidents Nixon and Carter have proposed a national health insurance system whereby all employers would be required to provide their employees with a minimum set of health insurance benefits. Evaluate this proposal in terms of the demand for different types of labor, the effects on federal revenues, and the effects on the prices of goods and services produced by different types of industries.

CHAPTER 21

1. Currently, the private market for long-term care insurance is small. Many persons believe that the growing number of aged, particularly those over 75 years of age, would justify a much more extensive demand for private long-term care insurance. What are some reasons for this market's slow development?

Index

Where the reference is in a footnote the page number is followed by n.